HANDBOOK

OF

SELF-REGULATION

D1204909

Handbook

of

Self-Regulation

Edited by

Monique Boekaerts
Leiden University
Center for the Study of Education and Instruction
Leiden, The Netherlands

Paul R. Pintrich
University of Michigan
Combined Program in Education and Psychology
Ann Arbor, Michigan

Moshe Zeidner
University of Haifa
Faculty of Education
Mount Carmel, Israel

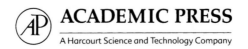

ACADEMIC PRESS
A Harcourt Science and Technology Company

San Diego   San Francisco   New York   Boston   London   Sydney   Tokyo

Elsevier Academic Press
30 Corporate Drive, Suite 400, Burlington, MA 01803, USA
525 B Street, Suite 1900, San Diego, California 92101-4495, USA
84 Theobald's Road, London WC1X 8RR, UK

This book is printed on acid-free paper. ∞

Copyright © 2000, 2005 Elsevier Inc. All rights reserved.

No part of this publication may be reproduced or transmitted in any form or by any means, electronic or mechanical, including photocopy, recording, or any information storage and retrieval system, without permission in writing from the publisher.

Permissions may be sought directly from Elsevier's Science & Technology Rights Department in Oxford, UK: phone: (+44) 1865 843830, fax: (+44) 1865 853333, E-mail: permissions@elsevier.co.uk. You may also complete your request on-line via the Elsevier homepage (http://elsevier.com), by selecting "Customer Support" and then "Obtaining Permissions."

Library of Congress Catalog Card Number: 99-62844

British Library Cataloguing in Publication Data
A catalogue record for this book is available from the British Library

ISBN 13: 978-0-12-369519-2
ISBN 10: 0-12-369519-8

For all information on all Elsevier Academic Press publications
visit our Web site at www.books.elsevier.com

Printed in the United States of America
05   06   07   08   09   10   9   8   7   6   5   4   3   2   1

Working together to grow
libraries in developing countries

www.elsevier.com | www.bookaid.org | www.sabre.org

ELSEVIER   BOOK AID   Sabre Foundation
              International

ACC Library Services
Austin, Texas

CONTENTS

1

SELF-REGULATION:
AN INTRODUCTORY OVERVIEW

MONIQUE BOEKAERTS, PAUL R. PINTRICH, AND MOSHE ZEIDNER

PART I

GENERAL THEORIES AND MODELS
OF SELF-REGULATION

2

ATTAINING SELF-REGULATION: A SOCIAL
COGNITIVE PERSPECTIVE

BARRY J. ZIMMERMAN

3

ON THE STRUCTURE OF BEHAVIORAL
SELF-REGULATION

CHARLES S. CARVER AND MICHAEL F. SCHEIER

4

ASPECTS OF GOAL NETWORKS: IMPLICATIONS FOR SELF-REGULATION

JAMES Y. SHAH AND ARIE W. KRUGLANSKI

5

A FUNCTIONAL-DESIGN APPROACH TO
MOTIVATION AND SELF-REGULATION:
THE DYNAMICS OF PERSONALITY
SYSTEMS AND INTERACTIONS

JULIUS KUHL

6

PERSONALITY, SELF-REGULATION,
AND ADAPTATION:
A COGNITIVE – SOCIAL FRAMEWORK

GERALD MATTHEWS, VICKI L. SCHWEAN, SIAN E. CAMPBELL,
DONALD H. SAKLOFSKE, AND ABDALLA A. R. MOHAMED

7

ORGANIZATION AND DEVELOPMENT OF
SELF-UNDERSTANDING AND SELF-REGULATION:
TOWARD A GENERAL THEORY

ANDREAS DEMETRIOU

8

THE ROLE OF INTENTION IN SELF-REGULATION:
TOWARD INTENTIONAL SYSTEMIC MINDFULNESS

SHAUNA L. SHAPIRO AND GARY E. SCHWARTZ

9

COMMUNAL ASPECTS OF SELF-REGULATION

TAMARA JACKSON, JEAN MACKENZIE, AND STEVAN E. HOBFOLL

PART II

DOMAIN-SPECIFIC MODELS AND RESEARCH ON SELF-REGULATION

10

SELF-REGULATION IN ORGANIZATIONAL SETTINGS: A TALE OF TWO PARADIGMS

JEFFREY B. VANCOUVER

11

SELF-REGULATION AND HEALTH BEHAVIOR: THE HEALTH BEHAVIOR GOAL MODEL

STAN MAES AND WINIFRED GEBHARDT

12

REGULATION, SELF-REGULATION, AND CONSTRUCTION OF THE SELF IN THE MAINTENANCE OF PHYSICAL HEALTH

SUSAN BROWNLEE, HOWARD LEVENTHAL, AND ELAINE A. LEVENTHAL

13

SELF-REGULATED LEARNING:
FINDING A BALANCE BETWEEN LEARNING
GOALS AND EGO-PROTECTIVE GOALS

MONIQUE BOEKAERTS AND MARKKU NIEMIVIRTA

14

THE ROLE OF GOAL ORIENTATION IN SELF-REGULATED LEARNING

PAUL R. PINTRICH

15

MOTIVATION AND ACTION IN SELF-REGULATED LEARNING

FALKO RHEINBERG, REGINA VOLLMEYER, AND WOLFRAM ROLLETT

16

MEASURING SELF-REGULATED LEARNING

PHILIP H. WINNE AND NANCY E. PERRY

PART III

INTERVENTIONS AND APPLICATIONS OF SELF-REGULATION THEORY AND RESEARCH

17

SELF-REGULATION AND DISTRESS IN CLINICAL PSYCHOLOGY

NORMAN S. ENDLER AND NANCY L. KOCOVSKI

18

SELF-MANAGEMENT OF CHRONIC ILLNESS

THOMAS L. CREER

19

SELF-REGULATION AND ACADEMIC LEARNING: SELF-EFFICACY ENHANCING INTERVENTIONS

DALE H. SCHUNK AND PEGGY A. ERTMER

20

TEACHER INNOVATIONS IN SELF-REGULATED LEARNING

JUDI RANDI AND LYN CORNO

21

SELF-REGULATION: A CHARACTERISTIC AND A GOAL OF MATHEMATICS EDUCATION

ERIK DE CORTE, LIEVEN VERSCHAFFEL, AND PETER OP 'T EYNDE

22

SELF-REGULATION INTERVENTIONS WITH A FOCUS ON LEARNING STRATEGIES

CLAIRE ELLEN WEINSTEIN, JENEFER HUSMAN,
AND DOUGLAS R. DIERKING

23

SELF-REGULATION: DIRECTIONS AND CHALLENGES FOR FUTURE RESEARCH

MOSHE ZEIDNER, MONIQUE BOEKAERTS, AND PAUL R. PINTRICH

FOREWORD

When I was a graduate student (1945–1948), Hullian behaviorism was the dominant theoretical position in psychology. Although Hullian behaviorism began to fade in the 1950s, Skinner's radical behaviorism surged to the fore in the late 1950s and early 1960s. But even in the heyday of behaviorism other research was indicating that behaviorist theories were not well suited to explaining much animal and human behavior. The cognitive maps of Tolman's rats, the Gestalt theorists' research on reasoning and problem solving, Lewin's field theory, and especially the vigorous motivational research of McClelland and Atkinson and their students on expectancies and values presaged the cognitive revolution in psychology. In the late 1960s and the 1970s the computer replaced the telephone switchboard as the major metaphor for psychological theory, and major advances were made in understanding perception, memory, and cognitive processes in general.

One of the consequences of the cognitive revolution was a greater emphasis on human cognition and greater acceptance of research in natural settings as well as in laboratories. Cognitive psychologists became interested in applications of cognitive theory to social psychology, organizational psychology, educational systems, and health behavior and systems. Reciprocal interactions between applied and laboratory research enriched both theory and practice.

In the late 1970s the term "metacognition" began to appear, as researchers and theorists discussed knowledge about knowledge and thinking about thinking. But what can one do with metacognition? Here the computer metaphor is less useful, and a number of the major cognitivists realized that in order to understand the use of knowledge and skills, theorists needed to deal with goals, motivation, and affect. If individuals were to plan how to use their knowledge of the conditions under which their knowledge and skills could be used most effectively, they needed to consider their goals. Thus motivation research, which had continued as a vigorous area through the decades, came to the fore.

Both expectancy-value and attribution theories of motivation recognized that the concept of "self" was an important motivational value. Enhancing one's self-concept and protecting it against threat influenced one's behavior in many situations. Bandura's monumental program of research on self-efficacy and Hazel Markus's research on possible selves are but two examples of the resurgence of the self as a major theme in theory and research.

Thus a handbook on self-regulation is timely. Self-regulation constructs nicely integrate the cognitive, motivational, social, and behavioral strands of theory and research. As this volume illustrates, self-regulation also takes account of cultural, organizational, and contextual variables that influence self-regulation. The attribute-treatment interaction research signaled by Cronbach's American Psychological Association presidential address. "The Two Disciplines of Scientific Psychology" (Cronbach, 1957), also resonates in research on individual differences in self-regulation in different situations.

I once chaired an address by Al Bandura. After his brilliant discussion of the wide-ranging power of self-efficacy in explaining behavior, I opened the floor for discussion by saying, "This was marvelous, but it is simply too good to be true. Nothing in psychology has ever been able to cover so much so well."

At times I have the same concerns about self-regulation. Certainly self-regulation is generally a good thing, but are there contexts in which it interferes with optimal performance? Does being mindful and self-regulating sometimes take capacity needed for basic information processing? Is it possible that excessive self-monitoring may be detrimental to the performance of automatized and nonconscious responses, much as in the classic anecdote of the centipede who tried to pay attention to his legs as he walked? The authors in this handbook recognize this possibility, but we still know little about how to discriminate between situations when mindfulness will be helpful and when it may be detrimental.

Bargh and Chartrand (1999) review extensive research showing that we are not conscious of the cues that control a great deal of our behavior. Such automatic processing is efficient most of the time. But often the behaviors that are automatized are not those that are most effective. Students come into my courses who habitually study their assignments by simply reading them and study for tests by rereading. I try to teach them to think about the material, to relate it to their own experience and prior knowledge, to ask questions, and to check their understanding. Old habits are hard to break and the new self-regulatory skills are difficult to perfect. But with practice these skills can become habitual.

But even such self-regulatory skills that are usually effective are not the best for every situation. We evolved consciousness because instinctive and habitual behavior gets us into trouble when we encounter new situations that differ in critical features from those in which our typical response is optimal. Conscious self-regulation is still needed. I believe that we need to train individuals in the use of self-regulatory skills to the point where appropriate self-regulation occurs without thought in most situations, but where the individual is able to take conscious self-regulatory measures when a situation poses new complications or uncertainties.

As research on self-regulation burgeons, one might expect this volume to be quickly superseded. I believe, however, that it will continue for some time to provide the perspectives needed by researchers if they are to build on what we now know and untangle the myriad complexities that still perplex us.

REFERENCES

Bargh, J. A., & Chartrand, T. L. (1999). The unbearable automaticity of being. *American Psychologist, 54*, 462–479.
Cronbach, L. J. (1957). The two disciplines of scientific psychology. *American Psychologist, 12*, 671–684.

W. J. McKeachie
The University of Michigan
Ann Arbor, Michigan

ABOUT THE EDITORS

Monique Boekaerts is Professor of Educational Psychology at Leiden University (The Netherlands) and chairs the Research Committee of the Faculty of Social Sciences. As a principal investigator, she is supervising a national school reform program in vocational schools. Her main field of interest is self-regulated learning with a focus on motivation, volitional control, coping with stress, and soliciting social support. President-elect of the European Association of Learning and Instruction and President of the Educational and Institutional Psychology division of the International Association of Applied Psychology, she has written over 100 scientific articles and book chapters. She serves as associate editor of *Learning and Instruction* and as reviewer for several international and European journals.

Paul R. Pintrich is Professor of Education and Psychology and Chair of the Combined Program in Education and Psychology at The University of Michigan, Ann Arbor. He also serves as Associate Dean for Research for the School of Education at Michigan. His research focuses on the development of motivation and self-regulated learning in adolescence and how the classroom context shapes the trajectory of motivation and self-regulation development. He has published over 80 articles, book chapters, and books, and currently serves as editor of the American Psychology Association (APA) journal for Division 15 (Educational Psychology), *Educational Psychologist*. A Fellow of the American Psychological Association (APA), he has previously been a National Academy of Education Spencer Fellow, and Program Chair for

the American Educational Research Association. He is currently President-Elect of Division 5-Educational and Instructional Psychology for
the International Association of Applied Psychology. Co-editor of the
book series *Advances in Motivation and Achievement*, he has edited
several other books on motivation and achievement, as well as being the
co-author of a graduate level text titled *Motivation in Education: Theory,
Research and Applications*.

Moshe Zeidner   is Professor of Educational and Social Psychology at the
University of Haifa, Israel. He serves as Director of the Center
for the Interdisciplinary Research on Emotions and Scientific Director
of the Laboratory for Cross-Cultural Research in Personality and Individual Differences. His main field of interest is personality and individual differences research, with particular concern for anxiety, stress and
coping, and the personality–intelligence interface. He is series editor
for two series: *Human Emotions*, and *Human Exceptionality*. He also
serves as Associate Editor of *Anxiety, Stress, and Coping: An International Journal* and as a reviewer for a number of APA journals. He is the
author of over 100 scientific papers and chapters and his recent books
include *Test Anxiety: The State of the Art* (1998), *Handbook of Coping,
Stress, Anxiety, and Coping in Academic Settings*, and *International
Handbook of Personality and Intelligence*.

CONTRIBUTORS

Numbers in parentheses indicate the pages on which the authors' contributions begin.

Monique Boekaerts (1, 417, 749) Center for the Study of Education and Instruction, Leiden University, NL-2300 Leiden, The Netherlands.

Susan Brownlee (369) Institute for Health, Health Care Policy, and Aging Research, Rutgers University, New Brunswick, New Jersey 08901.

Sian E. Campbell (171) Department of Psychology, University of Dundee, Dundee DD1 4HN, Scotland.

Charles S. Carver (41) Department of Psychology, University of Miami, Coral Gables, Florida 33146.

Lyn Corno (651) Teachers College, Columbia University, New York, New York 10027.

Thomas L. Creer (601) Department of Psychology, Ohio University, Athens, Ohio.

Erik De Corte (687) Department of Education, University of Leuven, B-3000 Leuven, Belgium.

Andreas Demetriou (209) Department of Educational Sciences, University of Cyprus, CY-1678 Nicosia, Cyprus.

Douglas R. Dierking (727) Department of Educational Psychology, University of Texas at Austin, Austin, Texas 78712.

Norman S. Endler (569) Department of Psychology, York University, North York, Ontario M3J 1P3, Canada.

Peggy A. Ertmer (631) School of Education, Purdue University, West Lafayette, Indiana 47907.

Winifred Gebhardt (343) Department of Clinical and Health Psychology, Leiden University, NL-2300 RB Leiden, The Netherlands.

Stevan E. Hobfoll (275) Applied Psychology Center, Kent State University, Kent, Ohio 44242.

Jenefer Husman (727) Department of Educational Psychology, University of Alabama, Tuscaloosa, Alabama 35487.

Tamara Jackson (275) Applied Psychology Center, Kent State University, Kent, Ohio 44242.

Nancy L. Kocovski (569) Department of Psychology, York University, North York, Ontario M3J 1P3, Canada.

Arie W. Kruglanski (85) Department of Psychology, University of Maryland, College Park, Maryland 20742.

Julius Kuhl (111) Department of Psychology, University of Osnabrück, D-49069 Osnabrück, Germany.

Elaine A. Leventhal (369) Department of Medicine, Robert Wood Johnson School of Medicine, University of Medicine and Dentistry of New Jersey, New Brunswick, New Jersey 08903.

Howard Leventhal (369) Institute for Health, Health Care Policy, and Aging Research, Rutgers University, New Brunswick, New Jersey 08901.

Jean Mackenzie (275) Applied Psychology Center, Kent State University, Kent, Ohio 44242.

Stan Maes (343) Department of Clinical and Health Psychology, Leiden University, NL-2300 RB Leiden, The Netherlands.

Gerald Matthews (171) Department of Psychology, University of Dundee, Dundee DD1 4HN, Scotland.

Abdalla A. R. Mohamed (171) Department of Psychology, University of Dundee, Dundee DD1 4HN, Scotland.

Markku Niemivirta (417) Department of Education, Helsinki University, Helsinki, The Netherlands.

Peter Op 't Eynde (687) Department of Education, University of Leuven, B-3000 Leuven, Belgium.

Nancy E. Perry (531) Department of Special Education and Educational Psychology, Faculty of Education, University of British Columbia, Vancouver, British Columbia V6T 1Z4, Canada.

Paul R. Pintrich (1, 451, 749)   Combined Program in Education and Psychology, The University of Michigan, Ann Arbor, Michigan 48109.

Judi Randi (651)   Teachers College, Columbia University, New York, New York 10027.

Falko Rheinberg (503)   Institut für Psychologie, University of Potsdam, D-14415 Potsdam, Germany.

Wolfram Rollett (503)   Institut fur Psychologie, University of Potsdam, D-14415 Potsdam, Germany.

Donald H. Saklofske (171)   Department of Educational Psychology, University of Saskatchewan, Saskatchewan, Saskatoon, Canada.

Michael F. Scheier (41)   Department of Psychology, Carnegie Mellon University, Pittsburgh, Pennsylvania 15213.

Dale H. Schunk (631)   School of Education, Purdue University, West Lafayette, Indiana 47907.

Gary E. Schwartz (253)   Department of Psychology, University of Arizona, Tucson, Arizona 85721.

Vicki L. Schwean (171)   Department of Education of Exceptional Children, University of Saskatchewan, Saskatoon, Saskatchewan, Canada S7N 0W0.

James Y. Shah (85)   Department of Psychology, University of Maryland, College Park, Maryland 20742.

Shauna L. Shapiro (253)   Department of Psychology, University of Arizona, Tucson, Arizona 85721.

Jeffrey B. Vancouver (303)   Department of Psychology, Ohio University, Athens, Ohio 45701.

Lieven Vershaffel (687)   Department of Education, University of Leuven, B-3000 Leuven, Belgium.

Regina Vollmeyer (503)   Institut für Psychologie, University of Potsdam, D-14415 Potsdam, Germany.

Claire Ellen Weinstein (727)   Department of Educational Psychology, University of Texas at Austin, Austin, Texas 78712.

Philip H. Winne (531)   Faculty of Education, Simon Fraser University, Burnaby, British Columbia, Canada V5A 156.

Moshe Zeidner (1, 749)   Faculty of Education, University of Haifa, Mount Carmel, 31905 Israel.

Barry J. Zimmerman (13)   Graduate School and University Center, City University of New York, New York, New York 10036.

1

SELF-REGULATION

AN INTRODUCTORY OVERVIEW

MONIQUE BOEKAERTS,* PAUL R. PINTRICH,[†]
AND MOSHE ZEIDNER[‡]

Leiden University, Leiden, The Netherlands
[†] *The University of Michigan, Ann Arbor, Michigan*
[‡] *The University of Haifa, Haifa, Israel*

In planning the *Handbook of Self-Regulation,* our aim was to provide an overview of a relatively new and increasingly important area in psychological research: self-regulation. Although self-regulation is a relative newcomer in the psychology journals, there is now a large but diverse body of research on this topic. In the 1980s, a large number of articles on self-regulation appeared, mainly in social psychology and personality journals. In the 1990s, the concept was broadened to include various aspects and application of self-regulation constructs, including self-regulated learning, self-control, and self-management. Publications began to appear in educational, organizational, clinical, and health psychology journals that used a number of related but different self-regulation constructs and labels.

Each of us was struck by the many different viewpoints on self-regulation that had been presented in the literature and by the broad range of phenomena that had been addressed by researchers involved in self-regulation research. We noticed that scholars from different areas of psychology had written about parallel but nonoverlapping phenomena and regretted that these articles were scattered throughout the many different psychological journals that reflected their own parochial interests and concerns. We felt that what was needed was a dialogue between researchers from these different fields within psychology. In our view, our understanding of the dynamics of self-regulation would profit a great deal from cross-area fertilization. A handbook offers the opportunity for schol-

Copyright © 2000 by Academic Press.
All rights of reproduction in any form reserved.

ars from the different areas to discuss their perspective on self-regulation, but to have these different viewpoints represented in one volume.

In this respect we wanted to echo Bruner's (1990) plea for less fragmentation and more coherence in psychological theory and research:

> I have written it (his book) at a time when psychology, the science of the mind as William James once called it, has become fragmented as never before in its history. It has lost its center and risks losing the cohesion needed to assume the internal exchange that might justify a division of labor between its parts. And the parts, each with its own organizational identity, its own theoretical apparatus, and often its own journals, have become specialties whose products become less and less exportable. Too often they seal themselves within their own rhetoric and within their own parish of authorities. This self-sealing risks making each part (and the aggregate that increasingly constitutes psychology's patchquilt whole) ever more remote from other inquiries dedicated to the understanding of mind and the human condition—inquiries in the humanities or the other social sciences. (pp. ix–x)

This quote can certainly be applied to research on self-regulation as it has been pursued by individuals working within the many different areas of psychology with a diversity of theories, models, constructs, and methodologies. Self-regulation theory and research in its many guises certainly deals with issues of the science of the mind. In fact, many of the specific issues William James was concerned with, such as willpower and behavior (e.g., his classic example of the difficulty of arising from a warm bed in the morning), are directly related to current topics in self-regulation.

However, the search for a general understanding of self-regulation has not been coherent given the diversity in the field. For example, researchers in one area, such as educational psychology, may not read articles on self-regulation produced by researchers working in a different area, such as health psychology. The main reason for this alienation may be that applied psychologists working within a particular context consider themselves a specific scientific community: They speak the same language, use their own conceptual models, and construct their own instruments and research designs to collect data about a specific aspect of self-regulation (e.g., about self-regulated learning, managing stress, regulation of one's health) in a specific context (e.g., homes, classrooms, health clinics, workplaces). This has resulted in large bodies of domain-specific knowledge about self-regulation, each covering specific aspects of self-regulation and using their own scientific terminology. A consequence of such domain or area specificity is that the information assembled about self-regulation is published in separate journals. Even more detrimental to the development of a common insight into the various phenomena of self-regulation is that a kaleidoscope of terms and labels exists and that these may sound unfamiliar, even alien, to researchers who are not in that particular area.

In our opinion, models and data collected from different vantage points with respect to the same or similar constructs are highly relevant to our efforts to achieve a science of the mind and a true understanding of what a complex construct such as self-regulation really means. These models and data can be the starting point for scholarly discussions which will promote reflection on one's own ideas and further one's understanding of the phenomena involving self-regulation. However, we are well aware that discussion and interaction of researchers who have drifted apart over the last few decades will be successful only if researchers have an open mind and are willing to question their own constructs and measurement instruments and are willing to extend and elaborate their own models.

Given this diversity, but armed with the goal of helping to reduce fragmentation and increase coherence in the field, we sought to bring together authors with different perspectives on self-regulation. To achieve this goal, we invited authors with an active program of research in a particular area of self-regulation to write a chapter for this handbook. We also wanted to include authors from outside the United States of America to avoid the traditional bias of much of American psychology, as well as to represent the diversity of international research on this topic. We explained to our authors that a book with a diversity of vantage points on self-regulation would help to identify cross-cutting themes that unite researchers in the different areas of psychology. We encouraged them to write a chapter that would allow for exploration of the similarities and dissimilarities in the conceptual frameworks, paradigms, and research methodologies of various research groups and to stimulate cross-fertilization of ideas in the field. We asked our authors to focus on the different ways individuals guide and direct their own behavior, cognition, and affect as well as the interactions among cognition, affect, and action. To our delight most of the authors we invited agreed to write a chapter, and we think they were successful in discussing and integrating these different aspects in their chapters.

In addition, we organized an expert meeting at Leiden University in The Netherlands. This expert meeting was sponsored by the Dutch National Foundation of Scientific Research (NWO) and we are very grateful for their support. For seven days, researchers from three applied fields of psychology met in Leiden to present their views on self-regulation and discuss the implications of their views, as well as to comment on the data and views presented by others. Many interesting questions were raised, the most prominent being whether the concepts used in health psychology, educational psychology, and organizational psychology represent similar ideas or whether quite different meanings are attached to these concepts in these different applied fields. Several chapters presented in this handbook grew out of these presentations and discussions.

The choice of the other topics for inclusion in the handbook was guided by our wish to include a wide range of contributors who together would enhance the breadth of paradigmatic perspectives relevant to self-regulation. We have not strived for genuine comprehensiveness: It is clearly impossible to cover the entire range of topics that constitute the phenomenon of self-regulation and do justice to each aspect. Consequently, some topics were left out of the book. For example, activity psychology and the vast domain of mood regulation are clearly missing. The range of topics that are included cover the use of self-regulation constructs in various areas of psychology, such as social, personality, clinical, developmental, educational, organizational, health, and community psychology.

It is clear from the diversity of the chapters in this handbook that self-regulation is a very difficult construct to define theoretically as well as to operationalize empirically. Nevertheless, the several years we worked together on the handbook have strengthened our conviction that self-regulation is an important topic that is highly relevant to the science of the mind and human behavior. At the same time, we are convinced that significant future progress is going to depend on our ability to clearly define the construct theoretically and to empirically distinguish it from other similar constructs. In this handbook many different definitions of self-regulation have been provided and a variety of explanations have been advanced to account for the observed effects of self-regulation on various outcome measures. We hope that the handbook will contribute to the cross-area conversations that are necessary to foster the much needed clarification of the term self-regulation and related constructs. The concluding chapter in this handbook provides a summary of the different definitions and future directions for theory and research as one attempt to stimulate the cross-area conversations.

The 23 chapters are organized into three sections. The chapters in Part I focus on general theories and models of self-regulation that can be applied to many different domains of human behavior. Part II includes chapters on domain specific applications of self-regulation theory and research in the areas of educational, health, and organizational psychology. Finally, the chapters in Part III concern the application of self-regulation constructs to improve practice in some way.

The chapters in Part I present an overview of the concept of self-regulation within psychology and some of the many constraints to its becoming a major construct within psychology. These chapters help us raise once again general questions about the nature of information processing, problem solving, motivation and decision making, as well as questions about the interaction between cognition and affect that cut across all areas of psychology. We hope that these chapters begin to address Bruner's concerns about fragmentation and they do suggest that self-regulatory constructs could be a cohesive force for integrating the different parochial areas of psychology.

The first three substantive chapters in this section take a more social psychological perspective on self-regulation. Zimmerman outlines the role of self-regulation as part of a general social cognitive theory of behavior. He argues that our regulatory skills, or lack thereof, are the sources of our perception of personal agency that lies at the core of our sense of self. He describes what is presently understood about the structure of the self-regulatory system, as well as the effect of the social and physical environmental context on self-regulation. Zimmerman also describes dysfunction in self-regulation and points to its development. Arguing that self-regulation is self-directed and feedback controlled, Carver and Scheier focus their chapter on hierarchicality among goals. These authors describe multiple paths to high-level goals and multiple meanings of concrete actions. The ideas discussed in their chapter have interesting implications for conceptualizing problem-solving behavior in various applied settings, including therapeutic behaviorial change. In the third chapter, Shah and Kruglanski present a structural theory of goal networks. They explain how goals and means relate to each other and the implications of these associations for a number of regulatory phenomena, such as goal commitment, choice of means, and means substitution. These authors also explicitly address individual differences in self-regulatory focus.

The next two chapters represent both social and personality perspectives on self-regulation. The chapter by Kuhl introduces a differentiated view of energy flow between personality systems and provides access to an additional category of determinants of goal-directed action. His theory of Personality Systems Interactions spells out the conditions under which cognitive performance is modulated by affect and relevant personality traits. Matthews, Schwean, Campbell, Saklofske, and Mohamed argue that styles of self-regulation are an integral aspect of personality. They emphasize the dynamic nature of self-knowledge and describe how traits such as neuroticism, introversion, and optimism–pessimism may be linked to various aspects of self-regulation.

Demetriou's chapter adds a developmental as well as systemic perspective to our understanding of self-regulation. He reviews research on the development of the self-concept, self-representations, self-monitoring, and self-modification. Demetriou presents a theory of cognitive change, focusing on the way children and adolescents self-monitor and how this important aspect of self-regulation develops. Shapiro and Schwartz continue with a more systemic model and address the possible implications of making intention explicit in self-regulation theory. They introduce the construct of "intention to systemic mindfulness," which refers to a broad self-regulatory focus that embeds the self and symptom in larger systems. Jackson,

Mackenzie, and Hobfoll also present a larger systemic view and draw attention to major biases that exist in traditional theories of psychology, including self-regulation theory. They argue that traditional models of self-regulation assume that behavior is determined by individual goals and needs with limited influence from others or the environmental context. They show how notions that are highly valued within a particular society, such as self-control, personal freedom, and accountability, are reflected in theories of self-regulation that researchers who grew up in that culture propose to the scientific community.

Part II includes chapters on paradigms that have emerged in research on self-regulation in specific areas. Domain-specific models of self-regulation that are used in organizational, health, and educational psychology are represented in this section. Vancouver describes two general approaches to understanding human behavior in industrial and organizational settings, and how they have been integrated in self-regulation models. Most importantly, he offers his own model for integrating the cybernetic or systems approach with the decision-making or problem-solving approach to organizational psychology. At the same time, the issues he discusses regarding the architecture of self-regulating systems is relevant to many areas of self-regulation, not just organizational models.

The next two chapters in Part II focus on models of self-regulation as applied to health behaviors. The chapter by Maes and Gebhardt concerns the promotion of health and healthy living. They review the major health behavior models and provide a general listing of the important components of these models such as goals, values, perceived competence, cost–benefit analysis, and mediating processes as well as more general personal and environmental characteristics that influence individual's health choices and behavior. After this review, they present their own integrated model, the health behavior goal model, which incorporates the important components from other models and ties them to various self-regulatory processes. The second chapter on health issues, by Brownlee, Leventhal, and Leventhal, focuses on health maintenance and coping with illness. They present their Common-Sense Model of self-regulation, which is based on the idea that the content of the domain or behavior is of great importance in determining the functioning of various self-regulation processes. They summarize their program of research on how content representations of illness and health influence the functioning of the cognitive and affective systems for coping with health problems. In addition, they discuss the role of social and contextual factors and how they influence individual representations of illness and health problems.

The next four chapters all discuss models of self-regulation in the context of educational settings. Boekaerts and Niemivirta discuss how school and classroom learning contexts and episodes can offer opportunities for self-regulation. At the same time, they point out that these opportunities can be appraised in different ways and that different goals, such as learning and ego-protective goals, promote and facilitate different ways of coping and learning in the classroom. Their Model of Adaptable Learning represents a systematic perspective on the role of goals and self-regulated learning in the classroom. In a similar manner, Pintrich discusses the role of personal goal orientations in facilitating and constraining self-regulated learning in the classroom. He provides a general taxonomy for conceptualizing self-regulated learning and links these various regulation processes to different goals students may adopt in the classroom. Finally, he suggests that the normative two-goal model of mastery and performance goals may be improved by adopting the approach–avoidance distinction and highlights how this model may result in a more differentiated view of the relationships between goals and self-regulated learning.

In contrast to the goal models of motivation in the previous two chapters, the chapter by Rheinberg, Vollmeyer, and Rollett represents an expectancy-value perspective on motivation and self-regulated learning in achievement settings. They refine and enlarge the various expectancy and value constructs that may play a role in self-regulated learning. In addition, they suggest how volitional processes can contribute to learning in achievement settings. Finally, Winne and Perry discuss issues related to the measurement of self-regulated learning in classroom contexts. In line with current psychometric theory, they present a general theoretical model of self-regulated learning and then consider issues of construct validity and measurement procedures in light of this model. Their chapter highlights the difficult conceptual and assessment issues that are endemic to research on self-regulated learning in classroom contexts.

Part III addresses theory and research that has transformed self-regulation theory into practice. Various researchers describe how they have created social settings in which self-regulation has been put to work or in which self-regulation had been formally taught or facilitated. The first two chapters in this section deal with general physical and mental health problems. Endler and Kocovski argue that strategies and techniques based on self-regulation models of human behavior can be used for the management of health problems and the treatment of clinical disorders. These authors extend the scope of self-regulation theory to addictive behaviors, coping with health problems, social anxiety, and depression. Creer illustrates that in the case of chronic disease, neither of the traditional definitions of self-regulation or self-management is appropriate. He explains that coining different terms for the same behavior is a way of avoiding the important issues. He provides a state-of-the-art glimpse of the development and application of self-management programs for chronic illness.

The next four chapters all concern issues of teaching or facilitating self-regulatory processes in educational contexts. Schunk and Ertmer focus on systematic interventions that are designed to teach skills and raise students' self-efficacy for learning. They follow a general social cognitive model and discuss how efficacy, goals, and strategies for self-monitoring and regulating can be taught in formal educational interventions. Randi and Corno's chapter moves away from generic strategy training programs and suggests the need for contextualized and embedded self-regulation instruction. They argue that teachers should try to connect aspects of self-regulation training explicitly with their own curriculum and their own classroom teaching environment. They use a case study of how self-regulation may be facilitated through the use of literature in a humanities curriculum and they suggest a need for a more collaborative model of how researchers and teachers might work together to improve self-regulation and learning in classrooms.

De Corte, Verschaffel, and Op't Eynde discuss the role of self-regulation in mathematics learning and instruction. They describe how self-regulatory processes are important in mathematics expertise and learning as well as the many difficulties students have in regulating their mathematics learning and problem solving. Their chapter also includes a discussion of how mathematics classrooms can be designed to facilitate the learning of important mathematical self-regulatory strategies. The chapter by Weinstein, Husman, and Dierking presents a systematic approach to the teaching of self-regulatory strategies for college learners. They present a model of strategic learning that incorporates skill, will, and self-regulatory components. Their chapter also discusses the important components for any formal intervention to teach self-regulatory strategies.

In the concluding chapter, we discuss the various themes and issues that emerge from a reading of all the chapters in the book. We do not offer any one solution to the many problems in this area, but we do think that identifying the common themes and issues will help start the conversation that should reduce the fragmentation and lack of cohesion in the field of self-regulation research. In the final chapter, we note that there are 12 general themes or overlapping issues the field must consider in future theory and research. These include:

1. Developing a common theoretical framework and nomenclature of constructs.
2. Clarifying the structures and processes of self-regulation.
3. Developing the nomological network of different self-regulation constructs and other related but distinct psychological constructs.
4. Constructing more refined and detailed models.
5. Refining and improving the measurement of self-regulation.
6. Improving and diversifying our research designs and methodology.

7. Exploring more fully the interactions between persons and contexts, including more attention to how self-regulation is situated and contextualized.
8. Attending to the processes of acquisition and transmission of self-regulatory processes in the course of normal development.
9. Investigating developmental differences in self-regulation.
10. Examining individual and cultural differences in self-regulation.
11. Generating applications of self-regulation to various domains of human behavior.
12. Improving formal training and instructional efforts to promote self-regulation.

We believe that the handbook addresses the clear need in the field to develop a broad and integrative perspective on theory and research in self-regulation. In thinking about the nature of self-regulation, the contributors to the handbook have drawn on disparate sources. The result is an aggregation of models, principles, and empirical data that together represent our best inferences about how self-regulation takes place and how it influences a diversity of psychological and behavioral outcomes. The conceptual picture is far from complete and many avenues await further empirical exploration.

We wish to thank our contributors for their generosity and willingness to participate in this project, particularly because we know they all had very busy schedules. Their patient and effective self-regulation of their own writing and revision of their chapters made it possible to complete the handbook in a fairly timely manner. We have certainly learned a great deal from this project and we hope that future readers will also profit from reading the chapters in this handbook. We hope this handbook is just the beginning of a sustained and productive conversation about the role of self-regulation in the science of the human mind and behavior.

REFERENCE

Bruner, J. (1990). *Acts of meaning*. Cambridge, MA: Harvard University Press.

General Theories and Models of Self-Regulation

2

ATTAINING

SELF-REGULATION

A SOCIAL COGNITIVE
PERSPECTIVE

BARRY J. ZIMMERMAN

City University of New York, New York, New York.

I. INTRODUCTION

Perhaps our most important quality as humans is our capability to self-regulate. It has provided us with an adaptive edge that enabled our ancestors to survive and even flourish when changing conditions led other species to extinction. Our regulatory skill or lack thereof is the source of our perception of personal agency that lies at the core of our sense of self. Understanding how this capability develops, its various subcomponents, and its functions has been a major thrust of social cognitive theory and research. Of equal importance is the explanation for common dysfunctions in self-regulatory functioning, such as biased self-monitoring, self-blaming judgments, and defensive self-reactions. This chapter will define self-regulation and will discuss the structure of self-regulatory systems, social and physical environmental context influences on self-regulation, dysfunctions in self-regulation, and self-regulatory development.

A. A TRIADIC DEFINITION OF SELF-REGULATION

A social cognitive perspective is distinctive in viewing self-regulation as an interaction of *personal, behavioral,* and *environmental* triadic processes (Bandura, 1986). More specifically, it entails not only behavioral skill in

---

Copyright © 2000 by Academic Press.
All rights of reproduction in any form reserved.
13

self-managing environmental contingencies, but also the knowledge and the sense of personal agency to enact this skill in relevant contexts. Self-regulation refers to self-generated thoughts, feelings, and actions that are planned and cyclically adapted to the attainment of personal goals. This definition, in terms of actions and covert processes whose presence and quality depends on one's beliefs and motives, differs from definitions emphasizing a singular trait, ability, or stage of competence. A process definition can explain why a person may self-regulate one type of performance but not another. This personal agency formulation also differs from metacognitive views of self-regulation that emphasize only knowledge states and deductive reasoning when, for example, choosing cognitive strategies. Although metacognition plays an important role, self-regulation also depends on self-beliefs and affective reactions, such as doubts and fears, about specific performance contexts (Zimmerman, 1995b). Aspiring chess players may try to emulate a well known defense strategy but often abandon it when their confidence falters during a competitive match. Contextually related self-processes, such as perceived efficacy, have been shown to be well suited to explaining variations in personal motivation to self-regulate one's performance (Bandura, 1997; Pajares & Miller, 1994; Zimmerman, 1995a). Self-efficacy refers to beliefs about one's capabilities to organize and implement actions necessary to attain designated performance of skill for specific tasks.

Self-regulation is described as cyclical because the feedback from prior performance is used to make adjustments during current efforts. Such adjustments are necessary because personal, behavioral, and environmental factors are constantly changing during the course of learning and performance, and must be observed or monitored using three self-oriented feedback loops (see Figure 1). *Behavioral self-regulation* involves self-observing and strategically adjusting performance processes, such as one's method of learning, whereas *environmental self-regulation* refers to observing and adjusting environmental conditions or outcomes. *Covert self-regulation* involves monitoring and adjusting cognitive and affective states, such as imagery for remembering or relaxing. The accuracy and constancy of learners' self-monitoring of these triadic sources of self-control directly influence the effectiveness of their strategic adjustments and the nature of their self-beliefs. These triadic feedback loops are assumed to be open. Unlike closed-loop views, which limit self-regulation to reducing performance discrepancies *reactively* against an unchanging standard (Locke, 1991), open-loop perspectives include *proactively* increasing performance discrepancies by raising goals and seeking more challenging tasks. For example, when chess players decide to move up to a new level of competition, they make success more difficult to achieve but use the outcome discrepancies as a way to motivate themselves to attain higher levels of

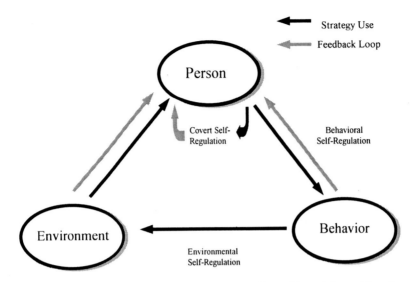

FIGURE 1   Triadic forms of self-regulation. *Note.* From "A social cognitive view of self-regulated academic learning," by B. J. Zimmerman, 1989, *Journal of Educational Psychology, 81,* p. 330. Copyright 1989 by the American Psychological Association. Adapted with permission.

skill. Thus, self-regulation involves triadic processes that are proactively as well as reactively adapted for the attainment of personal goals.

II. THE STRUCTURE OF SELF-REGULATORY SYSTEMS

It has been argued that every person attempts to self-regulate his or her functioning in some way to gain goals in life and that it is inaccurate to speak about un-self-regulated persons or even the absence of self-regulation (Winne, 1997). From this perspective, what distinguishes effective from ineffective forms self-regulation is instead the quality and quantity of one's self-regulatory processes. The most effective processes have been identified through a variety of empirical sources, including interviews with experts who are known for their self-discipline and success (e.g., Ericsson & Lehman, 1996; Zimmerman & Martinez-Pons, 1986, 1988), clinical studies of individuals experiencing self-regulatory dysfunctions (Watson & Tharp, 1993), and experimental research on personal methods of control during demanding performance tasks (Kanfer & Ackerman, 1989; Kuhl, 1985). An important issue is to understand how these processes are structurally interrelated and cyclically sustained.

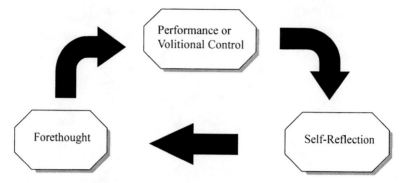

FIGURE 2   Cyclical phases of self-regulation. *Note.* From *Self-Regulated Learning: From Teaching to Self-Reflective Practice.* (p. 3), by D. H. Schunk and B. J. Zimmerman (Eds.), 1998, New York: Guilford. Copyright 1998 by Guilford Press. Reprinted with permission.

From a social cognitive perspective, self-regulatory processes and accompanying beliefs fall into three cyclical phases: forethought, performance or volitional control, and self-reflection processes (see Figure 2). Forethought refers to influential processes that precede efforts to act and set the stage for it. Performance or volitional control involves processes that occur during motoric efforts and affect attention and action. Self-reflection involves processes that occur after performance efforts and influence a person's response to that experience. These self-reflections, in turn, influence forethought regarding subsequent motoric efforts—thus completing a self-regulatory cycle.

A. FORETHOUGHT PHASE

There are two distinctive but closely linked categories of forethought: (1) task analysis and (2) self-motivational beliefs (see Table 1). A key form of task analysis involves the setting of goals. *Goal setting* refers to deciding

TABLE 1   Phase Structure and Subprocesses of Self-Regulation

Cyclical self-regulatory phases		
Forethought	Performance/volitional control	Self-reflection

Task analysis
  Goal setting
  Strategic planning
	Self-control
	  Self-instruction
	  Imagery
	  Attention focusing
	  Task strategies
		Self-judgment
		  Self-evaluation
		  Causal attribution

Self-motivation beliefs
  Self-efficacy
  Outcome expectations
  Intrinsic interest/value
  Goal orientation
	Self-observation
	  Self-recording
	  Self-experimentation
		Self-reaction
		  Self-satisfaction/affect
		  Adaptive-defensive

upon specific outcomes of learning or performance, such as solving a group of division problems in mathematics during a study session (Locke & Latham, 1990). The goal systems of highly self-regulated individuals are organized hierarchically, such that process goals operate as proximal regulators of more distal outcome goals. These process subgoals are not merely mechanical check points on the path to attaining highly valued outcomes; instead they become invested with personal meaning because they convey evidence of progress. For example, a pupil learning a tennis serve will feel an increasing sense of efficacy about mastering this stroke as components of it are acquired, such as the take back of the racket, the ball toss, and the follow-through. Bandura and Schunk (1981) reported evidence that as students pursued and attained proximal goals in mathematics, they developed greater self-efficacy and intrinsic interest in this topic.

A second form of task analysis is *strategic planning* (Weinstein & Mayer, 1986). For a skill to be mastered or performed optimally, learners need methods that are appropriate for the task and the setting. Self-regulative strategies are purposive personal processes and actions directed at acquiring or displaying skill (Zimmerman, 1989). Appropriately selected strategies enhance performance by aiding cognition, controlling affect, and directing motoric execution (Pressley & Wolloshyn, 1995). For example, key word or integrative image strategies are known to enhance the recall and use of information during motoric performance (Schneider & Pressley, 1997). The planning and selection of strategies requires cyclical adjustments because of fluctuations in covert personal, behavioral, and environmental components. No self-regulatory strategy will work equally well for all persons, and few, if any, strategies will work optimally for a person on all tasks or occasions. As a skill develops, the effectiveness of an initial acquisition strategy often declines to the point where another strategy becomes necessary, such as when a novice golfer shifts from a swing execution strategy to a ball flight aiming strategy. Thus, as a result of diverse and changing intrapersonal, interpersonal, and contextual conditions, self-regulated individuals must continuously adjust their goals and choice of strategies.

Self-regulatory skills are of little value if a person cannot motivate themselves to use them. Underlying forethought processes of goal setting and strategic planning are a number of key self-motivational beliefs: self-efficacy, outcome expectations, intrinsic interest or valuing, and goal orientation. As was noted earlier, *self-efficacy* refers to personal beliefs about having the means to learn or perform effectively, whereas *outcome expectations* refer to beliefs about the ultimate ends of performance (Bandura, 1997). For example, self-efficacy refers to the belief that one can attain a course grade of A, and outcomes refer to expectations about the consequences this grade will produce after graduation, such as a desirable job. A person's willingness to engage and sustain their self-regulatory efforts depends especially on their self-regulatory efficacy, which refers to beliefs about their capability to plan and manage specific areas of functioning. There is evidence that self-regulatory efficacy beliefs causally influence use of such regulatory processes as academic learning strategies (Schunk & Schwartz, 1993; Zimmerman, Bandura, & Martinez-Pons, 1992), academic time management (Britton & Tessor, 1991), resisting adverse peer pressures (Bandura, Barbaranelli, Caprara & Pastorelli, 1996b), self-monitoring (Bouffard-Bouchard, Parent, & Larivee, 1991), self-evaluation, and goal setting (Zimmerman & Bandura, 1994).

For example, self-efficacy beliefs influence goal setting in the following way: The more capable people believe themselves to be, the higher the goals they set for themselves and the more firmly committed they remain to those goals (Bandura, 1991; Locke & Latham, 1990). When people fall short of attaining their outcome goals, those who are self-efficacious increase their efforts, whereas those who are self-doubters withdraw (Bandura & Cervone, 1986). Goals can reciprocally affect self-efficacy beliefs. Self-regulated learners feel self-efficacious in part because they have adopted hierarchical process goals for themselves whose progressive mastery provides them with immediate satisfaction rather than requiring them to suspend any sense of success until a final outcome goal is attained. There is evidence that process goal attainment can become intrinsically motivating in its own right and can even outweigh attainment of superordinate outcome goals (Schunk & Schwartz, 1993; Zimmerman & Kitsantas, 1997).

With time, process goal seekers begin to see outcome rewards merely as milestones in a lifelong mastery process, such as when musicians see the ultimate value of their talent lies in performing masterfully rather than in winning a particular competition. In this way, process accomplishments provide a sense of *intrinsic* motivation or valuing that can complement and even surpass extrinsic outcomes (Deci, 1975; Lepper & Hodell, 1989). This self-regulatory process *goal orientation* also has been labeled a learning (Dweck, 1988), a mastery (Ames, 1992), or a task goal orientation (Nicholls, 1984), and has been shown to sustain motivation and improve acquisition and performance better than an outcome goal orientation (Pintrich & Schunk, 1996).

B. PERFORMANCE OR VOLITIONAL CONTROL PHASE

Two major types of performance or volitional control processes have been studied to date: self-control and self-observation. Self-control processes, such as self-instruction, imagery, attention focusing, and task strategies, help learners and performers to focus on the task and optimize their effort. *Self-instruction* involves overtly or covertly describing how to proceed as one executes a task, such as solving a mathematics problem or memorizing a formula, and research shows that such verbalizations can improve students' learning (Schunk, 1982). Meichenbaum (1977) has been at the forefront of efforts to enhance students' self-instruction during learning efforts, especially with learning disabled children. *Imagery* or the forming of mental pictures is another widely used self-control technique to assist encoding and performance. In a series of influential studies, Pressley and colleagues (Pressley 1977; Pressley & Levin, 1977) taught learners to mentally construct integrative images, such as a knife piercing a hat, to improve their recall of these two items. Sports psychologists have taught competitors, such as skaters, divers, or gymnasts, to imagine successful executions of their planned routines in order to enhance their performance (Garfield & Bennett, 1985).

A third form of self-control, *attention focusing*, is designed to improve one's concentration and screen out other covert processes or external events. Expert performers report using a wide variety of techniques to improve their attentional control, such as environmental structuring to eliminate diversions or slow-motion task execution to assist coordination (Mach, 1988). Kuhl and his colleagues (Kuhl, 1985) studied the use of volitional methods of control, such as ignoring distractions and avoiding ruminating about past mistakes, and found them to be effective. There is evidence that knowing how to concentrate and screen out other covert processes and external events is an essential strategy for effective studying (Corno, 1993; Weinstein, Schulte, & Palmer, 1987). *Task strategies* assist learning and performance by reducing a task to its essential parts and reorganizing the parts meaningfully. For example, when students listen to a history lecture, they might identify a limited number of key points and record them chronologically in brief sentences. The effectiveness of a wide variety of task strategies has been studied by Weinstein and Mayer (1986), Wood, Woloshyn, and Willoughby (1995), and Zimmerman and Martinez-Pons (1988) to guide learning efforts, and the effectiveness of these strategies is well documented. These included study strategies, such as note taking, test preparation, and reading for comprehension, as well as performance strategies, such as writing techniques, elocution, and problem solving.

The second type of volition or performance control process involves self-observation. This refers to a person's tracking of specific aspects of their own performance, the conditions that surround it, and the effects that it produces (Zimmerman & Paulsen, 1995). Although this skill may seem elemental, it is not, because the amount of information involved in complex performances can easily inundate naive self-observers and typically can lead to disorganized or cursory self-monitoring. Experts are able to track themselves selectively at a detailed process level when necessary, such as when concert pianists monitor their hand positions, which enables them to make more fine-grained adaptations than novices (Mach, 1988).

Setting hierarchical process goals during forethought facilitates selective self-observation because these goals focus on specific processes and proximal events.

There are a number of features of self-observation that can influence its effectiveness. The temporal proximity of one's self-observations is a critical variable (Bandura, 1986; Kazdin, 1974). Self-feedback that is delayed precludes a person from taking corrective action in a timely fashion, such as monitoring one's running time after the completion of a long distance track race rather than during it. A second feature of high quality self-observation is the informativeness of performance feedback. Practicing a skill in a standardized or structured setting can enhance informativeness of the results (Ericsson & Lehman, 1996). For example, practicing sprints on an official 100 meter track permits runners to see if changes in technique improve their competitive speed. A third qualitative feature is the accuracy of self-observations: Individuals who misperceive or distort their actions cannot correct them appropriately. For example, there is evidence that speakers of minority dialects needed special training to discriminate erroneous word pronunciations before they could practice in a self-corrective fashion on their own (Ellis, 1995). A fourth qualitative feature of self-observation involves the valence of the behavior. Monitoring negative aspects of one's functioning, such as cigarettes smoked or dietary failures, can diminish a persons' motivation to self-regulate these activities (Kirschenbaum & Karoly, 1977). Often it is possible to record performance accomplishments rather than deficits, such as days without smoking or the frequency of dietary success. Undoubtedly, feedback about deficits can lead to self-criticism.

Self-recording is a common self-observational technique that can increase greatly the proximity, informativeness, accuracy, and valence of feedback (Zimmerman & Kitsantas, 1996). Records can capture personal information at the point it occurs, structure it to be most meaningful, preserve its accuracy without need for intrusive rehearsal, and provide a longer data base for discerning evidence of progress. For example, asthmatics who keep records of their symptoms can discern their allergy triggers as well as the effectiveness of preventive medications (Bonner, Rivera, & Zimmerman, 1997).

Through observation of covert thought patterns and emotional reactions as well as overt performance, people begin to notice recurrent patterns in their functioning, such as when or where a smoker craves cigarettes or actually smokes them. If any regularities in pattern can be discerned, they can be used to identify influential features of their environment, such as consistently smoking after eating or in the presence of other smokers. For those individuals who can alter their behavior or modify their environment, these insights can lead to corrective courses of action, such as avoiding places where smokers congregate.

Self-observation can lead to cycles of *self-experimentation* (Bandura, 1991). When self-observation of natural variations in behavior does not provide decisive diagnostic information, people can engage in personal experimentation by systematically varying the aspects of their functioning that are in question. For example, when the urge to smoke may seem random and spontaneous, a smoker may test out various contextual hypotheses, such as the presence of stress, ash trays, or advertisements. In this way systematic self-observation can lead to greater personal understanding and to better performance or volitional control.

C. SELF-REFLECTION PHASE

Bandura (1986) has identified two self-reflective processes that are closely associated with self-observation: self-judgment and self-reactions. *Self-judgment* involves self-evaluating one's performance and attributing causal significance to the results. *Self-evaluation* refers to comparing self-monitored information with a standard or goal, such as a sprinter judging practice runs according to his or her best previous effort. Judging the adequacy of one's performance is relatively easy when it produces simple objective outcomes, such as being able to swim, drive an automobile, or solve a mathematical problem. However, high levels of expertise depend on the judgments using refined criteria, such as swimming 100 meters in a particular time period or faster than 98% of other swimmers. Ultimately, the adaptive quality of one's self-reactions depends on the sensitivity of his or her self-judgments (Zimmerman & Paulsen, 1995), and knowing this, experts set challenging criteria for themselves (Ericsson & Lehman, 1996).

There are four distinctive types of criteria that people use to evaluate themselves: mastery, previous performance, normative, and collaborative. Mastery criteria involve the use of a graduated sequence of tests or test scores ranging from novice to expert performance, such as the seven point system that tennis instructors use to rate players. Mastery hierarchies also have been used for testing and curriculum selection in schools, such as workbooks that are color coded for level of expertise. Mastery criteria have been advocated by Covington and Roberts (1994) because they highlight evidence of personal learning progress in the attainment, which usually occurs with continuing practice. The use of process goal hierarchies predisposes a person to adopt a mastery criterion for self-evaluation because the sequential order of the subgoals provides an ready index of mastery.

Previous performance or self-criteria involves comparisons of current performance with earlier levels of one's behavior, such as a baseline or the previous performance (Bandura, 1997). For example, smokers can judge their success in overcoming this habit by comparing cigarettes smoked currently with the previous day's level of consumption. Like mastery comparisons, self-comparisons involve within-subject changes in functioning, and as a result, they also highlight learning progress, which typically improves with repeated practice.

In contrast to mastery or previous performance criteria, normative criteria involve social comparisons with the performance of others, such as classmates or a national population that was tested. Awards are given at most competitions on the basis of social rankings, such as the gold medalist at the Olympics, who is the person who comes in first regardless of whether or not he or she breaks the existing world record. Normative criteria can be defended on the basis of the competitive nature of many human enterprises, such as employment and sales. In these circumstances, a person must be not only effective or skilled, but also must be better than a competitor. Among the drawbacks of using normative criteria for self-evaluative judgments is the fact they deemphasize selective self-observation and conversely heighten attention to social factors. Another shortcoming is that social comparisons often tend to emphasize negative aspects of functioning instead of the positive ones, such as when a person loses the race despite having improved his or her time in comparison to previous efforts. Learners who focus on outcome goals are predisposed to using normative criteria for self-evaluative judgments because outcomes are often competitively awarded and socially visible, such as grades in school.

Finally, a collaborative criterion is used primarily in team endeavors (Bandura, 1991). Under these common but more complex circumstances, success is defined in terms of fulfilling a particular role, such as the point guard on a basketball team. The criteria of success for a point guard are different than those used for the other team positions, and how well a point guard can work cooperatively with his or her teammates becomes the ultimate criterion of success.

Self-evaluative judgments are linked to *causal attributions* about the results, such as whether poor performance is due to one's limited ability or to insufficient effort. These attributional judgments are pivotal to self-reflection, because attributions of errors to a fixed ability prompt learners to react negatively and discourage efforts to improve (Weiner, 1979). There is recent evidence (e.g., Zimmerman & Kitsantas, 1996, 1997) that attributions of errors to learning strategies are highly effective in sustaining motivation during periods of subpar performance because strategy attributions sustain perceptions of efficacy until all possible strategies have been tested. Attributions are not automatic outcomes of favorable or unfavorable self-evaluations, but rather depend on cognitive appraisal of extenuating factors, such as perceptions of personal efficacy or mitigating environmental conditions (Bandura, 1991). For example, when workers receive a negative evaluation for their job performance, those who are self-efficacious are more likely to attribute it to insufficient effort or a poor task strategy than those who are self-doubters. Alternatively, workers who felt the evaluation occurred during atypical circumstances, such as when directed by a temporary supervisor, might attribute it to bad luck rather than inability.

Forethought processes also impact attributional judgments. People who plan to use a specific strategy during forethought and implement its use during performance are more likely to attribute failures to that strategy rather than low ability, which can be devastating personally (Zimmerman & Kitsantas, 1997). Because strategies are perceived as correctable causes, attributions to their use protect against negative self-reactions and foster a strategically adaptive course of subsequent action.

Self-evaluative and attributional self-judgments are linked closely to two key forms of self-reactions: self-satisfaction and adaptive inferences. *Self-satisfaction* involves perceptions of satisfaction or dissatisfaction and associated affect regarding one's performance, which is important because people pursue courses of action that result in satisfaction and positive affect, and avoid those courses that produce dissatisfaction and negative affect, such as anxiety (Bandura, 1991). When self-satisfaction is made conditional on reaching adopted goals, people give direction to their actions and create self-incentives to persist in their efforts. Thus, a person's motivation does not stem from the goals themselves, but rather from self-evaluative reactions to behavioral outcomes.

A person's level of self-satisfaction also depends on the intrinsic value or importance of the task. For example, people who greatly value their job will experience severe dissatisfaction and anxiety if they receive unfavorable performance ratings. However, individuals who view their position as only temporary employment and unworthy of serious consideration will not be overly distressed by unfavorable job ratings. Highly self-regulated people value their intrinsic feelings of self-respect and self-satisfaction from a job well done more highly than acquiring material rewards (Bandura, 1997).

Adaptive or defensive inferences are conclusions about how one needs to alter his or her self-regulatory approach during subsequent efforts to learn or perform. Adaptive inferences are important because they direct people to new and potentially better forms of performance self-regulation, such as by shifting the goals hierarchically or choosing a more effective strategy (Zimmerman & Martinez-Pons, 1992). In contrast, defensive inferences serve primarily to protect the person from future dissatisfaction and aversive affect, but unfortunately they also undermine successful adaptation. These defensive self-reactions include helplessness, procrastination, task avoidance, cognitive disengagement, and apathy. Garcia and Pintrich (1994) have referred to such defensive reactions as self-handicapping strategies, because, despite their intended protectiveness, they ultimately limit personal growth.

These self-reactions affect forethought processes cyclically and often dramatically impact future courses of action toward one's most important goals and away from one's deepest fears. For example, self-satisfaction reactions strengthen self-efficacy beliefs about eventually mastering the academic skill, learning goal orientations (Schunk, 1996), and intrinsic interest in the task (Zimmerman & Kitsantas, 1997). These enhanced self-motivational beliefs form the basis for peoples' sense of personal agency about continuing their cyclical self-regulatory efforts and eventually attaining their goals. In contrast, self-dissatisfaction reactions reduce one's sense of efficacy and intrinsic interest in pursuing the task further. Bandura (1997, in press) has discussed many examples of how a person's feelings of self-efficacy can dramatically alter his or her life path, such as when dissatisfaction with grades in a chemistry course undermines a premed student's sense of efficacy to continue in the program. Thus, a cyclical social cognitive model can explain the persistence and sense of self-fulfillment of achievers as well as the avoidance and self-doubts of nonachievers.

III. SOCIAL AND ENVIRONMENTAL INFLUENCES ON SELF-REGULATION

A key feature of a social cognitive model of self-regulation is the interdependent roles of social, environmental, and self influences. As was illustrated in Figure 1 regarding triadic feedback loops, environmental and personal (self) processes interact bidirectionally in naturalistic settings. Self-initiated processes alter one's social and physical environment, and are in turn affected by those changes, such as when a mother puts a note on the refrigerator (an environmental cue) to remind herself or other family members (a social resource) to buy milk. From a triadic perspective, people who neglect to use social and physical environmental resources or who view them as an obstacle to personal development will be less effective in regulating their lives. Internal views of self-regulatory functioning, such as will power beliefs, are often based on insufficient information about the social and environmental nature of skilled functioning (Ericsson & Charness, 1994; Newman, 1994; Thoresen & Mahoney, 1974).

Even with the seemingly solitary and highly personal craft of writing, there is abundant evidence (Zimmerman & Risemberg, 1997) of the value of social and physical environmental regulation techniques, such as emulating the styles of exemplary models, soliciting assistance from teachers or confidants, and restructuring the writing setting. Regarding the self-selected use of modeling, the famed publisher, scientist, and statesman Benjamin Franklin improved his writing style by imitatively practicing passages written by exemplary writers of his day. One of the most unusual forms of social assistance was reported by Victor Hugo, who enlisted the aid of a servant. Because this novelist had so much trouble resisting the temptations of tavern life while writing, he gave his clothing to his valet with strict orders not to return them until he had completed a manuscript. Writers have used an interesting assortment of methods to self-regulate their writing environment. For example, the French poet and novelist Cendrars wrote only in a small enclosed place to screen out visual distractions (Plimpton, 1965) and the French novelist Marcel Proust wrote in a cork-lined room he had constructed to block outside sounds (Barzon, 1964). In addition to these instances of modeling and environmental structuring, there is evidence (Zimmerman & Risemberg, 1997) that professional writers rely on many other social and environmental resources, such as record keeping, to assist them during forethought and self-control of their functioning.

The social milieu influences self-reflection processes in a similar fashion to forethought and performance phase processes. Youth often form standards for self-evaluative judgment on the basis of instruction, social feedback, and modeling from peers, parents, teachers, and coaches. For example, child prodigies often come from families where successful parents, siblings, or relatives model high standards of performance and self-judgment (Mach, 1988). Verbal self-criticism and pessimism or self-praise and optimism are often visible to others, and these vicarious cues can convey standards for self-reaction to an observer (Zimmerman & Ringle, 1981).

People can increase their self-reactions by using environmental supports, such as self-administered rewards or praise. Athletic coaches frequently advise their pupils to reward themselves with refreshment breaks for completing effective exercise or practice sessions or to "pump themselves up" by making self-congratulatory comments for scoring a winning point. A relatively common technique to motivate oneself to complete daily activities is to put off favored activities, such as relaxing breaks or recreational activities, until after completing less attractive ones. The writer Irving Wallace (1971) reports that novelists can increase the amount they write by making pursuit of other activities contingent upon attaining certain amounts or time periods of writing. Tangible self-rewards are designed to increase people's reactions to their performance and outcome expectations. There is evidence (Bandura & Kupers, 1964) that individuals who reward their own attainments accomplish more than those who perform the same activities without self-administered incentives.

Thus, the social and physical environment is viewed by social cognitive researchers as a resource for self-enhancing forethought, performance or volitional control, and self-reflection. Modeling and instruction serve as a primary vehicle through which parents, teachers, and communities socially convey self-regulatory skills, such as persistence, self-praise, and adaptive self-reactions to children. Conversely, when social models demonstrate impulsiveness, self-criticism, or defensive self-reactions, or when social groups reward or accept such actions, a wide array of personal dysfunctions often ensue.

IV. DYSFUNCTIONS IN SELF-REGULATION

The consequences of dysfunctions in personal regulation have been enormous, particularly in Western societies with their many freedoms. Low self-regulatory skill is associated with a wide range of personal problems. For example, there is evidence that students who have trouble self-regulating their academic studying achieve more poorly in school (Zimmerman and Martinez-Pons, 1986, 1988) and present more deportment problems for their teachers (Brody, Stoneman, & Flor, 1996). Poor regulation of one's health through an improper diet, failure to take needed medicines, and exposure to disease also has had a costly impact on lives. For example, people who cannot self-regulate the chronic disease of asthma display higher levels of symptoms, lower quality of life, and are hospitalized more frequently (Zimmerman, Bonner, Evans, & Mellins, 1999). The inability of girls to self-regulate their weight is a very prevalent health problem that often results in binge eating, anorexia, and bulimia. Similarly, boys' misguided regulatory efforts to develop a muscular body have often led to use of use of hazardous food additives or drugs, questionable forms of exercise, and a wide range of somatic problems. In addition to these difficulties, a major cause of death, injury, and sickness among youth and young adults is their failure to self-regulate a variety of dangerous behaviors, such as drinking alcohol, taking recreational drugs, engaging in unprotected sex, and driving with excessive speed. Even the incidence of misbehavior, aggression, and crime has been associated with low impulse control and disengagement of moral self-regulatory standards (Bandura, Barbaranelli, Caprara, & Pastorelli 1996a). These self-regulatory problems extend well beyond mere misinformation about dangerous or healthful personal practices; they stem from entrenched self-beliefs, habits, and styles of living (Prochaska, DiClemente, & Norcross, 1992). As a result, their solution often requires arduous changes in behavior, home and work settings, and, in some cases, even one's social groups. How can such changes be effected? What is the nature and cause of the underlying self-regulatory dysfunctions?

From a social cognitive perspective, dysfunctions in self-regulation are chiefly due to the ineffective forethought and performance control techniques, such as planning one's daily diet and self-recording the frequency of exercise to control weight (Bandura, 1991; Zimmerman, 1998). Instead of using these *proactive methods*, the poorly self-regulated rely primarily on *reactive methods* to manage personal outcomes, such as skipping meals when a scale reveals excess body weight. As previously mentioned, reactive methods of self-regulation are generally ineffective because they fail to provide the necessary goal structure, strategic planning, and sense of personal agency for students to progress consistently. Instead, dysfunctional self-regulators try to correct themselves using post hoc task outcomes, which are often delayed, difficult to interpret, and socially stigmatizing, such as gains in weight. Success is not an objective property of performance results, but rather depends on the criteria by which they are self-evaluated, such as self-comparisons with a fashion model's type of body (Bandura, 1991). Whereas reactive self-regulators lack specific process goals and baseline information, they must rely on social comparisons to evaluate their outcomes, which are frequently unfavorable and often lead to fixed ability attributions, self-dissatisfaction, and defensive self-reactions. Because of these adverse self-reactions to their task outcomes, reactive self-regulators experience not only a loss of self-efficacy about subsequent performance efforts, but also a decline in intrinsic interest in the academic task (Zimmerman & Kitsantas, 1996).

What types of experiential deficits or inherited personal limitations may predispose a person to rely on reactive methods of self-regulation? A *lack of social learning experiences* is the first important source of self-regulatory dysfunctions. Many forms of self-regulation are difficult to learn by individuals who grow up in homes or communities where they are not taught, modeled, or rewarded. Brody and his colleagues (Brody & Flor, in press; Brody, Stoneman, & Flor, 1996) have found that parental processes play an important role in children's self-regulatory development and that significant numbers of children lack sufficient self-regulatory skill to manage personal problems and achieve consistently in school. Children whose parents set clear "no nonsense" standards and closely monitor their school activity and achievement display not only greater self-regulation, but also higher levels of social and cognitive development.

A second personal limitation that leads to dysfunctions in self-regulation is motivational; namely, the presence of *apathy or disinterest*. Because the most effective self-regulatory techniques require anticipation, concentration, effort, and careful self-reflection, they are used only when the skill or its outcomes are highly valued. When a skill or its outcomes are not perceived as valuable, there is no incentive to self-regulate. For example, teachers report significant numbers of disengaged students who display apathy or disinterest regarding participation in class or completion of homework (Steinberg, Brown, & Dornbusch, 1996). Because of their low self-confidence and lack of intrinsic interest in school, apathetic students will resort to reactive methods of self-regulation when the academic outcomes become too punishing, such as joining deviant peer groups. There is evidence that parents' motives have an impact on their children's.

For example, parents' academic goals for their children significantly predict their youngsters' academic goal setting and academic achievement (Zimmerman et al., 1992). Although apathy is a very difficult problem to overcome with older children and adults, there is some evidence in the field of health that specially trained social change agents have been successful in prompting apathetic parents to self-record asthma symptoms of their children and, as a result, these parents increased their administration of preventive medications and perceived higher levels of self-efficacy (Bonner et al., 1997).

Mood disorders, such as mania or depression, are a third personal limitation that can cause major dysfunctions in self-regulation. For example, depressives typically exhibit a self-defeating bias, misperceive their performance attainments, or negatively distort their recollections of these attainments (Bandura, 1991). This bias stands in stark contrast to the self-enhancing optimism of nondepressives who remember their successes well, but recall fewer failures than they actually experienced (Nelson & Craighead, 1977). Depressives also set higher standards for themselves than nondepressives (Schwartz, 1974; Simon, 1979) and are quick to blame themselves for failures (Kuiper, 1978). Unfortunately, minimizing one's success only further exacerbates one's sense of despondency.

A fourth common dysfunction in self-regulation is associated with the presence of *learning disabilities*, such as cognitive problems in concentration, recall, reading, and writing. These personal limitations, which are widely believed to have neurological origins, lead to a number of self-regulatory dysfunctions (Borkowski & Thorpe, 1994). For example, learning disabled students set lower academic goals for themselves, have trouble controlling their impulses, and are less accurate in assessing their capabilities. They are also more self-critical and less self-efficacious about their performance and tend to give up more easily than nondisabled students. Fortunately, several efforts to teach the learning disabled compensatory self-regulatory methods for reading and writing dysfunctions have proven effective in teaching attentional and behavioral control, reading, and writing as well as other subject matter skills (Butler, 1998; Graham & Harris, 1994; Schunk, 1998). Thus, although cognitive, affective, and motivational problems produce a range of self-regulatory dysfunctions, there is increasing evidence that interventions that target these dysfunctions are helpful in compensating for them (Schunk & Zimmerman, 1998).

V. DEVELOPMENT OF SELF-REGULATORY SKILL

Although it is possible to develop self-regulatory competence by personal discovery, this path is often tedious, frustrating, and limited in its effectiveness. As Bandura (1986) humorously cautioned, Those who are foolish enough to try to learn dangerous skills, such as skiing or driving an automobile by trial-and-error, should first check their medical coverage! Fortunately, self-regulatory processes can be acquired from and are sustained by social as well as self sources of influence. Most important task skills, whether they are primarily motoric or cognitive, are initially acquired by observing, reading, or hearing about the performance of skilled models, such as parents, teachers, coaches, or peers with expertise, but how do socially conveyed skills become self-regulated?

According to a social cognitive perspective (Schunk & Zimmerman, 1997; Zimmerman & Bonner, in press), the acquisition of a wide range of task competencies, from personal care skills to academic learning strategies, emerge in a series of regulatory skill levels. As toddlers, children learn that they can acquire new skills or strategies most effectively by watching the performance of skilled adults or sibling models and listening to their verbal explanations and self-expressed beliefs. This awareness of the value of social models remains with them as new skills are acquired throughout life. An *observational level* of skill occurs when learners can induce the major features of the skill or strategy from watching a model learn or perform (see Table 2). In addition to strategic skill, models convey associated self-regulatory processes, such as performance standards, motivational orientations, and values that observers can use personally during subsequent developmental phases. For example, there is evidence (Zimmerman & Ringle, 1981) that the persistence of a model during complex problem solving affects the perseverence of observers. An observational level of proficiency can be assessed through strategy descriptions or vicarious performance predictions (Zimmerman & Blom, 1983). Perceived similarity to a model and vicarious consequences of a model's use of this skill will determine an observer's motivation to develop the skill further (Zimmerman & Rosenthal, 1974). Despite the value of this vicarious information, most learners also need to perform the strategies personally to incorporate them into their behavioral repertoires.

TABLE 2 Developmental Levels of Regulatory Skill

Level	Name	Description
1	Observation	Vicarious induction of a skill from a proficient model
2	Emulation[a]	Imitative performance of the general pattern or style of a model's skill with social assistance
3	Self-control	Independent display of the model's skill under structured conditions
4	Self-regulation	Adaptive use of skill across changing personal and environmental conditions

[a]This level was referred to as imitation in prior descriptions.

Efforts to enact a skill produce proprioceptive cues that must be integrated with vicarious ones. An *emulation level* of self-regulatory skill is attained when a learner's behavioral performance approximates the general strategic form of the model.[1] Seldom does a learner copy the exact actions of the model, but rather he or she emulates the general pattern or style of functioning, such as the type of question a model asks instead of the model's exact words (Rosenthal, Zimmerman, & Durning, 1970). The observer's accuracy can be improved further when a model adopts a teaching role and provides guidance, feedback, and social reinforcement during practice (Kitsantas, Zimmerman, & Cleary, 1999). The motoric and social consequences of the observer's use of this skill will determine the motivation to develop the skill further. It should be noted that the source of learning of regulatory skill is primarily social for these first two levels, but at more advanced levels, the locus shifts to self sources.

Acquiring the use of a skill on one's own usually requires more than exposure to a teacher or model; it also depends on extensive deliberate practice on one's own (Ericsson & Lehman, 1996). Deliberate practice involves performance that is structured (often by teachers) to enhance performance and self-observation. Attainment of a third, *self-controlled level* of self-regulatory skill occurs when learners master the use of a skill in structured settings outside the presence of models, such as when a pianist can play scales fluidly in the major and minor keys. At this level, a learner's use of a skill depends on representational standards of a model's performance (e.g., covert images or verbal recollections of a teacher's performance) rather than an overt social referent (Bandura & Jeffery, 1973). The learner's success in matching that covert standard during practice efforts will determine the amount of self-reinforcement he or she will experience. During this phase, learning strategies that focus on fundamental processes rather than outcomes are most beneficial in producing mastery.

A *self-regulated level* of task skill is achieved when learners can systematically adapt their performance to changing personal and contextual conditions. At this fourth level of skill, the learner can vary the use of task strategies and make adjustments based on outcomes. Such learners can choose a strategy and adapt its features with little or no residual depen-

---

[1]The word "imitation" has been used previously by me and my colleagues to describe level 2 in the development of skill in order to distinguish between the observer's role and the model's during social cognitive learning. Imitation was previously defined in terms of higher order changes in abstract pattern or style rather than individual response components. The word "emulation" will be used in this chapter to emphasize the generative nature of this process and avoid any semantic implication that vicarious learning is limited to mimicry or copying.

dence on the model. The motivation to sustain this level of skill depends on perceptions of self-efficacy. Skills during this phase usually can be performed with minimal process monitoring, and the learners' attention can be shifted toward performance outcomes without detrimental consequences. For instance, a tennis player's attention can be shifted from the execution of the serve to its effective use, such as placing it where it is likely to win a point.

In summary, this multilevel analysis of the development of self-regulatory competence begins with the most extensive social guidance at the first level, and this social support is systematically reduced as learners acquire underlying self-regulatory skill. However, level 4 functioning continues to depend on social resources on a self-selective basis, such as when a professional baseball player seeks advice from a coach during a batting slump. Because self-regulatory skill is context dependent, new performance problems can uncover limitations in existing strategies and require additional social learning experiences. Unlike developmental stage models, this formulation does not assume learners must advance through the four levels in an invariant sequence or that once the highest level is attained, it will be used universally. Instead, like learning hierarchy models, it assumes that students who master each skill level in sequence will learn more easily and effectively. Although level 4 learners have the competence to perform self-regulatively, they may not choose to do so because of the motivational or contextual factors that were discussed at the outset of this chapter. Intentional forethought, proactive performance effort, and self-reflection are mentally and physically demanding activities, and a person may decide to forego their use if he or she feels tired, disinterested, or uncommitted.

There is a growing body of evidence indicating that the speed and quality of learners' self-regulatory development can be enhanced significantly if learners proceed according to a multilevel developmental hierarchy. The sequentiality of the observational and emulation learning levels of self-regulatory development were studied by Kitsantas et al. (1999), who compared the acquisition of dart skill by novice learners who learned initially from modeling with that of learners who initially learned from enactment. In this research, an adult model demonstrated a multistep process dart throwing strategy for some of the high school students and provided social feedback on a selective basis. The results were consistent with a social cognitive view of self-regulatory development. Students who had the benefit of modeling significantly surpassed the dart skill of those who attempted to learn from performance outcomes only. Furthermore, students who received social feedback learned better than those who practiced on their own, but this feedback was insufficient to make up for the absence of vicarious experience. Students exposed to strategic modeling also showed higher levels of self-motivation according to an array of measures, such as self-efficacy and intrinsic interest, than students who relied on discovery and social feedback. These results confirmed the sequential advantages of engaging in observational learning before attempting enactive learning experiences.

Another study (Zimmerman & Kitsantas, 1997) tested the sequentiality of self-control and self-regulation skill levels by examining the effectiveness of shifting process goals to outcome goals during dart throwing practice. Recall that process goals were hypothesized to be optimal during the acquisition of self-control, but outcome goals were expected to be superior during the acquisition of self-regulation. Before being asked to practice on their own, all of the high school subjects were taught strategic components of the skill through observation and emulation (levels 1 and 2). The experiment compared the effects of process goals, outcome goals, and shifting goals as well as self-recording during self-controlled practice. The results were consistent with a multilevel hierarchical view of goal setting: Students who shifted goals developmentally from processes to outcomes after reaching level 4 (i.e., having achieved automaticity) surpassed classmates who adhered only to process goals or only to outcome goals in posttest dart throwing skill. In addition to their superior learning outcomes, students who shifted their goals displayed superior self-efficacy perceptions and intrinsic interest in the game. In support of a cyclical view of self-regulation, the students' self-reactions to dart throwing outcomes were highly predictive of their self-efficacy perceptions about dart skill and their intrinsic interest in the game.

VI. FUTURE RESEARCH DIRECTIONS

The social cognitive hypothesis that self-regulation of learning develops initially from social modeling experiences and progresses through increasing levels of self-directed functioning needs further validation in several important ways. First, research on the effects of goal shifting during self-controlled learning (Zimmerman & Kitsantas, 1997) needs to be extended to new tasks to determine whether these goal effects are a general or a task-specific phenomenon. It would be particularly impressive if the transfer task were cognitive in nature, such as an academic learning task, in order to ascertain whether the results generalized beyond motoric functioning. If the advantage of setting process goals before shifting to outcome goals does transfer to a cognitive task, it would further demonstrate the importance of the distinction between the self-control level and self-regulatory levels in this hierarchical model of learning.

Second, research also is needed to extend the distinction between the observational and emulation levels to determine if these vicarious learning effects are general or limited in scope (Kitsantas et al., 1999). As was recommended previously, it would most convincingly dispel concerns about the scope of existing motoric results if transfer were demonstrated with a cognitive learning task. An academic learning study showing that observers who discriminated and abstracted the strategic rule underlying a model's performance (level 1) learn to use an academic skill emulatively (level 2) more readily than those who failed to do so would validate the pedagogical importance of the distinction between the observational and emulation levels of regulatory skill.

Third, the distinction between the second (emulation) level and the third (self-control) level should be tested in future research. This would entail comparing the self-directed practice of learners who had the opportunity to learn through modeling with those who did not. From a social cognitive perspective, it is hypothesized that learners who acquire a high level of emulation accuracy with the support of a model form a motorically detailed representational standard to guide and self-monitor their practice efforts and experience a heightened sense of self-efficacy. These benefits of emulation would enable them to practice more effectively on their own than learners who had acquired only an observational level of skill. This result would demonstrate the pedagogical importance of comprehensive modeling training before engaging in self-controlled learning on one's own.

If these efforts to extend this social cognitive model are successful, they will indicate specifically how human self-regulatory development can be facilitated using social models. This is important because of evidence showing that self-organized learning without a teacher's social guidance can impede students' acquisition of knowledge and skill (Brown & Van Lehn, 1982; Weinert & Helmke, 1995). Teachers who model strategies and verbalize their thought processes as they perform tasks can enhance students' self-regulatory development greatly (Graham & Harris, 1989a, 1989b; Palincsar & Brown, 1984; Sawyer, Graham, & Harris, 1992). Although peer models have been be used as well as teachers to guide learning (Schunk, 1987), research is needed on the use of expert peers for instructional purposes during levels 1 and 2. This issue is especially important in future research because peer tutors are often available as a social resource. A key pedagogical issue regarding socially initiated self-regulatory training is when to withdraw the various forms of modeling support. Although social models are advantageous in conveying high quality methods of task skill, they may inhibit learners from assuming self-direction unless these models are phased out as soon as possible. A multilevel model of self-regulatory development seeks to provide teachers, peers, coaches, and learners with specific guidance regarding optimal timing of instructional shifts between each successive level in the hierarchy.

VII. A CONCLUDING COMMENT

Although there is considerable agreement about the importance of self-regulation to human survival, there has been disagreement about how it can be analyzed and defined in a scientifically useful way. A social cognitive perspective differs markedly from theoretical traditions that seek to define self-regulation as a singular internal state, trait, or stage that is genetically endowed or personally discovered. Instead it is defined in terms of context-specific processes that are used cyclically to achieve personal goals. These processes entail more than metacognitive knowledge and skill; they also include affective and behavioral processes, and a resilient sense of self-efficacy to control them. The cyclical interdependence of these processes, reactions, and beliefs was described in terms of three sequential phases: forethought, performance or volitional control, and self-reflection. An important feature of this cyclical model is that it can explain dysfunctions in self-regulation as well as exemplary achievements. Dysfunctions occur because of the unfortunate reliance on reactive methods of self-regulation instead of proactive methods, which can profoundly change the course of cyclical learning and performance.

An essential issue confronting all theories of self-regulation is how this capability or capacity can be developed or optimized. Social cognitive views place particular emphasis on the role of socializing agents in the development of self-regulation, such as parents, teachers, coaches, and peers. At an early age, children become aware of the value of social modeling experiences, and they rely heavily on them when acquiring needed skills. It was hypothesized that human skills become self-regulated in a series of levels that begin with an observational level of proficiency and then progress to an emulation level of proficiency, thereafter shifting to a self-controlled level, and finally reaching a self-regulated level. Although social support is systematically reduced from levels 1 to 4, it continues to be used as a resource when it is needed during the last two levels. These developmental levels of skill function are like learning hierarchies, and there is evidence that learners who master the skills in sequence display a higher level of skill and experience more satisfying self-reactions and higher perceptions of self-efficacy as well as increase intrinsic interest in the skill. Together these cyclical developments in self-belief are of particular theoretical importance because they suggest that students' attained levels of self-regulatory skill have profoundly altered their forethought, which according to Bandura (1991) is the ultimate source of human agency.

ACKNOWLEDGMENT

I thank Albert Bandura for helpful comments and suggestions on an earlier draft of this chapter. Correspondence regarding this chapter should be sent to Barry J. Zimmmerman, Doctoral Program in Educational Psychology, Graduate School and University Center, City University of New York, 365 Fifth Ave., New York, NY 10016 or bzimmerm@email.gc.cuny.edu.

REFERENCES

Ames, C. (1992). Achievement goals and the classroom motivational climate. In D. H. Schunk & J. L. Meece (Eds.), *Student perceptions in the classroom* (pp. 327–348). Hillsdale, NJ: Erlbaum.

Bandura, A. (1986). *Social foundations of thought and action: A social cognitive theory.* Englewood Cliffs, NJ: Prentice-Hall.

Bandura, A. (1991). Self-regulation of motivation through anticipatory and self-reactive mechanisms. In R. A. Dienstbier (Ed.), *Nebraska Symposium on Motivation*: (Vol. 38. *Perspectives on motivation* pp. 69–164). Lincoln: University of Nebraska Press.

Bandura, A. (1997). *Self-efficacy: The exercise of control.* New York: W. H. Freeman.

Bandura, A. (in press). Exploration of fortuitous determinants of life paths. *Psychological Inquiry.*

Bandura, A., Barbaranelli, C., Caprara, G. V., & Pastorelli, C. (1996a). Mechanisms of moral disengagement in the exercise of moral agency. *Journal of Personality and Social Psychology, 71*, 364–374.

Bandura, A., Barbaranelli, C., Caprara, G. V., & Pastorelli, C. (1996b). Multifaceted impact of self-efficacy beliefs on academic functioning. *Child Development, 67*, 1206–1222.

Bandura, A., & Cervone, D. (1986). Differential engagement of self-reactive influences in cognitive motivation. *Organizational Behavior and Human Decision Processes, 38*, 92–113.

Bandura, A., & Jeffrey, R. W. (1973). Role of symbolic coding and rehearsal processes in observational learning. *Journal of Personality and Social Psychology, 26*, 122–130.

Bandura, A., & Kupers, C. J. (1964). Transmission of patterns of self-reinforcement through modeling. *Journal of Abnormal and Social Psychology, 69*, 1–9.

Bandura, A., & Schunk, D. H. (1981). Cultivating competence, self-efficacy, and intrinsic interest through proximal self-motivation. *Journal of Personality and Social Psychology, 41*, 586–598.

Barzon, J. (1964). Calamaphobia, or hints towards a writer's discipline. In H. Hull (Ed.), *The writers book* (pp. 84–96). New York: Barnes & Noble.

Bonner, S., Rivera, R., & Zimmerman, B. J. (1997, May). Improving asthma management by focusing on families' self-regulatory phase. Poster presented at the annual meeting of the American Thoracic Society, San Francisco, CA.

Borkowski, J. G., & Thorpe, P. K. (1994). Self-regulation and motivation: A lifespan perspective on underachievement. In D. H. Schunk & B. J. Zimmerman (Eds.), *Self-regulation of learning and performance: Issues and educational applications* (pp. 45–73). Hillsdale, NJ: Erlbaum.

Bouffard-Bouchard, T., Parent, S., & Larivee, S. (1991). Influence of self-efficacy on self-regulation and performance among junior and senior high-school age students. *International Journal of Behavior Development, 14*, 153–164.

Britton, B. K., & Tessor, A. (1991). Effects of time management practices on college grades. *Journal of Educational Psychology, 83*, 405–410.

Brody, G. H., & Flor, D. L. (1998). Maternal resources, parenting practices and child competence in rural single-parent families. *Child Development, 69*, 803–816.

Brody, G. H., Stoneman, Z., & Flor, D. (1996). Parental religiousity, family processes, and youth competence in rural, two-parent African American families. *Developmental Psychology, 32*, 696–706.

Brown, J. S., & Van Lehn, K. (1982). Towards a generative theory of "bugs." In T. Romberg, T. Carpenter, & J. Moses (Eds.), *Addition and subtraction: Developmental perspectives* (pp. 117–135). Hillsdale, NJ: Erlbaum.

Butler, D. L. (1998). A strategic content learning approach to promoting self-regulated learning by students with learning disabilities. In D. H. Schunk & B. J. Zimmerman (Eds.), *Self-regulated learning: From teaching to self-reflective practice* (pp. 160–183). New York: Guilford.

Corno, L. (1993). The best-laid plans: Modern conceptions of volition and educational research. *Educational Researcher, 22*, 14–22.

Covington, M. V., & Roberts, B. (1994). Self worth and college achievement: Motivational and personality correlates. In P. R. Pintrich, D. R. Brown, & C. E. Weinstein (Eds.), *Student motivation, cognition, and learning: Essays in honor of Wilbert J. McKeachie* (pp. 157–187). Hillsdale, NJ: Erlbaum.

Deci, E. L. (1975). *Intrinsic motivation*. New York: Plenum.

Dweck, C. S. (1988). Motivational processes affecting learning. *American Psychologist, 41*, 1040–1048.

Ellis, D. (1995, April). *The role of discrimination accuracy in self-monitoring of dialect acquisition*. Paper presented at a meeting of the American Educational Research Association, San Francisco, CA.

Ericsson, A. K., & Charness, N. (1994). Expert performance: Its structure and acquisition. *American Psychologist, 49*, 725–747.

Ericsson, A. K., & Lehman, A. C. (1996). Expert and exceptional performance: Evidence of maximal adaptation to task constraints. *Annual Review of Psychology, 47*, 273–305.

Garcia, T., & Pintrich, P. R. (1994). Regulating motivation and cognition in the classroom: The role of self-schemas and self-regulatory strategies. In D. H. Schunk & B. J. Zimmerman (Eds.), *Self-regulation of learning and performance: Issues and educational applications* (p. 127–153). Hillsdale, NJ: Erlbaum.

Garfield, C. A., & Bennett, Z. H. (1985). *Peak performance: Mental training techniques of the world's greatest athletes*. New York: Warner Books.

Graham, S., & Harris, K. R. (1989a). Components analysis of cognitive strategy instruction: Effects on learning disabled students' compositions and self-efficacy. *Journal of Educational Psychology, 81*, 353–361.

Graham, S., & Harris, K. R. (1989b). Improving learning disabled students' skills at composing essays: Self-instructional strategy training. *Exceptional Children, 56*, 210–214.

Graham, S., & Harris, K. R. (1994). The role and development of self-regulation in the writing process. In D. H. Schunk & B. J. Zimmerman (Eds.), *Self-regulation of learning and performance: Issues and educational applications* (pp. 203–228). Hillsdale, NJ: Erlbaum.

Kanfer, R., & Ackerman, P. L. (1989). Motivation and cognitive abilities: An integrative aptitude-treatment interaction approach to skill acquisition. *Journal of Applied Psychology —Monograph, 74*, 657–690.

Kazdin, A. (1974). Self-monitoring and behavior changed. In M. J. Mahoney & C. E. Thoresen (Eds.), *Self-control: Power to the person* (pp. 218–246). Monterey, CA: Brooks/Cole.

Kirschenbaum, D. S., & Karoly, P. (1977). When self-regulation fails: Tests of some preliminary hypotheses. *Journal of Consulting and Clinical Psychology, 45,* 1116–1125.

Kitsantas, A., Zimmerman, B. J., & Cleary, T. (1999). *Observation and imitation phases in the development of motoric self-regulation.* Unpublished manuscript, Graduate School of the City University of New York.

Kuhl, J. (1985). Volitional mediators of cognitive behavior consistency: Self-regulatory processes and action versus state orientation. In J. Kuhl & J. Beckman (Eds.), *Action control: From cognition to behavior* (pp. 101–128). New York: Springer-Verlag.

Kuiper, N. A. (1978). Depression and causal attributions for success and failure. *Journal of Personality and Social Psychology, 36,* 236–246.

Lepper, M. R., & Hodell, M. (1989). Intrinsic motivation in the classroom. In C. Ames & R. Ames (Eds.), *Research on motivation in education* (Vol. 3, pp. 255–296). Hillsdale, NJ: Erlbaum.

Locke, E. A. (1991). Goal theory vs. control theory: Contrasting approaches to understanding work motivation. *Motivation and Emotion, 15,* 9–28.

Locke, E. A., & Latham, G. P. (1990). *A theory of goal setting and task performance.* Englewood Cliffs, NJ: Prentice-Hall.

Mach, E. (1988). *Great contemporary pianists speak for themselves.* Toronto, Canada: Dover Books.

Meichenbaum, D. (1977). *Cognitive-behavior modification: An integrative approach.* New York: Plenum.

Nelson, R. E., & Craighead, W. E. (1977). Selective recall of positive and negative feedback, self-control behaviors, and depression. *Journal of Abnormal Psychology, 86,* 379–388.

Newman, R. (1994). Academic help-seeking: A strategy of self-regulated learning. In D. H. Schunk & B. J. Zimmerman (Eds.), *Self-regulation of learning and performance: Issues and educational applications* (pp. 283–301). Hillsdale, NJ: Erlbaum.

Nicholls, J. (1984). Achievement motivation: Conceptions of ability, subjective experience, task choice, and performance. *Psychological Review, 91,* 328–346.

Pajares, F., & Miller, M. D. (1994). Role of self-efficacy and self-concept beliefs in mathematical problem solving: A path analysis. *Journal of Educational Psychology, 86,* 193–203.

Palincsar, A. S., & Brown, A. L. (1984). Reciprocal teaching of comprehension-fostering and comprehension-monitoring activities. *Cognition and Instruction, 1,* 117–175.

Pintrich, P. R., & Schunk, D. H. (1996). *Motivation in education: Theory, research and applications.* Englewood Cliffs, NJ: Prentice-Hall.

Plimpton, G. (Ed.). (1965). Ernest Hemingway. *Writers at work: The Paris Review interviews* (second series, pp. 215–239). New York: Viking Press.

Pressley, M. (1977). Imagery and children's learning: Putting the picture in developmental perspective. *Review of Educational Research, 47,* 586–622.

Pressley, M., & Levin, J. R. (1977). Task parameters affecting the efficacy of a visual imagery learning strategy in younger and older children. *Journal of Experimental Child Psychology, 24,* 53–59.

Pressley, M., & Woloshyn, V. & Associates (1995). *Cognitive strategy instruction that really improves children's academic performance* (2nd ed.). Cambridge, MA: Brookline Books.

Prochaska, J. O., DiClemente, C. C., & Norcross, J. C. (1992). In search of how people change: Applications to addictive behaviors. *American Psychologist, 47,* 1102–1114.

Rosenthal, T. L., Zimmerman, B. J., & Durning, K. (1970). Observationally-induced changes in children's interrogative classes. *Journal of Personality and Social Psychology, 16,* 631–688.

Sawyer, R. J., Graham, S., & Harris, K. R. (1992). Direct teaching, strategy instruction, and strategy instruction with explicit self-regulation: Effects on the composition skills and self-efficacy of students with learning disabilities. *Journal of Educational Psychology, 84,* 340–352.

Schneider, W., & Pressley, M. (1997). *Memory development between two and twenty.* Mahwah, NJ: Erlbaum.

Schunk, D. H. (1982). Verbal self-regulation as a facilitator of children's achievement and self-efficacy. *Human Learning, 1,* 265–277.

Schunk D. H. (1987). Peer models and children's behavioral change. *Review of Educational Research, 57,* 149–174.

Schunk, D. H. (1996). Goal and self-evaluative influences during children's cognitive skill learning. *American Educational Research Journal, 33,* 359–382.

Schunk, D. H. (1998). Teaching elementary students to self-regulate practice of mathematical skills with modeling. In D. H. Schunk & B. J. Zimmerman (Eds.), *Self-regulated learning: From teaching to self-reflective practice* (pp. 137–159). New York: Guilford.

Schunk, D. H., & Schwartz, C. W. (1993). Goals and progress feedback: Effects on self-efficacy and writing achievement. *Contemporary Educational Psychology, 18* (3), 337–354.

Schunk, D. H., & Zimmerman, B. J. (1997). Social origins of self-regulatory competence. *Educational Psychologist, 32,* 195–208.

Schunk, D. H., & Zimmerman, B. J. (1998). *Self-regulated learning: From teaching to self-reflective practice.* New York: Guilford.

Schwartz, J. L. (1974). Relationship between goal discrepancy and depression. *Journal of Consulting and Clinical Psychology, 42,* 309.

Simon, K. M. (1979). Self-evaluative reactions: The role of personal valuation of the activity. *Cognitive Therapy and Research, 3,* 111–116.

Steinberg, L., Brown, B. B., & Dornbusch, S. M. (1996). *Beyond the classroom.* New York: Simon & Schuster.

Thoresen, M. J., & Mahoney, M. J. (1974). *Behavioral self-control.* New York: Holt, Rinehart & Winston.

Wallace, I. (1971). *The writing of one novel.* Richmond Hill, Canada: Simon & Schuster of Canada (pocket book edition).

Watson, D. L., & Tharp, R. (1993). *Self-directed behavior: Self-modification for personal adjustment.* Pacific Grove, CA: Brooks/Cole.

Weiner, B. (1979). A theory of motivation for some classroom experiences. *Journal of Educational Psychology, 71,* 3–25.

Weinert, F. E., & Helmke, A. (1995). Learning from wise mother nature or big brother instructor: The wrong choice as seen from an educational perspective. *Educational Psychologist, 30,* 135–142.

Weinstein, C. E., & Mayer, R. E. (1986). The teaching of learning strategies. In M. C. Wittrock (Ed.), *Handbook of research on teaching* (pp. 315–327). New York: Macmillan.

Weinstein, C. E., Schulte, A. C., & Palmer, D. R. (1987). *LASSI: Learning and study strategies inventory.* Clearwater, FL: H. & H. Publishing.

Winne, P. H. (1997). Experimenting to bootstrap self-regulated learning. *Journal of Educational Psychology, 88,* 397–410.

Wood, E., Woloshyn, V. E., & Willoughby, T. (1995). *Cognitive strategy instruction for middle and high schools.* Cambridge, MA: Brookline Books.

Zimmerman, B. J. (1989). A social cognitive view of self-regulated academic learning. *Journal of Educational Psychology, 81,* 329–339.

Zimmerman, B. J. (1995a). Self-efficacy and educational development. In A. Bandura (Ed.), *Self-efficacy in changing societies* (pp. 202–231). New York: Cambridge University Press.

Zimmerman, B. J. (1995b). Self-regulation involves more than metacognition: A social cognitive perspective. *Educational Psychologist, 29,* 217–221.

Zimmerman, B. J. (1998). Developing self-fulfilling cycles of academic regulation: An analysis of exemplary instructional models. In D. H. Schunk & B. J. Zimmerman (Eds.), *Self-regulated learning: From teaching to self-reflective practice* (pp. 1–19). New York: Guilford.

Zimmerman, B. J., & Bandura, A. (1994). Impact of self-regulatory influences of writing course attainment. *American Educational Research Journal, 31*, 845–862.

Zimmerman, B. J., Bandura, A., & Martinez-Pons, M. (1992). Self-motivation for academic attainment: The role of self-efficacy beliefs and personal goal setting. *American Educational Research Journal, 29*, 663–676.

Zimmerman, B. J., & Blom, D. E. (1983). Toward an empirical test of the role of cognitive conflict in learning. *Developmental Review, 3*, 204–216.

Zimmerman, B. J., & Bonner, S. (in press). A social cognitive view of strategic learning. In C. E. Weinstein & B. L. McCombs (Eds.), *Strategic learning: Skill, will and self-regulation.* Hillsdale, NJ: Erlbaum.

Zimmerman, B. J., Bonner, S., Evans, D., & Mellins, R. (1999). Self-regulating childhood asthma: A developmental model of family change. *Health Education & Behavior, 26*, 55–71.

Zimmerman, B. J., & Kitsantas, A. (1996). Self-regulated learning of a motoric skill: The role of goal setting and self-monitoring. *Journal of Applied Sport Psychology, 8*, 69–84.

Zimmerman, B. J., & Kitsantas, A. (1997). Developmental phases in self-regulation: Shifting from process to outcome goals. *Journal of Educational Psychology, 89*, 29–36.

Zimmerman, B. J., & Martinez-Pons, M. (1986). Development of a structured interview for assessing students use of self-regulated learning strategies. *American Educational Research Journal, 23*, 614–628.

Zimmerman, B. J., & Martinez-Pons, M. (1988). Construct validation of a strategy model of student self-regulated learning. *Journal of Educational Psychology, 80*, 284–290.

Zimmerman, B. J., & Martinez-Pons, M. (1992). Perceptions of efficacy and strategy use in the self-regulation of learning. In D. H. Schunk & J. Meece (Eds.), *Student perceptions in the classroom: Causes and consequences* (pp. 185–207). Hillsdale, NJ: Erlbaum.

Zimmerman, B. J., & Paulsen, A. S. (1995). Self-monitoring during collegiate studying: An invaluable tool for academic self-regulation. In P. Pintrich (Ed.), *New directions in college teaching and learning: Understanding self-regulated learning* (No. 63, Fall, pp. 13–27). San Francisco, CA: Jossey-Bass.

Zimmerman, B. J., & Ringle, J. (1981). Effects of model persistence and statements of confidence on children's self-efficacy and problem solving. *Journal of Educational Psychology, 73*, 485–493.

Zimmerman, B. J., & Risemberg, R. (1997). Becoming a self-regulated writer: A social cognitive perspective. *Contemporary Educational Psychology, 22*, 73–101.

Zimmerman, B. J., & Rosenthal, T. L. (1974). Observational learning of rule governed behavior by children. *Psychological Bulletin, 81*, 29–42.

3

ON THE STRUCTURE OF
BEHAVIORAL
SELF-REGULATION

CHARLES S. CARVER* AND
MICHAEL F. SCHEIER[†]

*University of Miami, Coral Gables, Florida
[†]Carnegie Mellon University, Pittsburgh, Pennsylvania

We are interested in the structure of human behavior, broadly conceived. This interest has taken us into several specific research domains, including test anxiety, social anxiety, and self-regulation of health-related behavior. But in some respects the specific explorations in diverse areas of work have been in the service of a more general interest in the structure of behavior.

The questions underlying this interest are very abstract: What is the most useful way to think about how people create actions from intentions and desires? Once people have decided to do something, how do they stay on course? What processes account for the existence of feelings, as people make their way through the world? At the fore of our thinking over the past two decades is the idea that behavior is a self-regulatory event. It is an attempt to make something happen in action that is already in mind. This general idea forms the basis of this chapter.

This chapter is organized in terms of a series of conceptual themes that we've found useful. Some of them have been central in our thinking for a long time; others have been taken up only more recently. We start simple, with basic ideas about the nature of behavior and the organization of some of the processes by which we believe behavior is regulated. We then turn to consideration of emotion—how we think it is created and how certain classes of affects differ from each other. This is followed by a discussion of

Copyright © 2000 by Academic Press.
All rights of reproduction in any form reserved.

the fact that people sometimes are unable to do what they set out to do, and what follows from that problem. The next sections are more speculative. They deal with dynamic systems and catastrophe theory as models for understanding behavior and how these models may contribute to the ways in which people such as ourselves think about self-regulation.

I. BEHAVIOR IS GOAL DIRECTED AND FEEDBACK CONTROLLED

The view we take on behavior begins with the concept of goal and the process of feedback control. We see these ideas as intimately linked. Our focus on goals is very much in line with a growing reemergence of goal constructs (Austin & Vancouver, 1996; Elliott & Dweck, 1988; Miller & Read, 1987; Pervin, 1989). A variety of labels are used in this literature: for example, *current concern* (Klinger, 1975, 1977), *personal strivings* (Emmons, 1986), *life task* (Cantor & Kihlstrom, 1987), and *personal project* (Little, 1983). In all these theories, there is room for individualization. That is, a life task can be achieved in many ways. People choose paths that are compatible with other aspects of their life situations (many current concerns must be managed simultaneously) and other aspects of their personalities.

Two goal constructs that differ somewhat from those named thus far are the *possible self* (Markus & Nurius, 1986) and the *self-guide* (Higgins, 1987, 1996). These constructs are intended to bring a dynamic quality to conceptualization of the self-concept. In contrast to traditional views, but consistent with other goal frameworks, possible selves are future oriented. They concern how people think of their unrealized potential, the kind of person they might become. Self-guides similarly reflect dynamic aspects of the self-concept.

Theorists who use these various terms—and others—have their own emphases (for broader discussions, see Austin & Vancouver, 1996; Carver & Scheier, 1998), but many points are the same. All include the idea that goals energize and direct activities; these views implicitly (and sometimes explicitly) convey the sense that goals give meaning to people's lives (cf. Baumeister, 1989). In each theory there is an emphasis on the idea that understanding the person means understanding the person's goals. Indeed, in the view represented by these theories, it is often implicit that the self consists partly of the person's goals and the organization among them.

A. FEEDBACK LOOPS

How are goals used in behaving? Part of our answer is that goals serve as reference values for feedback loops. A feedback loop, the unit of cybernetic control, is a system of four elements in a particular organization (cf. Miller, Galanter, & Pribram, 1960): an input function, a reference value, a comparator, and an output function (Figure 1).

An input function is a sensor. We will treat this function as equivalent to perception. The reference value is a second bit of information (i.e., in addition to the input function). We'll treat the reference values in the loops we're interested in as goals. A comparator is a device that makes comparisons between input and reference value. The comparison yields one of two outcomes: either the values being compared are discriminably different from one another or they're not. The comparison can vary in sensitivity. Sometimes very small discrepancies are detected; sometimes only quite large ones.

Following the comparison is an output function. We will treat this as equivalent to behavior, although sometimes the behavior is internal. If the comparison yields a "no difference," the output function remains whatever it was. If the comparison yields "discrepancy," the output changes.

There are two kinds of feedback loops, corresponding to two kinds of goals (Figure 2). In a negative or discrepancy-reducing loop, the output function is aimed at diminishing or eliminating any detected discrepancy between input and reference value. It yields conformity of input to reference. This conformity is seen in the attempt to approach or attain a valued goal.

In this view, behavior isn't for the sake of behavior, but occurs in the service of creating and maintaining conformity of input to standard. Behavior can create conformity, but disturbances from outside also can create conformity. Although disturbances often change conditions ad-

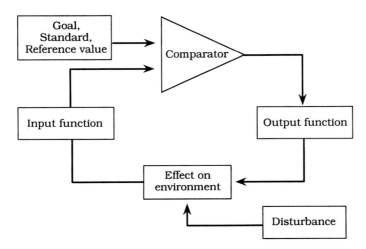

FIGURE 1   Schematic depiction of a feedback loop, the basic unit of cybernetic control. In such a loop, a sensed value is compared to a reference value or standard, and adjustments are made in an output function (if necessary) to shift the sensed value in the direction of the standard.

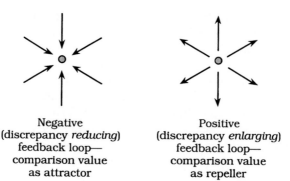

Negative
(discrepancy *reducing*)
feedback loop—
comparison value
as attractor

Positive
(discrepancy *enlarging*)
feedback loop—
comparison value
as repeller

FIGURE 2   Negative feedback loops cause sensed qualities to shift *toward* positively valenced reference points. Positive feedback loops cause sensed qualities to shift *away from* negatively valenced reference points. *Note.* From *On the self-regulation of Behavior*, by C. S. Carver and M. F. Scheier, 1998, New York: Cambridge University Press; Copyright 1998 by Cambridge University Press. Reprinted with permission.

versely (enlarging a discrepancy with the reference value), they also can change conditions favorably (diminishing a discrepancy). In the first case, recognition of a discrepancy prompts a change in output, as always. In the second case, the disturbance preempts the need for an output adjustment, because the system sees no discrepancy. Thus no output adjustment occurs.

The second kind of feedback loop is a positive or discrepancy-enlarging loop (Figure 2). The reference value here is not one to approach, but one to avoid. Think of this as an "anti-goal." A psychological high-level example is a feared possible self. Other, more concrete examples would be traffic tickets, public ridicule, and being fired from your job. A positive loop senses present conditions, compares them to the anti-goal, and tries to enlarge the discrepancy. For example, a rebellious adolescent who wants to be different from his parents senses his own behavior, compares it to his parents' behavior, and tries to make his own behavior as different from theirs as possible.

The action of discrepancy-enlarging processes in living systems is typically constrained in some way by discrepancy reducing loops (Figure 3). To put it differently, avoidance behaviors often lead into approach behaviors. An avoidance loop creates pressure to increase distance from the anti-goal. The movement away occurs until the tendency to move away is captured by the influence of an approach loop. This loop then serves to pull the sensed input into its orbit. The rebellious adolescent, trying to be different from his parents, soon finds other adolescents to *conform* to, all of whom are deviating from their parents.

Our use of the word orbit in the last paragraph suggests a metaphor that may be useful for anyone to whom these concepts do not feel terribly

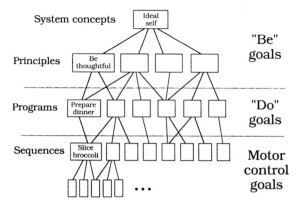

FIGURE 4   A hierarchy of goals (or of feedback loops). Lines indicate the contribution of lower level goals to specific higher-level goals. They also can be read in the opposite direction, indicating that a given higher order goal specifies more concrete goals at the next lower level. The hierarchy described in text involves goals of "being" particular ways, which are attained by "doing" particular actions. *Note:* From *On the Self-Regulation of Behavior*, by C. S. Carver and M. F. Scheier, 1998, New York: Cambridge University Press; Copyright 1998 by Cambridge University Press. Reprinted with permission.

are abstract (e.g., becoming more cultured), lower-level identifications get more and more concrete (e.g., attending a ballet, listening to sounds, and watching people move while you sit quiet and still). Low-level identifications tend to convey a sense of "how" an activity is done; high-level identifications tend to convey a sense of "why."

Although the Vallacher and Wegner (1985) model is hierarchical, it doesn't specify what qualities define various levels. It simply assumes that where there is a potential emergent property there is the potential for differing levels of identification. On the other hand, the examples used to illustrate the theory tend to map onto the levels of the Powers hierarchy: sequences of acts, programs of actions (with variations of smaller-scale and larger-scale programs), and principles of being. Thus, work on action identification tends to suggest the reasonableness of these particular levels of abstraction in thinking about behavior.

C. MULTIPLE PATHS TO HIGH-LEVEL GOALS, MULTIPLE MEANINGS IN CONCRETE ACTION

Although the hierarchy we are discussing is in some ways very simple, it has implications for several issues in thinking about behavior (for a broader treatment, see Carver & Scheier, 1998). It is implicit here that goals at any given level can often be achieved by a variety of means at lower levels. This flexibility is particularly apparent at upper levels of the hierarchy, where the goals are abstract. This permits one to address the fact that people sometimes shift radically the manner in which they try to reach a goal when the goal itself has not changed. This happens commonly when the emergent quality that is the higher order goal is implied in several lower order activities. For example, a person can be helpful by writing a donation check, picking up discards for a recycling center, volunteering for a charity, or holding a door open for someone else.

Just as a given goal can be obtained via multiple pathways, so can a specific act be performed in the service of diverse goals. For example, you could buy someone a gift to make him or her feel good, to repay a kindness, to put him or her in your debt, or to satisfy a perceived holiday-season role. Thus, a given act can have strikingly different meanings, depending on the purpose it's intended to serve. This is an important subtheme of this view on behavior: Behavior can be understood only by identifying the goals to which behavior is addressed. This isn't always easy to do, either from an observer's point of view (cf. Read, Druian, & Miller, 1989) or from the actor's point of view.

D. GOAL IMPORTANCE: GOALS AND THE SELF

Another point made by the notion of hierarchical organization concerns the fact that goals are not equivalent in their importance. The higher you go into the organization, the more fundamental to the overriding sense of self are the qualities encountered. Thus, goal qualities at higher levels would appear to be intrinsically more important than those at lower levels.

Goals at lower levels are not necessarily equivalent to one another in importance, however. Just as it's sometimes hard to tell what goal underlies a given behavior, it can also be hard to tell from a behavior how important is the goal that lies behind it. In a hierarchical system there are at least two ways in which importance accrues to a concrete goal. The more directly a concrete action contributes to attainment of some highly valued goal at a more abstract level, the more important is that concrete action. Second, an act that contributes to the attainment of several goals at once is more important than an act that contributes to the attainment of only one goal.

Relative importance of goals returns us to the concept of self. In contemporary theories the self-concept has several aspects: one is the structure of knowledge about your history; another is knowledge about who you are now; another is the self-guides or images of potential selves used to guide movement from the present into the future (which may also be working models). A broad implication of this sort of theory is that the self is partly the person's goals.

III. FEEDBACK CONTROL AND
CREATION OF AFFECT

We shift now to another aspect of human self-regulation: emotion. Here we add a layer of complexity to the feedback model which differs greatly from the complexity represented by hierarchicality. Again the fundamental organizing principle is feedback control, but now the control is over a different quality.

What are feelings and what makes them exist? Many have analyzed the information that feelings provide and situations in which affect arises (see, e.g., Frijda, 1986; Lazarus, 1991; Ortony, Clore, & Collins, 1988; Roseman, 1984; Scherer & Ekman, 1984). The question we address here is slightly different: What is the internal mechanism by which feelings arise?

A. THEORY

We have suggested that feelings arise as a consequence of a feedback process (Carver & Scheier, 1990). This process operates simultaneously with the behavior-guiding function and in parallel to it. One way to describe this second function is to say it's checking on how well the behavior loop is doing at reducing its discrepancies. Thus, the input for this second loop is a representation of the *rate of discrepancy reduction in the action system over time*. (We focus first on discrepancy-reducing loops, turning later to enlarging loops.)

We find an analogy useful here. Because action implies change between states, consider behavior analogous to distance. If the action loop deals with distance, and if the affect-relevant loop assesses the progress of the action loop, then the latter loop is dealing with the psychological equivalent of velocity, the first derivative of distance over time. To the extent this analogy is meaningful, the perceptual input to this loop should be the first derivative over time of the input used by the action loop.

We don't believe this input creates affect by itself, because a given rate of progress has different affective consequences under different circumstances. As in any feedback system, this input is compared against a reference value (cf. Frijda, 1986, 1988). In this case, the reference is an acceptable or desired rate of behavioral discrepancy reduction. As in other feedback loops, the comparison checks for a deviation from the standard. If there is one, the output function changes.

We suggest that the result of the comparison process at the heart of this loop (the error signal generated by the comparator) is manifest phenomenologically in two forms: one is a hazy and nonverbal sense of expectancy—confidence or doubt; the other is affect, feeling—a sense of positiveness or negativeness.

B. RESEARCH EVIDENCE

At least a little evidence has accumulated to support the idea that affect originates in a velocity function. Hsee and Abelson (1991), who came independently to this idea, reported two studies of velocity and satisfaction. In one, subjects read descriptions of paired hypothetical scenarios and indicated which one they would find more satisfying. For example, they chose whether they would be more satisfied if their class standing had gone from the 30th percentile to the 70th over the past 6 weeks or if it had done so over the past 3 weeks.

Some comparisons were of positive outcomes; some negative. Given positive outcomes, subjects preferred *improving* to a high outcome over a *constant* high outcome; they preferred a fast velocity over a slow one; and they preferred fast brief changes to slower larger changes. When the change was negative (e.g., salaries got worse), subjects preferred a constant low salary to a salary that started high and fell to the same low level; they preferred slow falls to fast falls; and they preferred large slow falls to small fast falls.

We conducted a study that conceptually replicates aspects of these findings, but with an event that was personally experienced rather than hypothetical (Lawrence, Carver, & Scheier, 1999). We manipulated success feedback on an ambiguous task over an extended period. The patterns of feedback converged such that block 6 was identical for all subjects at 50% correct. Subjects in a neutral condition had 50% on the first and last block, and 50% average across all blocks. Others had positive change in performance, starting poorly and gradually improving. Others had negative change, starting well and gradually worsening. All rated their mood before starting and again after block 6 (which they did not know ended the session). Those whose performances were improving reported better moods; those whose performances were deteriorating reported worse moods, compared to those with a constant performance.

Another study that appears to bear on this view of affect, although not having this purpose in mind, was reported by Brunstein (1993). It examined subjective well being among college students over the course of an academic term as a function of several perceptions, including perception of progress toward goals. Of particular interest at present, progress at each measurement point was strongly correlated with concurrent well being.

C. CRUISE CONTROL MODEL

Ours is essentially a "cruise control" model of affect. That is, the system we've postulated functions much the same as the cruise control on a car. If you're going too slowly toward some goal in your behavior, negative affect arises. You respond by putting more effort into your action, trying to speed up. If you're going faster than you need to, positive affect arises and you coast. A car's cruise control is very similar. You come to a hill, which slows you down. Your cruise control responds by feeding the engine more gas to bring the speed back up. If you come across the crest of a hill and roll downhill too fast, the system pulls back on the gas and drags the speed back down.

The analogy is intriguing in part because it concerns an electromechanical regulation of the very quality we believe the affect system is regulating: velocity. It is also intriguing to realize that this analogy incorporates a similar asymmetry in the consequences of deviating from the set point. That is, both in your car's cruise control system and in your behavior, going too slow requires investment of greater effort and resources. Going too fast does not. It requires only pulling back on resources. That is, your cruise control doesn't apply your brakes, it just cuts back on the gasoline. In this way it permits you to coast back to your velocity set point. In the same fashion, you don't respond to positive affect by trying to make it go away, but just by easing off.

Does positive affect lead people to withdraw effort? There is a little information on this, but not much. Melton (1995) found that people in a good mood performed worse than control subjects on syllogisms. A variety of ancillary data led him to the conclusion that the people in good moods did worse because they were expending less effort. To us, this looks like coasting.

D. AFFECT FROM DISCREPANCY-ENLARGING LOOPS

When we began this section we said we would restrict ourselves at first to discrepancy-reducing loops. Thus far we've done that, dealing only with issues that arise in the context of approach. Now we turn to attempts to distance oneself from a point of comparison, attempts to not be or not do, discrepancy-*enlarging* loops.

It should be apparent from our earlier discussion that behavior toward avoidance goals is just as intelligible as behavior toward approach goals. But what about the affective accompaniments to avoidance loops? The affect theory described here rests on the idea that positive affect results when a behavioral system is making rapid progress in *doing what it is organized to do*. The systems considered thus far are organized to close discrepancies. There's no obvious reason, however, why the principle shouldn't apply just as well to systems with the opposite purpose. If the system is making rapid progress doing what it's organized to do, the result should be positive affect. If the system is doing poorly at what it's organized to do, the result should be negative affect.

That much would seem to be fully comparable across the two types of systems. We see, however, a difference in the affect qualities involved (see

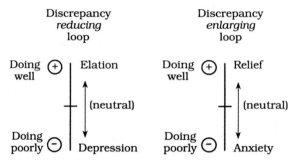

FIGURE 5   Two sorts of affect-creating systems and the affective dimensions we believe arise from the functioning of each. Discrepancy-reducing systems are presumed to yield affective qualities of sadness or depression when progress is below standard and happiness or elation when progress is above standard. Discrepancy-enlarging systems are presumed to yield anxiety when progress is below standard and relief or contentment when progress is above standard. *Note.* From *On the Self-Regulation of Behavior*, by C. S. Carver and M. F. Scheier, 1998, New York: Cambridge University Press; Copyright 1998 by Cambridge University Press. Reprinted with permission.

Figure 5). In each case there's a positive pole and a negative pole, but the positives aren't quite the same, nor are the negatives.

Our view of this difference derives partly from the insights of Higgins and his colleagues (Higgins, 1987, 1996). Following their lead, we suggest that the affect dimension relating to discrepancy reducing loops is (in its purest form) the dimension that runs from depression to elation. The affect dimension that relates to discrepancy-enlarging loops is (in its purest form) the dimension from anxiety to relief or contentment. As Higgins and his colleagues note, dejection-related and agitation-related affect may take several forms, but these two dimensions capture the core qualities behind them. The connections drawn in Figure 5 between affect quality and type of system are compatible not just with the Higgins model, but also with certain other theories. For example, Roseman (1984, p. 31) has argued that joy and sadness are related to appetitive (moving-toward) motives, whereas relief and distress are related to aversive (moving-away-from) motives.

E. MERGING AFFECT AND ACTION

How does the mechanism creating affect influence *action*? A more basic question (which takes us to the same end) is this: We've treated affect as the error signal of a feedback loop, but what's the *output function* of that loop? If the input function is a perception of rate of progress, the output function must be an *adjustment* in rate of progress.

Some adjustments are straightforward—go faster. Sometimes it's less so. The rates of many "behaviors" (higher order activities) aren't defined by the literal pace of physical action. Rather, they're defined in terms of

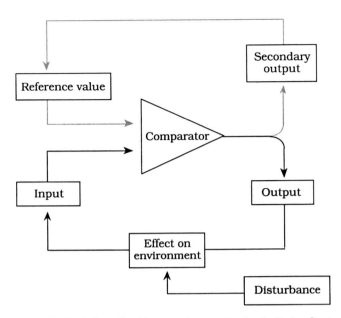

FIGURE 6   A feedback loop (in this case, the postulated velocity loop) acts to create change in the input function to shift it toward the reference value. Sometimes an additional process is in place as well (gray lines), which adjusts the reference value in the direction of the input. This additional process is presumed to be weaker or slower; thus, the reference value is stable relative to the input value. *Note.* From *On the Self-Regulation of Behavior*, by C. S. Carver and M. F. Scheier, 1998, New York: Cambridge University Press; Copyright 1998 by Cambridge University Press. Reprinted with permission.

It is also of interest (and once again counterintuitive) that these shifts in reference value (and the resultant effects on affect) imply a mechanism within the organism that functions to actively prevent the too frequent occurrence of positive feeling, as well as the too frequent occurrence of negative feeling. That is, the (bidirectional) shifting of the rate criterion over time would tend to control pacing of behavior in such a way that affect continues to vary in both directions around neutral, roughly the same as it had before.

Such an arrangement for changing the standard thus would not result in maximization of pleasure and minimization of pain. Rather, the affective consequence would be that the person experiences more or less the same range of variation in affective experience over extended periods of time and circumstances (cf. Myers & Diener, 1995). The organization as a whole would function as a gyroscope serving to keep us floating along within the framework of the affective reality we're familiar with. It would provide for a continuous recalibration of the feeling system across changes in situation. To use a different image, it would repeatedly shift the balance point of a psychic teeter-totter, so that rocking in both directions remains possible.

H. COMPARISON WITH BIOLOGICAL MODELS
OF BASES OF AFFECT

It is useful to compare this model with the group of biologically focused theories we mentioned earlier. The theories are quite similar to one another in many ways, but in other ways they differ. These theories all incorporate the idea that two systems (or more) are involved in the regulation of behavior. Many assume further that the two systems underlie affect. In situations with cues of impending reward, the activity of the approach system creates positive feelings. In situations with cues of impending punishment, the avoidance system creates feelings of anxiety.

Data from a variety of sources fit this picture. Of particular interest is work by Davidson and collaborators, involving EEG recordings assessing changes in activation in response to affective inducing stimuli. Among the findings are these: Subjects exposed to films inducing fear and disgust (Davidson, Ekman, Saron, Senulis, & Friesen, 1990) and confronted with possible punishment (Sobotka, Davidson, & Senulis, 1992) show elevations in *right* frontal activation. In contrast, subjects with a chance to obtain reward (Sobota et al., 1992), subjects presented with positive emotional adjectives (Cacioppo & Petty, 1980), and smiling 10-month-olds viewing their approaching mothers (Fox & Davidson, 1988) show elevations in *left* frontal activation. From findings such as these, Davidson (1992a, 1992b) concluded that neural substrates for approach and withdrawal systems (and thus positive and negative affect) are located in the left and right frontal areas of the cortex, respectively.

The logic of these models thus far resembles the logic of our model. At this point, however, theories diverge. The question on which they diverge concerns the regulatory processes involved in, and affects that result from, *failure to attain reward* and *successful avoidance of punishment*. Gray (1987b, 1990) holds that the avoidance system is engaged by cues of punishment and cues of frustrative nonreward. It thus is reponsible for negative feelings in response to either of these types of cues. Similarly, he holds that the approach system is engaged by cues of reward or cues of escape from (or avoidance of) punishment. It thus is responsible for positive feelings in response to either of these types of cues. In his view, then, each system creates affect of one hedonic tone (positive in one case, negative in the other), regardless of its source (see Figure 7). This view is consistent with a picture of two unipolar affective dimensions, each linked to a distinct behavioral system. A similar position has been taken by Lang, Bradley, and Cuthbert (1992).

Our position is different. It argues for an approach system and an avoidance system, in which—in each case—affect is a product of either doing well or doing poorly. Thus, it implies two bipolar dimensions: one tied to approach, the other to avoidance (Figure 7). We think the frustration and eventual depression that result from failure to attain desired goals involve the approach system (for similar predictions, see Clark, Watson, & Mineka, 1994, p. 107; Cloninger 1988, p. 103). Sadness and depression involve *reduced* activity in the approach system, as the pursuit of goals diminishes. A parallel line of reasoning suggests that relief, contentment, tranquility, and serenity relate to the avoidance rather than the approach system, reflecting low levels of activity in that system.

Less information exists about neurophysiological bases of these affects than about anxiety and happiness. With regard to relief–tranquility, we know of no data at all. With respect to depression, limited evidence exists. Henriques and Davidson (1991) found that clinically depressed persons had less activation in left frontal areas than nondepressed controls. In contrast, there was no evidence of a difference in right frontal activation. This pattern has since been replicated by Allen, Iacono, Depue, and Arbisi (1993). Recall that Davidson viewed baseline measures as representing susceptibility rather than ambient affect per se. Thus, this finding tenta-

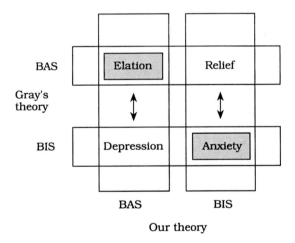

Our theory

FIGURE 7   Gray's view of affect (horizontal groupings) ties positive affects to the effects of a behavioral activation system (BAS), as results of occurrence of reward and avoidance of punishment. It ties negative affects to the effects of a behavioral inhibition system (BIS), as results of frustrative nonreward and occurrence of punishment. Our view (vertical groupings, as in Figure 5) ties the dimension of elation–depression to an approach system and the dimension of anxiety–relief to an avoidance system, each of which thus has properties somewhat different from those assumed by Gray. *Note.* From *On the Self-Regulation of Behavior*, by C. S. Carver and M. F. Scheier, 1998, New York: Cambridge University Press; Copyright 1998 by Cambridge University Press. Reprinted with permission.

tively seems to suggest that depressed persons are vulnerable to depression through deficits in their approach system. This set of findings seems quite compatible with our position.

IV. CONFIDENCE AND DOUBT, PERSISTENCE AND GIVING UP

In describing the genesis of affect, we suggested that one mechanism yields two subjective readouts: affect, and a hazy sense of confidence versus doubt. We turn now to a consideration of confidence and doubt—expectancies for the immediate future. We focus here on the *consequences* of this sense of confidence and doubt.

We've often suggested that when people experience adversity in trying to move toward their goals, they periodically experience an interruption of efforts, to assess in a more deliberative way the likelihood of a successful outcome (e.g., Carver & Scheier, 1981, 1990). In effect, people suspend the behavioral stream, step outside it, and evaluate in a more deliberated way than occurs while acting. This may happen once or often. It may be brief or it may take a long time. In this assessment, people presumably depend heavily on memories of prior outcomes in similar situations. They may also consider such things as additional resources they might bring to bear (cf. Lazarus, 1966) or alternative approaches to the problem. People use social comparison information (Wills, 1981; Wood, 1989) and attributional analyses of prior events (Wong & Weiner, 1981).

How do these thoughts influence the expectancies that emerge? In some cases, when people retrieve "chronic" expectancies from memory, the information already *is* expectancies, summaries of products of previous behavior. For some cases, however, people bring to mind possibilities for the situation's evolution. For these possibilities to influence expectancies, their consequences must be evaluated. We suggest they are briefly played through mentally as behavioral scenarios (cf. Taylor & Pham, 1996). This should lead to conclusions that influence the expectancy. ("If I try approaching it this way instead of that way, it should work better." "This is the only thing I can see to do, and it will just make the situation worse.")

It seems reasonable that this mental simulation engages the same mechanism as handles the affect creation process during actual overt behavior. When your progress is temporarily stalled, playing through a scenario that is confident and optimistic yields a higher rate of progress than is currently being experienced. The affect loop thus yields a more optimistic outcome assessment than is being derived from current action. If the scenario is negative and hopeless, it indicates a further reduction in progress and the loop yields further doubt.

A. ENGAGEMENT VERSUS GIVING UP

The expectancies that result, whatever their source, are reflected in behavior (Figure 8). If expectations are for a successful outcome, the person returns to effort toward the goal. If doubts are strong enough, the result is an impetus to disengage from further effort and potentially from the goal itself (Carver & Scheier, 1981, 1990, 1998, 1999; see also Klinger, 1975; Kukla, 1972; Wortman & Brehm, 1975). This theme—divergence in behavioral response as a function of expectancies—is an important one, applying to a surprisingly broad range of literatures (see Chapter 11 of Carver & Scheier, 1998).

Sometimes the disengagement that follows from doubt is overt, but disengagement sometimes takes the form of mental disengagement—off-task thinking, daydreaming, and so on. Although this sometimes can be useful (self-distraction from a feared stimulus may permit anxiety to abate), it also can create problems. If there is time pressure, mental disengagement can impair performance, as time is spent on task-irrelevant thoughts. Consistent with this, interactions between self-focus and expectancies have been shown for measures of performance (Carver, Peterson, Follansbee, & Scheier, 1983; Carver & Scheier, 1982).

Often mental disengagement can not be sustained, because situational cues force a reconfrontation of the task. In such cases, the result is a phenomenology of repetitive negative rumination, which often focuses on

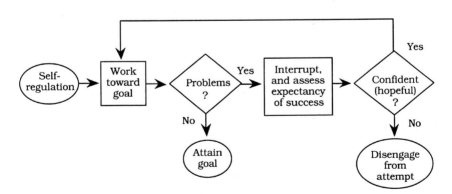

FIGURE 8 Flow-chart depiction of self-regulatory possibilities, indicating that action sometimes continues unimpeded toward goal attainment, that obstacles to goal attainment sometimes induce a sequence of evaluation and decision making, and that if expectancies for eventual success are sufficiently unfavorable, the person may disengage from further effort. *Note.* From *On the Self-Regulation of Behavior,* by C. S. Carver and M. F. Scheier, 1998, New York: Cambridge University Press; Copyright 1998 by Cambridge University Press. Reprinted with permission.

self-doubt and perceptions of inadequacy. This cycle is both unpleasant and performance impairing.

A number of writers—both from an earlier tradition of cognitive-attentional theories of anxiety (e.g., Sarason, 1975; Wine, 1971, 1980) and some more recent (Ingram, 1990)—have equated this phenomenology of negative rumination with the term "self-focus." We would argue that this label is misleading (see also Pyszczynski, Greenberg, Hamilton, & Nix, 1991). Why? Because self-focus does not always produce interference. As described earlier, self-focus is in many cases associated with *task* focus, as the experience of attention inward engages the feedback process underlying effort. Indeed, among confident subjects in the studies just mentioned, this is what occurred even under conditions of adversity. Self-focus led to better task effort, as manifest both in overt behavior and in contents of consciousness. Only among doubtful subjects did self-focus lead to performance impairment or to negative rumination.

B. IS DISENGAGEMENT GOOD OR BAD?

Is the disengagement tendency good or bad? The answer is that it is both and neither. On the one hand, disengagement (at some level, at least) is an absolute necessity. Disengagement is a natural and indispensable part of self-regulation. If we are ever to turn away from efforts at unattainable goals, if we are ever to back out of blind alleys, we must be able to disengage, to give up and start over somewhere else.

The importance of disengagement is particularly obvious with regard to concrete, low-level goals: We must be able to remove ourselves from literal blind alleys and wrong streets, give up plans that have become disrupted by unexpected events, even spend the night in the wrong city if we've missed the last plane home. The tendency is also important, however, with regard to more abstract and higher-level goals. A vast literature attests to the importance of disengaging and moving on with life after the loss of close relationships (e.g., Orbuch, 1992; Stroebe, Stroebe, & Hansson, 1993; Weiss, 1988). People sometimes must even be willing to give up values that are deeply embedded in the self, if those values create too much conflict and distress in their lives.

As with most processes in self-regulation, however, the choice between continued effort and giving up presents opportunities for things to go awry. It's possible to stop trying prematurely, thereby creating potentially serious problems for oneself (Carver & Scheier, 1998). It's also possible to hold onto goals too long and prevent oneself from taking adaptive steps toward new goals. However, both continued effort and giving up are necessary parts of the experience of adaptive self-regulation. Each plays an important role in the flow of behavior.

C. HIERARCHICALITY AND IMPORTANCE
CAN IMPEDE DISENGAGEMENT

Disengagement sometimes is precluded by situational constraints. However, another, broader aspect of this problem stems from the idea that behavior is hierarchically organized, with goals increasingly important higher in the hierarchy and thus harder to disengage from.

Presumably disengaging from concrete values is often easy. Lower order goals vary, however, in how closely they are linked to values at a higher level, and thus how important they are. To disengage from low-level goals that are tightly linked to higher-level goals causes discrepancy enlargement at the higher level. These higher order qualities are important, even central to one's life. One cannot disengage from them, or disregard them, or tolerate large discrepancies between them and current reality without reorganizing one's value system (Greenwald, 1980; Kelly, 1955; McIntosh & Martin, 1992; Millar, Tesser, & Millar, 1988). In such a case, disengagement from even very concrete behavioral goals can be quite difficult.

Now recall again the affective consequences of being in this situation. The desire to disengage was prompted by unfavorable expectancies. These expectancies are paralleled by negative affect. In this situation, then, the person experiences negative feelings (because of an inability to make progress toward the goal) and is unable to do anything about the feelings (because of an inability to give up). The person simply stews in the feelings that arise from irreconcilable discrepancies. This kind of situation—commitment to unattainable goals—seems a sure prescription for distress.

D. WATERSHEDS, DISJUNCTIONS, AND
BIFURCATIONS AMONG RESPONSES

An issue that bears some further mention is the divergence of the behavioral and cognitive responses to favorable versus unfavorable expectancies that is part of this model. We've long argued for a psychological watershed among responses to adversity (Carver & Scheier, 1981). One set of responses consists of continued comparisons between present state and goal, and continued efforts. The other set consists of disengagement from comparisons and quitting. Just as rainwater falling on a mountain ridge ultimately flows to one side of the ridge or the other, so do behaviors ultimately flow to one of these sets or the other.

Our initial reason for taking this position stemmed largely from the several demonstrations that self-focused attention creates diverging effects on both information seeking and behavior, as a function of expectancies of success (Figure 9). We aren't the only ones to have emphasized a disjunction among responses, however. A number of others have done so, for reasons of their own.

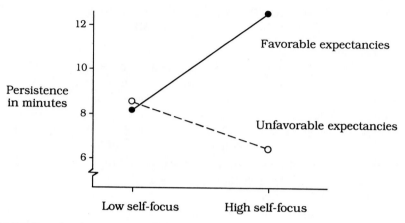

FIGURE 9   Persistence at an insoluble problem as a function of performance expectancy regarding the target task and self-directed attention. *Note.* Adapted by combining data from Experiments 1 and 2 from "Reassertion and Giving Up: The Interactive Role of Self-Directed Attention and Outcome Expectancy," by C. S. Carver, P. H. Blaney, & M. F. Scheier, 1979, *Journal of Personality and Social Psychology, 37,* pp. 1859–1870. Copyright 1979 by the American Psychological Association. Adapted with permission.

An early model that emphasized the idea of a disjunction in behavior was proposed by Kukla (1972). Another such model is the reactance–helplessness integration of Wortman and Brehm (1975): the argument that threats to control produce attempts to regain control and that perceptions of loss of control produce helpless. Brehm and his collaborators (Brehm & Self, 1989; Wright & Brehm, 1989) have more recently developed an approach to task engagement that resembles that of Kukla (1972), although their way of approaching the description of the problem is somewhat different. Not all theories about persistence and giving up yield this dichotomy among responses. The fact that some do, however, is interesting. It becomes more so a little bit later on.

V. DYNAMIC SYSTEMS AND HUMAN BEHAVIOR

Recent years have seen the emergence in psychology of new (or at least newly prominent) ideas about how to conceptualize natural systems. Several labels attach to these ideas: chaos, dynamic systems theory, complexity, catastrophe theory. A number of introductions to various aspects of this body of thought have been written, some of which include applications to psychology (e.g., Brown, 1995; Gleick, 1987; Thelen & Smith, 1994; Vallacher & Nowak, 1994, 1997; Waldrop, 1992). In this section we sketch some themes that are central to this way of thinking and indicate places where we think the themes apply meaningfully to subjects of our own interest.

Dynamic systems theory (or chaos theory) is deterministic (despite the contrary implication of the word chaos). It holds that the behavior of a system reflects the forces operating on (and within) it. It also emphasizes that the behavior of a complex system over anything but a brief time is very hard to predict. Why?

A. NONLINEARITY

One reason is that the system's behavior may be influenced by the forces operating on and within it in nonlinear ways. Thus, the behavior of the system—even though highly determined—can appear random. This determinism in principle but unpredictability in practice underlies the label *chaotic*.

Many people are used to thinking of relationships between variables as linear. Dynamic-systems thinking asserts that many relationships are not linear. Familiar examples of nonlinear relationships are step functions (ice turning to water and water turning to steam as temperature increases), threshold functions, and floor and ceiling effects. Other examples of nonlinearity are interactions (Figure 10). In an interaction, the effect of one predictor on the outcome differs as a function of the level of a second predictor. Thus the effect of the first predictor on the outcome is not linear. The second predictor is thereby acting as a *control parameter*—a factor "that hold[s] potential for changing the intrinsic dynamics of a system" (Vallacher & Nowak, 1997).

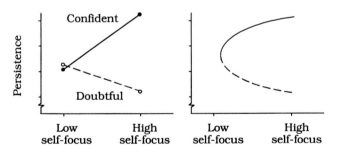

FIGURE 10   Interactions indicate that the effect of one variable differs as a function of the level of another variable. On the left is the interaction between self-focus and expectancy that was shown in Figure 9. This indicates that the effect of self-focus is nonlinear (right panel). Its impact reverses at some point along the distribution of the variable confidence–doubt. *Note.* From "Themes and issues in the Self-Regulation of Behavior" by C. S. Carver & M. F. Scheier, in R. S. Wyer, Jr. (Ed.), *Advances in Social Cognition*, 1999, Mahwah, NJ: Erlbaum. Copyright 1999 by Lawrence Erlbaum Associates. Reprinted with permission.

Obviously the interaction in Figure 10 is far from unique. Indeed, many psychologists think in terms of interactions much of the time. Threshold effects and interactions are nonlinearities that many people take for granted, though perhaps not labeling them as such. Looking intentionally for nonlinearities, however, reveals others. For example, many psychologists now think many developmental changes are dynamic rather than linear (Goldin−Meadow & Alibali, 1995; Siegler & & Jenkins, 1989; Ruble, 1994; Thelen, 1992, 1995; van der Maas & Molenaar, 1992).

B. SENSITIVE DEPENDENCE ON INITIAL CONDITIONS

Nonlinearity is one reason why it's hard to predict complex systems. Two more reasons why prediction over anything but the short term is difficult is that you never know all the influences on a system, and the ones you do know you never know with total precision. What you *think* is going on may not be quite what is going on. That difference, even if it's small, can be very important.

This theme is identified in the dynamic systems literature with the phrase *sensitive dependence on initial conditions*. This phrase means that a very small difference between two conditions of a system can lead to divergence, and ultimately the absence of any relation between the paths taken later on. The idea is (partly) that a small initial difference causes a difference in what the systems encounter next, which yields slightly different influences on the systems, producing slightly different outcomes (Lorenz, 1963). Through repeated iterations, the systems diverge, eventually leading the two systems to very different pathways. After a surprisingly brief period, they no longer have any noticeable relation to one another.

How does the notion of sensitive dependence on initial conditions relate to human behavior? Most generally, it suggests that a person's behavior will be hard to predict over a long period except in general terms. For example, although you might be confident that Joe usually eats lunch, you wouldn't be able to predict as well what time, where, or what he'll eat on the second Friday of next month. This does not mean Joe's behavior is truly random or unlawful (cf. Epstein, 1979). It just means that small differences between the influences you think are affecting him and the influences that are *actually* taking place will result in moment-to-moment behavior that's unpredicted.

This principle also holds for prediction of your own behavior. There's evidence that people don't plan very far into the future (Anderson, 1990, pp. 203−205), even experts (Gobet & Simon, 1996). People seem to have goals in which the general form of the goal is sketched out, but only a few program-level steps toward it have been planned. Even attempts at relatively thorough planning appear to be recursive and "opportunistic," changing—sometimes drastically—when new information becomes known (Hayes-Roth & Hayes-Roth, 1979).

The notion of sensitive dependence on initial conditions provides an explanation for this. It is pointless (and maybe even counterproductive) to plan too far ahead too fully (cf. Kirschenbaum, 1985), because chaotic forces in play (forces that are hard to predict because of nonlinearities and sensitive dependence) can render much of the planning irrelevant. Thus, it makes sense to plan in general terms, chart a few steps, get there, reassess, and plan the next bits. This seems a perfect illustration of how people implicitly take chaos into account in their own lives.

C. PHASE SPACE, ATTRACTORS, AND REPELLERS

Another set of concepts important in dynamic-systems thinking are variations on the terms *phase space* and *attractor* (Brown, 1995; Vallacher & Nowak, 1997). A *phase diagram* is a depiction of the behavior of a system over time. The system's states are plotted along two (sometimes three) axes, with time displayed as the progression of the line of the plot, rather than on an axis of its own. A phase space is the array of states that a system occupies across a period of time. As the system changes states over time, it traces a *trajectory* within its phase space—a path of the successive states it occupies across that period.

Phase spaces often contain regions called attractors. Attractors are areas the system approaches, occupies, or tends toward more frequently than other areas. Attractors seem to exert a metaphorical gravitational pull on the system, bringing the system into proximity to them. Each attractor has what is called a *basin*, the attractor's region of attraction. Trajectories that enter the basin tend to move toward that attractor (Brown, 1995).

There are several kinds of attractors, some simple, others more complex. In a *point attractor*, all trajectories converge onto some point in phase space, no matter where they begin (e.g., body temperature). Of greater interest are *chaotic attractors*. The pattern to which this term refers is an irregular and unpredictable movement around attraction points. The best known example is the Lorenz attractor (Figure 11), named for the man who first plotted it (Lorenz, 1963). It has two attraction zones. Plotting the behavior of this system yields a tendency to loop around both attractors, but unpredictably. Shifts in trajectory from one basin to the other seem random.

The behavior of this system displays sensitivity to initial conditions. A small change in starting point changes the specific path of motion entirely. The *general tendencies* remain the same—that is, the revolving around both attractors—but details such as the number of revolutions around one before deflection to the other, form an entirely different pattern. The

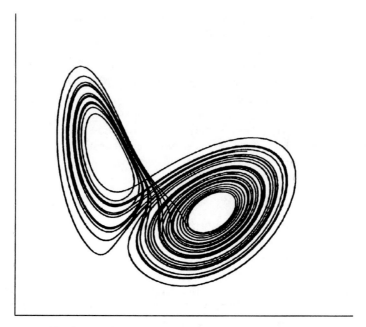

FIGURE 11   The Lorenz attractor, an example of what is known as a chaotic attractor or strange attractor. *Note*. From *On the Self-Regulation of Behavior*, by C. S. Carver and M. F. Scheier, 1998, New York: Cambridge University Press; Copyright 1998 by Cambridge University Press. Reprinted with permission.

trajectory over iterations shows this same sensitivity to small differences. As the system continues, it often nearly repeats itself, but never quite does, and what seem nearly identical paths can diverge abruptly, with one path leading to one attractor and the adjacent path leading to the other.

A phase space also contains regions called repellers, regions that are hardly ever occupied. Indeed, these regions seem to be actively avoided. That is, a minimal departure from the focal point of a repeller leads to a rapid escape from that region of phase space.

D. ANOTHER WAY OF PICTURING ATTRACTORS

The phase-space diagram gives a vivid visual sense of what an attractor "looks like" and how it acts. Another way that is often used to portray attractors is shown in Figure 12. In this view, attractor basins are basins or valleys in a surface (a more technical label for a basin is a *local minimum*). Repellers are ridges. This view assumes a metaphoric "gravitational" drift downward in the diagram, but other forces are presumed to be operative in all directions. (For simplicity, this portrayal usually is done as a two-dimen-

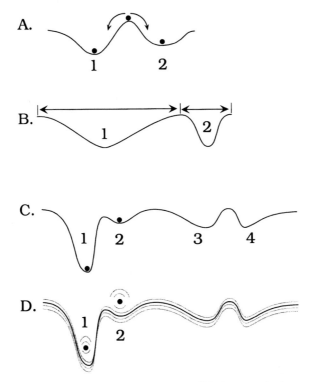

FIGURE 12 Another way to portray attractors. (A) Attractor basins as valleys in a surface (local minima). The behavior of the system is represented as a ball. If the ball is in a valley (point 1 or 2), it is in an attractor basin and will tend to stay there unless disturbed. If the ball is on a ridge (between points 1 and 2), it will tend to escape its current location and move to an attractor. (B) A wider basin (point 1) attracts more trajectories than a narrower basin (point 2). A steeply sloping basin (point 2) attracts more *abruptly* any trajectory that enters the basin than does a more gradually sloping basin (point 1) (C). A system in which attractor point 1 is very stable and the others are less stable. It will take more energy to free the ball from attractor point 1 than from the others. (D) The system's behavior is energized, much as the shaking of a metaphoric tambourine surface, keeping the system's behavior in flux and less than completely captured by any particular attractor. Still, more shaking will be required to escape from attractor point 1 than attractor point 2. *Note.* From *On the Self-Regulation of Behavior*, by C. S. Carver and M. F. Scheier, 1998, New York: Cambridge University Press; Copyright 1998 by Cambridge University Press. Reprinted with permission.

sional drawing, but keep in mind that the diagram often assumes the merging of a large number of dimensions into the horizontal axis.)

The behavior of the system at a given moment is represented as a ball on the surface. If the ball is in a valley (points 1 and 2 in Figure 12A), it's in an attractor basin and will tend to stay there unless disturbed. If it's on a hill (between 1 and 2), any slight movement in either direction will cause it to escape its current location and move to an adjacent attractor.

A strength of this portrayal is that it does a good job of creating a sense of how attractors vary in robustness. The breadth of a basin indicates the diversity of trajectories in phase space that are drawn into it. The broader the basin (point 1, in Figure 12B), the more trajectories are drawn in. The narrower the basin (Figure 12B, point 2), the closer the ball has to come to its focal point to be drawn to it. The steepness of the valley indicates how *abruptly* a trajectory is drawn into it. The steeper the slope of the wall (Figure 12B, point 2), the more sudden is the entry of a system that encounters that basin.

The depth of the valley indicates how firmly entrenched the system is, once drawn into the attractor. Figure 12C represents a system of attractors with fairly low stability (most of the valleys are shallow). In Figure 12C, one attractor represents a stable situation (valley 1), whereas the others are less so. It will take a lot more "energy" to free the ball from valley 1 than from the others.

There's a sense in which both breadth and depth suggest that a goal is important. Breadth does so because the system is drawn to the attractor from widely divergent trajectories. Depth does so because the system that's been drawn into the basin tends to stay there.

A weakness of this picture, compared to a phase-space portrait, is that it isn't as good at giving a sense of the erratic motion from one attractor to another in a multiple-attractor system. You can regain some of that sense of erratic shifting, however, if you think of the surface in Figure 12 as a tambourine, with a certain amount of shaking going on all the time (Figure 12D). Even a little shaking causes the ball to bounce around in its well, and may jostle it from one well to another, particularly if the attractors are not highly stable. An alternative would be to think of the ball as a jumping bean, hopping and bouncing. These two characterizations are analogous to jostling that comes from situational influences and jostling from internal dynamics, respectively.

E. GOALS AS ATTRACTORS

The themes of dynamic systems thinking outlined here have had several applications in personality–social and even clinical psychology (Vallacher & Nowak, 1997). An easy and intuitive application of the attractor concept to human behavior is to link it with the goal concept. Goals are points around which behavior is regulated. That is, people spend much of their time doing things that keep their behavior in close proximity to their goals. It seems reasonable to suggest, then, that a goal represents a kind of attractor. Furthermore, if an attractor represents a goal, it seems reasonable that a repeller represents an anti-goal.

The idea of attractors and trajectories within phase space provides an interesting complement and supplement to the idea that behavior is guided by feedback processes regarding goals and anti-goals. However, we don't think the ideas about phase space *replace* the ideas about feedback and goals. Rather, the ideas mesh. Each provides something the other lacks. Movement toward a goal is not really an automatic gravitational drift, once the goal is identified (no matter how convenient that image). The feedback model provides a mechanism through which goal directed activity is managed, a mechanism that isn't in the phase-space model. The phase-space model, however, suggests ways of thinking about how goals diverge and how people shift among multiple goals over time, issues that aren't dealt with as easily in terms of feedback processes.

That is, think of the landscape of chaotic attractors, but think about there being *many* different basins attracting behavior rather than just two or three. This seems to capture rather well the sense of human behavior. Because no attractor basin in this system ever becomes a point attractor, behavior tends toward one goal, then another, never being completely captured by any goal. The person does one thing for a while, then something else. The goals are all predictable—in the sense that they all have an influence on the person over time—an influence that is highly predictable when aggregated across time. However, the shifts from one to another occur unpredictably (thus are chaotic).[1]

VI. CATASTROPHE THEORY

Another set of ideas that has been around for a while but seems to be reemerging in influence is catastrophe theory, a mathematical model focusing on creation of discontinuities, bifurcations, or splittings (Brown, 1995; Saunders, 1980; Stewart & Peregoy, 1983; van der Maas & Molenaar, 1992; Woodcock & Davis, 1978; Zeeman, 1977). A catastrophe occurs when a small change in one variable produces an abrupt (and usually large) change in another variable.

An abrupt change implies nonlinearity or discontinuity. This focus on nonlinearity is one of several themes that catastrophe theory shares with dynamic systems theory, although the two bodies of thought have different origins (and, indeed, some view them as quite different from each other-see Chapter 2 of Kelso, 1995). The discontinuity that is the focus of catastrophe theory can be seen as reflecting "the sudden disappearance of one attractor and its basin, combined with the dominant emergence of another attractor" (Brown, 1995, p. 51).

---

[1]Although our greatest interest in the themes of dynamic systems is in their application to the goal construct, several other possibilities have also been suggested. Treatment of these possibilities is beyond the scope of this chapter, however (for broader consideration see Carver & Scheier, 1998; Nowak & Vallacher, 1998; Vallacher & Nowak, 1994).

Though several types of catastrophe exist (Brown, 1995; Saunders, 1980; Woodcock & Davis, 1978), the one that has been considered most frequently regarding behavior is the *cusp catastrophe*, in which two control parameters influence an outcome. Figure 13 portrays its three-dimensional surface, where x and z are the control parameters and y is the outcome. At low values of z, the surface of the figure expresses a roughly linear relationship between x and y. As x increases, so does y. As z (the second control parameter) increases, the relationship between x and y becomes less linear. It first shifts toward something like a step function. With further increase in z, the x–y relationship becomes even more clearly discontinuous—the outcome is either on the top surface or on the bottom. Thus, changes in z cause a change in the way x relates to y.

Another theme that links catastrophe theory to dynamic systems is the idea of sensitive dependence on initial conditions. The cusp catastrophe model displays this characteristic nicely. Consider the portion of Figure 13 where z has low values and x has a continuous relation to y, the system's behavior. Points 1 and 2 on x are nearly identical, but not quite. As z increases and we follow the movement of these points forward on the surface, for a while they track each other closely, until suddenly they begin

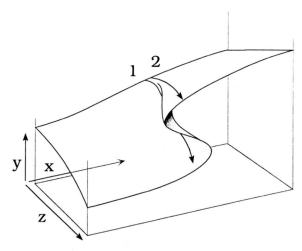

FIGURE 13   Three-dimensional depiction of a cusp catastrophe. Variables x and z are control parameters; y is the system's "behavior," the dependent variable. The catastrophe shows sensitive dependence on initial conditions. Where z is low, points 1 and 2 are nearly the same on x. If you project these points forward on the surface (with increases in z), you find that they move in parallel until the cusp begins to emerge. The lines are separated by the formation of the cusp and project to completely different regions of the surface. *Note.* From *On the Self-Regulation of Behavior*, by C. S. Carver and M. F. Scheier, 1998, New York: Cambridge University Press; Copyright 1998 by Cambridge University Press. Reprinted with permission.

to be separated by the fold in the catastrophe. At higher levels of z, one track ultimately projects to the upper region of the surface, the other projects to the lower region. Thus, a very slight initial difference results in a substantial difference farther along.

A. HYSTERESIS

The preceding description also hinted at an interesting and important feature of a catastrophe known as *hysteresis*. There are several ways to get a handle on what this term means. A simple characterization is that at some levels of z, there's a kind of foldover in the middle of the $x-y$ relationship. A region of x exists in which there is more than one value of y. Another way to characterize the hysteresis is that two regions of this surface are attractors and one is a repeller (Brown, 1995). This unstable area is illustrated in Figure 14. The dashed-line portion of Figure 14 that lies between values a and b on the x axis—the region where the fold is going backward—repels trajectories (Brown, 1995), whereas the areas near values c and d attract trajectories. To put it more simply, you can't *be* on the dashed part of this surface.

Yet another way of characterizing hysteresis is captured by the statement that the system's behavior depends on the system's recent history (Brown, 1995; Nowak & Lewenstein, 1994). That is, as you move into the zone of variable x that lies between points a and b in Figure 14, it matters

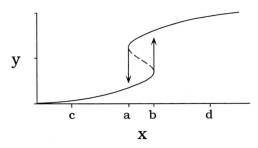

FIGURE 14 A cusp catastrophe exhibits a region of hysteresis (between values a and b on the x axis) in which x has two stable values of y (the solid lines) and one unstable value (the dotted line that cuts backward in the middle of the figure). The region represented by the dotted line repels trajectories, whereas the stable regions (those surrounding values c and d on the x axis) attract trajectories. Traversing the zone of hysteresis from the left of this figure results in an abrupt shift (at value b on the x axis) from the lower to the upper portion of the surface (right arrow). Traversing the zone of hysteresis from the right of this figure results in an abrupt shift (at value a on the x axis) from the upper to the lower portion of the surface (left arrow). Thus, the disjunction between portions of the surface occurs at two different values of x, depending on the starting point. *Note.* From *On the Self-Regulation of Behavior*, by C. S. Carver and M. F. Scheier, 1998, New York: Cambridge University Press, Copyright 1998 by Cambridge University Press. Reprinted with permission.

which side of the figure you're coming from. If the system is moving from point c into the zone of hysteresis, it stays on the bottom surface until it reaches point b, where it jumps to the top surface. If the system is moving from d into the zone of hysteresis, it stays on the top surface until it reaches point a, where it jumps to the bottom surface.

B. SOME APPLICATIONS OF CATASTROPHE THEORY

How does catastrophe theory apply to the human behaviors of most interest to personality and social psychologists? Several applications of these ideas have been made in the past decade or so, and others seem obvious candidates for future study.

The first serious application of catastrophe theory by a social psychologist apparently came in an article published nearly two decades ago by Tesser (1980). He described there two potential influences on a romantic relationship: attraction toward the partner and social pressures against the partner (e.g., when the partner is the "wrong" race, social class, or religion). When social pressures are low, dating-related behavior is at the back plane of the catastrophe figure. The extent of dating activity shows a generally linear increase with attraction.

When social pressures against the relationship are high, however, dating-related behavior is at the forward plane of the figure. When attraction is low to moderate (z is low), the social pressure keeps dating activity low. When attraction (z) is high, the social pressure is resisted and dating activity is high. In the middle range of attraction, the behavior that emerges depends on the system's prior history. When attraction that once was high fades, the model predicts that dating-related behavior will continue until (and unless) attraction slips too low. When attraction that once was low increases, the model predicts that dating-related behavior will remain low unless attraction increases beyond the region of hysteresis.

Other candidates for examination in terms of catastrophes are easy to find. Here are a few more: Consider latitudes of acceptance and rejection in persuasion. When a persuasive message deviates from the recipient's opinion but remains within the opinion range that the recipient is willing to consider (the latitude of acceptance), it has a persuasive influence. If the message is too deviant (the latitude of rejection), it will be rejected out of hand. The fact that there's a break between these two latitudes suggests a discontinuity. But is there also a region of hysteresis? Would an initially acceptable message continue to be seen as such, even when it actually had gone outside that range? Would an initially rejected message continued to be taken as such, even when it had shifted to be within the acceptable range?

Another potential application is suggested by Martin and Tesser's (1996) analysis of rumination. They argued that rumination constitutes implicit problem solving, which occurs in the service of an eventual discrepancy reduction. This argument leads to the further idea that there is a balance between action and rumination, such that they tend to occur in different circumstances. Action dominates when there are no obstacles or when obstacles are manageable. Rumination dominates when the action is fully thwarted. Presumably there is a grey area where each might go on. Again, an interesting question is whether this grey area displays hysteresis. Is a person who's stuck in rumination more likely to remain there when the situation changes to where action is more effective? Is a person who's struggling to overcome obstacles likely to keep struggling past the point where it would make more sense to step back and think things over?

C. EFFORT VERSUS DISENGAGEMENT

What we think is another potentially important application of the catastrophe concept concerns the bifurcation between engagement in effort and giving up. Earlier we pointed to a set of theories that assume such a disjunction (Brehm & Self, 1989; Kukla, 1972; Wortman & Brehm, 1975). In all those models (as in ours), there is a point at which effort seems fruitless and the person stops trying. Earlier we simply emphasized that the models all assumed a discontinuity. Now we look at the discontinuity more closely and suggest that the phenomena addressed by these theories may embody a catastrophe.

Figure 15 shows a slightly relabeled cross section of a cusp catastrophe, similar to what was seen earlier in Figure 14. This figure displays a region of hysteresis in the engagement versus disengagement function. In that region, where task demands are close to people's perceived limits to perform, there should be greater variability in effort or engagement, because some people are on the top surface of the catastrophe and others

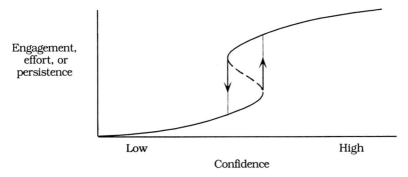

FIGURE 15 A catastrophe model of effort versus disengagement. *Note.* From *On the Self-Regulation of Behavior*, by C. S. Carver and M. F. Scheier, 1998, New York: Cambridge University Press; Copyright 1998 by Cambridge University Press. Reprinted with permission.

are on the bottom surface. Some people would be continuing to exert efforts, at the same point where others would be exhibiting a giving-up response.

Recall that the catastrophe figure also conveys the sense that the history of the behavior matters. A person who enters the region of hysteresis from the direction of high confidence (who starts out confident but confronts many cues indicating otherwise) will continue to display efforts and engagement, even as the situational cues imply less and less basis for confidence. A person who enters that region from the direction of low confidence (who starts out doubtful but confronts cues indicating otherwise) will continue to display little effort, even as the situational cues imply more and more basis for confidence.

This model helps indicate why it can be so difficult to get someone with strong and chronic doubts about success in some domain of behavior to exert real effort and engagement in that domain. It also suggests why a confident person is so rarely put off by encountering difficulties in the domain where the confidence lies. To put it in terms of broader views about life in general, it helps to show why optimists tend to stay optimistic and pessimists tend to stay pessimistic, even when the current circumstances of the two sorts of people are identical (i.e., in the region of hysteresis).

Figure 16 shows a slightly simplified version of the Wortman and Brehm (1975) model (oriented horizontally to be on a scale that's directionally similar to that of Figure 15) and the Brehm and Self (1989) model (which, for this discussion, is the same as the Kukla, 1972, model).[2] These functions both show bifurcations between two classes of response. As drawn by their authors, neither has a region of hysteresis. Is that feature—missing from the diagrams—present in the phenomena addressed by the theories? We think a plausible case can be made that it is.

We suspect that a person who enters the situation portrayed in the Wortman–Brehm model with a belief of no control will continue to show little effort even when control begins to emerge. We suspect that a person struggling with a threat to control will continue to struggle even when control is lost. These effects of behavioral history would create a hysteresis, rendering this function very similar to the catastrophe.

The Brehm and Self model (Figure 16B) differs in a number of ways from Figure 16A and from Figure 15, but we think a case can be made that a region of hysteresis may exist here as well. The critical issue here may be

[2] It should be noted that the x axes of these various models do not represent quite the same variables, although the variables are related to one another. Perceived task difficulty influences confidence (Brehm & Self, 1989), as does perceived facility at the task (Kukla, 1972) and extent of threat to control (Wortman & Brehm, 1975). Although none of these variables is a *complete* determinant of confidence, they all are related to confidence closely enough to warrant our treating them as equivalent for the purposes of this exercise.

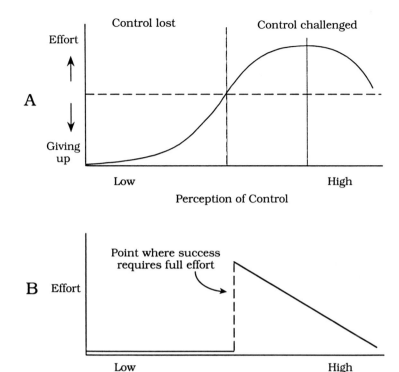

FIGURE 16 Slightly modified depictions of (A) Wortman and Brehm's (1975) model of helplessness and reactance and (B) Brehm and Self's (1989) model of effort (which for this purpose is essentially the same as Kukla's 1972 model). *Note.* From *On the Self-Regulation of Behavior,* by C. S. Carver and M. F. Scheier, 1998, New York: Cambridge University Press; Copyright 1998 by Cambridge University Press. Reprinted with permission.

the ambiguity of the situation the person is facing. The figure assumes the person knows the point at which maximum effort is required, but this is unlikely to always be true. A person who begins with a task that's far too hard to perform won't engage in serious effort. But if the task changes so that success is now possible, how will the person know it, if only minimal effort is being exerted? Not knowing, why would the person try harder? A person who begins with a task that's challenging but doable will exert strong effort. But how will this person know if the task demands change so that they exceed his or her maximum effort, unless he or she continues to try? In short, it appears there is good potential here for a region of hysteresis.

Two further points about these figures. First, no one has studied the processes of effort and disengagement in a truly parametric manner that would allow plotting the full range of the figures. Most work on the

Wortman–Brehm (1975) model has chosen two points in the range of threat to control. Brehm, Wright, and co-workers have typically chosen three points on the range of task difficulty: easy, demanding-but-possible, and too hard to bother with. The exact shape of the function represented by these figures still is not well known.

Second, keep in mind that the catastrophe cross section (Figure 15) is the picture that emerges under catastrophe theory *only once a clear region of hysteresis has begun to develop*. Farther back, the catastrophe model is more of a step function. An implication is that it's important to engage the control variable that's responsible for bringing out the bifurcation in the catastrophe surface (that is, axis z in Figure 13). It may be that in research bearing on this set of issues, this variable is only at a low to moderate level. If so, the hysteresis would be less observable, even if the research procedures were otherwise suitable to observe it.

What *is* the control variable that induces the bifurcation? We think that in the motivational models under discussion—and perhaps much more broadly—the control parameter is *importance*. Tesser (1980) pointed to social pressure as a control variable. Social pressure is one force that can make a behavior or a decision important, but we think social pressure is only one of a broader set of pressures. Importance arises from several sources, but there is a common thread among events seen as important: They demand mental resources. We suspect that almost any strong pressure that demands resources (time pressure, self-imposed pressure) will induce similar bifurcating effects.

VII. CONCLUDING COMMENT

In this chapter we sketched a set of ideas that we think are important in conceptualizing human self-regulation. We believe that behavior is goal directed and feedback controlled, and that the goals underlying behavior form a hierarchy of abstractness. We believe that the experience of affect (and of confidence versus doubt) also arises from a process of feedback control, but a feedback process that takes into account more explicitly temporal constraints. We believe that confidence and doubt yield patterns of persistence versus giving up and that these two responses to adversity form a dichotomy in behavior. These ideas have been part of our work for some time.

We have also recently begun to consider some newer ideas, which we addressed in the latter parts of the chapter. In those sections we described ideas from dynamic systems theory and catastrophe theory, and suggested that they represent useful tools for the analysis and construal of behavior. Our view is that they supplement rather than replace the tools now in use (though not everyone will agree on this point). We see many ways in which

those ideas mesh with the ideas presented earlier, although space constraints limited us to discussing only a few of them.

In thinking about the structure of self-regulation, we have drawn on
ideas from disparate sources. At the same time, however, we've tried to
continue to follow the thread of the logical model from which we started.
The result is an aggregation of principles that we think have a good deal to
say about how behavioral self-regulation takes place. The conceptual
model surely is not complete, and many avenues exist for further work. For
example, although a few studies have provided evidence bearing on the
affect portion of the model, the implications of those ideas thus far have
been explored only superficially.

Another area of thought that certainly will receive further attention
over the next few years comprises the ideas of dynamic systems and
catastrophe theory. Many people are becoming intrigued by dynamic
systems thinking and are exploring the implications of these ideas in
several ways. Some people believe these conceptual tools, and the new
angles they give us on the human experience, will force us to change not
just the ways we conceptualize behavior, but also the ways we study
behavior. Whether this will be true or not remains to be seen. The answer
will be played out in the methods that people find to explore the ideas.

There are also some additional ideas—not discussed here—that we
think are likely to receive further attention in the years to come. Some of
these ideas come from connectionist models of thought, which are starting
to have an influence on personality and social psychology (Anderson, 1995;
Read, Vanman, & Miller, 1997; Sloman, 1996; Smith, 1996; Smolensky,
1988; Thagard, 1989). Other ideas of potentially great value come from the
literature of robotics (Beer, 1995; Brooks & Stein, 1994; Maes, 1994).
These literatures push thinking in a variety of directions beyond the ideas
that were discussed in this chapter, injecting new ideas and fresh viewpoints (see Carver & Scheier, 1998, Chapter 17).

Finally, we believe that the ideas discussed in this chapter also have
interesting implications for conceptualizing both problems in self-regulation and therapeutic behavior change (see Carver & Scheier, 1998).
Although there was not space to consider such issues here in any detail,
there are several ways in which the concepts addressed here bear on
problems. For example, we suspect that many of the problems in people's
lives are, at their core, problems of disengagement versus engagement and
the failure to disengage adaptively. As another example, it may be useful
to conceptualize problems as being less-than-optimal adaptations in a
multidimensional phase space, which require some jostling to bounce the
person to a new attractor (Hayes & Strauss, 1998).

These are just some of the ways in which we think the ideas under
discussion are likely to be explored in the immediate future. Doubtlessly
there will be others. The next generation of attempts to understand the

self-regulation of human behavior can be expected to create an ever-evolving landscape of ideas, as has the current generation. There are sure to be some surprises, as well. We look forward to seeing them.

ACKNOWLEDGMENT

This chapter was adapted from more extensive discussions elsewhere (Carver & Scheier, 1998, 1999). Preparation of this chapter was facilitated by NCI grants CA64710 and CA64711.

REFERENCES

Allen, J. J., Iacono, W. G., Depue, R. A., & Arbisi, X. (1993). Regional EEG asymmetries in bipolar affective disorder before and after phototherapy. *Biological Psychiatry, 33*, 642–646.

Anderson, J. A. (1995). *An introduction to neural networks*. Cambridge, MA: MIT Press.

Anderson, J. R. (1990). *The adaptive character of thought*. Hillsdale, NJ: Erlbaum.

Austin, J. T., & Vancouver, J. B. (1996). Goal constructs in psychology: Structure, process, and content. *Psychological Bulletin, 120*, 338–375.

Baumeister, R. F. (1989). The problem of life's meaning. In D. M. Buss & N. Cantor (Eds.), *Personality psychology: Recent trends and emerging directions* (pp. 138–148). New York: Springer-Verlag.

Beer, R. D. (1995). A dynamical systems perspective on agent–environment interaction. *Artificial Intelligence, 72*, 173–215.

Brehm, J. W., & Self, E. A. (1989). The intensity of motivation. *Annual Review of Psychology, 40*, 109–131.

Brooks, R. A., & Stein, L. A. (1994). Building brains for bodies. *Autonomous Robots, 1*, 7–25.

Brown, C. (1995). *Chaos and catastrophe theories: Vol. 107. Quantitative applications in the social sciences*. Thousand Oaks, CA: Sage.

Brunstein, J. C. (1993). Personal goals and subjective well-being: A longitudinal study. *Journal of Personality and Social Psychology, 65*, 1061–1070.

Cacioppo, J. T., & Petty, R. E. (1980). The effects of orienting task on differential hemispheric EEG activation. *Neuropsychologia, 18*, 675–683.

Cantor, N., & Kihlstrom, J. F. (1987). *Personality and social intelligence*. Englewood Cliffs, NJ: Prentice-Hall.

Carver, C. S. (1979). A cybernetic model of self-attention processes. *Journal of Personality and Social Psychology, 37*, 1251–1281.

Carver, C. S., & Humphries, C. (1981). Havana daydreaming: A study of self-consciousness and the negative reference group among Cuban Americans. *Journal of Personality and Social Psychology, 40*, 545–552.

Carver, C. S., Peterson, L. M., Follansbee, D. J., & Scheier, M. F. (1983). Effects of self-directed attention on performance and persistence among persons high and low in test anxiety. *Cognitive Therapy and Research, 7*, 333–354.

Carver, C. S., & Scheier, M. F. (1981). *Attention and self-regulation: A control-theory approach to human behavior*. New York: Springer-Verlag.

Carver, C. S., & Scheier, M. F. (1982). Outcome expectancy, locus of attributions for expectancy, and self-directed attention as determinants of evaluations and performance. *Journal of Experimental Social Psychology, 18*, 184–200.

Carver, C. S., & Scheier, M. F. (1990). Origins and functions of positive and negative affect: A control-process view. *Psychological Review, 97*, 19–35.

Carver, C. S., & Scheier, M. F. (1998). *On the self-regulation of behavior*. New York: Cambridge University Press.

Carver, C. S., & Scheier, M. F. (1999). Themes and issues in the self-regulation of behavior. In R. S. Wyer, Jr. (Ed.), *Advances in social cognition*. Mahwah, NJ: Erlbaum.

Clark, L. A., Watson, D., & Mineka, S. (1994). Temperament, personality, and the mood and anxiety disorders. *Journal of Abnormal Psychology, 103,* 103–116.

Cloninger, C. R. (1987). A systematic method for clinical description and classification of personality variants. *Archives of General Psychiatry, 44,* 573–588.

Cloninger, C. R. (1988). A unified biosocial theory of personality and its role in the development of anxiety states: A reply to commentaries. *Psychiatric Developments, 2,* 83–120.

Davidson, R. J. (1992a). Anterior cerebral asymmetry and the nature of emotion. *Brain and Cognition, 20,* 125–151.

Davidson, R. J. (1992b). Prolegomenon to the structure of emotion: Gleanings from neuropsychology. *Cognition and Emotion, 6,* 245–268.

Davidson, R. J., Ekman, P., Saron, C. D., Senulis, J. A., & Friesen, W. V. (1990). Approach–withdrawal and cerebral asymmetry: Emotional expression and brain physiology I. *Journal of Personality and Social Psychology, 58,* 330–341.

Depue, R. A., & Iacono, W. G. (1989). Neurobehavioral aspects of affective disorders. *Annual Review of Psychology, 40,* 457–492.

Depue, R. A., Krauss, S. P., & Spoont, M. R. (1987). A two-dimensional threshold model of seasonal bipolar affective disorder. In D. Magnusson & A. Öhman (Eds.), *Psychopathology: An interactional perspective* (pp. 95–123). Orlando, FL: Academic Press.

Elliott, E. S., & Dweck, C. S. (1988). Goals: An approach to motivation and achievement. *Journal of Personality and Social Psychology, 54,* 5–12.

Emmons, R. A. (1986). Personal strivings: An approach to personality and subjective well being. *Journal of Personality and Social Psychology, 51,* 1058–1068.

Epstein, S. (1979). The stability of behavior: I. On predicting most of the people much of the time. *Journal of Personality and Social Psychology, 37,* 1097–1126.

Fowles, D. C. (1980). The three arousal model: Implications of Gray's two-factor learning theory for heart rate, electrodermal activity, and psychopathy. *Psychophysiology, 17,* 87–104.

Fox, N. A., & Davidson, R. J. (1988). Patterns of brain electrical activity during facial signs of emotion in 10-month old infants. *Developmental Psychology, 24,* 230–236.

Frijda, N. H. (1986). *The emotions*. Cambridge, UK: Cambridge University Press.

Frijda, N. H. (1988). The laws of emotion. *American Psychologist, 43,* 349–358.

Gleick, J. (1987). *Chaos: Making a new science*. New York: Viking Penguin.

Gobet, F., & Simon, H. A. (1996). The roles of recognition processes and look-ahead search in time-constrained expert problem solving: Evidence from grand-master-level chess. *Psychological Science, 7,* 52–55.

Goldin-Meadow, S., & Alibali, M. W. (1995). Mechanisms of transition: Learning with a helping hand. In D. Medin (Ed.), *The psychology of learning and motivation* (Vol. 33, pp. 115–157). San Diego, CA: Academic Press.

Gray, J. A. (1982). *The neuropsychology of anxiety: An enquiry into the functions of the septohippocampal system*. New York: Oxford University Press.

Gray, J. A. (1987a). Perspectives on anxiety and impulsivity: A commentary. *Journal of Research in Personality, 21,* 493–509.

Gray, J. A. (1987b). *The psychology of fear and stress*. Cambridge, UK: Cambridge University Press.

Gray, J. A. (1990). Brain systems that mediate both emotion and cognition. *Cognition and Emotion, 4,* 269–288.

Greenwald, A. G. (1980). The totalitarian ego: Fabrication and revision of personal history. *American Psychologist, 35*, 603–618.

Hayes, A. M., & Strauss, J. L. (1998). Dynamic systems theory as a paradigm for the study of change in psychotherapy: An application to cognitive therapy for depression. *Journal of Consulting and Clinical Psychology, 66*, 939–947.

Hayes-Roth, B., & Hayes-Roth, F. (1979). A cognitive model of planning. *Cognitive Science, 3*, 275–310.

Henriques, J. B., & Davidson, R. J. (1991). Left frontal hypoactivation in depression. *Journal of Abnormal Psychology, 100*, 535–545.

Higgins, E. T. (1987). Self-discrepancy: A theory relating self and affect. *Psychological Review, 94*, 319–340.

Higgins, E. T. (1996). Ideals, oughts, and regulatory focus: Affect and motivation from distinct pains and pleasures. In P. M. Gollwitzer & J. A. Bargh (Eds.), *The psychology of action: Linking cognition and motivation to behavior* (pp. 91–114). New York: Guilford.

Higgins, E. T., Bond, R., Klein, R., & Strauman, T. J. (1986). Self-discrepancies and emotional vulnerability: How magnitude, accessibility and type of discrepancy influence affect. *Journal of Personality and Social Psychology, 41*, 1–15.

Higgins, E. T., & Tykocinski, O. (1992). Self-discrepancies and biographical memory: Personality and cognition at the level of psychological situation. *Personality and Social Psychology Bulletin, 18*, 527–535.

Hsee, C. K., & Abelson, R. P. (1991). Velocity relation: Satisfaction as a function of the first derivative of outcome over time. *Journal of Personality and Social Psychology, 60*, 341–347.

Ingram, R. E. (1990). Self-focused attention in clinical disorder: Review and a conceptual model. *Psychological Bulletin, 107*, 156–176.

Kelly, G. A. (1955). *The psychology of personal constructs*. New York: W. W. Norton.

Kelso, J. A. S. (1995). *Dynamic patterns: The self-organization of brain and behavior*. Cambridge, MA: MIT Press.

Kirschenbaum, D. S. (1985). Proximity and specificity of planning: A position paper. *Cognitive Therapy and Research, 9*, 489–506.

Klinger, E. (1975). Consequences of commitment to and disengagement from incentives. *Psychological Review, 82*, 1–25.

Klinger, E. (1977). *Meaning and void: Inner experience and the incentives in people's lives*. Minneapolis: University of Minnesota Press.

Kukla, A. (1972). Foundations of an attributional theory of performance. *Psychological Review, 79*, 454–470.

Lang, P. J., Bradley, M. M., & Cuthbert, B. N. (1992). A motivational analysis of emotion: Reflex–cortex connections. *Psychological Science, 3*, 44–49.

Lawrence, J. W., Carver, C. S., & Scheier, M. F. (1999). Velocity and affect in immediate personal experience. Unpublished manuscript.

Lazarus, R. S. (1966). *Psychological stress and the coping process*. New York: McGraw-Hill.

Lazarus, R. S. (1991). *Emotion and adaptation*. NewYork: Oxford University Press.

Little, B. R. (1983). Personal projects: A rationale and methods for investigation. *Environment and Behavior, 15*, 273–309.

Lorenz, E. N. (1963). Deterministic nonperiodic flow. *Journal of Atmospheric Science, 20*, 130–141.

Maes, P. (1994). Modeling adaptive autonomous agents. *Artificial Life, 1*, 135–162.

Markus, H., & Nurius, P. (1986). Possible selves. *American Psychologist, 41*, 954–969.

Martin, L. L., & Tesser, A. (1996). Some ruminative thoughts. In R. S. Wyer, Jr. (Ed.), *Advances in social cognition* (Vol. 9, p. 1–47). Mahwah, NJ: Erlbaum.

McIntosh, W. D., & Martin, L. L. (1992). The cybernetics of happiness: The relation of goal attainment, rumination, and affect. In M. S. Clark (Ed.), *Review of personality and social psychology: Volume 14. Emotion and social behavior* (pp. 222–246). Newbury Park, CA: Sage.

Melton, R. J. (1995). The role of positive affect in syllogism performance. *Personality and Social Psychology Bulletin*, *21*, 788–794.

Millar, K. U., Tesser, A., & Millar, M. G. (1988). The effects of a threatening life event on behavior sequences and intrusive thought: A self-disruption explanation. *Cognitive Therapy and Research*, *12*, 441–458.

Miller, G. A., Galanter, E., & Pribram, K. H. (1960). *Plans and the structure of behavior*. New York: Holt, Rinehart, & Winston.

Miller, L. C., & Read, S. J. (1987). Why am I telling you this? Self-disclosure in a goal-based model of personality. In V. J. Derlega & J. Berg (Eds.), *Self-disclosure: Theory, research, and therapy* (pp. 35–58). New York: Plenum.

Myers, D. G., & Diener, E. (1995). Who is happy? *Psychological Science*, *6*, 10–19.

Nowak, A., & Lewenstein, M. (1994). Dynamical systems: A tool for social psychology. In R. R. Vallacher & A. Nowak (Eds.), *Dynamical systems in social psychology* (pp. 17–53). San Diego, CA: Academic Press.

Nowak, A., & Vallacher, R. R. (1998). *Dynamical social psychology*. New York: Guilford.

Orbuch, T. L. (Ed.). (1992). *Close relationship loss: Theoretical approaches*. New York: Springer-Verlag.

Ortony, A., Clore, G. L., & Collins, A. (1988). *The cognitive structure of emotions*. New York: Cambridge University Press.

Pervin, L. A. (Ed.). (1989). *Goal concepts in personality and social psychology*. Hillsdale, NJ: Erlbaum.

Powers, W. T. (1973). *Behavior: The control of perception*. Chicago: Aldine.

Pyszczynski, T., Greenberg, J., Hamilton, J., & Nix, G. (1991). On the relationship between self-focused attention and psychological disorder: A critical reappraisal. *Psychological Bulletin*, *110*, 538–543.

Read, S. J., Druian, P. R., & Miller, L. C. (1989). The role of causal sequence in the meaning of action. *British Journal of Social Psychology*, *28*, 341–351.

Read, S. J., Vanman, E. J., & Miller, L. C. (1997). Connectionism, parallel constraint satisfaction processes, and Gestalt principles: (Re)introducing cognitive dynamics to social psychology. *Review of Personality and Social Psychology*, *1*, 26–53.

Roseman, I. J. (1984). Cognitive determinants of emotions: A structural theory. In P. Shaver (Ed.), *Review of personality and social psychology* (Vol. 5, pp. 136). Beverly Hills, CA: Sage.

Ruble, D. N. (1994). A phase model of transitions: Cognitive and motivational consequences. In M. Zanna (Ed.), *Advances in experimental social psychology* (Vol. 26, pp. 163–214). San Diego, CA: Academic Press.

Sarason, I. G. (1975). Anxiety and self-preoccupation. In I. G. Sarason & C. D. Spielberger (Eds.), *Stress and anxiety* (Vol. 2, pp. 27–44). Washington, DC: Hemisphere.

Saunders, P. T. (1980). *An introduction to catastrophe theory*. Cambridge, UK: Cambridge University Press.

Scheier, M. F., & Carver, C. S. (1983). Self-directed attention and the comparison of self with standards. *Journal of Experimental Social Psychology*, *19*, 205–222.

Scherer, K. R., & Ekman, P. (Eds.). (1984). *Approaches to emotion*. Hillsdale, NJ: Erlbaum.

Siegler, R. S., & Jenkins, E. A. (1989). *How children discover new strategies*. Hillsdale, NJ: Erlbaum.

Sloman, S. A. (1996). The empirical case for two forms of reasoning. *Psychological Bulletin*, *119*, 3–22.

Smith, E. R. (1996). What do connectionism and social psychology offer each other? *Journal of Personality and Social Psychology*, *70*, 893–912.

Smolensky, P. (1988). On the proper treatment of connectionism. *Behavioral and Brain Sciences*, *11*, 1–23.

Sobotka, S. S., Davidson, R. J., & Senulis, J. A. (1992). Anterior brain electrical asymmetries in response to reward and punishment. *Electroencephalography and Clinical Neurophysiology*, *83*, 236–247.

Stewart, I. N., & Peregoy, P. L. (1983). Catastrophe theory modeling in psychology. *Psychological Bulletin, 94,* 336–362.

Stroebe, M. S., Stroebe, W., & Hansson, R. O. (Eds.). (1993). *Handbook of bereavement: Theory, research, and intervention.* Cambridge, UK: Cambridge University Press.

Taylor, S. E., & Pham, L. B. (1996). Mental stimulation, motivation, and action. In P. M. Gollwitzer & J. A. Bargh (Eds.), *The psychology of action: Linking cognition and motivation to behavior* (pp. 219–235). New York: Guilford.

Tesser, A. (1980). When individual dispositions and social pressure conflict: A catastrophe. *Human Relations, 33,* 393–407.

Thagard, P. (1989). Explanatory coherence. *Behavioral and Brain Sciences, 12,* 435–467.

Thelen, E. (1992). Development as a dynamic system. *Current Directions in Psychological Science, 1,* 189–193.

Thelen, E. (1995). Motor development: A new synthesis. *American Psychologist, 50,* 79–95.

Thelen, E., & Smith, L. B. (1994). *A dynamic systems approach to the development of cognition and action.* Cambridge, MA: MIT Press.

Tomarken, A. J., Davidson, R. J., Wheeler, R. E., & Doss, R. C. (1992). Individual differences in anterior brain asymmetry and fundamental dimensions of emotion. *Journal of Personality and Social Psychology, 62,* 676–687.

Vallacher, R. R., & Nowak, A. (Eds.). (1994). *Dynamical systems in social psychology.* San Diego, CA: Academic Press.

Vallacher, R. R., & Nowak, A. (1997). The emergence of dynamical social psychology. *Psychological Inquiry, 8,* 73–99.

Vallacher, R. R., & Wegner, D. M. (1985). *A theory of action identification.* Hillsdale, NJ: Erlbaum.

van der Maas, H. L. J., & Molenaar, P. C. M. (1992). Stagewise cognitive development: An application of catastrophe theory. *Psychological Review, 99,* 395–417.

Waldrop, M. (1992). *Complexity: The emerging science at the edge of order and chaos.* New York: Simon & Schuster.

Weiss, R. S. (1988). Loss and recovery. *Journal of Social Issues, 44,* 37–52.

Wills, T. A. (1981). Downward comparison principles in social psychology. *Psychological Bulletin, 90,* 245–271.

Wine, J. D. (1971). Test anxiety and direction of attention. *Psychological Bulletin, 76,* 92–104.

Wine, J. D. (1980). Cognitive-attentional theory of test anxiety. In I. G. Sarason (Ed.), *Test anxiety: Theory, research, and application* (pp. 349–378). Hillsdale, NJ: Erlbaum.

Wong, P. T. P., & Weiner, B. (1981). When people ask "why" questions, and the heuristics of attributional search. *Journal of Personality and Social Psychology, 40,* 650–663.

Wood, J. V. (1989). Theory and research concerning social comparisons of personal attributes. *Psychological Bulletin, 106,* 231–248.

Woodcock, A., & Davis, M. (1978). *Catastrophe theory.* New York: E. P. Dutton.

Wortman, C. B., & Brehm, J. W. (1975). Responses to uncontrollable outcomes: An integration of reactance theory and the learned helplessness model. In L. Berkowitz (Ed.), *Advances in experimental social psychology* (Vol. 8, pp. 277–336). New York: Academic Press.

Wright, R. A., & Brehm, J. W. (1989). Energization and goal attractiveness. In L. A. Pervin (Ed.), *Goal concepts in personality and social psychology* (pp. 169–210). Hillsdale, NJ: Erlbaum.

Zeeman, E. C. (1977). *Catastrophe theory: Selected papers 1972–1977.* Reading, MA: Benjamin.

4

ASPECTS OF GOAL

NETWORKS

IMPLICATIONS FOR

SELF-REGULATION

JAMES Y. SHAH AND ARIE W. KRUGLANSKI

University of Maryland, College Park, Maryland

Psychologists have long recognized the importance of goals in understanding how our desires affect our specific actions. In defining a "desirable future state of affairs," goals serve as concrete points of reference for directing our actions in fulfillment of our needs. Everyday self-regulation however, involves the pursuit of many different goals. Indeed, our lives are frequently "juggling acts" of important but disparate everyday concerns such as getting enough sleep, teaching, and writing this chapter. Complicating self-regulatory matters further, psychologists have long appreciated that just as we have many different goals, we usually have more than one road to these psychological destinations (Heider, 1958; McDougal, 1923). For instance, many of us may have the intention of "staying healthy," but have very different ways of pursuing this goal. On some days we may choose to play sports, but occasionally we may opt to work out or to run. Certainly the manner in which this goal is pursued can vary across different individuals and different situations, but whatever one's particular preferences, we commonly are faced with a choice among a number of different activities, all of which are means to attain our health goal.

Clearly, goals can become associated with other goals and with a wide range of specific behaviors designed to bring about their attainment. Moreover, the number and strength of these associations can vary as a function of the specific goal or individual involved.

Copyright © 2000 by Academic Press.
All rights of reproduction in any form reserved.

The notion that goals relate to each other and to a wide range of substitutable behaviors gives rise to a number of important self-regulatory issues such as (1) how these associations affect our commitment to any given goal, (2) how a specific attainment behavior, or means, is chosen among those associated with a specific goal, (3) how this behavior is experienced with respect to the goal, and finally (4) how it will be replaced with another behavior if it proves ineffectual for attaining the goal.

The purpose of this chapter, then, is to address these important self-regulatory issues by considering the basic ways in which goals and means can differ in their associations with each other. To illustrate these differences, we adopt a connectionist perspective by assuming that an individual's goals and means can be viewed as a network of cognitive associations that vary in complexity. We first describe *how* these goal networks may differ. That is, we examine the fundamental characteristics of goal networks. In doing so, we show how consideration of these structural properties differs from other current perspectives on goals, and may help shed additional light on the important self-regulatory challenges mentioned above. Finally, we consider *why* goal networks differ. We consider how individual differences in motivational orientation, goal content, and regulatory experience may influence the associations between goals and means.

I. A STRUCTURAL ANALYSIS OF GOAL NETWORKS

Goals are knowledge structures (Kruglanski, 1996) and, as such, should follow similar principles of acquisition, activation, change, and organization that have been articulated in reference to all knowledge structures regardless of content (e.g., Higgins, 1996). Like other knowledge structures, goals can vary in the number and strength of their connection to other knowledge structures. However, because goals represent a specific type of knowledge structure, one that defines a future positive state, they should come to be associated particularly with those constructs that facilitate their attainment (i.e., means).

For this reason, goals are commonly thought to be organized hierarchically, with relatively few abstract goals served by a larger number of concrete means, or subgoals (Miller, Galanter, & Pribram, 1960; Powers, 1973, 1989). These means are themselves served by lower order means, and this pattern of associations continues downward to levels below conscious control.

With this in mind, consider the hypothetical goal network depicted in Figure 1 in which goal 2, goal 3, and goal 4 are served by more concrete means. Activation of any goal is assumed to spread *downward* to lower

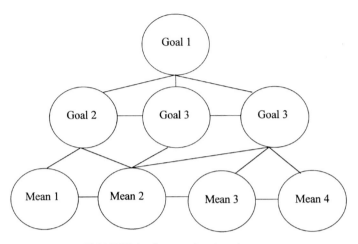

FIGURE 1   System of goals and means.

order means, defined as activities whose completion brings about goal attainment. The strength of the association between a given goal and means is defined as the likelihood that activation of the given goal will result in the use of the given means. It is assumed that the more likely the means is to lead to goal attainment, the stronger is the association created between the goal and the means.

We (Shah & Kruglanski, 1999b) tested this assumption in a recent study in which a computer program asked participants to describe four different attributes that they desired to possess. We regarded these attributes as goals to which our participants aspired. The participants were also asked to list one activity they could perform to attain each of the attributes. We regarded these as means to those particular goals. After completing the initial procedure, the computer prompted the participants to list all the activities they could think of that would help them possess each attribute-goal. Finally, participants completed a lexical decision procedure in which they were asked to determine whether or not a target word was an attribute or activity. Before making each determination, participants first saw a prime word for 3 seconds. The four attributes listed by the participant and the first attainment means listed for each attribute were randomly included in the presented set of prime and target words. The link between attribute and means could be assessed, then, by examining reaction times when the attribute was the prime for the means or the means was the prime for the attribute (see Figure 2). These times were found to be significantly quicker than reaction times when participants' attributes

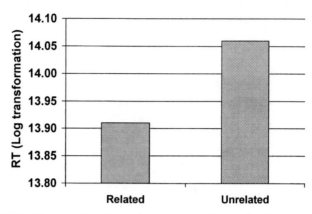

FIGURE 2   Reaction time when primes are related or unrelated goals and means.

primed means unrelated to those attributes or participants' means primed
their unrelated attributes. This finding is consistent with the notion that
goals and means are cognitively associated with each other.

A. EQUIFINALITY AND THE GOALS–MEANS ASSOCIATION

As mentioned earlier and is evident in Figure 1, goals have the property
of equifinality: that is, they typically can be attained through a number of
different actions. In this respect, however, all goals are not created equal.
Some (e.g., pleasing one's parents) may be attained readily by a wide
variety of actions (e.g., behaving politely, doing well in school, excelling in
athletics), whereas others (e.g., demonstrating intelligence) may be accomplished only through one class of behaviors (e.g., getting high grades in
school). Figure 3 shows how differences in equifinality may be represented
graphically.

Goals may vary not only in the number of different ways they can be
attained, but in how strongly they invoke each particular means (i.e., the
strength of their association with each available means). Yet, if one
assumes that each available means is sufficient to attain the superordinate
goal, the strength of the association between a goal and a means should
decrease as more alternative means become available, holding other
determinants of this association strength constant. We refer to this phenomenon as "means disassociation" because it suggests that a goal's
association with a single means is weakened by the presence of other
available means. Indeed, in the study described earlier, the attribute–means
link also was found to be significantly negatively related to the average
number of means listed for possessing each attribute. So the more subsequent attainment means listed for each attribute, the weaker the associa-

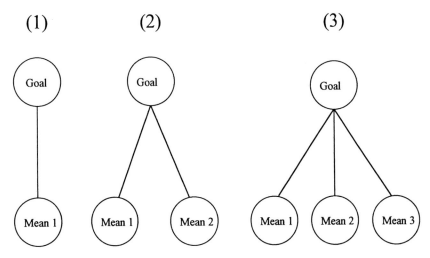

FIGURE 3   Differences in equifinality.

tion between the attribute and the first means listed ($F(1,41) = 5.2$, $p < .05$).

B. MULTIFINALITY AND THE MEANS–GOALS ASSOCIATION

Just as goals can have more than one means of attainment, any one means may serve more than one goal. We refer to this property as *multifinality*. Like equifinality, this property can vary as a function of motivational orientation, goal content, and one's past experiences with specific goals. The simple act of walking, for instance, can be viewed as a means of transportation in one context and a means of exercising in another. Alternatively, consider the significant psychological phenomenon of intergroup bias. Although many researchers have seen it as a means for attaining self-esteem, Shah, Kruglanski, and Thompson (1998) have found that it also may serve as a means for attaining cognitive closure: A favorable appreciation of one's reference group upholds the social reality to which it subscribes, thus promoting the sense of cognitive closure embodied in such reality. Figure 4 graphically illustrates how means may differ in their association with different goals.

Just as with the association of a single goal with several means, the number of associations between a single means and several goals should be negatively related to the strength of any single goal–means association. So, if one strongly associates the act of jogging with the goal of getting in shape, one may be less likely to consider it as a means for getting to school. This notion of "goal dissociation" refers to the weakening of association between an activity and a given goal due to its association with

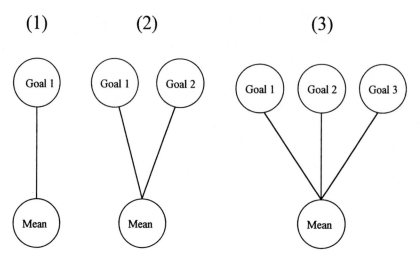

FIGURE 4   Differences in mean multifinality.

other goals. To take an example from the intrinsic motivation literature, consider the well-studied phenomenon that offering a reward for engaging in an interesting activity can undermine subsequent motivation when the reward is removed (for reviews, see Deci, 1975; Deci & Ryan, 1985; Lepper, Greene, & Nisbett, 1973). From our structural perspective, linking an activity with a tangible reward may create an association between the activity and an extrinsic goal (e.g., a tangible reward) to the detriment of any prior association of the activity to other intrinsic goals, such as mastery or competence. When the tangible reward is ultimately withdrawn, the tendency to engage in the activity is reduced because the activity's original association with a given goal has been diminished. The work of Higgins, Lee, Kwon, and Trope (1995) suggests that this goal dissociation is not limited to situations involving the association of an activity with a new extrinsic goal. Goal dissociation may, in fact, occur even when both goals are intrinsic, suggesting that this phenomenon may have more to do with the strength of the association between goals and means as such rather than with differences in specific goal contents (see also Higgins & Trope, 1990).

C. "LATERAL" ASSOCIATIONS WITHIN GOAL NETWORKS

Finally, different goals can differ in their "lateral" associations with other goals and different means can differ in their lateral associations with other means. To illustrate the latter, think of the decision one may make about how to get home. Pondering whether to walk might lead (by dint of prior association) to thoughts of jogging, but not so readily lead one to consider taking a cab, although all three are seen as means to travel. Of course means may relate to each other indirectly via their common goal. With this in mind, one reason that means may differ in their relationship to each other is that they differ in the number of different goals they commonly serve. For instance, when trying to get home, walking and jogging may be related more directly to each other because they both additionally serve as means of "getting some fresh air."

As knowledge structures, however, means can differ also in their degree of direct association. Figure 5 illustrates this point graphically.

As discussed subsequently, such a direct or "lateral" degree of association between means may play a significant role in determining means substitution should one's original means fail to attain its purpose.

Of course goals also can differ in their direct associations with other goals. To the degree that this association is based on the fact that attainment of either goal would facilitate attainment of the other, this association should increase overall goal progress. However, as will be discussed, goals may be associated with each other for other reasons as well. As knowledge structures, they may be associated because they are semantically similar or because their activations commonly co-occur. The very different goals of relaxing and studying, for instance, may come to be associated if one commonly studies in the bedroom, thereby creating a situation in which the same situational cue that activates a goal to study also may activate a goal to rest. As we also discuss subsequently, the

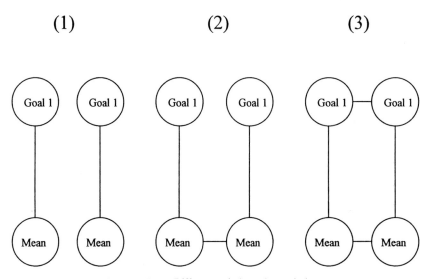

FIGURE 5   Differences in lateral associations.

degree of association between goals can affect one's singular commitment to either goal by creating a situation of goal conflict.

In summary, then, we have suggested that goal networks differ (1) in the degree to which goals are directly associated with other goals and (2) with various attainment means. We have also proposed that these networks differ (3) in the degree to which means are directly associated with other means and (4) are associated with various goals. Having provided an initial sketch of some structural properties of goal networks and how they differ from other goal qualities, we now address their implications for a number of significant regulatory issues.

II. SELF-REGULATORY CONSEQUENCES OF GOAL NETWORK STRUCTURE

A. GOAL COMMITMENT

Is the association of goals with means an important determinant of goal commitment? As the work of Gollwitzer and his colleagues has shown (e.g., Gollwitzer & Brandstatter, 1997), the accessibility of an attainment means is a crucial determinant of whether one follows through with goal attainment. Some question remains, however, about the added benefit of multiple attainment means. Roese (1994) showed that after failing on a task, considering additive counterfactuals (i.e., different things one *could* have tried) increased subsequent performance on the same task. This suggests that although the presence of different means for goal attainment may decrease the likelihood that any one means will be used consistently, it may, in fact, increase overall goal commitment by raising the overall perceived likelihood of goal attainment. To test this idea, we (Shah & Kruglanski, 1999b) asked participants to list four attributes they would like to possess. Half were then asked to list three means for attaining the first two attributes and one means for attaining the remaining two. The other half reversed this order, listing one means for attaining their first two attributes and three means for their remaining two. All participants also rated the likelihood that they would possess all four attributes. Those attributes for which three means were requested subsequently were rated as significantly easier to attain than those attributes for which only one means was requested (see Figure 6). Thus, it appears that the salience of multiple attainment means reduces the perceived difficulty of attainment or the risk of failure.

On the other hand, the degree to which goal activation activates other goals, rather than means, should be detrimental to goal commitment, especially if these goals are in conflict with each other. To test this idea, we had participants complete a computer program that asked them to

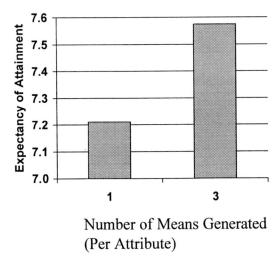

Number of Means Generated
(Per Attribute)

FIGURE 6   Number of means generated in positively related to perceived goal expectancy.

perform a lexical decision task by determining whether a presented letter string was a word or not after first seeing a prime word. Randomly distributed among the set of prime words and target words, participants were presented with common attribute-goals, that is, goals most persons in our culture may subscribe to (e.g., of being "educated," "caring," "strong," and "outgoing"), and attainment means for these attributes (e.g., "study," "volunteer," "exercise," and "socialize"). All possible combinations of means and attributes as primes and targets were presented.

After completing the word recognition task, participants rated on a 9-point scale ranging from "not at all" to "extremely" the degree to which they would ideally like to possess each of the presented attributes and the extent to which they thought it was their duty or obligation to possess them. These two ratings were combined to form one overall measure of attribute commitment (see Table 1). The goal–means association was calculated by summing the times it took a participant to complete the lexical decision task with regard to a given mean: that is, to decide whether it was or was not a word when the prime word was an attribute that, a priori, had been thought to be facilitated by this mean. The goal–non-means association was calculated by summing the times to identify a means as a word when the prime word was an attribute that, a priori, had been thought not to be facilitated by this activity. Similarly, the goal–goal association was calculated by summing the times to identify an attribute goal as word when the prime word was another attribute goal. A regression analysis of these variables indicated that overall goal commitment was

TABLE 1   Partial Correlations of Goal–Goal Association and Goal–Mean Association on Goal Commitment for Normative Goals and Personal Goals

Type of association	Goal commitment	
	Normative goals	Personal goals
Goal–goal	−.34*	−.37*
Goal–means	.44**	.34*
	($n = 47$)	($n = 49$)

*$p < .05$.
**$p < .01$.

significantly positively related to the strength of the goal–means association, but negatively related to the goal–goal connection, suggesting that the degree of association between goals hinders commitment to any individual goal. A second study tested this same idea using participants' own idiosyncratic goals and means, rather than common or normative goals and means as used in our previous study. In most other respects, however, the procedure was similar to the first study and a regression analysis of the same set of variables again indicated that overall goal commitment was positively related to the strength of the goal–means connection, but negatively related to the goal–goal connection.

Overall goal commitment, then, may depend not only on qualities of the goal itself, but also on the strength of its relationship to other goals and to other means. A strong association between goals often may bring about goal conflict, which is aversive to the individual and hence may lower commitment to all the goals involved. Of course, the amount of conflict may vary depending on the degree to which attaining one goal serves as a means for attaining the other (see Sheldon & Emmons, 1995; Sheldon & Kasser, 1995). To the degree that it does, the conflict may be attenuated and goal commitment actually may be enhanced.

B. CHOICE OF MEANS

Equifinality, that is, the association of several means with the same goal, poses the problem of means choice. Presumably, individuals strive to choose the best available means for attaining the goal. This formulation, however, begs the question of how "best" is defined. In fact, the number of criteria whereby a means could be assessed as "best" could be quite considerable. To give a few examples, a means could be regarded as best because it most easily comes to mind, because it is most likely to bring about goal attainment, because it requires the least amount of effort, because it promises the most immediate attainment, or because it promises the most enduring satisfaction. So when is each criterion applied? To answer this question, one must acknowledge that goals are rarely pursued in isolation. While phenomenally, an individual may be pursuing a single "focal" goal, the pursuit occurs within the context of fulfilling other activated goals that may or may not escape awareness and that represent a hidden or overt agenda the individual is also pursuing. Consider a situation in which the individual "chooses" between a simple and a complex message argument as two possible routes to persuasion. When the individual is fatigued, time pressed, or otherwise low on cognitive resources, he or she might opt for the simple heuristic over the complex argument, thus applying the "least effort" criterion. The simple heuristic in this case not only advances the focal goal of forming a judgment, but also advances the background goal of "conserving cognitive resources."

In a classic study by Nisbett and Wilson (1977), passersby at a department store chose among four different nightgowns of similar quality or four identical pairs of nylon stockings. A strong *position effect* was found such that the rightmost object in the array was heavily overchosen. Nisbett and Wilson (1977) suggested that participants carried into the judgment task the consumers' habit of "shopping around," holding off on choice of *early-seen garments on the left* in favor of *later-seen garments on the right*. In other words, participants may have had two goals in this situation: (1) making a reasonable choice (this is a "focal" goal that would have been satisfied by any of the four objects in the array) and (2) reaching quick closure *after* the full array had been examined (this constituted a "background" goal). Both goals are satisfied by the rightmost object in the array, which indeed ends up being overchosen by a large margin. Interestingly, participants reported little, if any, awareness of this background goal, implying that background goals need not be salient to affect choice of means.

More generally, then, the means chosen is often that which *maximizes* attainment within the entire goal system: that is, a means characterized by *multifinality*. Note that a similar notion appears in Ajzen's (1985, 1991) theory of reasoned action or planned behavior, namely, that a behavioral intention to perform a given activity is partially determined by the degree to which the activity is seen to advance various positive goals or promote various positive consequences. Indeed, the number of associations between a single activity and the attainment of different goals should determine the overall value of pursuing this activity This should be especially true when the activity is connected to the attainment of goals with *unique* value: that is, goals that are not themselves linked to the same higher order goal.

Recently, we (Shah and Kruglanski, 1999b) asked students to list two important attributes that could be attained by studying. They were then asked to assess the degree to which these attributes represented distinct goals. Controlling for the total subjective value of these attributes, it was found that the degree to which these attributes represented different goals was positively related to participants' reported commitment to studying, suggesting that this commitment was strongest when studying was linked to different goals.

In a related study, we presented participants with the opportunity to play a hypothetical lottery in which they had a chance to win two prize packages (see Figure 7). The overall content of the prize packages were exactly the same, but in one condition the prizes were divided in such a way as to strongly invoke two different goals (i.e., one of the prize packages consisted entirely of items relating to fitness and the other consisted of items relating entirely to entertainment). In the other condition, the prizes were divided in such a way that neither goal was strongly invoked (i.e., each package contained a mixture of items relating to fitness and entertainment).

Participants were significantly more likely to play the lottery in the condition where two goals were strongly invoked by the manner in which the prizes were divided, even though the overall content of both prize packages was the same in both conditions and the participants understood that winning the lottery meant winning both packages.

In short, what constitutes the best means to a goal may be defined collectively in terms of the entire system of currently active goals. So, the more goals an activity is seen to fulfill, the more likely it is to be chosen. An intriguing implication of this notion is that as the set of active

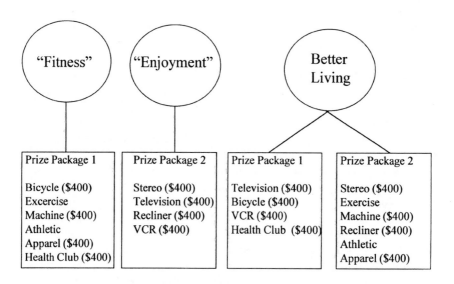

FIGURE 7   Lottery study prize packages.

background goals may shift imperceptibly from one context to the next, so may, *unwittingly*, the choice of the "best" means to a given "focal" goal or indeed the choice of a criterion for deciding what is "best" in a given context.

If one's choice and commitment to a means is dependent on both its connection to the focal goal and its connection to background goals, then the association between these goals could become a strong determinant of means choice. Specifically, if the focal goal is strongly associated with background goals, then its activation frequently would lead to activation of these other goals. The "best" means, then, often would be defined in terms of its fulfillment of the same set of background goals.

To illustrate the potential effects of these different associations, consider the following hypothetical experiment. In this study, participants initially are led to associate the goal of exercising with the goal of being social and the goal of looking good. At a later time they are asked to name their favorite way to exercise in a room with a pinup poster of an attractive person of the opposite sex (presumably invoking a personal appearance goal) or a poster relating to same-sex camaraderie (presumably invoking a "social bonding" goal). In the room with the pinup poster, participants may be more likely to choose an option such as lifting weights, whereas in the room with the "camaraderie" poster, they more readily may choose to name a team sport. Although both choices presumably do not involve conscious recognition of the influence of the poster, this effect may be moderated by the degree to which thinking about exercising is associated with a personal appearance goal versus a social bonding goal. In short, the association of a given means with focal as well as background goals and the activation of the background goals by the focal goal may all combine to affect the means choice, due to their prior association.

C. HOW MEANS ARE EXPERIENCED

The association between goals and means also may influence how a chosen means is experienced. This experience would be drawn primarily from the focal goal served by the means. Certainly, the strength of the association between the means and the focal goal increases the overall positivity of succeeding at the activity and the negativity of failing. The association between an activity and goal attainment is assumed to lend the activity positive value in proportion to goal magnitude, and the degree of association between an activity and attainment–failure will lend the activity negative value, again proportionate to goal magnitude. However, the association between goal and means may affect more than the general positivity or negativity of the means: it also may affect the type or quality of experienced affect while pursuing the given means. That is, specific emotional experiences associated with goal attainment or attainment failure may be *transferred* to the means that serve these goals.

One example of this value transfer comes from work on promotion and prevention framing mentioned earlier. Higgins, Shah, and Friedman (1997) demonstrated that the same task, solving anagrams, can relate to different emotional experiences when associated with a promotion goal versus a prevention goal. A memory task was framed to relate to either a goal of promotion or a goal of prevention. In the promotion condition, participants were told that they would receive a payment of $5 for their participation, but they possibly could gain an additional $1. They would receive the extra $1 if their performance exceeded or equaled the 70th percentile of students who had participated in the study. In the prevention condition, participants were told that they would receive a payment of $6 for their participation, but they possibly could lose $1. They would not lose the $1 if their performance exceeded or equaled the 70th percentile of students who had participated in the study. Participants' level of happiness, dejection, quiescence, and agitation were measured before participants' completed the memory task and after completing the task and randomly receiving either success or failure feedback.

As shown in Table 2, success or failure at the anagram task led to more happiness or dejection, respectively, when it was associated with a promotion goal, but to more quiescence or agitation, respectively, when the task was associated with a prevention goal. How an activity was experienced, then, was a function of the regulatory qualities of the goal with which it was associated.

The strength of the association between goal and means also should affect the means' perceived intrinsicality, usually defined as the attribution that one is performing the activity for its own sake (see Deci, 1975; Deci & Ryan, 1985). The greater the association is between a goal and an activity, the more likely engagement in the activity will be seen as "the end itself," that is, the more likely it is that activity engagement will be experienced as goal fulfillment. This should be likely especially when the activity is not associated with other goals and the goal has no other means of attainment because, as noted earlier, the more singular the association between goal and means, the stronger this connection. These particular theoretical

TABLE 2   Feedback Consistent Emotional Change as a Function of Regulatory Focus Framing and Emotion Dimension

Regulatory focus framing	Cheerfulness– dejection	Quiescence– agitation
Promotion	1.07	– .52
Prevention	.78	.68

predictions, however, remain speculative at present and are in need of further empirical validation.

D. MEANS SUBSTITUTION

Thomas Edison once commented on how often we are forced to consider other means to our goals: he claimed that he had never failed, but had just found 10,000 ways that did not work. Indeed, we are frequently thwarted in our initial efforts at goal attainment forcing us to resort to other means. In some respects, how we choose a substitute means is similar to how we chose the original means. In exercising choice, we select a specific activity out of several potential means to the same goal. In performing substitution, we initiate an alternate activity from the same set of original means after the original means has failed. In another sense, however, choice and substitution are quite different. The issue of choice depends on how the activities *differ*, so that a rational selection among them is possible. By contrast, substitution revolves on how the activities are *the same*, so that we can replace one with another.

Lewin (1935) addressed this latter issue when he specified the principles that guide our selection of replacements. He observed that the substitution of one activity for another was possible only if both arose from the same goal tension system. That is, both must ease the tension caused by the need underlying goal pursuit. According to Lewin, the "substitute value" of one task for another, then, depends on their dynamic connection within this system. From our structural perspective, the choice of a replacement means depends on its common association with goal attainment. Despite differences in content, an activity will be considered a substitute to the extent that it is associated with fulfillment of the same focal goal. So, activities that are very different in content (e.g., playing golf and sky diving) nevertheless would be seen as substitutable to the extent that they relate to the same goal (e.g., exercising). Likewise, activities that are very similar in some sense (e.g., showering and swimming) may, in fact, not replace each other when they are thought to relate to different goals (e.g., hygiene and fitness). What makes this particularly interesting is that the association between activities and goals is a matter of perception or mental representation, and thus it is highly sensitive to contextual variations, possibly altering the substitutability relationships between the same activities.

To illustrate this point empirically, we framed two instances of the same activity as relating to the same goal or to different goals. We then attempted to demonstrate that subsequent performance on the same task following initial success or failure would vary as a function of whether each instance was framed to relate to the same goal or different goals. Thus, two anagram sets were framed as having *either* the same regulatory focus (i.e., a promotion focus or a prevention focus) or different regulatory foci (i.e., one task having a promotion focus and the second a prevention focus, or vice versa). Participants either succeeded or failed on the first task. Performance on the second task, controlling for actual performance on the first, served as the dependent measure. As you can see in Figure 8, success on the first task *decreased* performance on the second only when the second had the same regulatory focus framing, but not when the second had a different regulatory focus framing. Similarly, failure on the first task *increased* performance on the second when the second had the same regulatory focus framing, but not when it had a different focus framing, indicating that the substitutability of two instances of the same activity still depended on an association to the same underlying goal. This dependency raises the intriguing possibility that behaviors formerly found to be substitutable could, under certain circumstances, lose their substitutability. For instance, the work of Steele and Lui (1983) and that of Tesser, Martin, and Cornell (1996) suggest that various psychological phenomena such as dissonance and self-affirmation are, in fact, substitutable means for attaining or maintaining self-esteem (see Figure 9). This is so presumably because the abstract goal of self-esteem maintenance is activated for participants in this research. However, is the self-esteem goal invariantly activated for all individuals? Our analysis that views goals as knowledge structures (Kruglanski, 1996) suggests that this need not be the case and that the activation of any given goal could vary from context to context.

According to this analysis, it should be possible in principle to activate just the concern with dissonance reduction or just the concern with self-affirmation without activating the abstract, self-esteem maintenance

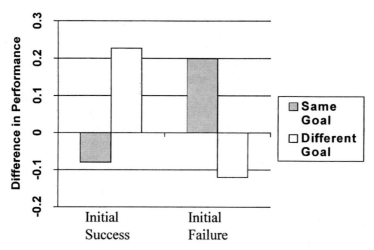

FIGURE 8   The effect of substitutability and success/failure on anagram performance.

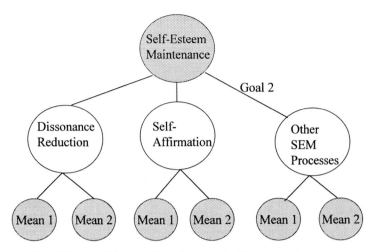

FIGURE 9   Substitutability of means of self-esteem maintenance.

goal (see Figure 10). This should reduce the substitutability relationship among all of these phenomena. That is, the range of substitutable mechanisms should be reduced to those relating to the more concrete subgoal rather than all the mechanisms relating to the abstract goal of self-esteem maintenance. These possibilities as well could be profitably explored in future research.

Having identified the range of substitutable alternatives based on their common connection to the focal goal, the specific choice one makes among these alternatives also may depend on their lateral association with the

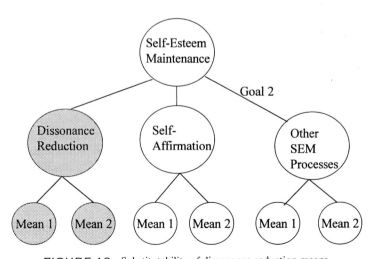

FIGURE 10   Substitutability of dissonance reduction means.

initial choice and on their association to the same background goals fulfilled by the initial choice. Returning to an earlier example, if one chooses to go home by jogging, but cannot find her running shoes, she may opt to walk rather than take a cab because the former option also satisfies the background goal of "getting some air."

III. INDIVIDUAL DIFFERENCES IN THE STRUCTURE OF GOALS AND MEANS

Having discussed the manner and consequences of differences in the structure of goal networks, we now turn to why these differences arise. That is, what factors may lead individual goal structures to differ from one another? We consider three such factors: (1) differences in motivational orientation, (2) differences in goal content, and (3) differences in regulatory experiences.

A. DIFFERENCES IN MOTIVATIONAL ORIENTATION

Goals can be seen as the cognitive link between our general motives and specific behaviors. In fact, goals mediate the fulfillment of many different needs (for a review, see Austin & Vancouver, 1996). These needs, in turn, may give rise to quite different goal structures. For instance, the goals that arise to fulfill our need for achievement may be much more complexly structured than the goals that arise to fulfill our need for basic safety concerns.

Individuals also can differ in their chronic orientation toward fulfilling these different needs. So while one individual may consistently focus on fulfilling his or her need for achievement, another may focus on his or her need for safety. These differences in orientation may result in chronic differences in individuals' goal structure.

Differences in Regulatory Focus

As one example of how motivational orientation may affect goal structure, consider how individuals might differ in terms of their focus on promotion versus prevention. According to regulatory focus theory (Higgins, 1996), an individual is thought to have both a promotion goal system consisting of "ideal" goals pursued for the sake of gaining rewards or attaining nurturance, and a prevention goal system of "ought" goals pursued to gain safety or security.

We (Shah and Kruglanski, 1999c) explored how this fundamental distinction in the regulatory purpose of goals affects their association to each other and to the means by which they would be attained.

Because oughts goals involve issues of safety and security, it was suspected that they should be less relatively substitutable by other ought goals than ideal goals would be with other ideals. As a consequence of their greater substitutability and hence activation in the same circumstances, ideals could come to be associated more strongly with other ideals than may oughts with other oughts. After all, when it comes to security, one is only as safe as his or her weakest link and therefore must cover all bases rather than substitute one responsibility for another. To provide a concrete example, one could not expect that fulfilling one of the biblical commandments could substitute for failing to obey another. It was suspected additionally that because duties and obligations may be perceived as necessities that need to be attained, one might be hesitant to try new means of attainment, because to do so would entail some risk. Instead one may choose to fulfill these goals by "tried and true" methods, resulting in less associations between these goals and different activities.

By contrast, promotion goals or ideals are all aimed at attaining a sense of nurturance or well-being; hence, they should be relatively substitutable for each other. Furthermore, because ideals may not be experienced as dire necessities the way oughts may be, they may allow exploration and hence come to be associated with a greater number of means potentially leading to their attainment.

In short, we predicted that "ideal" goals would be associated more strongly with other ideals than would oughts be associated with other oughts, and that, additionally, ideal goals typically would be linked to a greater number of means than would ought goals. To test these notions, we asked participants in one study to list two important ideals and two important obligations that they currently were pursuing and indicate their degree of success in accomplishing each of those pursuits. Participants then listed all the different ways they could attain each of the two ideals and each of the two oughts. Finally, participants completed a lexical decision procedure, identical to the one described earlier, in which, after first seeing a prime word, they were asked to determine whether or not a target word was an attribute or an activity. The participants' stated ideals and oughts were included as both prime words and target words. We found that reaction times when ideals primed other ideals were quicker than when obligations primed other obligations and when a control word primed an ideal or an ought (see Figure 11). We also found that participants listed more different ways to attain their ideal goals than their ought goals (see Figure 12).

Higgins and his colleagues (Higgins et al., 1997; Shah, Higgins, & Friedman, 1998) also proposed that individuals differ in their general orientation toward fulfilling their prevention and promotion goals. Given our results, it is likely that these differences in chronic regulatory focus

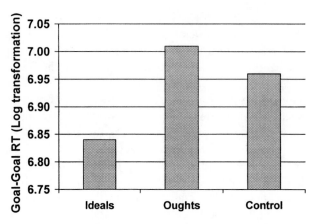

FIGURE 11   Goal–goal reaction time for ideals and oughts.

would be manifest in the structure of individuals' chronically accessible goals. This intriguing idea awaits future study.

Differences in Epistemic Motivation

Another motivational orientation that may influence goal structure is the need for closure (Kruglanski, 1989, 1990). The need for (nonspecific) cognitive closure is defined as a desire for a definite answer, any firm answer, rather than uncertainty, confusion, or ambiguity. The strength of this desire is a function of the benefits associated with possessing closure and the costs associated with lacking it. The need for closure, like other motivations, can vary across individuals and situations. The need for answers can be applied to the regulatory decisions inherent in goal pursuit: specifically, one's choice of means. If one assumes that means choice

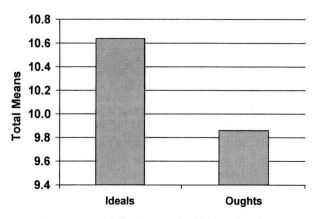

FIGURE 12   Total means for ideals and oughts.

becomes more difficult as more options are available, a need for closure may decrease the number of attainment options considered for goal attainment. Individuals with a high need for closure, then, may have goal networks with fewer attainment options that allow for quicker and more permanent regulatory decisions. Indeed, Shah and Kruglanski (1999a) found that individuals high in dispositional need for closure (see Webster and Kruglanski, 1994) list significantly fewer different means for attaining their personal goals.

B. DIFFERENCES IN PERSONAL GOAL CONTENT

The content of individuals' personal goals may differ on a number of different fundamental dimensions. For instance, a given individual may set higher (i.e., harder) goals than another or may have goals to attain more immediately or with less effort. All of these differences may have implications for how goals are structured. Take, for example, the issue of goal difficulty. Multiple means for goal attainment may be useful when goal attainment is uncertain, but distracting when goal attainment is relatively easy. An individual with difficult goals may, therefore, be more motivated to generate multiple attainment means.

In another study, we asked students to list several life goals and to rate them on difficulty of attainment. When asked to generate as many means as they could think of to attain each goal, we found that the number of means was positively related to their initial ratings of goal difficulty. Apparently, the more difficult the goal, the greater the participants' tendency to generate a larger set of means as a "backup" in case any one of them fails.

C. DIFFERENCES IN REGULATORY EXPERIENCE

Many goals, especially important ones, are not attained immediately, and much can be learned from one's goal attainment efforts. Indeed, as one continues to work toward a goal despite initial failure, he or she may become aware of other options or paths to success. One may learn, then, from post regulatory experiences, which would allow one to see other attainment means not initially recognized. This may be particularly true when one has had little history of success in working toward goal attainment. For instance, researchers have noted that a greater number of counterfactuals (i.e., possible means) are generated in response to task failure as opposed to task success (Roese & Hur, 1997; Sanna & Turley, 1996). Thus, individuals with long histories of striving for a specific goal may be expected to have connections to more possible attainment means than individuals who have adopted this goal only recently.

IV. COMPARISON TO OTHER PERSPECTIVES
ON GOAL NETWORKS

As we have implied, the proposed goal network model is consistent with other cybernetic perspectives on goal system, but extends them to consider the fundamental ways in which goal systems differ. For instance, although Carver and Scheier (1981) proposed a hierarchical goal model of self-regulation, they are largely silent on the self-regulatory implications of individual differences in the structure of this hierarchy (see also Powers, 1973, 1989; Thagard & Millgram, 1995).

A number of researchers, however, have assumed that, like one's self-concept (Barron, 1953; Linville, 1982, 1986), one's personal goal system can differ in complexity, and these differences can have implications for how goal attainment or failure is experienced emotionally. For instance, Neidenthal, Setterlund, and Wherry (1992) found that personal goal complexity mediated affective reactions to evaluative feedback about future goals in much the same manner as self-complexity mediated reactions to feedback about one's present self. That is, the more differentiated one's goal system, the more tempered one's emotional reactions. Emmons and King (1992) elaborated on this notion of differentation by distinguishing differentation within goals from differentation between goals. Whereas differentiation within goals was defined as the number of different ways a goal could be attained, differentiation between goals was defined as the degree to which goals within a system are similar to each other, or help attain one another. Emmons and King (1989) suggested that both structural differences were important for predicting emotional experience, finding that emotional extremity was positively associated with differentiation within goals, but negatively associated with differentiation between goals.

These approaches are similar to the present model in that they consider the nature and consequences of structural differences in personal goal systems. However, the present model expands on these earlier perspectives in three significant ways: (1) Our model considers a wider range of possible goal–means associations such as the distinction between the goal–means association and the means–goal association. (2) It more broadly defines the reasons for these associations. That is, although associations between goals or between means may arise because of perceptions of similarity or mutual facilitation, they also may arise for other reasons that link cognitive structures such as their simultaneous activation in common situations (e.g., relaxing and studying are both things one can do when home). Finally, (3) our model considers how these associations have consequences that precede the emotional experience of goal attainment or failure. By considering how these associations affect issues such as means choice and substitution, the model illustrates the effects of goal structure on multiple levels of goal regulation.

V. FUTURE DIRECTIONS: INTERPERSONAL GOALS

It is also of interest to consider the potential social psychological implications of our goal networks theory. It is often the case, for instance, that other people constitute the *goals* of our strivings in some sense or, in other cases, they may represent *means* to further goals. We may, for example, strive for the *respect* or the *affection* of our parents or for a special "other" to find us attractive. To attain these ends, we may perform various activities: for example, strive for academic success to please our parents or work out at the gym to become more attractive to other people.

Again, the abstractness of our social goal should define the range of substitutable behaviors. For instance, if one's goal was to be more attractive generally, such a goal might be activated by the presence of any member of the opposite sex, whereas if one's goal was specific to a certain significant other, it might be activated only in their presence or impending arrival.

Beyond representing interpersonal goals, other people often may constitute the means to goal attainment. For example, other people may be the means to attaining one's objectives of feeling "powerful," "gifted," or "appealing"; they may constitute social mirrors that reflect one's various desired attributes and thus serve as comparison standards to assess progress. Depending on various goal attributes, one could generate several or only a few such means, and this could have important implications for their substitutability or perceived interchangeability. For example, a rather abstract goal such as being "friendly" could be gratified by virtually any person one might encounter, whereas a more specific (concrete) goal of "having a circle of friends" may be gratified by a much more restricted set of people. In turn, the greater the number of people seen as potential means of gratifying one's goal, the greater their "functional equivalence" or mutual substitutability and the less their unique attachment to the goal. The present theory of goal network, then, may furnish a useful conceptual tool not only for understanding individual goal pursuit, but also for gaining insights into our interpersonal relationships with others by addressing our significant interpersonal goals or significant means to goal attainment.

VI. CONCLUSION

Our structural theory of goal networks attempts to illustrate how goals and means may relate to each other and the implications of these associations for a number of important regulatory phenomena. Specifying the fundamental ways in which goals may differ in content has proven very useful for understanding the subjective experience of specific goal attainment or discrepancy (see Cantor et al., 1987; Dweck & Legget, 1988;

Higgins et al., 1997; Ryan, Sheldon, Kasser, & Deci, 1996). We believe that the structural level of analysis lends new insights into how goals are chosen, pursued, experienced, and replaced that are not readily explained by differences in goal content alone. Whereas previous treatments and theories have alluded to issues of equifinality, substitution, choice, etc. (e.g., Fein & Spencer, 1997; Festinger, 1957; Freud, 1920/1948; Lewin, 1935; Solomon, Greenberg, & Pyszczynski, 1991), they typically have done so in the context of specific motivational concerns or specific goals an individual may choose to pursue. In contrast, our structural analysis attempts to consider the properties of goal networks that transcend specific differences in motivation or goal content.

A promise of this general approach, therefore, lies in its integrative potential and in the general understanding it may foster for a wide range of significant and seemingly disparate psychological phenomena.

REFERENCES

Ajzen, I. (1985). From intentions to actions: A theory of planned behavior. In J. Kuhl & J. Beckmann (Eds.), *Action control: From cognition to behavior* (pp. 11–39). Berlin, Germany: Springer-Verlag.

Ajzen, I. (1991). The theory of planned behavior. *Organizational Behavior and Human Decision Processes, 50*, 179–211.

Austin, J. T., & Vancouver, J. B. (1996). Goal constructs in psychology: Structure, process, and content. *Psychological Bulletin, 120*, 338–375.

Barron, F. (1953). Complexity-simplicity as a personality dimension. *Journal of Abnormal and Social Psychology, 48*, 163–172.

Cantor, N., Norem, J. K., Niedenthal, P. M., Langston, C. A., & Brower, A. M. (1987). Life tasks, self concept ideals and cognitive strategies in a life transition. *Journal of Personality and Social Psychology, 53*, 1178–1191.

Carver, C. S., & Scheier, W. F. (1981). *Attention and self-regulation: A control theory approach to human behavior.* New York: Springer-Verlag.

Deci, E. L. (1975). *Intrinsic motivation.* New York: Plenum.

Deci, E. L., & Ryan, R. M. (1985). *Intrinsic motivation and self determination in human behavior.* New York: Plenum Press.

Dweck C. S., & Legget, E. L. (1988). A social-cognitive approach to motivation and personality. *Psychological Review, 95*, 256–273.

Emmons. R. A., & King, L. A. (1989). Personal striving complexity and affective reactivity. *Journal of Personality and Social Psychology, 56*, 478–484.

Fein, S., & Spencer, S. J. (1997). Prejudice as self-image maintenance: Affirming the self through derogating others. *Journal of Personality and Social Psychology, 73*, 31–44.

Festinger, L. (1957). *A theory of cognitive dissonance.* Stanford, CA: Stanford University Press.

Freud, S. (1948). *Beyond the pleasure principle.* London: Hogarth. (Original work published in 1920.)

Gollwitzer, P. M., & Brandstatter, V. (1997). Implementation intentions and effective goal pursuit. *Journal of Personality and Social Psychology, 73*, 171–183.

Heider, F. (1958). *The psychology of interpersonal relations*. New York: Wiley.

Higgins, E. T. (1996). Knowledge activation: Accessibility, applicability, and salience. In E. T. Higgins & A. W. Kruglanski (Eds.), *Social psychology: Handbook of basic principles* (pp. 133–168). New York: Guilford Press.

Higgins, E. T., Lee, J., Kwon, J., & Trope, Y. (1995). When combining intrinsic motivations undermines interest: A test of activity engagement theory. *Journal of Personality and Social Psychology, 68,* 749–767.

Higgins, E. T., Shah, J. Y., & Friedman, R. (1997). Emotional responses to goal attainment: Strength of regulatory focus as moderator. *Journal of Personality and Social Psychology, 72,* 515–525.

Higgins, E. T., & Trope, Y. (1990). Activity engagement theory: Implications of multiply identifiable input for intrinsic motivation. In E. T. Higgins & R. M. Sorrentino (Eds.), *Handbook of motivation and cognition: Foundations of social behavior* (Vol. 2, pp. 229–264). New York: Guilford Press.

Kruglanski, A. W. (1989). *Lay epistemics and human knowledge. Cognitive and motivational bases*. New York: Plenum.

Kruglanski, A. W. (1990). Motivation for judging and knowing: Implications for causal attribution. In E. T. Higgins & R. M. Sorrentino (Ed.), *The handbook of motivation and cognition: Foundation of social behavior* (Vol. 2, pp. 333–368). New York: Guilford Press.

Kruglanski, A. W. (1996). Goals as knowledge structures. In P. M. Gollwitzer & J. A. Bargh (Eds.), *The psychology of action: Linking cognition and motivation to behavior.* (pp. 599–619). New York: Guilford Press.

Lepper, M. R., Greene, D., & Nisbett, R. E. (1973). Undermining children's intrinsic interest with extrinsic reward: A test of the overjustification hypothesis. *Journal of Personality and Social Psychology, 28,* 129–137.

Lewin, K. (1935). *A dynamic theory of personality: Selected papers* (D. E. Adams & K. E. Zener, Trans.). New York: McGraw-Hill.

Linville, P. W. (1982). Affective consequences of complexity regarding the self and others. In M. S. Clark & S. T. Fiske (Eds.), *Affect and cognition* (pp. 79–109). Hillsdale, NJ: Erlbaum.

Linville, P. W. (1987). Self complexity as a cognitive buffer against stress related illness and depression. *Journal of Personality and Social Psychology, 52,* 663–676.

McDougal, W. (1923). *Outline of psychology*. New York: Scribners.

Miller, G. A., Galanter, E., & Pribram, K. H. (1960). *Plans and the structure of behavior*. New York: Holt.

Niedenthal, P. M., Setterlund, M. B., & Wherry, M. B. (1992). Possible self-complexity and affective reactions to goal-relevant evaluation. *Journal of Personality and Social Psychology, 63,* 5–16.

Nisbett, R. E., & Wilson, T. D. (1977). Telling more than we can know: Verbal reports on mental processes. *Psychological Review, 84,* 231–259.

Powers, W. T. (1973). *Behavior: The control of perception*. Chicago: Aldine.

Powers, W. T. (1989). *Living control systems*. Gravel Switch, KY: Control Systems Group.

Roese, N. J. (1994). The functional basis of counterfactual thinking. *Journal of Personality and Social Psychology, 66,* 805–818.

Roese, N. J., & Hur, T. (1997). Affective determinants of counterfactual thinking. *Social Cognition, 15,* 333–350.

Ryan, R. M., Sheldon, K. M., Kasser, T., & Deci, E. L. (1996). All goals are not created equal. In P. M. Gollwitzer & J. A. Bargh (Eds.), *The psychology of action: Linking cognition and motivation to behavior* (pp. 7–26). New York: Guilford Press.

Sanna, L. J., & Turley, K. J. (1996). Antecedents to spontaneous counterfactual thinking: Effects of expectancy violation and outcome valence. *Personality and Social Psychology Bulletin, 22,* 906–919.

Shah, J. Y., Higgins, E. T., & Friedman, R. (1998). Performance incentives and means: How regulatory focus influences goal attainment. *Journal of Personality and Social Psychology, 74,* 285–293.

Shah, J. Y., Kruglanski, A. W., & Thompson, E. P. (1998). Membership has its (epistemic) rewards: Need for closure effects on ingroup favoritism. *Journal of Personality and Social Psychology, 75,* 383–393.

Shah, J. Y., & Kruglanski, A. W. (1999a). *Knowing what to do: Epistemic determinants of the content and structure of goals.* Manuscript in preparation.

Shah, J. Y., & Kruglanski, A. W. (1999b). *Goal structure and goal regulation.* Manuscript in preparation.

Shah, J. Y., & Kruglanski, A. W. (1999c). *Regulatory focus and goal structure.* Manuscript in preparation.

Sheldon, K. M., & Emmons, R. A. (1995). Comparing differentiation and integration within personal goal systems. *Personality and Individual Differences, 18,* 39–46.

Sheldon, K. M., & Kasser, T. (1995). Coherence and congruence: Two aspects of personality integration. *Journal of Personality and Social Psychology, 68,* 531–543.

Solomon, S., Greenberg, J., & Pyszczynski, T. (1991). A terror management theory of social behavior: The psychological functions of self-esteem and cultural worldviews. In M. P. Zanna (Ed.), *Advances in experimental social psychology* (Vol. 24, pp. 91–159). New York: Academic Press.

Steele, C. M., & Liu, T. J. (1983). Dissonance processes as self-affirmation. *Journal of Personality and Social Psychology, 45,* 5–19.

Tesser, A., Martin, L. L., & Cornell, D. P. (1996). On the substitutability of self-protective mechanisms. In P. M. Gollwitzer & J. A. Bargh (Eds.), *The psychology of action: Linking cognition and motivation to behavior.* (pp. 48–68). New York: Guilford Press.

Thagard, P., & Millgram, E. (1995). Inference to the best plan: A coherence theory of decision. In A. Ram & D. B. Leake (Eds.), *Goal-driven learning* (pp. 439–454). Cambridge, MA: MIT Press.

Webster, D. M., & Kruglanski, A. W. (1994). Individual differences in need for cognitive closure. *Journal of Personality and Social Psychology, 67,* 1049–1062.

5

A FUNCTIONAL-DESIGN APPROACH TO MOTIVATION AND SELF-REGULATION

THE DYNAMICS OF PERSONALITY SYSTEMS INTERACTIONS

JULIUS KUHL

University of Osnabrück, Osnabrück, Germany

I. INTRODUCTION

This chapter explores the mechanisms underlying motivation and self-regulation from a functional-design perspective. Traditional approaches emphasize the mediating role of beliefs and other cognitive contents. An example of this approach is classical expectancy-value theory according to which a student's motivation to invest time and effort depends on his or her expectation of success and on the perceived value of good achievement (Atkinson & Feather, 1966; Heckhausen, 1977, 1991). In a similar vein, the degree to which students are able to self-regulate the enactment of their work-related intentions is attributed to their self-efficacy beliefs; that is, their beliefs that they will be able to initiate and successfully perform the intended behavior (Bandura, 1977; Peterson, Maier, & Seligman, 1993). This chapter is based on a different approach: Instead of focusing on

Copyright © 2000 by Academic Press.
All rights of reproduction in any form reserved.

cognitive *content*, such as beliefs, expectations, or causal attributions, the basic properties of the functional architecture underlying motivation and self-regulation are analyzed.

Learned helplessness is a practical example that illustrates the difference between content-based and functional explanations: After exposure to uncontrollable failure, many people lose their motivation and show impaired performance just as depressed patients do in response to adverse life conditions (Peterson et al., 1993). According to traditional theorizing, those motivational and cognitive deficits are attributable to negative beliefs, such as pessimistic beliefs about one's own abilities (e.g., Seligman, Nolen-Hoeksema, Thornton, & Thornton, 1990). In contrast, according to a functional account, pessimistic beliefs and motivational deficits are consequences rather than causes of performance deficits that occur when people are confronted with uncontrollable failure: Experimental evidence shows that generalized pessimistic control beliefs typically occur after, not before, people develop symptoms of helplessness and depression (Kuhl, 1981; Lewinsohn, Steinmetz, Larson, & Franklin, 1981). According to these findings, learned helplessness and depression cannot be remedied through making people believe in their abilities as attempted in cognitive therapy (Bandura, 1977; Beck, 1979; Peterson et al., 1993) until one has established the necessary abilities. Specifying the mechanisms that underlie self-regulatory abilities has been the target of functional approaches to self-regulation (Kuhl, 1984; Mischel & Mischel, 1983). In the first part of this chapter, mechanisms that affect self-regulation irrespective of the content of thought are analyzed in the context of action control theory (Kuhl, 1984, 1992). Examples of relevant mechanisms that may cause symptoms of helplessness and other self-regulatory deficits are impaired mood regulation (emotion control), impaired control of unwanted thoughts (attention control), impaired ability to restore one's motivation (motivation control), especially under frustrating or threatening conditions (state orientation), and impaired access to holistic (implicit) self-representations (e.g., representations of one's own needs, values, feelings, and action alternatives available).

Searching for functional mechanisms underlying motivation and self-regulation is, of course, not incompatible with the notion that the content of thought such as cognitive beliefs can have a functional significance. Even if many cognitive beliefs merely reflect functional deficits after they develop, there is no reason to disclaim the possibility that sometimes beliefs do have a causal impact on behavior as discussed in other chapters of this volume. The functional framework described in this chapter is meant to extend rather than replace content-based approaches: It spells out the mechanisms that affect self-regulatory behavior over and above the self-regulatory effects of cognitive beliefs and strategies in the ways explained in other chapters of this volume.

As suggested by the examples described in the preceding paragraph, self-regulation is not a homogeneous entity that can be described by global concepts such as self-efficacy or willpower. Instead, several forms of self-regulation can be distinguished, each of which can be decomposed into several functions. Each self-regulatory mode can be described in terms of a characteristic configuration of certain macrosystems that form the building blocks of motivation and self-regulation. As will be pointed out in this chapter, these basic building blocks are not identical to the ones used in cognitive science, such as working memory, long-term memory, and executive control (e.g., Baddeley, 1986). Moreover, self-regulation does not depend only on various configurations of cognitive macrosystems, but also on certain "subcognitive" mechanisms that can be related to classical concepts of energy and motivation. Because these dynamic concepts are especially important for some poorly understood components of self-regulation, I will discuss them in detail in this chapter.

A. COGNITIVE VERSUS DYNAMIC CONCEPTS OF MOTIVATION

Motivation is sometimes regarded as the problem child of psychology. Compared to her cognitive brothers and sisters, she does not receive much attention and support, and she does not always seem to pamper her parents with great accomplishments. Some cognitive observers do not even regard motivation as a legitimate member of the family. During the shift from "folk to science" in cognitive psychology (Stich, 1983), one investigator put a common opinion this way: "Motivation is a derived phenomenon" (Norman, 1980). This is to say that cognitive mechanisms, such as perception, attention, memory, and consciousness, suffice to explain goal-directed behavior. Once the dominant knowledge structures of an individual are known, we can explain his or her behavior: "Tell me what goals a person has and I will tell you what this person will be doing." The amount of attention and other cognitive resources that are devoted to a goal presumably determines the extent to which it guides behavior. Cognitive psychologists like the concept of goal because, compared to other motivational concepts, it seems best suited for a cognitive reinterpretation of motivation: Goals can be considered a special category of cognitive representations. No wonder that goals have become a preferred topic in research on human motivation: They seem to enable us to study motivation by taking advantage of the methodological advances in cognitive science.

There is more to motivation than goals or other cognitive representations, such as expectations, beliefs, and values. The focus of this chapter is on noncognitive aspects of motivation. Some of them may be called *subcognitive*; others could be classified as *supra-* or *metacognitive*.

This chapter has four parts. Following a brief summary of action control theory, I first discuss some dynamic concepts of motivation proposed in

Freud's and Kurt Lewin's theories. The most famous operationalization of the dynamic concepts of needs and intentions is Bluma Zeigarnik's demonstration of superior recall of information related to uncompleted intentions. As a second step, I analyze some of the reasons why these dynamic concepts fell short of providing a sufficient theoretical and methodological paradigm for motivational psychology. This will take us back to the roots of motivational concepts: Ancient philosophy has explicated many concepts underlying our commonsense conceptions of motivation. I use Aristotle's (1975) concept of motivation as an illustration of the roots of a type of dynamic concept that forms an antithesis to Lewin's conception. After making these steps "ahead by going back" to the past, I try to point out a way back to the future in the third part, where I report some ideas that I developed in my search for a synthesis of the ancient and commonsense concepts of motivation, on the one hand, and dynamic concepts proposed by classical motivational psychology, on the other hand. I illustrate this attempted synthesis with an outline of my theory of personality systems interactions (PSI theory). PSI theory specifies the differences between the concepts of motivation and self-regulation, and integrates them within a coherent framework. In the fourth part, I conclude with some reflections about future directions in motivational research. This outlook amounts to a critique of what I call content-based explanations of self-regulated behavior. According to my view, content-based explanations will be extended more and more, sometimes even replaced by functional accounts when motivational psychology learns to identify the basic mechanisms of motivation.

B. THE THEORY OF ACTION CONTROL

The introductory remarks about learned helplessness illustrate a functional-design alternative to traditional content-based accounts. My basic assumption (Kuhl, 1981) that the primary cause of helplessness phenomena may be a functional deficit rather than a particular type of cognitive content (e.g., pessimistic control beliefs) was the starting point for the development of a theory of action control, which extended classical motivation theory to incorporate self-regulatory processes. According to this theory, a person can believe in his or her self-efficacy or can be highly motivated and still might not be able to enact intentions he or she is committed to if self-regulatory abilities are insufficient. The term "action control" was chosen to avoid the term "self-regulation," which could not be explicated in functional-design terms at that time. The concept of action control emphasizes the assumed effects of the processes described: It summarizes all processes that facilitate the enactment of intended actions. According to action control theory (Kuhl, 1984), these processes are based on various mechanisms or strategies that help maintain a difficult intention active in memory and shield it from competing action tendencies (Kuhl, 1984). Examples are strategies like *attention control* (e.g., focusing on information related to an uncompleted intention rather than to distracting information), *motivation control* (e.g., enhancing the subjective attractiveness of an intended action), *emotion control* (e.g., disengaging from a sad mood if it renders enactment of an intention difficult), and *coping with failure* (e.g., using failure as self-corrective information rather than responding to it with self-handicapping emotionality).

In recent years, this theory could be extended to incorporate a functional account of the self and its role in action control (Kuhl, 1996, 1998, in press). Originally, action control strategies were conceived of as consciously controlled processes that enhance the activational strength of intention-related cognitions and emotions, and suppress processes that would strengthen competing action tendencies. As will be pointed out later in this chapter, the conscious form of action control, which is based on suppression of nonintended processing, is only one of two fundamentally different forms of central (i.e., volitional) control of motivational processes. The second mode of volition is called *self-regulation*. It is described in terms of largely implicit (unconscious) processes that integrate as many subsystems and processes as possible for the support of a chosen action. In contrast, the conscious form of action control, which is called *self-control*, is based on suppression of many subsystems and processes to reduce the risk that any competing action tendency takes over and jeopardizes the enactment of a difficult intention. An example of self-control is a student who attempts to enact his or her intention to study by inhibiting all thoughts related to attractive alternatives such as talking with friends or going to the movies. Self-regulation is characterized by a different approach: The student would pay attention to all his or her needs, emotions, and thoughts, and find a way for each of them to be taken care of either simultaneously (e.g., study with friends) or successively. This openness to self-related thoughts and feelings that is characteristic of self-regulation can be compared to an inner democracy, whereas self-control can be described in terms of an inner dictatorship. In the first case, the self forms the basis or "agent" of self-regulation, providing cognitive and emotional support for self-generated goals and actions. In the second case, the self is the target of self-control; that is, self-related thoughts and feelings are suppressed to reduce the risk that any self-related thought or feeling that might be incompatible with the current conscious intention could take over.

At this point of theory development, many theoretical questions arise. What is the self and how can it be explained in functional terms. What are the conditions that determine whether self-control or self-regulation is activated? What role do positive and negative affects play in this process? How are motivational processes that provide the energy for the enactment of intentions affected by volitional processes? These questions require a substantially broader theoretical framework than the original theory of action control. In the remainder of this chapter, I describe the theory of personality systems interactions (PSI theory), which was developed to answer the questions raised by the extended theory of action control. I begin with one of the most challenging (and most neglected) questions regarding the concept of motivational energy: What does it mean in functional terms when a student says, "I want to study, but I do not have the energy to do so"? How can the energy necessary for volitional action be conceptualized and how does it affect the interaction among cognitive systems involved in volitional action?

II. DYNAMIC CONCEPTS IN CLASSICAL THEORIES OF MOTIVATION

The first problem arising at the cognition–motivation interface concerns the divergent nature of cognition versus motivation: Classical concepts of motivation are subcognitive.[1] The impulses originating in Freud's id were not endowed with cognitive insights. Freud's concept of libido as the universal energy underlying all motivated behavior left little room for higher forms of intelligence. In Lewin's (1935) theory, needs were described in terms of tension systems that do not release their energy until an appropriate goal is attained. He called these systems *dynamic systems* to express the waxing and waning properties of what he considered the driving forces of motivation. According to this view, a person can reflect intensely about an aspired goal state without necessarily performing any appropriate action: In addition to a cognitive representation of a goal, some subcognitive driving force seems to be necessary to move the organism toward the goal. Atkinson & Birch (1970) developed a mathematical model of similar dynamic aspects of motivation three decades ago. This model and the theory underlying it was ahead of its time for at least two reasons: First, psychology was busy elaborating a scientific basis for the assessment and analysis of cognitive processes. Second, the specific type of theorizing proposed by Atkinson and Birch would have required a

---

[1]The term "subcognitive" describes nonrepresentational processes. A common example is global arousal, which relates to a process that does not represent some aspect of the external or internal world, but can affect the activational strength of representations. Affects (but not emotions) are conceptualized as subcognitive processes as well. The terms "metacognitive" and "supracognitive" relate to representations about representations. Although virtually any cognitive representation is a "metarepresentation" in the sense that it aggregates more elementary representations, I use the term in the sense of some knowledge that represents a combination of subcognitive and cognitive states (e.g., a representation of a wish to buy a car, where wish has a subcognitive component, such as a positive affect associated with the cognitive representation of a car).

paradigm shift: Their model assumed bidirectional causal relationships among motivational variables at a time when everyone was eager to apply the unidirectional logic of classical experimental methodology and the analysis of variance model derived from it.

Today we have less reason to avoid dynamic concepts: We can handle the mathematical intricacies of nonlinear bidirectional causality as exemplified by models on fractals, deterministic chaos, and synergetics (Haken, 1981). In an application of a simple chaos model, I found support for the capacity that a model allowing for bidirectional (nonlinear) causality had for explaining level of aspiration data (Kuhl, 1985).

Besides the neglect of bidirectional causality, there are two additional causes of the difficulty to integrate dynamic concepts in motivational research: The neglect of subcognitive mechanisms and the conceptual underspecification of dynamic concepts.

A. NEGLECT OF SUBCOGNITIVE MECHANISMS

Compared to the theoretical and methodological advances made in cognitive research, dynamic concepts still have the aura of sunken Freudian vessels (perhaps of *Titanic* dimensions) that are buried in the deep waters of the unconscious, unable to make contact with the daylight where they easily could be observed and examined. Fortunately, new perspectives for examining dynamic processes are emerging today. First, advances made in the neurosciences make a strong case for subcognitive processes. One of the well-known examples is LeDoux's (1995) research on two neurobiological routes from perception toward affect generation: A direct route reaching affect-generating structures (e.g., the amygdala) without a cognitive loop and an indirect route that enables cognitive structures to modulate affect-generating subcortical mechanisms.

The neurobiological evidence for a direct mechanism that generates affect without the intervention of higher-order cognitive processes (presumably mediated by the cortex) provides a strong argument against cognitive reductionism (cf. Zajonc, 1980): Affective reactions to a situation cannot be explained fully on the basis of what a person thinks or believes. The term "subcognitive" denotes the component of affectivity that is not mediated by higher-order cognitive processing. Motivation and self-regulation depend on the type of affective response characteristic of an individual (Atkinson, 1958; Heckhausen, 1991; Klinger, 1977; Kuhl, 1984, 1992). The introductory remarks concerning the relationship between the content of thought and motivation are corroborated by neurobiological evidence (LeDoux, 1995): Exploring people's beliefs and other cognitive contents does not suffice to explain the affective basis of motivation and volition. A student may have problems experiencing positive affect and intrinsic motivation with a task and enacting his or her intentions to work on it even if he or she has been made to believe that he or she can handle the task.

B. UNDERSPECIFICATION OF DYNAMIC CONCEPTS

The evidence for subcognitive processes underlying affect generation suggests that there is more to motivation than cognitive contents such as goals, expectations, and other beliefs. However, this evidence does not tell us much about the specific features of dynamic mechanisms. Some theorists have specified motivational energy in terms of a mechanism that "channelizes" available undirected neuronal energy in favor of some goal representation (Klinger, in press; Nuttin, 1984). Cognitive theories use dynamic concepts in some sense; for instance, when referring to the activational strengths of specific or global memory structures (Anderson, 1983; Kahneman, 1973). However, when motivational psychologists speak of dynamic properties such as "energy," they do not mean quite the same that cognitive psychologists describe in terms of activation or arousal. This leads us to central questions of motivation: What exactly does the dynamic component add to the system? What does it mean in functional terms when we say that a student is motivated (e.g., beyond saying that he or she has increased arousal or positive control beliefs)?

According to Lewin's dynamic theory of motivation, the dynamic component can be described as a certain form of motivational energy that is necessary to maintain uncompleted intentions active in memory and that facilitates their performance under certain conditions. The motivational energy that facilitates initiation of study behavior and persistent efforts toward achieving relevant goals increases with increasing strengths of underlying needs and attractiveness of the goal; energy decreases when the goal has been attained or substitute goals have been achieved (e.g., when one has succeeded on an alternative task that is sufficiently similar to the one originally attempted).

Similar ideas about dynamic properties of the organism are reflected in many theories of motivation (Atkinson & Birch, 1970; Freud, 1938/11989; Heckhausen, 1991; Lewin, 1935; McClelland, Atkinson, Clark, & Lowell, 1953; Murray, 1938). How can we make progress in explaining such intuitive concepts of motivational dynamics contained in classical theories? The scientific status of the dynamic concepts contained in those theories critically depends on the extent to which they can be operationalized. Zeigarnik (1927) used superior recall of uncompleted compared to completed tasks as a measure of the degree of tension energizing an intentional system: When participants were asked at the end of her experiments which tasks they recalled, they reported more uncompleted than completed tasks. This finding was interpreted in terms of Lewin's hypothesis that uncompleted tasks relate to intentions that are kept in a state of tension until they are completed. Unfortunately, this intention-superiority effect did not replicate as a main effect (Atkinson, 1953; van Bergen, 1968). Zeigarnik had her participants work on several tasks and interrupted them on half of the tasks. A typical finding that demonstrates an interaction rather than the main effect expected on the basis of Lewin's theory is shown in Figure 1: In this study, the Zeigarnik effect, that is, superior recall of uncompleted compared to completed tasks, was obtained in a group of depressed students, whereas nondepressed participants showed the opposite effect (Johnson, Petzel, Hartney, & Morgan, 1983). This interaction between personality and the intention-superiority effect appears paradoxical in the context of classical theorizing about dynamic processes: Why should depressed individuals, who typically suffer from a lack of energy, be characterized by increased activation of their intentions? As I point out later, I believe that this paradox contains the key to understanding the subcognitive mechanisms working at the interface of motivation and self-regulation. Both cognitive and traditional motivational approaches reach their limits in accounting for this paradoxical interaction.

Another problem relates to a methodological issue: Free recall had been criticized as a measure of the activational status of intention-related

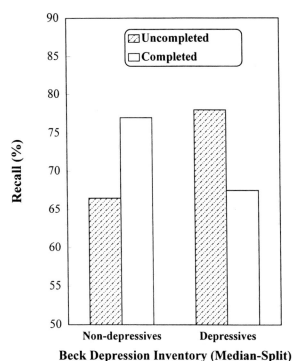

FIGURE 1   Recall of completed versus uncompleted tasks as a function of degree of depression. After Johnson et al., 1983.

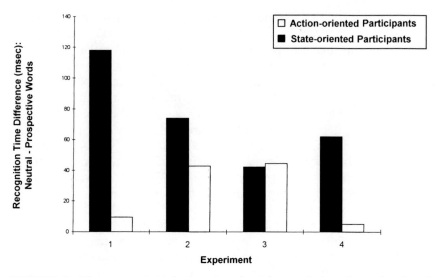

FIGURE 2 Memory superiority for intention-related (prospective) words as a function of a personality disposition for self-regulatory recruitment of energy for the enactment of intended actions. After Goschke and Kuhl (1993).

information because of several methodological shortcomings (Heckhausen, 1991, p. 125ff). However, Goschke and Kuhl (1993) obtained a similar pattern of results in a series of studies using recognition latencies as a measure of subthreshold activation of words related to uncompleted intentions compared to activation of neutral words. In the four experiments summarized in Figure 2, a personality disposition that can be regarded as a nonpathological analog of depression (i.e., prospective state orientation) was associated consistently with an intention-superiority effect, that is, shorter recognition latencies for words related to an uncompleted intention, (i.e., prospective words) as compared to neutral words (Figure 2). Prospective state orientation is assessed by a self-report scale that describes examples of hesitation and lack of energy to initiate intended behaviors. This construct is especially interesting in the context of self-regulation: As pointed out in a later section, research findings suggest that the basic mechanism underlying this construct can be described in terms of the ability for *self-motivation* (i.e., the ability to generate positive affect or other states that facilitate volitional action without the support of external prompts).[2] The findings from Goschke and Kuhl's (1993) experiments

---

[2] The special status of intention-related information in memory also has been demonstrated in research on prospective memory, although this research typically ignores individual differences (Brandimote, Einstein, & McDaniel, 1996). Although not explained in the text, the failure to find individual differences in the intention-superiority effect in Experiment 3 (Figure 2) was theoretically predicted on the basis of a critical feature in which this experiment differed from the other three studies (i.e., self-initiation rather than external control of enactment).

confirm the paradoxical findings from the Johnson et al. (1983) study (Figure 1): A personality disposition (i.e., state orientation) that can be regarded as a nonpathological component of depression in terms of reduced behavioral energy or "hesitation" (Kuhl & Helle, 1986) was associated with an increased activation of intention-related information (as indicated by faster recognition times for prospective words).

III. ARISTOTLE'S DYNAMIC CONCEPTS

The paradoxical interaction between personality and prospective memory highlights the limitations of classical dynamic concepts. What is wrong with these concepts? In my view, classical approaches specified the functional locus of motivational energy in too global terms. According to Lewin, the locus of energization was in structures underlying needs and *quasi needs* (which he called intentions to express his assumption that intentions had dynamic properties that were similar to those of needs). This assumption directly leads to the paradox mentioned: How can it be true that people characterized by a lack of energy observable in terms of behavioral inhibition (e.g., depressed or state-oriented individuals) show indications of heightened energization when measures of prospective memory (i.e., memory for intentions) are obtained? We clearly need a more differentiated model of dynamic aspects of motivation, a model that describes the flow of energy across various subsystems. In Lewin's theory, flow of energy was confined to the within-system exchange among similar intentions. What are the conditions that control energy flow between intention memory and systems relevant for the control of intended behavior? What are the functional characteristics of systems among which motivational energy flows? In search for an answer to these questions, I found this conclusion that Aristotle drew two and a half milleniums ago in his *Nicomachean Ethics*: "It is not thought as such that can move anything, but thought which is for the sake of something and is practical."

According to Aristotle's insight, we cannot expect cognition to instigate behavior all the time. As I show later, this assumption is not easily compatible with cognitive models of human behavior that are based on the idea that, to predict behavior, it suffices to study cognitive contents and mechanisms supporting them as, for instance, the resources allocated to goal representations activated in an organism at a given point in time. Aristotle maintained that additional conditions have to be met until thoughts can move anything; that is, until they have motivational significance. Note that the roots of the term "motivation" are related to the word "move," the term Aristotle used in what amounts to an abbreviated formulation of a model of human motivation.

A. FUNCTIONAL EXPLANATION OF ARISTOTLE'S THEORY OF MOTIVATION

Today we prefer a more functional language to express assumptions about psychological mechanisms. I already suggested that Aristotle's term "thought" can be understood in terms of motivationally significant cognitive representations, specifically representations of goals and cognitive representations of appropriate instrumental behavioral routines (i.e., intentions). When can we say that motivationally significant cognitions are "for the sake of something"? In my view, this term can be interpreted in terms of the meaningfulness of a goal or an action considered within the broader context of an individual's needs, values, and social environments. A goal or an action is meaningful, it is "for the sake of something," to the extent that it is compatible with an individual's needs, values, interpersonal relationships, and other aspects of what is called the self and its social context. Aristotle's statement emphasizes a second requirement for a cognitively represented goal to be able to instigate behavior: A thought has to be practical before it can move anything. What does Aristotle's additional determinant of motivation, *practicality*, mean in functional terms? A goal or an action is practical to the extent that it can be translated into behavioral routines available to the organism. Accordingly, my translation of Aristotle's model of motivation into functional language reads as follows:

> Cognitive representations of goals and anticipated instrumental activities are not endowed with dynamic properties, that is, they do not energize or facilitate behavior until their compatibility with a personal meaning structure (e.g., the self) has been established and/or until they have been translated into specific behavioral routines available to the organism.

In my view, this functional account of Aristotle's model of motivation entails the chance to make some progress in solving the problems left by the dynamic concepts contained in the theories of Freud, Lewin, Zeigarnik, and Atkinson. Global concepts of energy, dynamic forces, or motivational tendencies can be decomposed into more specific concepts. Motivational energy (i.e., activation of mental structures contributing to the instigation of goal-directed behavior) can come from various subsystems. According to my functional account of Aristotle's distinctions, the sources of motivational energy (i.e., behavioral facilitation) he refers to can be described in terms of energy flowing to and from the three subsystems depicted in Figure 3: (1) a subsystem that generates self-representations and self-compatible goals (i.e., goals that are "for the sake of something"; not necessarily conscious), (2) a subsystem that generates explicit, consciously accessible representations of intended actions (i.e., motivational thoughts), and (3) a subsystem that generates specific behavioral routines (i.e., thoughts that are practical). Adding a perceptual system specialized to

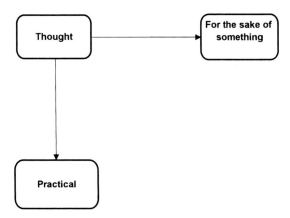

FIGURE 3   Aristotle's theory of volitional action.

the identification and recognition of objects in various modalities to this table, we have a list of what I consider the minimum number of macrosystems that have to be distinguished to arrive at a differentiated theory of energy flow among systems relevant for goal-directed action: (1) a system that provides extended (holistic) representations of internal and external contexts, including integrated self-representations (EM); (2) a system that supports explicit, sequential, and analytical operations for problem solving, including an explicit memory for difficult intentions (IM); (3) a system that controls the performance of intuitively available behavioral routines (IBC); and (4) a system that recognizes familiar "objects" perceived in the inner or outer world (OR) and identifies novel objects on the basis of mismatches between representations of familiar objects and new objects encountered.

B. SYSTEMS INTERACTIONS: MODULATION OF CONNECTIVITY AMONG SUBSYSTEMS

There is another, even more subtle implication in Aristotle's model. This aspect of his concept of motivation relates to the definition of dynamic properties; that is, the properties of a system that facilitate overt action. Aristotle did not say that strength of motivation is a function of the activational strength of a thought, nor did he describe motivation as a function of the activational strength of "practicality" (his term for appropriate habits or behavioral programs). Instead, he considered the *relationships* between a thought and whatever makes it practical and whatever makes it be for the sake of something as the essential condition for its motivational significance; that is, for its ability to move anything.

To put it in more functional language, it is the connectivity among systems that is the essence of the dynamic properties of a thought: The connectivity between systems that generate anticipated (intended) actions, on the one hand, and systems that generate self-representations (that tell the individual whether an action anticipated in thought is for the sake of something) as well as systems that control appropriate behavioral routines, on the other hand. This view dramatically contrasts with classical and modern approaches to motivation. According to Freud and Lewin, it is the "steam" accumulated in the motivational engine that makes it move. The dynamics of motivation are described in terms of the energy level of the total system or of some critical subsystem. In contrast, Aristotle's model implies that the degree to which a thought can move the individual critically depends on the connectivity this thought has with subsystems that control the motivational meaning and with subsystems that control the execution of actions intended by that thought (Figure 3). Birch, Atkinson, and Bongort (1986) developed a similar model when they described the functional significance of thought for the instigation of behavior.

The theoretical significance of this definition of dynamic properties hardly can be overestimated. In my view, virtually all concepts we use, including motivational or even dynamic concepts, do not denote intersystemic connectivity. Instead, they describe the dynamic properties of single systems. Our dynamic concepts, like arousal, motivation, and memory activation, typically describe properties of single entities rather than relationships among entities. Well-known examples in personality research are constructs such as introversion, neuroticism, and anxiety. According to Eysenck (1967), introverts are not very sociable because they typically are overaroused and they avoid social contacts because they would boost their level of arousal beyond the optimum medium level. Neuroticism and anxiety are identified with the sensitivity of the limbic mechanism; for example, sensitivity of the punishment system (Gray, 1987).

There are some cognitive and some neurobiological approaches that differentiate global concepts of arousal, for instance, into sensory arousal versus motor activation (e.g., Pribram & McGuiness, 1992). There are also models that focus on connectivities among subsystems, for example, interactions between anterior and posterior attentional networks (Posner & Rothbart, 1992). However, none of these approaches takes into account anything similar to Aristotle's concept of motivation, which I interpret in terms of the modulation of connectivities among various subsystems through subcognitive mechanisms. Dynamic parameters that describe the connectivity among subsystems are not common in psychology. The construct of action versus state orientation that I mentioned is an exception: It describes an intersystemic modulation parameter. Prospective action orientation describes the extent to which a thought can become practical or, in functional terms, the extent to which the pathway between intention memory (i.e., the assumed locus of an action-related thought) and subsystems storing appropriate behavioral routines is energized or inhibited. A global form of arousal that activates all mental systems indiscriminately cannot explain the dynamic paradox suggested by the findings described in Figures 1 and 2: Why can goal representations or intentions be highly energized (as indicated by superior memory performance) without mechanisms controlling appropriate behaviors being energized as well? How can the passivity associated with depression or prospective state orientation be explained despite the high activational status of intentions in those individuals?

Activation of a system like intention memory can be strong and still the activation of its connection with other systems can be weak. A person can strongly intend to engage in a course of action, but lack the motivational energy to keep on track because the intention is not sufficiently connected with systems that provide meaning and/or practicality. In personality research, we should search not only for individual differences in the arousability of subsystems, but also for personality dispositions that affect the arousability of systems connections. As I point out later, the dissociability between the two types of arousability (i.e., arousability of systems versus arousability of the connection between systems) also can be explained on the basis of differential developmental conditions that affect arousability of systems versus arousability of systems connections (Kuhl, in press; Kuhl & Völker, 1998).

What are the specific mechanism terms like "energy flow" or "activation" referring to? We are talking about an intermediate level of analysis between the level of microactivations of cognitive contents (e.g., through priming) and the global level of arousal of the total system or of specific subsystems. How can we describe the mechanisms underlying motivational dynamics on this intermediate level? What are the rules according to which the relative activations of the pathways among the four macrosystems I mentioned are controlled? How can the functional characteristics of the four macrosystems be described in detail? How can we operationalize the dynamics of motivation, that is, the temporal changes of activation of each macrosystem? Finally, how can a theory of motivational dynamics resolve paradoxes like the one I mentioned (i.e., the finding that people suffering from an energy deficit such as depression or state-orientation seem to have more energy available for the activation of their goals and intentions)? I will now provide a brief outline of the theory of personality systems interactions (PSI theory) that I have developed to find some answers to these questions.

IV. PERSONALITY SYSTEMS INTERACTION THEORY

Before explaining some details of this theory, I should mention one important point in which it departs from traditional theorizing on human motivation. Traditionally, motivational psychology has been concerned with the determinants of goal-directed behavior rather than with the mechanics of the system that enables an organism to move toward aspired objects. Cognitive psychologists sometimes have criticized their motivational colleagues because the latter do not deal with the mechanisms underlying the control of behavior. The reason why motivational psychologists have not considered cognitive mechanisms essential to their work can be illustrated by the following example: When somebody has the task to predict the itineraries of a traveling salesman, he or she does not take the engine of the salesman's car apart to figure out how it works. This example illustrates the traditional partition of labor between cognitive and motivational psychology: Cognitive psychologists study the mechanics of the mental machinery, whereas motivational psychologists study its purposive aspects; that is, the determinants of goal-directed behavior.

According to my view, there is a fundamental flaw in this type of reasoning. If we want to develop a deeper understanding of motivation and volition, we have to part with this segregation of purpose and mechanism. The reason for this statement follows from my previous analysis: To the extent that a differentiated concept of motivational dynamics amounts to the changes in activation of cognitive macrosystems, we can no longer ignore those macrosystems. The point I wish to make is this: We cannot investigate the dynamics of motivation unless we develop some understanding of the cognitive macrosystems whose dynamic interactions we wish to explore. The transition from global concepts of energy to more specific concepts of energy flow among mental macrosystems forces us to abandon the traditional partition of labor. Specifically, we need to develop an understanding of some functional characteristics of the two elementary macrosystems that support object recognition and performance of behavioral routines, and the two high-level macrosystems that support implicit self-representations, on the one hand, and explicit representations of behavioral intentions, on the other hand. We cannot accomplish a better understanding of the energy flow among these systems without developing a better understanding of their nature.

How much can we learn from cognitive science about the four systems? The first pair of systems relates to phenomena investigated in various cognitive fields (i.e., object recognition and intuitive behavior control). Compared to them, the second pair of systems [i.e., intention memory (including explicit commitments and ideals) and extension memory (including self-representations and motives)] is located on a high level of integration addressed in the areas of personality and motivation rather than in cognitive science. However, in contrast to the cognitive approach, it is uncommon in the area of personality psychology to talk about high-level concepts such as the self in terms of systems whose mechanisms are to be analyzed. The concept of self (Baumeister & Tice, 1986; Kihlstrom & Klein, 1997; Markus & Nurius, 1986) is a good example for a hypothetical construct of personality theory that usually is not identified with a concrete mechanism, let alone with a neurobiological system. In PSI theory, both the two low-level and the two high-level systems are conceptualized in terms of cognitive–motivational macrosystems whose functional characteristics can be specified in some detail. Table 1 summarizes functional characteristics associated with each of the four motivationally relevant macrosystems. Each of these characteristics is supported by experimental research (see Kuhl, 1998) for an overview of relevant research) and is further discussed in the following section.

A. ELEMENTARY SYSTEMS: INTUITIVE BEHAVIOR CONTROL AND OBJECT RECOGNITION

What can we say about the functional characteristics of each of the four macrosystems? What do we know about the low-level system controlling object recognition and about the system controlling behavioral routines on an intuitive basis, that is, with little or no intervention of conscious intentions? Some functional characteristics of intuitive behavior control can be found in research on motor control (e.g., Jeannerod, 1994). Interesting details stem from research on organisms whose behavior is under

TABLE 1   Functional Characteristics of Four Cognitive Macrosystems

	Behavioral systems	Experiential systems
High-inferential systems	Intention memory (IM)/thinking (left hemispheric) • Analytical (critical feature) • Sequential • Vulnerable • Slow • Accurate • Decoupling from emotions	Extension memory (EM)/feeling (right hemispheric) • Holistic (family resemblance) • Parallel • Robust • Fast • Impressionistic • Close interaction with autonomic reactions
Low-inferential systems	Intuitive behavior control (IBC) • Contextual • Cross-modal • Presence and future oriented • Anticipation • Holistic • Robust	Object recognition (OR) • Decontextualized • Modality specific • Past oriented • Recognition • Analytical • Vulnerable

the control of intuitive mechanisms because they do not have explicit intentionality: Developmental research on motor learning in infants has yielded interesting insights into the functional details of mechanisms underlying intuitive control of behavior. One of the earliest intuitive behavior programs is already observable in neonates: It regulates emotional contagion and imitation of emotional expression (Meltzhoff & Moore, 1989, 1994). These programs seem to be an essential prerequisite for the later development of intuitive programs for social interaction (Keller, Gauda, Miranda, & Schölmerich, 1985; Papoušek & Papoušek, 1987). High integration of contextual information from within and across various modalities is one of the characteristics in which systems underlying intuitive behavior control differ from object perception systems (Table 1): Whereas systems supporting intuitive behavior integrate information from various modalities and context information within modalities, systems underlying object recognition keep information from various modalities separate and yield object representations that are rather independent of and constant across various contextual variations (e.g., recognizing the identity of an object independent of its distance, its color, or its luminance).

The focus on recognition of objects that are identical to templates that have been stored in the past is the reason why object recognition is characterized by an orientation toward the past, whereas intuitive behavior control is characterized by present and future orientations (Table 1). The mechanisms underlying parallel distributed processing in on-line sensorimotor control are rather robust (Table 1): Degraded input can be handled as long as it has some family resemblance with the procedural knowledge available (Rumelhart & McClelland, 1986).

B. HIGH-LEVEL SYSTEMS: INTENTION MEMORY AND ANALYTICAL THINKING VERSUS EXTENSION MEMORY AND INTUITIVE FEELING

Analytical Thinking and the Memory for Explicit Intentions

What can we say about the functional characteristics of high-level macrosystems such as intention memory and self-representations? Interestingly, the dualism of intuitive and analytical styles also occurs on the level of higher-order cognitive processing: Analytical thinking shares its precision-oriented nature with object perception, whereas holistic feeling has the global and holistic type of processing in common with intuitive behavior control. A particularly important component of analytical thinking relates to the ability to form explicit representations of intended actions. Research demonstrating a neurobiological basis of intention memory shows that a memory for intended actions (set) can be separated from working memory (Fuster, 1995). According to the PSI theory, intention memory stores explicit, consciously accessible representations of anticipated action sequences, whereas working memory typically stores sensory information that includes cues that signal opportunities for executing intentions. Explicit representation of sequences of intended actions are attributed to left-hemispheric (prefrontal) processing (Knight & Grabowecky, 1995).

In a recent series of studies exploring additional characteristics that intention memory does not share with working memory, we came to the conclusion that intention memory is characterized by a special mechanism that controls facilitation and inhibition of the pathway between its analytical or verbal representations of intended actions and systems that control behavioral routines for performing such actions (Kuhl & Kazén, in press). In a broader context, we can regard intention memory as a pivotal part of a network of subsystems that underlie analytical thinking, verbal processing, and other functions that support planning (Shallice, 1988). Planning and explicit representation of an intended action are necessary whenever intuitive programs are not available to reach a goal; that is, whenever a problem needs to be solved or when the system has to delay responding until an appropriate situation for performing an intended action is encountered. In these situations, it is useful to maintain an explicit representation of an intended action active in memory until it can be performed; that is, until the difficulty to enact the intention is removed. I have called this condition for volitional control of action *difficulty of enactment* (Kuhl, 1984). Inhibition of the pathway between intention memory and the intuitive behavior control system now can be explained as an inherent function of intention memory: Because this memory system is designed for situations in which an intended action cannot (or should not) be carried out yet, inhibition of the pathway to behavior control systems can be considered to be an integral functional component of intention memory.

Feeling and the Implicit Memory for Self-Representations

The second high-level macrosystem has been widely neglected in psychological research. Like intuitive behavior control, it relates to the concept of intuition. Personality psychologists have claimed for many decades that there is a form of unconscious information processing that differs from analytical thinking: Freud's primary as opposed to secondary process, Jung's "feeling" as opposed to "thinking," McClelland's (1985) implicit versus explicit motives, and Epstein's distinction between experiential and analytical thinking styles (Epstein, Pacini, Denes-Raj, & Heier, 1996) are examples of intuitive processing. However, these concepts do not go very far to spell out the specific mechanisms in which the two types of processes differ, let alone specify differences among high-level versus low-level intuitive systems.[3] A few decades ago, cognitive psychologists did not see any reason to distinguish the mechanisms underlying intuition

---

[3]It can be shown that the experiential system of Epstein et al. (1996) relates to an elementary intuitive system rather than to the high-level system called feeling here (cf. Kuhl, 1998a).

from analytical problem solving that could be simulated on a computer: Intuitive problem solving was considered nothing else but fast, automatized analytical problem solving (Simon & Simon, 1978). I challenged that position at a time when there were no tools for modeling intuition in computer models and when experimental techniques for studying intuition were very limited (Kuhl, 1983).

Both limitations have been overcome in recent research on what is called *parallel-holistic processing* (e.g., Beeman et al., 1994; Smith & Shapiro, 1989) and *implicit learning* (Goschke, 1997; Nissen & Bullemer, 1987; Reber & Squire, 1994). Moreover, advances made in computer modeling of parallel-distributed processing (Rumelhart & McClelland, 1986) enable us today to spell out the differences between sequential-analytical thinking and intuitive-holistic processing in great detail. On the basis of these models, we can explain why intuitive processing (on both elementary and higher-order levels of processing) is faster than analytical processing and why intuitive processing nonetheless integrates much more information, is much more robust (e.g., in dealing with incomplete input), and is more flexible than analytical processing (see Kuhl, 1998a, for a discussion of this research in the context of PSI theory).

Even the neurobiological mechanisms underlying these functional distinctions are being investigated today: Functional and even neuroanatomical differences between the left and right hemispheres of the brain help explain why the two types of processing are so different (Bradshaw, 1989). The neuroanatomical organization of the left hemisphere is comparable to an ensemble of many highly specialized "experts" rather than a global network that integrates information from a vast variety of input systems: Compared to the right hemisphere, the left hemisphere consists of a greater number of rather small neuronal networks, each having a higher dentritic arborization than the more extended right hemispheric networks (Scheibel et al., 1985). High specialization, combined with low integration is also a feature that characterizes analytical people whose left hemisphere dominates cognitive processing. Analytical thinking is characterized by high competition between rather than integration of alternatives: An object is either good or bad, useful or useless, whereas holistic processing is better equipped to integrate seemingly contradictory aspects of an object or a person.

How can high-level and low-level intuitive processing be distinguished? In the context of a theory of personality, I have especially emphasized one aspect in which high-level intuitive processing (i.e., feeling) differs from the low-level intuitive system discussed earlier (i.e., intuitive behavior control): According to my view, high-level intuitive-holistic processing forms the basis of implicit *self-representations*; that is, integrated representations of internal states such as needs, emotions, somatic feelings (e.g., muscle tensions), and values. This assumption breaks with traditional views in personality psychology: It adds a highly sophisticated nonconscious system to Freud's and Jung's rather archaic unconscious, and it differs from current conceptions of self in its implicit nature: Whereas approaches to the concept of self that can be found in current personality and social psychology relate to explicit beliefs about the self, PSI theory postulates an implicit or "intuitive" knowledge base that integrates an extended network of representations of own states, including personal preferences, needs, emotional states, options for action in particular situations, and past experiences involving the self (cf. the concept of autonoetic consciousness: Tulving, 1985; Wheeler, Stuss, & Tulving, 1997).[4]

Because of the extended nature of the networks underlying self-representations, the memory system that supports implicit self-representations is called *extension memory* (Table 1): Whenever this system participates in decision making and action, one can be sure that a great number of needs, preferences, values, and other self-aspects are taken into account on the basis of multiple-constraint satisfaction principles that describe parallel processing (see Smith, 1996, for a summary of PDP models applicable to personality research). That right-hemispheric processing provides more extended semantic networks was demonstrated in an elegant experiment on "summation priming" (Beeman et al., 1994): Three words that had weak pairwise semantic relationships, but were highly associated when taken as a whole (e.g., foot; cry; glass) were contrasted with word triples that did not have such a configurational or summation effect (e.g., dog, church, phone). The configurational triples yielded a priming effect on a subsequent target word that was related to the configurational meaning of the triple: The target word (e.g., cut) was identified faster when it was preceded by the configurational triple than when it was preceded by a control triple. Most importantly, the summation priming was substantially stronger when the target word was shown in the left visual field; that is, when the right hemisphere had a processing advantage. This finding confirms the assumption that, compared to the left hemisphere, the right hemisphere provides more extended semantic networks, resulting in superior detection of holistic and configurational relationships between a pattern of objects perceived. From a motivational perspective, this capacity can help an individual confronted with a new situation to find, within milliseconds, an action that is in accordance with a variety of self-aspects, without the necessity to check explicitly each particular self-aspect in a

---

[4]Tulving and his associates explored episodic memory and autonoetic consciousness in terms of consciously accessible information about autobiographical experiences (Wheeler et al., 1997). The connection I propose between high-level implicit self-representations and autonoetic consciousness is based on the assumption that conscious representations of self-related experiences are based on an unconscious background or "context" memory (cf. Baars, 1988). The relationship between this implicit context memory, which places constraints on what can become conscious, bears some similarity to Freud's concept of the preconscious.

sequential way. This is to say that access to an implicit self-system enables self-determined action in the sense described by humanistic psychology (Maslow, 1970; Rogers, 1961) and, more recently, in self-determination theory (Deci & Ryan, 1991).

Extension Memory and Self-Regulation of Affect

As a final comment on the functional characteristics of extension memory and the self-system, I would like to emphasize its close connectedness with the autonomic system (Table 1). In fact, the right hemisphere of the brain is much better equipped to elicit and inhibit emotional reactions than the left hemisphere (Dawson & Schell, 1982; Gainotti, 1989). Presenting a romantic movie to the right hemisphere by keeping it in the left visual field elicits a considerably higher amplitude of autonomic responses (e.g., changes in blood pressure) than producing a left-hemispheric advantage in processing the movie (Wittling, 1990). I use the term "feeling" to express this additional aspect of the mechanism underlying implicit self-representations and other contents of extension memory. This term (which Jung used as one of his rational functions) nicely combines the cognitive and the emotional components of the particular type of implicit knowledge to which I wish to refer. Besides its reference to emotional states, the term "feeling" denotes tacit knowledge. When we cannot explain how we perform a certain task or how we arrived at a particular solution, we refer to an intuitive feeling (I don't know how I did it, I just feel it is right this way). In clinical practice, the asymmetry between the two hemispheres in its connectedness with affect-generating systems provides an explanation of the fact that explaining an emotional problem analytically usually does not suffice to cope with the emotional reactions associated with it: To the contrary, because the left hemisphere is characterized by a high degree of decoupling between cognition and emotion (Wittling, 1990), analyzing a problem without transforming the outcome of this analysis into "felt experience" can make it even more difficult to cope with emotionally (Perls, 1973).

The most important implication of the assumption that self-representations are based on implicit, right-hemispheric processes relates to self-regulation of affect. The close interaction between right-hemispheric activity and emotional processes explains a multitude of findings that suggest that access to differentiated self-representations (e.g., Linville, 1987) and intrinsically motivated self-determined action based on such representations (Deci & Ryan, 1991) are positively related to emotional support of self-determined action in educational, marital, and many other settings, which in turn is positively related to indices of psychological and physical well-being (Brunstein, 1993; Ryan, Kuhl, & Deci, 1997; Sheldon & Kasser, 1998). The capacity for affect regulation associated with the feeling system is important for another reason: It is one of the functional properties in which the two intuitive systems differ. Although intuitive behavior control and feeling share the characteristics of parallel-distributed processing (e.g., speed, robustness), the former does not have the affect regulation capacity associated with the latter. On the basis of this and several other arguments, it can be shown that the holistic-experiential (as opposed to analytical) system of Epstein et al. (1996) seems to capture a component of intuitive behavior control rather than feeling: Their measure of "intuitive style" is associated with naive and esoteric thinking patterns (Epstein et al., 1996, Table 3) and is not associated with measures of active, action-oriented emotional coping.

The Neurobiological Basis of Self-Relaxation

The neurobiological mechanisms underlying the important relationships between self-determination and psychological as well physical well-being are being revealed in current research on the stress-reducing function of the hippocampus (Sapolsky, 1992). There is an increasing consensus among neuroscientists that the common aspect to the various functions of the hippocampus relates to its capacity to form an enormous number of instantaneous and organized associations among sensations from the external and internal world (Jacobs & Nadel, 1985; Sutherland & Rudy, 1989). Tolman's concept of cognitive maps nicely expresses the holistic characteristics of hippocampal functions. According to recent research and connectionistic modeling, the hippocampus supports all cognitive (neocortical) systems that integrate many isolated pieces of information into a coherent representation that provides an organized overview of perceptual, spatial, and cognitive representations (McClelland, Mc-Naughton, & O'Reilly, 1995; Squire, 1992). It seems plausible to assume that the coherence-producing function of the hippocampus relates not only to the representation of external, but also of internal environments. Integrated self-representations can be regarded as holistic representations of "inner environments" (emotions, needs, values etc.). This extrapolation of the findings concerning hippocampal functions has the advantage that it explains why activation of self-representations facilitates downregulation[5] of negative affect and other adverse correlates of threatening and stressful experiences (Linville, 1987; Ryan, 1995; Sheldon & Kasser, 1998): Activa-

[5]The term "downregulation" denotes an active, self-regulatory process through which affect intensity is reduced. Throughout this chapter, this term is preferred to more common terms (e.g., controlling anger or coping with sadness) because the latter often are interpreted in terms of conscious attempts to control emotions, whereas downregulation relates to largely unconsciously operating mechanisms. The term "downregulation" per se is not confined to a particular mechanism through which negative affect is reduced. The second modulation assumption refers only to one of several mechanisms that serve this purpose (i.e., reducing negative affect through activation of relevant self-representations). Another example of a mechanism that reduces negative affect is an acquired disposition to replace negative affect by positive affect without accessing relevant self-representations.

tion of the hippocampus causes a downregulation of cortisol concentration in response to stress (Sapolsky, 1992). To the extent that hippocampal activity is needed for construing an on-line model of self-interests (as for many other configurational representations), we can understand why activation of self-representations reduces stress and its many adverse consequences. Moreover, findings that demonstrate inhibition of hippocampal activity when stress levels exceed a critical threshold (Pavlides, Watanabe, Magarinos, & McEwen, 1995) might shed some light upon the neurobiological mechanisms underlying the second modulation assumption of PSI theory, which states that critical levels of negative affect that cannot be downregulated inhibit access to self-representations. These modulation assumptions that form the core of PSI theory are explained now.

C. AFFECT–COGNITION MODULATION

Now that I have provided a rough sketch of the four most important macrosystems involved in the mechanics of goal-directed action, the interrupted task of developing a differentiated view of energy flow can be resumed. As can be seen from Figure 4, the energy flow among the four macrosystems is described in terms of mutual antagonistic relationships: Like the muscles enabling a human arm to bend and stretch, the four macrosystems work together on the basis of reciprocal antagonisms (depicted by dashed lines in Figure 4): The more strongly one system is activated, the more strongly it inhibits the activation of adjacent systems. To keep the presentation simple, not all antagonistic effects are depicted

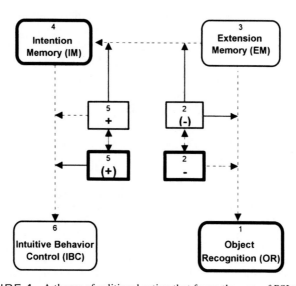

FIGURE 4   A theory of volitional action that forms the core of PSI theory.

in the figure: The figure shows top-down inhibition (indicated by dashed lines) of intuitive behavior control as a function of the activational strength of intention memory (delayed responding or impulse control), top-down inhibition of object recognition as a function of activational strength of extension memory and integrated self-representations (repression of unwanted perceptions), and a suppression of intention memory as a function of the strength of extension memory (EM) activation (e.g., refraining from conscious goal pursuit and planning after activation of implicit self-representations in EM). The reverse antagonisms (not depicted in Figure 4) also hold (if included in the figure, the modulatory effects from affective states also would have to be reversed). For example, the more strongly someone focuses on an explicit goal by maintaining its representation active in intention memory, the more difficult it can become to access extension memory. Inhibition of intuitive behavior control (IBC) through activation of intention memory explains the introductory paradox: Prospective state orientation and, to a much stronger extent, depression, are associated with frequent failure to initiate intended actions, because explicit representations of uncompleted intentions are excessively maintained active in intention memory. According to this interpretation, depression is attributable to the excessive operation of a mechanism that is normally adaptive because it helps maintain a difficult intention in mind and delay action until a problem is solved or a good opportunity is encountered: The inhibition of the pathway between intention memory and its intuitive output system normally helps avoid premature action. The antagonistic relationship between intention and extension memories (Figure 4) explains rigidity: Alternative goals or actions are difficult to perceive in the case of a strong activation of intention memory, because intention memory causes an underactivation of extension memory, that is, of the system that normally provides extended networks of possible actions and possible selves: As a result, people who focus too hard on explicit goals or intentions cannot think easily of alternative actions should the chosen path fail.

What role do positive and negative affects play in this dynamic flow of activation among cognitive macrosystems? There is a wide consensus in psychology concerning the process of affect generation: Affects arise either on the basis of innate or acquired needs and conditioned responses to a variety of stimuli that need not even be consciously processed (Zajonc, 1980) or they are generated on the basis of elaborated cognitive evaluation of an event in terms of predictability and controllability (Lazarus, 1984). As mentioned before, these two sources of affect generation can be integrated (Kuhl, 1983; LeDoux, 1995). According to PSI theory, affects modulate the (antagonistic) dynamic relationships between macrosystems, quite in the sense that I have defined the term "dynamic" in the context of Aristotle's theory of motivation: In addition to the content-specific effects of affects in regulating approach and avoidance motivation (Atkinson &

Birch, 1970; Elliot & Church, 1997; Lewin, 1935), affects also have a dynamic significance because they strengthen or release inhibitory activational relationships among macrosystems. The two core assumptions of PSI theory describe this dynamic significance of affective processes in terms of the subcognitive mechanisms that modulate the changes in activation of the pathways among macrosystems.

1. First Modulation Assumption (Volitional Facilitation Assumption). Positive affect (A+) releases the inhibition of the pathway between intention memory (IM) and the intuitive behavior control (IBC) system, whereas downregulated (inhibited) positive affect [A(+)] facilitates maintenance of intentions in IM by strengthening the inhibitory relationship between IM and IBC.

2. Second Modulation Assumption (Self-Facilitation Assumption). Downregulation of negative affect [A(−)] facilitates access to integrated self-representations and other contents of extension memory (EM) by strengthening the inhibitory effect extension memory has on sensory input stemming from unexpected or unwanted information provided by the object recognition system (OR).

Unconscious Volition

PSI theory specifies the conditions that determine the energy level of each cognitive macrosystem and the conditions facilitating information exchange among antagonistic systems. For example, information flow from intention memory (IM) to its output systems (IBC) is facilitated if an affective change from low positive affect to positive affect takes place. This affect-modulated flow of information among systems is not assumed to be dependent on conscious control of behavior. Therefore, PSI theory extends action control theory (Kuhl, 1984) by spelling out unconscious components of volitional processes. This is to say that the extended theory departs from everyday conceptions of willful action (volition) by postulating several unconscious components of what we normally consider a largely conscious process, according to our daily introspections: Accessing extension memory and integrated self-representations (e.g., through downregulation of negative affect) is regarded as a largely unconscious process, activating intuitively available programs to enact intentions (e.g., through activation of positive affect) does not require a conscious process, and so forth.

Besides descriptions of the functional profiles of the four macrosystems, PSI theory contains five additional modulation assumptions. It is beyond the scope of this presentation to provide a detailed description of these assumption and the phenomena explained by them (see Kuhl, 1998a, for a more detailed account). A brief overview may suffice (Table 2). In a

TABLE 2   Modulation Assumptions of PSI Theory and Some Applications[a]

Modulation assumptions	Applications (explained throughout the chapter)	Relevant studies
1. Volitional facilitation: A + → [IBC * IM]	Interaction: Personality × Zeigarnik Stroop removal	Atkinson (1953); Johnson et al. (1983) Kuhl & Kazén (in press)
2. Self facilitation (vs. inhibition of access to self-representations and other components of EM through A −):	Alienation Self-infiltration	Klinger (1977); Kuhl & Beckmann (1994b) Kuhl & Kazén (1994a)
A(−) → [EM/OR]	Interaction: Personality × Yerkes−Dodson	Atkinson (1974); Eysenck (1967)
3. Volitional inhibition: IM → A(+)	Self-discrepancy Intention superiority Procrastination [cf. entry 1]	Higgins (1987) Goschke & Kuhl (1993) Beswick & Man (1994)
4. Self-relaxation (vs. emotional sensitization): EM → A(−)	Uncontrollable Rumination [See also entry 2]	Kuhl & Baumann (in press); Martin & Tesser, 1989; Nolen−Hoeksema et al. (1994)
5. Self-motivation: EM → A +	Intrinsic motivation Incentive escalation	Deci & Ryan (1991) Beckmann & Kuhl (1984)
6. Systems conditioning (Figure 5)	Development of self-regulation of affect	Kuhl & Völker (1998); Kuhl (1998)
7. Self-actualization: A + ← EM & IM → A(+)	Emotional dialectics Volitional efficiency	Oettingen (1997); Fuhrmann
A − ← IM & EM → A(−)	Self-growth	& Kuhl (1998)

[a]Symbols: A + = positive affect; A(+) = inhibition of positive affect; A − = negative affect; A(−) = inhibition of negative affect (downregulation); IM = intention memory; EM = extension memory; IBC = intuitive behavior control; OR = object recognition; → = increases; ← = is increased by; ↔ = increases and is increased by; [X * Y] = facilitatory pathway connecting system X and system Y; [X/Y] = inhibitory pathway between system X and Y.

nutshell, the additional assumptions describe reversals and extensions of the first two modulation assumptions.

   3. Volitional Inhibition.   The third modulation assumption is the reversal of the first: Activation of intention memory reduces positive affect (volitional inhibition). This part of PSI theory provides a possible mechanism underlying Higgins's (1987) findings, which showed that confronting individuals with information related to ideal self-aspects reduced their positive affective states: Thinking of ideal self-aspects (i.e., something one would like to be) should increase the risk that intention memory is overloaded with unrealistic intentions, which in turn should reduce positive affect, according to the volitional inhibition assumption (Table 2). Kuhl & Helle's (1986) finding that state-oriented as well as depressed participants enacted fewer intentions after induction of an uncompleted intention is attributed to the same mechanism.

4. Self-Relaxation. The fourth modulation assumption is the reversal of the second: It describes downregulation of negative affect through the activation of extension memory mentioned earlier. This self-relaxation assumption can explain the therapeutical (i.e., distress-reducing) effect of engaging in creative work or of finding meaning in one's previous, present, or future life (Frankl, 1981; Klinger, 1977, in press; Perls, 1973): Any activity that capitalizes on the extended semantic networks provided by extension memory and the feeling system supported by it can help down-regulate negative affect. Finding meaning amounts to a search for config-urational information not unlike the type of processing studied in the aforementioned experiments on summation priming (Beeman et al., 1994): Finding a deeper meaning in a difficult personal experience (e.g., the death of a loved person) can be described in terms of constructing relationships between this experience and a variety of self-aspects (e.g., one's needs, one's strengths and weaknesses, and one's aspirations for the future), and discovering new personal implications that emerge from the configuration of all the self-aspects encountered. A great number of research findings are consistent with the view that the right hemisphere supports the global and extended type of information processing that also is associated with implicit self-representations, according to PSI theory (Bradshaw, 1989; Hellige, 1990; Tucker & Williamson, 1984). The prefrontal region of the right hemisphere seems to be especially relevant for the self-representa-tional portion of extension memory, including integrated memories of personal experiences (autonoetic consciousness: Wheeler, et al., 1997). I already mentioned some of the evidence that demonstrates how strongly the right hemisphere is involved in the control of emotional responses, as reflected, for example, in right-hemispheric superiority in the control of cardiovascular responses (Posner & Rothbart, 1992; Wittling, 1990) and skin conductance (Dawson & Schell, 1982). In light of the theoretical and empirical arguments that suggest a close interaction between the hip-pocampus and neocortical systems involved in the construction of configu-rational knowledge (McClelland et al., 1995; Sutherland & Rudy, 1989), the stress-reducing function of the hippocampus (Sapolsky, 1992) can become associated indirectly with the activation of those neocortical systems as well.

For the present purposes, it is not necessary to analyze the details of the complex processes involved in these systems interactions. However, it is important to acknowledge these findings from cognitive and neuroscience research because they define constraints for the formulation of psychologi-cal models of affect regulation: The accessibility of an extended semantic network that provides integrated representations of external and internal (self-related) contexts (i.e., extension memory) should be considered an important determinant of the capacity for self-relaxation. Empirical research is consistent with this assumption. For example, in a study by Linville (1987), the interaction between life stress and self-complexity as assessed, for instance, on the basis of the number of distinct features with which participants described themselves was a significant predictor of subsequent indices of subjective stress, psychosomatic complaints, and depressive symptoms. Other examples for this type of coping can be found in research on mastery orientation (Dweck, 1986) and in the study of active coping styles that transform threats to one's self-esteem aroused by difficult tasks into the experience of challenges that are associated with moderate degrees of negative emotionality and with facilitation of performance. The second modulation assumption provides an explanation of these facilitatory effects: The very system that helps reduce negative affect (i.e., extension memory) provides extended semantic networks that facilitate performance, especially in tasks that draw upon remote associations and creative solutions.

5. Self-Motivation. The fifth modulation assumption describes self-motivation, that is, the generation of positive affect associated with a goal or an activity on the basis of activation of appropriate self-representations (e.g., values associated with the activity). The mechanism described in this assumption provides an explanation of the positive effects of intrinsic motivation and self-determination on emotional well-being (Deci & Ryan, 1991; Kuhl, in press; Sheldon & Elliot, in press): According to the self-motivation assumption, intrinsic motivation critically depends on the accessibility of the self-system. There are many empirical findings that demonstrate that the value or positive affect associated with an object increases once a decision for that object has been made. For example, Langer (1975) found that people who were given free lottery tickets and later were asked to sell them requested considerably higher prices for them (i.e., an average of $8.67) if they had been given a free choice to select their ticket compared to a group who had received an experimenter-selected ticket ($1.96). Similar increases in value were obtained in quite different settings provided the conditions were conducive to the activation of the self-system, for example, through free choice like in Langer's experiment (Festinger & Walster, 1964) or through other conditions: Participants accepted the arguments of a message more (e.g., rate them more positively) if they were induced to argue in favor of them in a role play (Janis & King, 1954). According to PSI theory, these and many similar phenomena can be attributed to a common self-regulatory mechanism: The top-down generation of positive affect toward an object once its relevance for an activated self-aspect has been detected (self-motivation).

This is to say that one common mechanism can explain a diversity of phenomena that have been attributed to quite different mechanisms such as "illusion of control" (Langer, 1975) or reductions of cognitive dissonance (Festinger & Walster, 1964).

PSI theory extends the range of conditions that facilitate self-motivation to any situation that activates the self. According to the second modulation assumption (self-facilitation), arousal of negative affect (conscious or not) should activate the self as long as it can be downregulated by the individual. Experiments (Festinger & Carlsmith, 1959) that show increases in perceived value (increased liking of a boring experiment) after induction of insufficient justification (e.g., receiving low pay for participation) can be interpreted in this way. According to this view, people increased their evaluation of a boring activity not to reduce the cognitive dissonance between contradictory beliefs (e.g., I have participated in this experiment for little money versus the experiment is boring), but because being underpaid induces a mild increase in negative affect, whose downregulation activates the self system (including all mechanisms associated with it such as self-motivation). Self-motivation not only helps people to become involved in tasks that are not attractive in themselves, but it also facilitates decision making: Beckmann and Kuhl (1984) found that participants who scored high on prospective action orientation (i.e., low on hesitation), showed gradual increases of a tentatively preferred apartment during the decision-making process, even though no new information concerning the apartments offered for rent was introduced. This finding confirms the theoretical interpretation of prospective action orientation mentioned earlier: Apparently, initiative is related to a mechanism that actively recruits facilitatory energy once a self-based decision to do something has been made.

6. *Systems Conditioning.*   How does the degree of participation of the self-system in action control develop? According to the systems-conditioning assumption of PSI theory, whenever two subsystems are repeatedly activated within a time window, the pathway between the two systems is strengthened. This generalization from classical conditioning to the conditioning of intersystemic pathways is to explain the development of self-relaxation and self-motivation, the two major forms in which the self-system modulates affect and behavior. How can systems conditioning be compared to classical conditioning? The analogy is based on two assumptions. First, the expression of negative or positive affect is associated with an activation of the self-system. Second, there are external cues that have a "prewired" (unconditioned) effect on affect regulation: A mother's encouraging vocalizations or her initiation of eye contact facilitates positive affect, whereas her reassuring vocalization and her touching the baby inhibits negative affect. Whenever maternal responses that downregulate

or arouse negative or positive affects, respectively, follow the child's expression of negative or positive affect supposedly mediated by an activation of the self-system (e.g., when the child is bothered by or interested in an object), the association between the child's self-system and downregulation or arousal of affect is strengthened (Figure 5). As a result, the child acquires the capacity to downregulate negative affect or activate positive affect without external stimulation of affect-generating systems.

In a similar way, positive affect gradually comes under the control of the self-system when positive self-expressions (e.g., the baby is looking toward an interesting object or the first-grader shows interest in the first words he or she can write) are answered promptly and adequately by another person. The positive affect that is automatically elicited by the

Classical Conditioning:
Formation of new S-R Associations

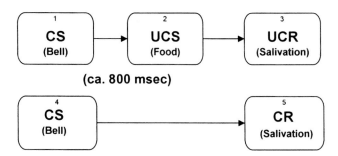

Systems Conditioning:
Formation of New Associations Among Systems

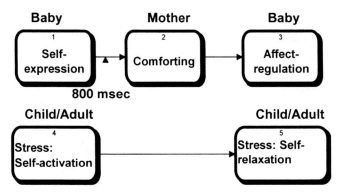

FIGURE 5   The systems-conditioning model.

friendly gesture of an interaction partner becomes conditioned upon the self-system provided the self was activated shortly before and the response semantically matches the self-expression. A positive treatment that does not occur in response to a self-expression cannot have this effect. In other words, during development, whenever a sufficient number of opportunities are encountered for associating activation of the self with the elicitation of positive or the downregulation of negative affect, the self acquires the capacity to control positive and negative affects, respectively. To the extent that the self-system participates in the regulation of positive affect, more aspects of an individual's needs, values, affects, and so forth are taken into consideration whenever he or she is pursuing a goal. According to this model, an excessive tendency toward non-self-determined extrinsic motivation (e.g., striving for money, status symbols, or other material goals) can be attributed to a weak connectivity between the self-system and subcognitive systems involved in the generation of positive affect (Gray, 1987).

The systems-conditioning model specifies the functional basis of autonomy-supporting conditions, which presumably facilitate self-determined action (Ryan, 1995): These conditions can now be characterized by temporally contingent and behaviorally adequate responding to the self-expressions of the child. Similar assumptions are described by the concept of responsivity in attachment research (Bowlby, 1969) or by the psychoanalytical concept of mirroring the child's self-expressions (Kohut, 1985). Parental reliance on controlling conditions (that undermine self-determination and intrinsic motivation; Deci & Ryan, 1991) can be regarded as a special case of a failure to respond adaquately and contingently to the child's self-expressions: When caretakers induce or force a child to do something, they do not respond to the child's self-expressions. In connection with the sixth assumption (Table 2), which describes how the connectivity between the self-system and affect-generating subcognitive systems develops in early childhood (i.e., the systems-conditioning assumption), the self-motivation assumption explains why "money does not make happy" (as a German proverb says): A rather short-lived and shallow satisfaction is typically associated with goal attainment that is not mediated through self-activation; in other words, with goal attainment that is "extrinsically" motivated according to the terminology of self-determination theory (Deci & Ryan, 1991), because the satisfaction is confined to the concrete goal at hand unless it is integrated in an implicit self-representational structure connecting it with various needs of the organism. A model that describes part of the extended network of self-aspects that underlie self-determination was proposed by Sheldon and Kasser (1995). Whenever goals are perceived to be integrated in and supported by an individual's self-representational system, people invest more time and effort, feel less exhausted, are more persistent, and are more successful in pusuing their goals (Sheldon & Elliot, 1998).

How can the beneficial effects of self-determination be explained from a functional design point of view? PSI theory provides a simple explanation based on the operation of a common mechanism. Whenever the self-system does not participate in the selection and performance of behavior, the affective consequences of goal attainment are rather local, that is, they are confined to a brief consummatory episode related to goal attainment: In this case, every affective response requires another goal attainment episode. In contrast, participation of the self-system in the instigation of behavior provides a more extended activation of associated affect, temporally and motivationally. This double extendedness of the affective consequences of self-determined behavior can be derived from the two major functional characteristics of the self-system: According to PSI theory, the self-system is conceived of (1) as an implicit background monitoring system whose operation is not confined to conscious episodes (e.g., those elicited by attainment of explicitly represented goals) and (2) as being supported by an extended network of needs, values, and many other self-aspects. This explains the greater satisfaction derived from intrinsic, self-determined goals: Participation of the self-system in goal selection and performance provides access to a great variety of self-aspects, each of which can contribute positive affect to the activity in question. Finally, the satisfaction derived from a self-determined activity should last longer than satisfaction derived from attainment of an extrinsic goal (temporal extension of satisfaction), and self-determined activity should reach deeper into the need and values structure of the organism (spatial extension of satisfaction). Both the temporal and the spatial extendedness of the positive affect can be attributed to the operational characteristics of extension memory and self-representations that are considered part of it: Extension memory is a background monitoring system that provides temporally persisting connections with a great variety of even remote (deep) structures.

Preference for Symbiotic Relationships

In a similar vein, the systems-conditioning assumption combined with the self-relaxation assumption explains why some people have problems accepting their partners' emotional autonomy or why some students need more emotional support from their teachers than others. In accordance with predictions derived from PSI theory, personality styles characterized by an impaired capacity for self-relaxation (i.e., impaired downregulation of negative feelings like frustration or loneliness) are associated with problems in relationships, because of a preference for symbiotic forms of interactions; that is, interactions that do not leave much room for the partners' emotional autonomy. The partner is not allowed to have his or her own emotions because he or she is needed as an external regulator of the other partner's emotional well-being. In positive cases in which a person's need for external mood regulation is met by the responsiveness of a loving partner or an understanding teacher, deficits in affect regulation acquired during childhood should be remedied as common wisdom suggests (e.g., the fairy tale prince who rescues the neglected young girl). In a recent study (Gunsch, 1996), a particular form of state orientation that is related to uncontrollable rumination after exposure to aversive events (i.e., failure-related state orientation or preoccupation) was among the personality styles associated with symbiotic preferences, that is, preferences for the partner not to have emotions and emotional developments of his or her own. This aspect of state orientation is assessed on the basis of reports of uncontrollable ruminations. The self-relaxation assumption also explains, in combination with the second modulation assumption, why the same type of individuals suffer from uncontrollable intrusive thoughts and have an increased tendency to mistake others' expectations and preferences as their own (self-infiltration; Kuhl & Kazén, 1994a): To the extent that these individuals cannot downregulate the negative affect associated with aversive events, stressful life events make them lose access to integrated self-representations that are necessary to identify and reject self-alien (unwanted) thoughts or social demands.

Rumination versus Repression

Unimpeded access to the self-system also is needed to inhibit unwanted perceptions and thoughts effectively, that is, before they reach conscious awareness. Self-reports of frequent uncontrollable ruminations are used to assess a second form of state orientation that can interfere with volitional action in addition to the hesitation form of state orientation already discussed (Kuhl & Beckmann, 1994a). Suppression of unwanted thoughts through conscious mechanisms seems to be far less effective (Wegner, 1994) than repression through the activation of implicit self-representations at early stages of processing. The assumption that individuals that have a good self-relaxation ability (i.e., action-oriented individuals) repress unwanted thoughts before they reach consciousness was corroborated in a recent study: When aversive words (remindful of painful life events) were shown briefly before presentation of a task, action-oriented participants showed particular components of event-related potentials as early as 180 and 600 ms after word onset; that is, at stages of processing at which conscious attempts to suppress the word cannot be performed (Haschke & Kuhl, 1994). Our hypothesis that these components were related to action-oriented individuals' tendency to disregard unwanted information at early stages of processing was corroborated by the finding that these components disappeared when participants were instructed to pay explicit attention to the aversive material. The short time window of an event-related potential (ERP) associated with the downregulation of negative affect fits surprisingly well into the time range expected on the basis of the systems-conditioning model (Figure 5): Conditioning works best when the interval between UCS (here, self-expression) and CS (here, external cues regulating affect) is rather short, that is, below 1 s (Mazur, 1990). Evidence from attachment research highlights the importance of prompt (< 1 s) succession of maternal reactions to an infants self-expressions for the former to be effective (Papoušek & Papoušek, 1987). Children whose mothers consistently failed to respond to eye contact initiated by them when they were babies (10 to 14 weeks) within a time window of 800 ms cannot easily downregulate negative emotions later in childhood (Keller & Gauda, 1987).

To the extent that self-regulation of affect is based on a systems-conditioning mechanism that amounts to an internalization of a process that originally features prompt (responsive) external regulation of affect, it should be expected that the affect regulation process (i.e., self-relaxation or self-motivation) controlled by the self-system should happen within a similar time window. The ERP findings cited are consistent with this expectation: Action-oriented participants showed a strong response (P600) 600 ms after the onset of words that reminded them of negative life events: The strong response disappeared when the participants were asked to continue reflecting about those experiences once reminded of them (Haschke & Kuhl, 1994). In contrast, state-oriented individuals (who reported uncontrollable ruminations in everyday life) did not show the P600 response when instructed to suppress experiences aroused by the words or when instructed to focus upon such experiences. In accordance with the self-facilitation assumption (Table 2), another study (Rosahl, Tennigkeit, Kuhl, & Haschke, 1993) confirmed that action-oriented individuals showed superior performance after negative compared to neutral words when a complex memory task followed 3 s after exposure to the word. This is what should be expected if downregulation of negative affect facilitates the activation of self-representations and other contents of extension memory (that were presumably needed for the memory scanning task used in the Rosahl et al., 1993, study).

7. Self-Actualization.   Finally, the seventh modulation assumption (cf. Table 2) specifies *affective change* (i.e., the ability to switch between positive and negative affects associated with an object) as the basis for self-actualization with its two basic components: (1) *self-development* (i.e., integrating new experiences into a coherent self-representational system) and (2) *volitional efficiency* (enacting one's intentions). Self-development requires frequent shifts between negative states (e.g., allowing feelings of pain, weakness, or guilt to occur) and downregulation of negative states through activation of relevant self-structures (e.g., former experiences and needs or values that are relevant for the negative event encountered). According to the second modulation assumption, perseverating periods of unattenuated negative affect inhibit self-access. In addition to keeping the self-system from repressing new experiences that may be unexpected or even unwanted, inhibited self-access is expected to render integration of painful experiences within a coherent self-representational system difficult. This implication of the second modulation assumption explains why traumatic experiences can lead to dissociation of related memories from relevant self-representations: The individual cannot retrieve those experiences easily because they are encoded like unconnected "islands" that cannot be retrieved when relevant self-representations are activated. On the other hand, without occasional states of negative emotionality, the self-system would be active all the time (i.e., making a self-assertive personality), but it would have no opportunity to grow by integrating new experiences (a deficit that is associated with the antisocial personality disorder). Without occasional downregulation of negative affect, the system also would be unable to grow, but for a different reason: Isolated needs, preferences, affects, and other sensations constantly would be accumulated without being integrated in a coherent self-representation (resulting in a personality characterized by low self-esteem and fragmentation rather than integration of the many isolated self-experiences accumulated).

In sum, the basis for self-development is the capacity for emotional change as illustrated by the ability to shift between positive and negative sides of an object, of a personal experience, or of a goal on the basis of relevant self-representations (i.e., self-driven emotional dialectics). Personality styles or disorders associated with a tendency to avoid negative affect through generating positive affect in threatening situations (e.g., histrionic personality disorder) or through actionism (e.g., compulsive personality disorder) should be associated with retarded self-growth, according to the self-actualization assumption, just as personality styles or disorders presumably associated with an excessive tendency to activate self-representations for repressing negative emotions (e.g., antisocial and paranoid personality). A questionnaire assessing these and other personality styles that may be regarded as nonpathological analogs of personality disorders was used recently to test assumptions derived from a model that defines each style or disorder in terms of a combination of high or low sensitivity for positive and negative affect, respectively, and the dominant macrosystem expected on the basis of the modulation assumptions (Kuhl & Kazén, 1997). Consistent with expectations, styles associated with high sensitivity for negative affect (e.g., avoidant and dependent) were negatively correlated with the ability to think of some positive aspect of personality features that had been rated as negative beforehand; moreover, these styles also were associated with a reduced capacity to form consistent and valid representation for one's own or one's partner's preferences. Reduced ability for positive reframing confirms the hypothesized fixation on negative affect, whereas impaired knowledge of self or others (alienation) confirms inhibited access to extension memory as predicted by the second modulation assumption.

Applying the self-actualization assumption to the action-control side of the model (i.e., the left half of Figure 4) relates affective change to volitional efficiency. According to the first modulation assumption, maintenance of a difficult intention in intention memory requires downregulation of positive affect, whereas its enactment requires the generation of positive affect at an appropriate time. Emotional fixation on positive affect or its inhibition developed in early childhood or later should interfere with the enactment or with the maintenance component, respectively. Constantly low positive affect should be associated with an (over-) efficient maintenance of difficult intentions (e.g., high ideals) in intention memory, but a low ability to act upon those intentions, whereas constantly high positive affect (conscious or not) should be associated with the opposite pattern. Hyperactivity can be regarded as an example for the latter case. Hyperkinetic children's difficulty maintaining a chosen course of action (through maintaining the relevant intention active in intention memory and inhibiting premature action) can be attributed to their inability to downregulate positive affect aroused when interesting action alternatives are encountered (Barkley, 1997). On the other hand, depressed individuals who have problems generating positive mood have no problems maintaining uncompleted intentions and self-ideals active in memory (Higgins, 1987), but they do have problems acting according to their intentions (Kammer, 1994; Kuhl & Kazén, 1994b). According to the self-actualization assumption, an efficient cooperation of the two antagonistic systems involved in the enactment of difficult intentions (i.e., IM and IBC systems) requires a change between positive affect (e.g., through focusing on the attractive sides of a goal) and its downregulation (e.g., through focusing on the difficulties to be overcome). In accordance with (but unaware of) this derivation, Oettingen (1997) found in a series of studies that participants enacted more of their intentions when they were instructed to switch between positive fantasies about goal attainment and a focus on the difficulties of enactment (compared to control groups that were instructed to focus either on positive fantasies or on difficulties).

D. MICROANALYTIC TESTING OF DYNAMIC MODULATION EFFECTS

Despite the empirical research mentioned that supports the modulation assumptions, new methods have to be developed to assess modulation effects more and more directly. Miguel Kazén and I developed a method for examining the effects of brief (i.e., phasic) activations of personality systems such as affect generators and intention memory. Specifically, we modified the familiar Stroop task to investigate the microdynamics of personality systems interactions (Kuhl & Kazén, in press). In the familiar version of this task, response times are increased when individuals are asked to name the color of the ink in which an incongruent color word is printed (e.g., to say "green" when the word RED is printed in green ink), compared to a control condition in which the color of neutral stimuli (e.g., XXXX) is to be named. We chose this task because it requires participants to perform the two central operations addressed in the first modulation assumption: (1) maintain a difficult intention active in memory (i.e., name the color of the ink rather than read the color word) and (2) establish the connection between intention memory and relevant output systems. According to the volitional facilitation assumption (i.e., the first modulation assumption), the connection between intention memory and relevant output systems should be facilitated by positive affect. To the extent that intention memory is loaded with the difficult intention to name the color of the ink rather than perform the simpler response of reading the color word, brief presentation of positive words prior to the onset of the incongruent color word should facilitate performance. The data confirmed this reasoning. In fact, after presentation of positive words (e.g., love and success), participants often were even faster in the difficult condition (i.e., naming the ink color of incongruent color words) than in the easy condition (i.e., naming the color of XXXX). In other words, the well-known Stroop interference effect replicated in hundreds of experiments can be completely removed simply by using positive words as warning stimuli to announce the onset of the color words, provided special measures are taken to ensure that intention memory is loaded (Kuhl & Kazén, in press). Cognitive models of Stroop interference do not suffice for a full description of the processes involved. According to PSI theory, affective modulation of the pathways between cognitive macrosystems must be taken into account (Kuhl & Kazén, in press).

V. BACK TO THE FUTURE: FROM CONTENTS TO MECHANISMS

In this final section, I discuss several applications of the theory that may help delineate a perspective for future research on motivation and self-regulation. What opportunities does the dynamic theory I have outlined provide for future research? How does it explain familiar phenomena such as success-oriented individuals' preferences of intermediate risks, changes in cognitive beliefs induced in experiments on cognitive dissonance, or mood effects on attitude change through persuasion? What perspectives are opened by dynamic reinterpretations of familiar phenomena? After contrasting explanations based on mechanisms with traditional content-based explanations, I conclude with a description of new techniques for the assessment of self-regulatory functions.

A. REINTERPRETATION OF FAMILIAR PHENOMENA

Preference for Intermediate Risks

One of the basic findings of achievement motivation research relates to risk preference: Success-oriented individuals typically prefer intermediate levels of difficulty, whereas individuals who score high on fear of failure do not show this preference consistently (Atkinson & Feather, 1966; Heckhausen, 1977; Schneider, 1973). According to most theories, this phenomenon is attributable to some content of success-oriented individuals' beliefs. For example, people prefer intermediately difficult tasks because they believe that these tasks provide a realistic compromise between desirability, which is highest at very difficult tasks, and attainability of success, which is highest at easy tasks (Atkinson & Feather, 1966). According to another content-based interpretation, people prefer moderate risks because they believe that intermediate difficulty levels yield the maximum information about their ability (Trope & Brickman, 1975). Another example can be found in attribution theory: Preference for intermediate risks occur because people believe that intermediately difficult tasks provide the best opportunities to attribute success to one's own efforts (Weiner, 1974). Common to these competing theories is the assumption that it is the content of people's beliefs that determines their action.

What explanation has PSI theory to offer? It should be noted first that content-based explanations are fully compatible with PSI theory: The theory presupposes transfer of information among macrosystems. Consequently, it expects effects of the content of information processed within and across macrosystems. As pointed out at the outset, the many examples that illustrate how the content of beliefs and strategies people use may affect their self-regulation and other behaviors are perfectly compatible with PSI theory. However, PSI theory offers an additional causal factor that affects behavior control. This factor is based on mechanisms rather than contents. Specifically, the additional explanation is based on the dynamic changes of energy flowing among macrosystems. According to this view, an additional cause of the observed preferences of intermediate risks in success-oriented individuals is related to their ability to switch among the activation of intention memory and the activation of intuitive behavioral control system. In other words, people characterized by strong positive achievement needs are able to initiate the changes themselves that Oettingen (1997) found to be so effective when externally controlled: Successive changes from (1) positive affective anticipations (e.g., basking in anticipated success) and (2) focusing on the difficult aspects of challenging goals and vice versa resulted in a higher rate of enactment of intended activities than positive anticipations or focusing on difficulties of enactment alone. Individuals scoring high on fear of failure scales would be expected to prefer either difficult or easy tasks: For example, difficult tasks should be preferred by individuals who are fixated on low positive mood states in achievement situations that would result in a biased activation of intention memory in combination with its inhibitory influence on the activation of the behavioral output system (IBC). Recall that intention memory is designed for the maintenance of difficult intentions. Hence the preference for difficult tasks would result simply from the overactivation of the system designed for difficult tasks, irrespective of the content of the beliefs activated at the time.[6]

Attitude Change

Whereas risk preference relates to the left-hand side of the model (Figure 4), attitude change in response to persuasive attempts is more closely related to the right-hand side of the model: According to this view, attitude change depends on the dynamics between existing self-representations and new input processed by the object perception system. The practical importance of attitude change research can be seen in many situations in which people are to be motivated or persuaded. Examples are not restricted to the domain of attitude change per se (e.g., health campaigns and political campaigns). The success of parents' attempts to exert influence on their children or teachers' efforts to motivate their students depends on the degree to which the messages communicated elicit attitude change. Improvement of educational efforts depends on the degree to which we make progress in understanding the processes underlying attitude change. Should parents and teachers create a happy or a more serious (reflective) atmosphere before they communicate important messages? Under what conditions would they have to invest much effort in providing strong arguments? Answers to such question critically depend on how the processes underlying attitude change are explained. According to common theorizing, attitude change is affected mainly by cognitive contents such as people's beliefs about the credibility and status of the source, their thoughts about the soundness of the arguments, and so forth. PSI

---

[6] Nonetheless, preference for high difficulties also can be mediated by beliefs people form after they perceive their behavior (whose primary cause would be low positive affect and excessive activation of intention memory resulting from it). Subjects seem to form such beliefs that produce an optimal fit with the behavior they observe in themselves (Bem, 1967; Festinger, 1957). Such beliefs can intensify the preferences they make. The extent to which a given preference (e.g., for difficult tasks) is mediated by a cognitive belief (e. g., I like difficult tasks because I do not have to be ashamed if I fail on them) or by a content-free mechanism (low positive affect leading to high activation of intention memory) cannot be estimated on introspective data alone (see Goschke & Kuhl, 1993 and Kuhl & Kazén, in press, for a method for the nonreactive assessment of the activation of intention memory).

theory provides additional possible causes for observed effects that go beyond content-based explanations.

Many examples of the latter explanations can be found in the literature. An example is the attribution of attitude change to beliefs concerning the credibility or status of the person communicating a persuasive message (Petty, Cacioppo, & Goldman, 1981) or the attribution of attitude change to the informational content of feelings (Schwarz, Bless, & Bohner, 1991). According to the latter view, happy moods make people believe that the environment is safe, leading them to conclude that it is not necessary to scrutinize information in that environment. How does this "mood-as-information" model explain the finding that attitude change is enhanced after induction of a happy mood when the message contains weak arguments, but is reduced when message arguments are strong (Petty, Wells, & Brock, 1976)? According to the model, happy people believe that there is not much good reason for thinking about the arguments of a message (because they feel safe). As a result, strong arguments cannot unfold their strengths, whereas the unconvincing nature of weak arguments is less likely to be detected. The amount of thinking is operationalized in this research by the persuasion superiority of strong over weak arguments. According to PSI theory, we can use a similar argument without having to refer to the content of people' beliefs. People need not have any beliefs about the low usefulness of thinking in safe situations, because the dampening effect of positive mood on the activation of thinking works independent of the content of thought. According to the first modulation assumption, the dampening of thinking through positive mood can be attributed to the dynamics of personality systems interactions. If enhanced thinking is the basis of the effectiveness of strong arguments, reduced effectiveness of such arguments in happy people could be explained without referring to particular belief contents.

It should be noted, however, that PSI theory leaves open the question of whether or not the persuasion superiority effect is based on enhanced thinking. Another possibility is that people are less persuaded by weak compared to strong arguments when their self-representations are activated, which should facilitate rejection of weak arguments. The more one has access to one's self-representations, the easier it should be to reject arguments that are not compatible with the self (which should be especially true for weak arguments). This mechanism is not very likely to occur, however, when people are exposed to depressing and/or counterattitudinal messages as in the cited experiments. According to the second modulation assumption, self-activation is more likely to occur when negative affect is reduced, for example, by an uplifting rather than a depressing message. Uplifting message contents have been investigated in the context of another content-based model of mood-persuasion interactions that is called the *hedonic-contingency model* (Wegener, Petty, & Smith, 1995).

According to this model, happy people did not think much about the message provided in earlier experiments because the message typically was counterattitudinal and/or depressing. In other words, happy people avoid thinking about a message only if it is likely to destroy their good mood; for example, when it is challenging their own beliefs or has a depressing content. Consistent with this prediction, Wegener et al. (1995) found indications of persuasion superiority of strong arguments (interpreted as an indication of good thinking), even after induction of a happy mood, provided the message had an uplifting rather than a depressing hedonic content.

As mentioned, there is an alternative to explaining the superiority of strong arguments on the basis of people's beliefs about the usefulness of thinking with regard to their hypothetical mood maintenance goals. According to the second modulation assumption of PSI theory, uplifting information activates self-representations because it helps downregulate negative affect (in the cited study, the uplifting message described a political plan to reduce tuition). To the extent that, compared to sad mood, happy mood provides better grounds for downregulation of negative affect (presumably associated with paying tuition in this experiment), one would expect greater rejection of weak arguments in happy participants. The results reported by Wegener et al. (1995) are consistent with this derivation.

This example illustrates that PSI theory suggests another factor involved in the dynamics of attitude change: Strong and weak arguments differ not only in cognitive aspects, for example, in the logical soundness of their message. In addition, they may differ in their affective qualities. For example, strong arguments sometimes can elicit more positive affective reactions than weak arguments. Compared to the typical mood induction procedures, these effects should be rather short-lived (phasic) affective changes that need not even reach conscious awareness. PSI theory suggests paying as much attention to such phasic subconscious affective changes as to the tonic effects of mood induction procedures. If the dynamics of the activation of self-representations affect attitude change, one can derive interesting predictions regarding individual differences. In light of the evidence that indicates that action-oriented people have a good ability to downregulate negative affect (Kuhl & Beckmann, 1994a), one should expect that they should be more inclined to reject a persuasive attempt if they are confronted with weak arguments that elicit a rather short-lived negative affect.

According to the second modulation assumption, negative affect elicited by weak arguments should activate self-representations in action-oriented individuals because of their tendency to downregulate negative affect. As outlined before, access to self-representations should facilitate rejection of weak arguments. This prediction was confirmed in a study by Ciupka

(1991) in which managers were exposed to persuasive attempts of an experimenter who played the role of the boss trying to talk the manager out of a previously made personnel decision (Figure 6). As expected, the discussion time that elapsed until managers gave in (e.g., by admitting that there was some truth to the counterarguments) was higher in action-compared to state-oriented participants if the experimenter started with weak arguments (according to the manager's own ratings obtained at an earlier occasion). Presumably, weak arguments lead to an enhanced activation of self-representations (e.g., as if one were asking oneself, "What is my own opinion") in action-oriented participants because they downregulated the negative affect associated with the weak arguments (recall that the activation of the self system is an integral part of the downregulation process, according to the self-relaxation assumption; Table 2). Consistent with this explanation, state-oriented individuals showed the opposite effect: They gave in earlier in a condition in which the discussion started with weak arguments. Presumably, state-oriented participants could not downregulate the negative affect elicited by weak arguments and, as a result, had more difficulties accessing self-representations, according to the second modulation assumption. If the interpretation is correct that action-oriented participants' greater resistance to persuasion after initial exposure to weak arguments was mediated by an extra activation of their self-system (expected as a result of their downregulating negative affect),

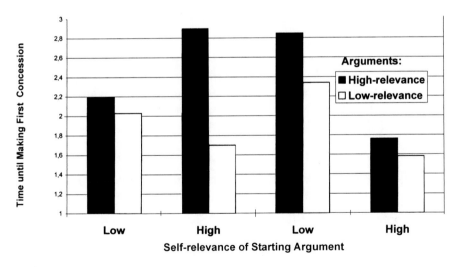

FIGURE 6   Resistance to persuasion as a function of self-relevance of arguments, relevance of starting argument, and personality.

this group should have higher ratings of self-esteem in the weak-start condition, but not in the condition that began with strong arguments. This pattern was indeed obtained in Ciupka's study. Interactions similar to the one shown in Figure 6 were reported in studies using a personality measure to assess uncertainty orientation (Sorrentino, Bobocel, Gitta, & Olson, 1988). Uncertainty-oriented individuals approach uncertain situations because they are confident they can reduce uncertainty by seeking information. The similarity between action orientation and uncertainty orientation is obvious: Both constructs describe dispositions toward using complex information processing resources that are especially suited for mastering mildly threatening (challenging) situations.

The results obtained in this persuasion study can be derived from PSI theory if one makes the assumption that weak arguments not only differ from strong ones in content, but also in their affective quality. A direct test of the assumption that the interaction between mood and personality affects persuasibility was conducted in a series of studies based on Asch's (1956) experiment on conformity (Beckmann, 1997). In these studies, participants were confronted with false perceptual judgments of other individuals (confederates of the experimenter) who maintained that the length of a line was equal to that of a standard line (which, in reality, had a different length). In an experimental condition that was intended to induce a negative mood state (extended pretreatment with a boring and monotonous task), state-oriented participants (scoring high on the preoccupation component of state orientation) displayed considerably more conformity than did action-oriented participants. In the control condition that did not involve any manipulation of mood, the former showed conformity as low as action-oriented participants. According to the explanation suggested by PSI theory, state-oriented individuals are less efficient than action-oriented ones to downregulate negative affect induced in the experimental condition. As a result, they are subject to a weaker activation of the self-system, which is needed for rejection of unacceptable suggestions from others.

B. DECOMPOSING SELF-REGULATION: NEW SELF-REPORT AND OBJECTIVE ASSESSMENT TECHNIQUES

The applications of PSI theory just described illustrate how well-known phenomena can be explained in a new way. Energy flow among the four motivationally relevant macrosystems is modulated by affective states and affects the extent to which each of the four macrosystems participates in volitional action and subjective experience. Affective states also modulate volitional processes: The explicit, self-suppressive type of volitional action (i.e., self-control) emphasized in the original theory of action control (Kuhl, 1984) should be facilitated by negative affect, whereas positive affect presumably facilitates the implicit, self-driven type of action control (i.e., self-regulation) mentioned in the first part of this chapter. The implications of the dynamics of personality systems interactions for self-regulation assessment now can be summarized. Global concepts of self-efficacy or will-power should be decomposed into many specific functions. Arno Fuhrmann and I developed a new self-report instrument that decomposes self-regulation in up to 30 functions (Kuhl & Fuhrmann, 1998). The instrument is called the *volitional components inventory* (VCI) and is available in a checklist (VCC) and in a traditional questionnaire format (VCQ). Because of space limitations I can provide only a brief summary of the structure of the VCI. At the first level of analysis, four modes of volition are distinguished. Two modes are facilitatory and two modes, are inhibitory. Self-regulation and self-control are the two facilitating modes, whereas volitional inhibition and inhibition of self-access are the inhibitory modes. Positive affect facilitates self-regulation and reduces volitional inhibition, whereas negative affect increases inhibition of self-access (unless downregulated) and facilitates the self-control mode. This set of formal statements summarizes the basic assumptions of the theory of volition that can be derived from PSI theory.

The formal statements come to life when one illustrates the four modes in terms of the system configurations that are characteristic of each of them. Specifically, self-regulation can be compared to an "inner democracy" as illustrated by the following scenario: A student is confronted with a difficult task that initially arouses some uncertainty as to whether he or she is able to solve it. Like many other forms of challenge, uncertainty should arouse a mild degree of negative affect (conscious or not). The student is able to downregulate this negative affect and feels an increase in self-esteem (presumably resulting from increased access to extension memory including self-representations that downregulation produces according to the second modulation assumption). Increased access to extension memory facilitates task performance, especially where new and creative solutions have to be found. Access to extension memory not only facilitates task performance, but also intrinsic motivation. Because the self-system is repeatedly activated during task performance (as a result of downregulation of negative affect that is sometimes needed when a new difficulty arises), the various mechanisms depending on self-activation also are facilitated, especially self-motivation. Intrinsic motivation is increased because of the many positively valued self-aspects that can be experienced (not necessarily conscious) during task performance, because the self-system is activated with each episode of downregulated negative affect. This amounts to a functional account of the democracy metaphor. The system behaves as if it were taking votes: Each time extension memory is activated, a great number of self-aspects are accessible and contribute whatever affective responses are associated with them. If the majority of self-aspects are associated with positive affect, the self system supports the ongoing activity emotionally and further stabilizes the positive emotional state through repeated self-motivational episodes. If the majority of self-aspects elicited by the task contribute negative affects and this balance cannot be changed by self-motivation, the self system would reject the current path, or even the subgoal or the task at hand. On a more formal level, this scenario can be succinctly described by the system configuration listed in the first line of Table 3.

Data that show that the VCI scales that presumably assess the various components of self-regulation can predict objective measures of self-regulatory efficiency are reported by Kuhl and Fuhrmann (1998). Significant correlations between a standardized measure of resistance to temptation and VCI scale values (> .50) were obtained for four subscales employed to assess functional components of the self-regulation mode (i.e., self-directed attention, self-determination, impulse control, and initiative). The standardized measure of resistance to temptation was an adult version of the computer-aided Self-Regulation and Concentration Test for Children (SRTC). This test decomposes various volitional functions involved in resistance to temptation (e.g., self-regulation versus self-control and attentional deficit versus self-regulatory deficit) during a simple, but monotonous, task that is occasionally accompanied by a distracting tree-climbing competition that appears in another sector of the screen. Individuals cannot control the outcome of that race, but they are tempted to

TABLE 3   Configuration of Subsystems Characterizing Various Volitional Modes or Functions[a]

	Level of		Relative activation of	
Mode or function	Positive affect	Negative affect	High-inferential systems	Elementary systems
1) Self-regulation	$A + \gtrless A(+)$	$A(-) > A -$	$EM > IM$	$IBC > OR$
2) Self-control	$A(+) \gtrless A +$	$A - > A(-)$	$EM < IM$	$IBC < OR$
3) Volitional inhibition (hesitation)	$A(+) \gg A +$	$A - > A(-)$	$EM \ll IM$	$IBC < OR$
4) Inhibited self-access (preoccupation)	$A(+) > A +$	$A - \gg A(-)$	$EM < IM$	$IBC \ll OR$

[a]Symbols: $A +$ = positive affect; $A(+)$ = inhibition of positive affect; $A -$ = negative affect; $A(-)$ = inhibition of negative affect (downregulation); IM = intention memory; EM = extension memory; IBC = intuitive behavior control; OR = object recognition; $\rightarrow$ = increases; $\leftrightarrow$ = increases and is increased by; $>$ = is more activated than; $\gg$ = is chronically much more activated than; $<$ = is less activated than; $\ll$ = is chronically less activated than; $\gtrless$ = is sometimes more and sometimes less activated than ("affective flexibility").

watch it because, depending on its outcome, they receive or lose extra points in their accounts. Even small drops in speed or increases in the variance of response times can be used as indicators of failures to resist the temptation to glance across the screen from the task field to the racing grounds (cf. Kuhl & Kraska, 1989, 1992).

As can be seen from line 2 in Table 3, the situation would change dramatically if negative affect could not be downregulated actively through an activation of extension memory. This volitional mode, which is called self-control, can be compared to an inner dictatorship: Access to the self is suppressed now (EM < IM). This is to say that both the cognitive resources of extension memory for finding new and unusual solutions are blocked together with the self-motivational resources that depend on self-access. In other words, in this self-control mode, a student would behave very self-disciplined, would not become easily distracted by alternative interests (because they are buried in the deactivated self), and would be able to perform well as long as told what to do (the left-hemispheric verbal abilities and memory for explicit intentions are even strongly activated), but would have difficulties as soon as unusual solutions were required. Easy external control is enhanced because the self system cannot "protest" against (i.e., inhibit) unwanted suggestions. It cannot check even the compatibility of an instruction with the self because the self-representational system is inhibited (EM < IM). This aspect of the system configuration assumed for self-control explains why self-disciplined people score higher on authoritarianism.

Increased conformity and inclination to introject self-alien expectations of others also was found in state-oriented individuals of the preoccupation type (Kuhl & Beckmann, 1994b). According to the analysis illustrated in Table 3, state orientation can be interpreted as a chronified version of inhibiting self-access (preoccupation) or volitional action (hesitation) under conditions of threat or frustration, respectively. If high negative affect cannot be downregulated for long periods (see line 4 in Table 3), uncontrollable rumination is expected because the object recognition system is especially sensitive in this case and the self-system can no longer check whether a thought or a feeling is wanted or whether it should be ignored (Table 3, line 4). To the extent that activation of the self system is a prerequisite for checking self-compatibility, it becomes more and more difficult to identify, let alone suppress thoughts, feelings, or wishes that would not "win an election" if the self system could take a vote across all self-aspects, no matter whether these self-alien elements come from within the system or from others. When the self system is inhibited, there is an increased risk to get stuck with an activity or thought that satisfies the isolated interest of a local operator (e.g., the wish to think about a past failure), but is not in accordance with the decision made on the level of the integrated self (e.g., to concentrate on the task at hand).

Health Behavior

I now illustrate the explanatory usefulness of this account with one example. In a study of university students' abilities to enact new intentions to improve their nutritional behavior, Fuhrmann and Kuhl (1998) found that students leaning more toward the self-regulation mode enacted more of their intentions than students who had higher scores on self-control scales of the VCC. A somewhat counterintuitive finding was that this pattern was obtained only in a condition in which participants were instructed to set easy goals and reward themselves even for small successes when filling in their daily self-monitoring sheets. In a self-punishment condition in which participants were instructed to (mildly) punish themselves for failures, should they detect any during self-monitoring, differences in volitional efficiency were completely reversed: Now participants leaning toward self-control outperformed their self-regulation friends in the number of intended behavioral changes that actually were performed (e.g., eat more broccoli). Obviously, this striking finding qualifies intervention programs that typically are biased toward self-reward strategies.

How can PSI theory explain this interaction? Why did self-controlled individuals' abilities to stick to their intentions deteriorate when they were instructed to reward themselves for their successes? With a self-control style, extension memory and self-representations are notoriously inhibited (Table 3). This should impair the ability to integrate new goals into the existing self-representational system (i.e., whole-heartedly endorse them and identify with them). Positive affect associated with self-reward should reduce the impairment and help release the inhibition of self-access that normally results from increased negative emotionality in these individuals, according to the model in Table 3 (line 2). As a result, many task-irrelevant self-interests, but not the new goals, are activated with enhanced self-access (because the latter are less likely to be integrated in the self system in individuals leaning toward the self-suppressive self-control mode). In other words, once an individual has employed self-control strategies for some time, he or she becomes dependent on negative emotionality to maintain volitional efficiency. Only a prolonged period of training for the release of inhibition of self-access and the integration of self-compatible goals into the self (after extensive self-compatibility checking) can restore the ability to put the self back into the service of self-selected goals. Recall that successful self-actualization consists of both self-awareness (i.e., uninhibited self-access) and volitional facilitation. A balanced coordination of these two aspects of self-actualization requires emotional flexibility; that is, the ability to shift from positive to negative affect and vice versa.

VI. CONCLUSION

Let me come to some conclusions. I hope I have shown that a differentiated view of energy flow between personality systems provides access to an additional category of determinants of goal-directed action. PSI theory challenges cognitive approaches to the explanation of goal-directed action by spelling out the conditions under which cognitive performance is modulated by affect and relevant personality dispositions. Admittedly, compared to sophisticated cognitive reasons for action, the dynamics of action described in PSI theory may hurt our need to view ourselves as purely rational human beings. We do not like to see ourselves driven by blind energies moving forth and back among macrosystems in the brain. However, there is no reason to identify PSI theory with such a passive conception of humans. The energy flow among personality systems merely forms the constraints under which even the most differentiated cognitive contents can unfold their power. Taking these constraints seriously will increase our degrees of freedom rather than reduce them to blind flows of energies. Examples are efforts toward improving personality training, toward optimizing conditions for personal development and self-growth, and even for therapy (Fuhrmann & Kuhl, 1998; Hartmann & Kuhl, in press): Taking into account the dynamics of systems interactions opens new opportunities wherever traditional attempts at changing critical behaviors or cognitive beliefs reach their limits. In my research on learned helplessness and depression, I found evidence for this conclusion: Whenever people show impairments of performance or volitional action that cannot fully be explained by cognitive beliefs (e.g., low perceived self-efficacy) or by the lack of task-oriented intentions (Kuhl, 1981), interventions designed to change the affective basis of systems interactions can remove helplessness effects even in state-oriented individuals whose performance normally declines following failure experiences (Kuhl & Weiss, 1994).

The most important implications of the theory that describes the dynamic flow of energy among the four motivationally relevant macrosystems can be summarized by the following six conclusions. PSI theory not only challenges reductionistic cognitive approaches, it also differentiates traditional motivational concepts in at least six ways:

1. *Dynamic versus content-based explanations.* PSI theory adds dynamic interpretations based on energization of subsystems to approaches that explain behavior on the basis of cognitive contents. Obviously, cognitive contents of thought can have a causal effect on goal-directed action. The dynamic mechanisms described by PSI theory simply can be added to content-based processes. Whenever we are dealing with individual exemplars of the system we are studying, contents of thoughts and feelings quickly can become more important than the general content-free laws of

energy flow among subsystems. A child can be motivated only if we understand the content of her or his thoughts and feelings and respond to them promptly and adequately. Nonetheless, the general mechanisms of energy flow might place some constraints on what can be achieved by attempts to change cognitive contents and strategies.

2. *Modulatory versus motivational effects of incentives.* The second of my conclusions relates to the fact that PSI theory calls attention to dynamic effects of incentives that work over and above the motivational effects attributed to them by classical theorizing: Positive incentives not only elicit approach behavior, but also modulate the interaction between intention memory and its output systems. Negative affect not only elicits avoidance behavior, but also modulates the interaction between integrated self-representations and unexpected or unwanted object perceptions including unwanted ruminations or unwanted recommendations by others (Kuhl & Baumann, in press; Kuhl & Kazén, 1994a).

3. *Action control: Specific rather than global activation.* PSI theory elaborates the dynamics underlying intentional action. Lewin's conception of tension systems could not explain the interactions between personality and the Zeigarnik effect (e.g., Atkinson, 1953; Johnson et al., 1983). According to PSI theory, excessive superiority of explicit memory for uncompleted intentions does not occur in people who do not easily develop long-lasting periods of reduced positive affect or an enhanced focus on unrealistic ideals (i.e., it is not expected in action-oriented, nondepressed individuals). Note that implicit memory for uncompleted intentions can be intact for both action and state-oriented individuals (Goschke & Kuhl, 1998).

4. *Performance deficits: Impaired self-relaxation rather than understimulation.* The fourth implication the flow-of-energy model has for motivation relates to the relationship between negative affect and performance. Whereas the action-related part of PSI theory differentiates the Zeigarnik effect, the experience-related part differentiates the second pillar of classical motivation theory reflected in interactions between arousal (or negative affect) and personality (Atkinson, 1974; Eysenck, 1967; Yerkes & Dodson, 1908): Performance deficits that result from aversive experiences are expected only in individuals whose capacity for self-based downregulation of negative affect is overtaxed by a threatening experience. Moreover, performance deficits are confined to tasks that place considerable demands on extension memory and/or integrated self-representations.

5. *Functional separation of personality constructs.* As a fifth contribution of PSI theory, I showed how the distinction between activation of systems and activation of connections between systems helps explain the communalities and differences between overlapping personality constructs such as state orientation, introversion, neuroticism, and anxiety. Whereas introversion, neuroticism, and anxiety can be interpreted in terms of the arousability of affect generation systems (i.e., inhibition of positive affect, arousal,

and negative affect, respectively), state orientation relates to the capacity for the self-regulation of such affective states.

6. *Motives: Beyond the travelling salesman analogy.* Finally, a sixth implication relates to the concept of motives. If we want to understand the way motives energize and direct behavior, we cannot ignore the machinery of the system any longer. The traveling salesman analogy has been misleading. Purpose and design cannot be separated nicely as suggested by classical philosophy. How do basic needs and motives interact with the extended cognitive machinery? PSI theory addresses not only the dynamic changes of activation of the four macrosystems that seem to be most relevant for goal-directed action, but it also integrates what we know from cognitive research about the functional characteristics of each of these macrosystems. From an evolutionary point of view, there is no reason to expect that different motives are expressed in behavior through the same macrosystem. Each system seems to be designed for a different motive. For example, affiliative needs critically rely on intuitive behavior control and are frustrated easily with too much explicit intentionality and planning (Papoušek & Papoušek, 1987). On the other hand, the satisfaction of needs for competence and achievement should benefit from explicit intentionality and planning. Explicit memory for difficult intentions is the prerequisite for planning and problem solving in achievement contexts. The need for autonomy, self-assertiveness, and power may benefit most from uninhibited access to integrated self-representations and intention memory. It follows from this analysis that a fixation on inhibited positive affect (or on negative affect), acquired in childhood and/or genetically prepared (e.g., in schizoid personality disorders), should be especially harmful for establishing healthy social relationships, whereas a fixation on positive affect (e.g., in histrionic personality disorders) should be harmful for the development of healthy achievement motivation. Likewise, exaggerated sensitivity for negative affect should be difficult for the conflict-free development of the need for autonomy and power (e.g., in avoidant, dependent, or borderline personalities), whereas a strong bias toward downregulation of negative affect should interfere with attachment behavior based on the need for security (e.g., in paranoid, narcissistic, or antisocial personality disorders).

Motive-Cognition Coalitions

According to PSI theory, these prototypical coalitions between each motive and its optimal macrosystem configuration are mediated by affective dispositions. The coalition between affiliative needs and intuitive behavior control (IBC) requires a disposition toward positive affect to develop during early parent–child interactions, the coalition between the achievement motive and explicit intentionality and planning requires the ability to tolerate frustration and states of inhibited positive affect, and, finally, the coalition between the needs for self-expression and power and integrated self-representations require the early development of competence for self-relaxation as described in the systems-conditioning model (Kuhl, 1998; Kuhl & Völker, 1998). It can be concluded from this account that developmental conditions departing from these ideal profiles can produce other coalitions between motives and the cognitive machinery. These coalitions may be useful to adapt to special environments: A coalition of planning and affiliative needs can be adaptive when social approval can be attained through personal achievements, manipulation, or even cheating, whereas a coalition between power-related needs and inhibited self-access (resulting from a low ability for self-relaxation) can be useful to adapt to an environment that does not allow for direct expression of self-related concerns as, for instance, when a child learns to support the needs of the family at the expense of personal needs. Obviously, such nonprototypical coalitions between motives and affect-modulated cognitive systems can turn out to be maladaptive if the environmental conditions change later in life.

The important methodological conclusion from this account relates to motive measurement: A motive no longer should be assessed without simultaneously assessing the system configuration with which it is associated. My colleagues and I have developed new tests to assess the degree to which each of the three motives tends to be expressed through each of the four macrosystems. Separate instruments to assess motive–cognition coalitions have been developed for people's explicit representations of their needs (i.e., the Motives-Enactment-Test; Kuhl, 1997) and for implicit motives (i.e., the Projective Multi-Motive Test; Kuhl & Scheffer, 1998).

Aristotelian Thinking Reconsidered

As a final remark, I would like to resume my introductory reflections concerning motivation being the problem child of psychology. I think this problem child is about to grow up. There is no longer a reason for her to copy her cognitive brothers and sisters who can do the things they do so efficiently. We do not have to copy the architectures they prefer; for example, the one consisting of short-term memory, long-term memory, and executive control. There is no need for us to reduce motivation to goal representations and cognitive mechanisms. The essence of motivation lies in the inarticulate forms of energy flow among personality-relevant macrosystems that establishes the connections among those systems. It is an interesting irony that we can find the roots of this holistic view of motivation in the work of an ancient philosopher who was criticized by Zeigarnik's teacher for offering content-based rather than dynamic explanations (Lewin, 1935). According to my analysis, we kept the problematic parts (i.e., the focus on intentional contents as the basis of motivation) and disposed of the promising parts of Aristotle's theory of motivation (i.e., his definition of motivation in terms of connections among psychological states or systems). In his famous article proposing a shift from Aristotelian to Galilean thinking in psychology, Lewin (1935) correctly identified the problematic part of Aristotle's approach to motivation and to science in general (i.e., the focus on content-based properties of the objects whose behavior is to be explained). However, Lewin failed to identify what I consider the roots of a differentiated approach to what Lewin (1935) established as the conceptual platform of motivation theory: The dynamic waxing and waning of systems that mediate the behavioral enactment of motivational forces.

ACKNOWLEDGMENT

This chapter is based on a series of grants supported by the German Science Foundation (DFG).

REFERENCES

Anderson, J. R. (1983). *The architecture of cognition.* Cambridge, MA: Harvard University Press.
Aristotle (1975). *Nichomachean Ethics* (H. G. Apostle, Trans.). Boston: Reidel.
Asch, S. E. (1956). Studies of independence and conformity: A minority of one against an unanimous majority. *Psychological Monographs, 70,* 416.
Atkinson, J. W. (1953). The achievement motive and recall of interrupted and completed tasks. *Journal of Experimental Psychology, 46,* 381–390.
Atkinson, J. W. (Ed.). (1958). *Motives in fantasy, action, and society.* Princeton, NJ: Van Nostrand.
Atkinson, J. W. (1974). Strength of motivation and efficiency of performance. In J. W. Atkinson & J. O. Raynor (Eds.), *Motivation and achievement* (pp. 193–218). New York: Wiley.
Atkinson, J. W., & Birch, D. (1970). *The dynamics of action.* New York: Wiley.
Atkinson, J. W., & Feather, N. T. (Eds.). (1966). *A theory of achievement motivation.* New York: Wiley.
Baars, B. J. (1988). *A cognitive theory of consciousness.* Cambridge, UK: Cambridge University Press.
Baddeley, A. (1986). *Working memory:* Oxford, UK: Oxford University Press.
Bandura, A. (1977). Self-efficacy: Toward a unifying theory of behavioral change. *Psychological Review, 84,* 191–215.
Barkley, R. A. (1997). Behavioral inhibition, sustained attention, and executive functions: Constructing a unifying theory of ADHD. *Psychological Bulletin, 121,* 65–94.
Baumeister, R. F., & Tice, D. M. (1986). Four selves, two motives and a substitute process self-regulation model. In R. F. Baumeister (Ed.), *Public self and private self* (pp. 63–97). New York: Springer-Verlag.
Beck, A. T. (1979). *Cognitive therapy of depression.* New York: Guilford Press.
Beckmann, J. (1997). *Alienation and conformity.* Unpublished manuscript, Max-Planck-Institute for Psychological Research, Munich, Germany.

Beckmann, J., & Kuhl, J. (1984). Altering information to gain action control: Functional aspects of human information processing in decision-making. *Journal of Research in Personality*, *18*, 223–279.

Beeman, M., Friedman, R. B., Grafman, J., Perez, E., Diamond, S., & Lindsay, M. B. (1994). Summation priming and coarse coding in the right hemisphere. *Journal of Cognitive Neuroscience*, *6*, 26–45.

Bem, D. J. (1967). Self-preception: An alternative view of cognitive dissonance phenomena. *Psychological Review*, *74*, 183–200.

Beswick, G., & Man, L. (1994). State orientation and procrastination. In J. Kuhl & J. Beckmann (Eds.), *Volition and personality: Action versus state orientation* (pp. 391–396). Göttingen, Germany: Hogrefe.

Birch, D., Atkinson, J. W., & Bongort, K. (1986). Cognitive control of action. In J. Kuhl & J. W. Atkinson (Eds.), *Motivation, thought, and action* (pp. 252–264). New York: Praeger.

Bowlby, J. (1969). *Attachment and loss* (Vol. 1). New York: Basic Books.

Bradshaw, J. L. (1989). *Hemispheric specialization and psychological function*. Chichester, UK: Wiley.

Brandimonte, M., Einstein, G. O., & McDaniel, M. A. (Eds.). (1996). *Prospective memory: Theory and applications*. Mahwah, NJ: Erlbaum.

Brunstein, J. C. (1993). Personal goals and subjective well-being: A longitudinal study. *Journal of Personality and Social Psychology*, *65*, 1061–1070.

Ciupka, B. (1991). *Selbstregulation und Entscheidungen von Führungskräften* [Self-regulation and decision-making in a group of managers]. Unpublished thesis, University of Osnabrück.

Dawson, M. E., & Schell, A. M. (1982). Electrodermal responses to attended and nonattended significant stimuli during dichotic listening. *Journal of Experimental Psychology: Human Perception and Performance*, *8*, 315–324.

Deci, E. L., & Ryan, R. M. (1991). A motivational approach to self: Integration in personality. In R. Dienstbier (Ed.), *Nebraska Symposium on Motivation: Vol. 38. Perspectives on motivation* (pp. 237–288). Lincoln: University of Nebraska Press.

Dweck, C. (1986). Motivational processes affecting learning. *American Psychologist*, *41*, 1040–1048.

Elliot, A. J., & Church, M. A. (1997). A hierarchical model of approach and avoidance achievement motivation. *Journal of Personality and Social Psychology*, *72*, 218–232.

Epstein, S., Pacini, R., Denes-Raj, V., & Heier, H. (1996). Individual differences in intuitive-experiential and analytical-rational thinking styles. *Journal of Personality and Social Psychology*, *71*, 390–405.

Eysenck, H. J. (1967). *The biological basis of personality*. Springfield, IL: Charles C. Thomas.

Festinger, L. (1957). *A theory of cognitive dissonance*, Evanston, IL: Row & Peterson.

Festinger, L., & Carlsmith, J. M. (1959). Cognitive consequences of forced compliance. *Journal of Abnormal and Social Psychology*, *58*, 203–210.

Festinger, L., & Walster, E. (1964). The post-decision process. In L. Festinger (Ed.), *Conflict, decision, and dissonance* (pp. 100–112). Stanford, CA: Stanford University Press.

Frankl, V. E. (1981). *Die Sinnfrage in der Psychotherapie* [The problem of meaning in psychotherapy]. Munich, Germany: Piper.

Freud, S. (1938/1989). *Abriß der Psychoanalyse* [Summary of psychoanalysis]. Frankfurt, Germany: Fischer.

Fuhrmann, A., & Kuhl, J. (1998). Maintaining a healthy diet: Effects of personality and self-reward versus self-punishment on commitment to and enactment of self-chosen and assigned goals. *Psychology and Health*, *13*, 651–686.

Fuster, J. M. (1995). Memory and planning: Two temporal perspectives of frontal lobe function. In H. H. Jasper, S. Riggio, & P. S. Goldman-Rakic (Eds.), *Epilepsy and the functional anatomy of the frontal lobe* (pp. 9–18). New York: Raven Press.

Gainotti, G. (1989). The meaning of emotional disturbances resulting from unilateral brain injury. In G. Gainotti & C. Caltagirone (Eds.), *Emotions and the dual brain* (pp. 147–167). Heidelberg, Germany: Springer-Verlag.

Goschke, T. (1997). Implicit learning of perceptual and motor sequences: Evidence for independent learning systems. In M. Stadler & P. Frensch (Eds.), *Handbook of implicit learning* (pp. 401–444). Thousand Oaks, CA: Sage.

Goschke, T., & Kuhl, J. (1993). The representation of intentions: Persisting activation in memory. *Journal of Experimental Psychology: Learning, Memory, and Cognition, 19,* 1211–1226.

Goschke, T., & Kuhl, J. (1996). Remembering what to do: Explicit and implicit memory for intentions. In M. Brandimonte, G. O. Einstein, & M. A. McDaniel (Eds.), *Prospective memory: Theory and applications* (pp. 53–91). Mahwah, NJ: Erlbaum.

Gray, J. A. (1987). *The psychology of fear and stress* (2nd ed.). Cambridge, UK: Cambridge University Press.

Gunsch, D. (1996). *Selbstbestimmung und Persönlichkeitsstile in Zweierbeziehungen* [Self-determination and personality styles in intimate relationships]. Unpublished thesis, University of Osnabrück.

Haken, H. (1981). *Synergetics: An introduction.* Heidelberg, Germany: Springer-Verlag.

Hartmann, K., & Kuhl, J. (in press). Der Wille in der Verhaltenstherapie. [The will in behavior therapy]. In K. Grawe, E. Wiesenhüter, & H. Petzold (Eds.), *Der Wille in der Psychotherapie* [The will in psychotherapy]. Paderborn, Germany: Junfermann.

Haschke, R., & Kuhl, J. (1994). Action control and slow potential shifts. *Proceedings of the 41st International Congress of Aviation and Space Medicine.* Bologna, Italy: Monduzzi.

Heckhausen, H. (1977). Achievement motivation and its constructs: A cognitive model. *Motivation and Emotion, 1,* 283–329.

Heckhausen, H. (1991). *Motivation and action.* Heidelberg, Germany: Springer-Verlag.

Hellige, J. B. (1990). Hemispheric asymmetry. *Annual Review of Psychology, 41,* 55–80.

Higgins, E. T. (1987). Self-discrepancy: A theory relating self and affect. *Psychological Review, 94,* 319–340.

Jacobs, W. J., & Nadel, L. (1985). Stress-induced recovery of fears and phobias. *Psychological Review, 92,* 512–531.

Janis, I. L. & King, B. (1954). The influence of role-playing on opinion change. *Journal of Abnormal and Social Psychology, 49,* 211–218.

Jeannerod, M. (1994). The representing brain: Correlates of motor intention and imagery. *Behavioral and Brain Sciences, 17,* 187–245.

Johnson, J. E., Petzel, T. P., Hartney, L. M., & Morgan, R. A. (1983). Recall of importance ratings of completed and uncompleted tasks as a function of depression. *Cognitive Therapy and Research, 7,* 51–56.

Kahneman, D. (1973). *Attention and effort.* Englewood Cliffs, NJ: Prentice-Hall.

Kammer, D. (1994). On depression and state orientation: A few empirical and theoretical remarks. In J. Kuhl & J. Beckmann (Eds.), *Volition and personality: Action versus state orientation* (pp. 351–362). Göttingen, Germany: Hogrefe.

Keller, H., & Gauda, G. (1987). Eye contact in the first months of life and its developmental consequences. In H. Rau & H.C. Steinhauser (Eds.), *Psychobiology and early development* (pp. 129–143). Amsterdam: Elsevier.

Keller, H., Gauda, G., Miranda, D., & Schölmerich A. (1985). Die Entwicklung des Blickkontaktverhaltens im ersten Lebensjahr. [The development of eye-contact during the first year]. *Zeitschrift für Entwicklungspsychologie und Pädagogische Psychologie, 17,* 258–269.

Kihlstrom, J. F., & Klein, S. B. (1997). Self-knowledge and self-awareness. *Annals of the New York Academy of Sciences, 818,* 5–17.

Klinger, E. (1977). *Meaning and void: Inner experience and the incentives in people's lives.* Minneapolis, MN: University of Minnesota Press.

Klinger, E. (in press). The search for meaning in evolutionary perspective and its clinical implications. In P. T. P Wong & P. S. Fry (Eds.), *The human quest for meaning: Theory, research and application*. Mahwah, NJ: Erlbaum.

Knight, R. T., & Grabowecky, M. (1995). Escape from linear time: Prefrontal cortex and conscious experience. In M. S. Gazzaniga (Ed.), *The cognitive neurosciences* (pp. 1357–1371). Cambridge, MA: MIT Press.

Kohut, H. (1985). *Self psychology and the humanities*. New York: Norton.

Kuhl, J. (1981). Motivational and functional helplessness: The moderating effect of state vs. action orientation. *Journal of Personality and Social Psychology, 40*, 155–170.

Kuhl, J. (1983). Emotion, Kognition und Motivation: II. Die funktionale Bedeutung der Emotionen für das problemlösende Denken und für das konkrete Handeln [Emotion, Cognition, and Motivation: II. The functional significance of emotions for problem-solving and action]. *Sprache und Kognition, 4*, 228–253.

Kuhl, J. (1984). Volitional aspects of achievement motivation and learned helplessness: Toward a comprehensive theory of action-control. In B. A. Maher (Ed.), *Progress in experimental personality research* (Vol. 13. pp. 99–171). New York: Academic Press.

Kuhl, J. (1985). Volitional mediators of cognitive-behavior consistency: Self-regulatory processes and actions versus state orientation. In: J. Kuhl & J. Beckmann (Eds.), *Action control: From cognition to behavior* (pp. 101–128). Heidelberg, Germany: Springer-Verlag.

Kuhl, J. (1992). A theory of self-regulation: Action versus state orientation, self-discrimination, and some applications. *Applied Psychology: An International Review, 41*, 95–173.

Kuhl, J. (1996). Who controls whom when "I control myself"? *Psychological Inquiry, 7*, 61–68.

Kuhl, J. (1997). *Der Motiv-Umsetzungs-Test* [The motiv-enactment test].Unpublished questionnaire, University of Osnabrück.

Kuhl, J. (1998a). *A functional design approach to personality and motivation: Central versus local organization of dynamic interactions among affective and cognitive systems*. Unpublished manuscript, University of Osnabrück.

Kuhl, J. (in press). A theory of self-development: Precursors and effects of affective fixation. In J. Heckhausen (Ed.), *Motivational psychology of human development*. Amsterdam: Elsevier.

Kuhl, J., & Baumann, N. (in press). Rumination and impaired self-regulation. In W. Perrig & A. Grob (Eds.), *Control of human behavior mental processes and consciousness: Essays in honor of the 60th birthday of August Flammer*. New York: Wiley.

Kuhl, J., & Beckmann, J. (1994a). *Volition and personality: Action versus state orientation*. Göttingen, Germany: Hogrefe.

Kuhl, J., & Beckmann, J. (1994b). Alienation: Ignoring one's preferences. In J. Kuhl & J. Beckmann (Eds.), *Volition and personality: Action versus state orientation*. Göttingen, Germany: Hogrefe.

Kuhl, J., & Fuhrmann, A. (1998). Decomposing self-regulation and self-control: The volitional components checklist. In J. Heckhausen & C. Dweck (Eds.), *Life span perspectives on motivation and control* (pp. 15–49). Mahwah, NJ: Erlbaum.

Kuhl, J., & Helle, P. (1986). Motivational and volitional determinants of depression: The degenerated-intention hypothesis. *Journal of Abnormal Psychology, 95*, 247–251.

Kuhl, J., & Kazén, M. (1994a). Self-discrimination and memory: State orientation and false self-ascription of assigned activities. *Journal of Personality and Social Psychology, 66*, 1103–1115.

Kuhl, J., & Kazén, M. (1994b). Volitional aspects of depression: State orientation and self-discrimination. In J. Kuhl & J. Beckmann (Eds.), *Volition and personality: Action versus state orientation* (pp. 297–315). Göttingen, Germany: Hogrefe.

Kuhl, J., & Kazén, M. (1997). *Das Persönlichkeits-Stil-und-Störungs-Inventar (PSSI): Manual*. [The personality styles and disorders inventory: Manual]. Göttingen, Germany: Hogrefe.

Kuhl, J., & Kazén, M. (in press). Volitional enactment of difficult intentions: Joint activation of intention memory and positive affect removes stroop interference. *Journal of Experimental Psychology: General*.

Kuhl, J., & Kraska, K. (1989). Self-regulation and metamotivation: Computational mechanisms, development, and assessment. In R. Kanfer, P. L. Ackerman, & R. Cudeck (Eds.), *Abilities, motivation, and methodology: The Minnesota Symposium on individual differences* (pp. 343–368). Hillsdale, NJ: Erlbaum Associates.

Kuhl, J., & Kraska, K. (1992). *Der Selbstregulations- und Konzentrationstest für Kinder (SRKT-K)* [The self-regulation and concentration test for children]. Göttingen, Germany: Hogrefe.

Kuhl, J., & Scheffer, D. (1998). *Der Pojektive Multi-Motiv-Test* (PMMT) [The projective-multimotive test]. Unpublished test, University of Osnabrück.

Kuhl, J., & Völker, S. (1998). Entwicklung und Persönlichkeit [Development and personality]. In H. Keller (Ed.), *Lehrbuch der Entwicklungspsychologie* (pp. 207–240). Bern, Switzerland: Huber.

Kuhl, J., & Weiss, M. (1994). Performance deficits following uncontrollable failure: Impaired action control or global attributions and generalized expectancy deficits? In J. Kuhl & J. Beckmann (Eds.), *Volition and personality: Action versus state orientation.* Göttingen, Germany: Hogrefe.

Langer, E. (1975). The illusion of control. *Journal of Personality and Social Psychology, 32,* 311–328.

Lazarus, R. S. (1984). On the primacy of cognition. *American Psychologist, 39,* 124–129.

LeDoux, J. E. (1995). Emotion: Clues from the brain. *Annual Review of Psychology, 46,* 209–235.

Lewin, K. (1935). *A dynamic theory of personality: Selected papers.* New York: McGraw-Hill.

Lewinsohn, P. M., Steinmetz, J. L., Larson, D. W. & Franklin, J. (1981). Depression-related cognitions: Antecedent or consequence? *Journal of Abnormal Psychology, 40,* 213–219.

Linville, P. (1987). Self-complexity as a cognitive buffer against stress-related illness and depression. *Journal of Personality and Social Psychology, 52,* 663–676.

Markus, H., & Nurius, P. (1986). Possible selves: Personalized representations of goals. *American Psychologist, 41,* 954–969.

Martin, L. L., & Tesser, A. (1989). Toward a motivational and structural theory of ruminative thought. In J. S. Uleman & J. A. Bargh (Eds.), *Unintended thought* (pp. 306–326). New York: Guilford.

Maslow, A. H. (1970). *Motivation and personality* (2nd ed.). New York: Harper & Row.

Mazur, J. E. (1990). *Learning and behavior.* Englewood Cliffs, NJ: Prentice-Hall.

McClelland, D. C. (1985). *Human motivation.* Glenview, IL: Scott, Foresman & Co.

McClelland, D. C., Atkinson, J. W., Clark, R. A., & Lowell, E. L. (1953). *The achievement motive.* New York: Appleton-Century-Crofts.

McClelland, J. L., McNaughton, B. L., & O'Reilly, R. C. (1995). Why there are complementary learning systems in the hippocampus and neocortex: Insights from the successes and failures of connectionist models of learning and memory. *Psychological Review, 102,* 419–457.

Meltzhoff, A. N., & Moore, M. K. (1989). Imitation in newborn infants: Exploring the range of gestures imitated and the underlying mechanisms. *Developmental Psychology, 25,* 954–962.

Meltzhoff, A. N., & Moore, M. K. (1994). Imitation, memory, and the representation of persons. *Infant Behavior, 17,* 83–100.

Mischel, H. N., & Mischel, W. (1983). The development of children's knowledge of self-control strategies. *Child Development, 54,* 603–619.

Murray, H. A. (1938). *Explorations in personality.* New York: Oxford University Press.

Nissen, M. J., & Bullemer, P. (1987). Attentional requirements of learning: Evidence from performance measures. *Cognitive Psychology, 19,* 1–32.

Nolen-Hoeksema, S., Parker, L., & Larson, J. (1994). Ruminative coping with depressed mood following loss. *Journal of Personality and Social Psychology, 67,* 92–104.

Norman, D. A. (1980). Twelve issues for cognitive science. *Cognitive Science, 4,* 1–32.

Nuttin, J. (1984). *Motivation, planning, and action. A relational theory of behavior dynamics.* Hillsdale, NJ: Erlbaum.

Oettingen, G. (1997). *Psychologie des Zukunftsdenkens* [The psychology of future orientation]. Göttingen, Germany: Hogrefe.

Papoušek, H., & Papoušek, M. (1987). Intuitive parenting: A dialectic counterpart to the infant's integrative competence. In J. D. Osofsky (Ed.), *Handbook of infant development* (2nd ed., pp. 669–720). New York: Wiley.

Pavlides, C., Watanabe, Y., Magarinos, A., & McEwen, B. (1995). Opposing roles of type I and type II adrenal steroid receptors in hippocampal long-term potentiation. *Neuroscience, 68*, 387–394.

Perls, F. (1973). *The Gestalt approach and eye witness to therapy.* Palo Alto, CA: Science and Bahavior Books.

Peterson, C., Maier, S. F., & Seligman, M. E. P. (1993). *Learned helplessness: A theory for the age of control.* New York: Oxford University Press.

Petty, R. E., Cacioppo, J. T., & Goldman, R. (1981). Personal involvement as a determinant of argument-based persuasion. *Journal of Personality and Social Psychology, 41*, 847–855.

Petty, R. E., Wells, G. L., & Brock, T. C. (1976). Distraction can enhance or reduce yielding to propaganda: Thought disruption versus effort justification. *Journal of Personality and Social Psychology, 64*, 5–20.

Posner, M. I. & Rothbart, M. K. (1992). Attentional mechanisms and conscious experience. In A. D. Milner & M. D. Milner & M. D. Rugg (Eds.), *The neuropsychology of consciousness.* (pp. 91–111). New York: Academic Press.

Pribram, K. H., & McGuiness, D. (1992). Attentional and para-attentional processing: Event-related brain potentials as tests of a model. *Annals of the New York Academy of Sciences, 658*, 65–92.

Reber, P. J., & Squire, L. R. (1994). Parallel brain systems for learning with and without awareness. *Learning and Memory, 1*, 217–229.

Rogers, C. R. (1961). *On becoming a person: A therapist's view of psychotherapy.* Boston: Houghton Mifflin.

Rosahl, S. K., Tennigkeit, M., Kuhl, J., & Haschke, R. (1993). Handlungskontrolle und langsame Hirnpotentiale: Untersuchungen zum Einfluß subjektiv kritischer Wörter (Erste Ergebnisse). [Action control and slow brain potentials: Studies on the influence of subjectively critical words (first results)]. *Zeitschrift für Medizinische Psychologie, 2*, 1–8.

Rumelhart, D. E., & McClelland, J. L. (1986). *Parallel distributed processing: Explorations in the microstructure of cognition* (Vol. 1). Cambridge, MA: MIT press.

Ryan, R. (1995). Psychological needs and the facilitation of integrative processes. *Journal of Personality, 63*, 397–427.

Ryan, R. M., Kuhl, J., & Deci, E. L. (1997). Nature and autonomy: An organizational view of social and neurobiological aspects of self-regulation in behavior and development. *Development and Psychopathology, 9*, 701–728.

Sapolsky, R. M. (1992) *Stress, the aging brain, and the mechanism of neuron death.* Cambridge, MA: MIT Press.

Scheibel, A. B., Freid, I., Paul, L., Forsythe, A., Tomiyasu, U., Wechsler, A., Kao, A., & Slotnick, J. (1985). Differentiating characteristics of the human speech cortex: A quantitative Golgi study. In D. F. Benson & E. Zaidel (Eds.), *The dual brain.* New York: Guilford.

Schneider, K. (1973). *Motivation unter Erfolgsrisiko.* [Motivation under risk]. Göttingen, Germany: Hogrefe.

Schwarz, N., Bless, H., & Bohner, G. (1991). Mood and persuasion: Affective states influence the processing of *persuasive* communications. In M. P. Zanna (Ed.), *Advances in experimental social psychology.* (Vol. 24, pp. 161–201). San Diego: CA: Academic Press.

Seligman, M. E. P., Nolen-Hoeksema, S., Thornton, N., & Thornton, K. M. (1990). Explanatory style as a mechanism of disappointing athletic performance. *Psychological Science, 1*, 143–146.

Shallice, T. (1988). *From neuropsychology to mental structure.* Cambridge, UK: Cambridge University Press.

Sheldon, K. M., & Elliot, A. J. (1998). Not all personal goals are personal: Comparing autonomous and controlled reasons for goals as predictors of effort and attainment. *Personality and Social Psychology Bulletin, 24*, 546–557.

Sheldon, K. M., & Kasser, T. (1995). Coherence and congruence: Two aspects of personality integration. *Journal of Personality and Social Psychology, 68*, 531–543.

Sheldon, K. M., & Kasser, T. (1998). Pursuing personal goals: Skills enable progress, but not all progress is beneficial. *Personality and Social Psychology Bulletin, 24*, 1319–1331.

Simon, D. P., & Simon, H. A. (1978). Individual differences in solving physics problems. In R. S. Siegler (Ed.), *Children's thinking: What develops*. Hillsdale, NJ: Erlbaum.

Smith, E. R. (1996). What do connectionism and social psychology offer each other? *Journal of Personality and Social Psychology, 70*, 893–912.

Smith, J. D., & Shapiro, J. H. (1989). The occurrence of holistic categorization. *Journal of Memory and Language, 28*, 386–399.

Sorrentino, R. M., Bobocel, D. R., Gitta, M. Z., & Olson, J. N. (1988). Uncertainty orientation and persuasion: Individual differences in the effects of personal relevance on social judgments. *Journal of Personality and Social Psychology, 55*, 357–371.

Squire, L. R. (1992). Memory and the hippocampus: A synthesis from findings with rats, monkeys, and humans. *Psychological Review, 99*, 195–231.

Stich, S. (1983). *From folk psychology to cognitive science*. Cambridge, MA: MIT Press.

Sutherland, R. W., & Rudy, J. W. (1989). Configurational association theory: The role of hippocampal formation in learning, memory and amnesia. *Psychobiology, 17*, 129–144.

Trope, Y., & Brickman, P. (1975). Difficulty and diagnosticity as determinants of choice among tasks. *Journal of Personality and Social Psychology, 31*, 918–925.

Tucker, D. M., & Williamson, P. A. (1984). Asymmetric neural control systems in human self-regulation. *Psychological Review, 91*, 185–215.

Tulving, E. (1985). How many memory systems are there? *American Psychologist, 40*, 495–501.

van Bergen, A. (1968). *Task interruption*. Amsterdam: North-Holland.

Wegener, D. T., Petty, R. E., & Smith, S. M. (1995). Positive mood can increase or decrease message scrutiny: The hedonic contingency view of mood and message processing. *Journal of Personality and Social Psychology, 69*, 5–15.

Wegner, D. M. (1994). Ironic processes of mental control. *Journal of Personality and Social Psychology, 101*(1), 34–52.

Weiner, B. (1974). *Achievement motivation and attribution theory*. Morristown, NJ: General Learning Press.

Wheeler, M. A., Stuss, D. T., & Tulving, E. (1997). Toward a theory of episodic memory: The frontal lobes and autonoetic consciousness. *Psychological Bulletin, 121*, 331–354.

Wittling, W. (1990). Psychophysiological correlates of human brain asymmetry: Blood pressure changes during lateralized presentation of an emotionally laden film. *Neuropsychologia, 28*, 457–470.

Yerkes, R. M., & Dodson, J. D. (1908). The relation of strength of stimulus to rapidity of habit-formation. *Journal of Comparative and Neurological Psychology, 18*, 459–482.

Zajonc, R. B. (1980). Feeling and thinking: Preferences need no inferences. *American Psychologist, 35*, 151–175.

Zeigarnik, B. (1927). Über das Behalten erledigter und unerledigter Handlungen [On remembering completed and uncompleted actions]. *Psychologische Forschung, 9*, 1–85.

6

PERSONALITY, SELF-REGULATION, AND ADAPTATION

A COGNITIVE – SOCIAL FRAMEWORK

GERALD MATTHEWS,[*] VICKI L. SCHWEAN,[†]
SIAN E. CAMPBELL,[*] DONALD H.SAKLOFSKE,[‡]
AND ABDALLA A. R. MOHAMED[*]

[*]*Department of Psychology, University of Dundee, Dundee, Scotland*
[†]*Department for the Education of Exceptional Children,*
University of Saskatchewan, Saskatoon, Canada
[‡]*Department of Educational Psychology, University of Saskatchewan,*
Saskatoon, Canada

I. FRAMEWORKS FOR PERSONALITY AND SELF-REGULATION RESEARCH

Integration of research on personality traits and self-regulation requires a resolution of two conflicting world views. The trait approach views personality as stable across time and across different situations. In contrast, much of the literature on self-regulation adopts a social–cognitive perspective that conceptualizes personality as the outcome of idiographic, contextually sensitive cognitive processes (Schwean & Saklofske, 1995). In this chapter, we outline a synthesis of these two perspectives that emphasizes stable cognitive knowledge structures as both a basis for personality traits and as an important influence on context-bound self-regulative cognitions. We conceptualize self-regulation as a generic umbrella term

---

Copyright © 2000 by Academic Press.
All rights of reproduction in any form reserved.

for the set of processes and behaviors that support the pursuit of personal goals within a changing external environment. Self-regulative constructs overlap to a large degree with constructs derived from the transactional theory of stress, such as appraisal and coping (Lazarus & Folkman, 1984).

We begin with definitions of constructs and a description of a cognitive architecture for self-regulation that specifies how self-knowledge influences appraisal and coping processes. We show that the architecture is compatible with both social–cognitive and trait perspectives. Next, we provide a general overview of empirical findings, that links various traits to individual differences in self-regulative processing and in self-knowledge. Then, we look at how the cognitive–social framework may be applied to three different research areas. Within each research area, we identify personality traits that relate to adaptive outcome and self-regulative processes that may mediate these associations. The first research area is that of reactions to life stressors. Traits associated with vulnerability to stress may influence appraisal and coping processes. The second area is performance of demanding tasks: traits and coping strategies are related to the cognitive psychology of attention. The third area is aggressive behavior, with a mainly developmental focus. Individual differences in aggression may reflect distorted appraisals of others and deficiencies in cognitive control. We conclude by summarizing the traits most closely related to self-regulation, and the cognitive structures and processes that may relate to those traits.

A. CONSTRUCTS OF THE COGNITIVE–SOCIAL FRAMEWORK

Cognitive models are vulnerable to overproliferation of constructs. Before describing our theoretical framework in detail, we outline some of the main distinctions made by cognitive theories of self-regulation and stress. Cognitive theories are based on an *architecture* that describes key processes and the flow of information between them. Processes have parameters or attributes: A schema may be activated to varying degrees or a stimulus evaluation process might output a code for "dangerous" or "harmless." Often, attributes of distinct processes tend to be correlated. For example, perceiving oneself as lacking control might be associated with activation of intrusive thoughts and choosing to avoid direct action. Sets of correlated process attributes define cognitive syndromes. Processes that contribute to the self-regulative architecture include the following.

Cognitive Stress Processes.   The transactional theory of stress describes information processing elicited by demanding encounters: appraisal and selection, and regulation of coping (Lazarus & Folkman, 1984). *Appraisal* is defined as the evaluation of a person's transactions with the environment, whereas *coping* refers to active, voluntary attempts to adapt to perceived demands. Appraisal may be variously directed toward the personal significance of external events (primary appraisal), evaluation of personal competence (secondary appraisal), and internal thoughts (metacognition) and emotions (mood awareness). Appraisals of other people are important to both real-life distress and to aggressive behavior. Coping may be directed either toward internal processing and states (emotion focused) or toward external action (task focused). Some types of coping are explicitly social in nature, such as constructive social problem solving and using confrontive or coercive actions against other people. Appraisal and coping reflect both dispositional factors and situationally dependent processing.

The syndrome of *worry* binds together appraisal and coping processes of special importance to self-regulation. In states of worry, a person's awareness of intrusive, predominantly negative ideation is supported by (1) metacognitive beliefs relating to the personal significance of intrusive or negative thoughts and (2) coping through perseverative rumination, as a form of problem solving (Matthews & Wells, 1996).

Knowledge Structures.   Long-term memory holds a library of items of self-referent information and "programs" for self-referent processing, which incorporate motivational information. Self-knowledge often is thought to be represented in organized, schematic form (Beck, 1967). It also includes normative information on personal and societal standards (Higgins, 1990). Cognitive stress processes (i.e., appraisal and coping) are influenced by this prior knowledge.

Outcome Variables.   The outcome of exposure to demanding or challenging events may be various symptoms of suboptimal adaptation, such as negative affect, health problems, performance impairment, or social dysfunction. We focus on outcomes appropriate to the research areas we review: general chronic distress in the case of life events, transient mental states in the case of performance environments, and aggressive behaviors.

Traits.   Traits are stable personality attributes, which may be divided into two categories: broad traits, and narrower self-referent traits. *Broad traits*, such as those of Eysenck, Costa, and McCrae, derive from comprehensive dimensional models of personality and relate to various psychological and physiological processes. This chapter is concerned with broad traits such as neuroticism that may be related closely to individual differences in self-knowledge. *Self-referent traits* are constructed specifically to measure some aspect of self-knowledge or self-regulative processing. Generalized self-efficacy, self-esteem, and optimism–pessimism describe the typical content of a person's thoughts, whereas dispositional self-consciousness, metacognitive style, and trait worry describe styles of information processing. Table 1 summarizes some of these trait measures.

TABLE 1   Brief Definitions of Some "Self-Regulative" Traits

Trait	Definition
Generalized self-efficacy	Beliefs that actions leading to desired outcomes can be performed successfully
Self-esteem	Beliefs of personal and social self-worth
Optimism–pessimism	Generalized expectancy of positive outcomes
Dispositional self-consciousness	Self-preoccupation and attention to various aspects of the self
Metacognitive style	Typical metacognitive beliefs and processes; i.e., typical appraisals of one's own thoughts
Trait worry	Tendency to engage in thought characterized by predominantly negative cognitions of the self and personal problems

B. A COGNITIVE ARCHITECTURE FOR SELF-REGULATION

Integration of personality trait and social–cognitive perspectives requires a specification of how the various aspects of processing just described are interrelated within a common cognitive architecture for self-regulation. The Wells and Matthews (1994, 1996) Self-Regulative Executive Function (S-REF) model of emotional dysfunction distinguishes three levels of cognition: a stimulus-driven lower-level network of interacting processing units, a supervisory executive implementing voluntary control, and self-knowledge held in long-term memory. The executive (the S-REF) is the core of the system and, in keeping with the cybernetic approach to self-regulation (Carver & Scheier, 1981), it operates to minimize self-discrepancy (defined as mismatch between a representation of the status of the self) and some normative representation (Higgins, 1990). S-REF activity is initiated by input from the lower-level network, which might be generated either by an external stimulus, such as an overt threat, or by internal cycles of processing, such as "automatic thoughts" (Beck, 1967). Executive processing of intrusions is influenced by self-knowledge and conceptualized as a library of "plans" or generic proceduralized knowledge (cf. Anderson, 1982). The executive accesses a plan or plans from long-term memory and modifies the plan to formulate and implement a coping strategy appropriate to (appraisals of) current circumstances. In states of severe distress, S-REF functioning is associated with perseverative worry; that is, a syndrome of self-focused attention, negative self-appraisals, ruminative coping, and impairment of attention to the external world. Appraisals of one's own cognitions (metacognitions) are an especially important influence on the maintenance of worry (Cartwright-Hatton & Wells, 1997).

The consequences of self-regulation depend on the coping and appraisal processes initiated by self-discrepancy. The two types of processes roughly correspond to the distinction traditionally made in research on the self, between an active conception of the self as doer and a more passive representation of the self as object (Smith, 1950). However, the transactional approach (Lazarus & Folkman, 1984) emphasizes the interplay rather than the distinctiveness of active and passive aspects of the self. Changes in appraisal of the self may be both a cause and a consequence of a person's active attempts to deal with external demands. For example, reappraisal of the success of active coping efforts may lead to a change in self-knowledge. Conversely, the S-REF model also emphasizes the role of self-knowledge as an influence on self-regulative processing and choice of coping strategy. The model also describes processing that is internally directed but active in nature, such as management of disturbing internal stimuli by monitoring or suppressing them, and active restructuring or transformation of self-knowledge.

Figure 1 summarizes the cognitive architecture that supports the S-REF. Note that the processing components distinguished in the figure may have various attributes, and syndromes such as worry cannot be localized at any single process. Stress outcomes reflect both the functioning of the system as a whole (e.g., negative affect) and specific coping responses (e.g., performance change, aggressive behavior). Traits are conceptualized as relating to stable individual differences in the various processing components, especially properties of self-knowledge. Typically, traits relate to attributes or parameters of multiple processes: In a sense, a trait is a cognitive syndrome frozen across time.

C. SELF-REGULATION AND SOCIAL COGNITION

Self-regulation often is conceptualized in terms of idiographic processing routines and knowledge structures shaped by social interaction and culture. Markus and Cross (1990) described various representations of the self, including the ideal self, and possible and future selves. Such representations may include a strong motivational component, as expressed by constructs such as life tasks, projects, or strivings (e.g., Emmons, 1992). Self-regulation then performs the functions of monitoring and promoting attainment of a person's idiosyncratic goals. Lavallee and Campbell (1995) showed that personal goal-related daily events elicited stronger self-regulatory responses than other events. From the S-REF perspective, self-constructs emerge from the plans relevant to different aspects of the self. For example, there is no single plan or schema labeled "future self." Instead, a person's sense of future self is distributed across various plans relevant to future adaptation, such as those for monitoring life trajectory and making preparations for future career and family needs. Clinical evidence illustrates how an individual's idiosyncratic self-beliefs shape specific (maladaptive) self-regulative processing (Wells, 1997).

D. TRAITS AND STABLE INDIVIDUAL DIFFERENCES
IN SELF-REGULATION

The personality trait construct appears superficially to be antagonistic to the fluid, dynamic nature of self-regulative processing. However, as Matthews and Deary (1998) argued, social processes are too important to be left to social psychologists. There are several areas of contact between trait psychology and social–cognitive theory. First, broad traits such as neuroticism relate to self-regulation, social cognition, and the personal meanings individuals attach to social interactions (Matthews & Deary, 1998). Second, the self-regulative traits listed in Table 1 are nomothetic constructs that predict individual differences in self-regulative behavior. It follows that self-regulation must have nomothetic as well as idiographic qualities. Third, the role of self-knowledge in maintaining the stability of personality traits has been neglected. Depression, for example, may be an expression of stable self-schemas, with not only idiosyncratic content, but also commonalities that drive the errors in reasoning typical of the disorder (Beck, 1967). In normal populations, traits relate (necessarily) to commonalities in self-appraisal and, perhaps more interestingly, to other aspects of cognition. Trait-anxious individuals give more pessimistic self-evaluations in various specific contexts such as performance and social interaction (Wells & Matthews, 1994). Matthews (1997, 1999) described a *cognitive–adaptive framework* for personality in which self-knowledge plays an important role in maintaining the stability of personality. Self-beliefs promote consistency in choice of environments and adaptive goals, and foster acquisition of objective skills required for adaptive specialization.

Finally, personality relates to attentional processes that constrain the operation of self-regulation. A key property of S-REF function is that attention is self-focused, biasing the system toward registration of self-relevant intrusions and toward accessing self-discrepancies. In states of worry, self-referent processing functions withdraw attentional resources from other mental activities, leading to performance decrements on attentionally demanding tasks. This process is described as *cognitive interference* (Sarason, Sarason, & Pierce, 1995). Hence, regardless of the idiographic content of self-regulative processing, system operation reflects the capacity of the cognitive architecture to handle concurrent task- and self-related processing. Worry may interfere not only with task performance (Sarason et al., 1995), but also with other self-regulative functions such as attentionally demanding coping strategies and modification of self-knowledge (Matthews & Wells, 1996).

Specifications of the cognitive architecture and adaptive significance of self-regulation provide a general framework that accommodates both the idiographic content of self-knowledge and stable, nomothetic qualities of self-regulation related to personality traits. Studies of individual differences in self-regulation allow personality traits to be linked to the various processes shown in Figure 1. Next, we review some of the evidence on traits and self-regulation.

II. SELF-REGULATION, TRAITS, AND COGNITIVE STRESS PROCESSES

To develop the cognitive–social model of personality, it is important to determine the underlying knowledge structures and self-regulative processes linked to traits. One of the difficulties here is that the research cannot assess knowledge structures directly. Instead, we must infer processing from behavior (including verbal report) and then infer knowledge structures from processing. This section comprises brief reviews of the relationships between traits and coping and appraisal processes, including the self-referent appraisals of one's own cognition (metacognition) and affect (mood awareness). It concludes by relating neuroticism and trait anxiety to worry.

A. COPING

Coping is closely linked to self-regulation in that choice of coping strategy reflects evaluation of personal competence to deal with the problem at hand, or "secondary appraisal" (Lazarus & Folkman, 1984). Lazarus and Folkman distinguished problem- (or task-) focused coping, directed toward changing external reality, from emotion-focused coping, which seeks to change feelings and thoughts about the source of stress. Endler and Parker (1990) added a third basic dimension of avoidance of the stressor. There are some difficulties with both taxonomies, especially the diverse nature of "emotion focus" (Carver, Scheier, & Weintraub, 1989; Summerfeldt & Endler, 1996). Endler and Parker's (1990) dimension relates primarily to self-criticism and wishful thinking, whereas Lazarus and Folkman (1984) also discussed rather different emotion-focused strategies including self-control and positive reappraisal.

The self-regulative theory outlined in the preceding text suggests a three-way conceptual distinction between *palliative* coping, producing temporary respite from distress, *ruminative problem-solving* attempts such as self-criticism and self-reflection, and *self-transformation* by modification of self-knowledge in long-term memory. Palliative coping covers various attempts at self-distraction (e.g., through fantasy or engaging in other activities), and attempts to suppress or deny stress symptoms. The person seeks to terminate S-REF operation without directly addressing the problem at hand. Coping through ruminating on the problem or one's faults are

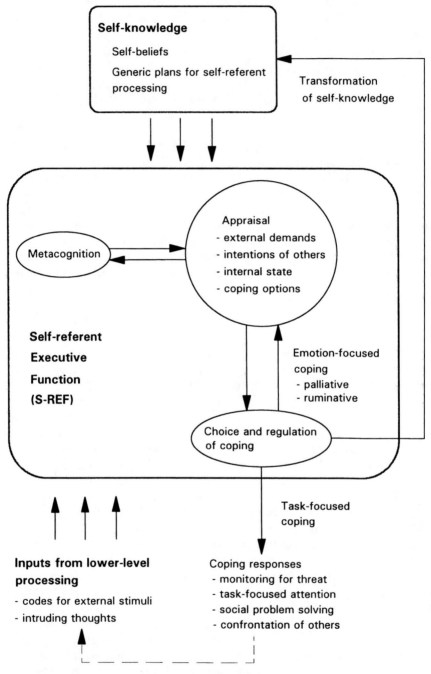

FIGURE 1   Cognitive architecture of the Wells and Matthews (1994) S-REF model.

instances of (usually) maladaptive problem solving, which involves protracted S-REF activity. People who engage in self-criticism, rumination, and similar forms of worry-related coping believe these forms of coping will provide solutions to their problems, although, as clinical evidence shows, this is rarely the case (Wells & Matthews, 1994). In fact, it seems that rumination and worry tend to block access to self-knowledge and so prevent the deeper modification of self-beliefs we describe as self-transformation (Morgan, Matthews, & Winton, 1995). The idea of adaptive restructuring of self-knowledge is common in clinical psychology (e.g., Wells, 1997), but it is poorly represented by existing coping measures. The Roger, Jarvis, and Najarian (1993) "detached coping" scale may assess one of its aspects; facilitation of coping through assessing the problem without feeling personally involved or threatened. It may be difficult to effect significant changes in self-representation simply by reflecting on the self; assistance from others or transforming life experiences may be required.

There is extensive evidence on personality correlates of coping (see Costa, Somerfield, & McCrae, 1996; Matthews et al., 1998b, for summaries). Coping may be assessed either through measures of general style of coping with life events or through context-specific measures. Both types of study tend to implicate neuroticism (N) as the broad trait most strongly related to coping tendencies, especially ruminative emotion-focused strategies. Neuroticism seems to be more weakly related to higher avoidance (palliative coping) and reduced task focus (Endler & Parker, 1990). Other broad personality factors are implicated to a lesser degree: both extroversion (E) and conscientiousness (C) have been linked to task focus, for example (Deary et al., 1996; Endler & Parker, 1990). A variety of narrower traits theoretically linked to self-regulation also are found to predict individual differences in coping. Trait anxiety has coping correlates similar to N (e.g., Bolger, 1990). Several traits, including optimism, locus of control, and hardiness, relate to use of task focus in preference to emotion focus (Scheier & Carver, 1992), although there are doubts about the extent to which such relationships may be mediated by the substantial correlations between these traits and neuroticism (Schaubroeck & Ganster, 1991). Self-regulative traits also correlate with coping. Dispositional self-consciousness, or self-focus of attention, tends to relate to a more passive style of coping (Matthews & Wells, 1996). Jerusalem and Schwarzer (1989) reported that both self-efficacy and self-esteem were associated with more use of instrumental coping (task focus) and less emotional coping.

B. APPRAISAL

Lazarus and Folkman (1984) identified threat, loss, and challenge as important aspects of situational demands. In addition, appraisals of control describe a person's overall appraisal of his or her ability to cope with demands. Generally, neurotic and trait-anxious individuals appraise them-

180   PART I. GENERAL THEORIES AND MODELS OF SELF-REGULATION

selves as especially vulnerable to threat and as lacking in the personal qualities required for successful coping (Wells & Matthews, 1994). Such biases have been shown in situations where the level of threat is experimentally controlled (e.g., Kennedy & Craighead, 1988), implying that the plans for interpreting the place of the self in the world available to neurotic individuals are negatively biased. Sometimes, emotionally stable individuals may be biased toward overoptimism, as depressive realism phenomena (Alloy & Abramson, 1979) show. Other broad and narrow traits may relate to individual differences in appraisal. Extroversion has been linked to challenge appraisals (Gallagher, 1990) and optimism has been linked to control appraisals in stressful situations (Carver, Scheier, & Pozo, 1992). Appraisal and coping biases may be interrelated, in that people choose coping strategies that match the appraised demands of the situation and that they believe they can implement personally.

Appraisals of social functioning are also biased by traits. Neurotic individuals underestimate the amount of social support available to them (Stokes, 1985), for example. Social anxiety is quite substantially correlated with N and relates to various negative social appraisals, such as low self-ratings of interpersonal abilities, which may lead to shyness and loneliness (Jones, Rose, & Russell, 1990). Shyness relates to both neuroticism and introversion. It is associated with low self-esteem in a variety of different contexts, including some that are not overtly social, such as academic and physical abilities (Cheek & Melchior, 1990). Negative self-beliefs in social settings contribute to socially oriented negative cognitive–affective states of guilt, shame, and embarrassment (Klass, 1990). Negative self-appraisals may constitute a self-fulfilling prophecy, in that shy persons may be appraised by others as aloof, and lonely individuals tend to be seen as lacking in self-esteem and social skills (Jones et al., 1990). In general, difficulties in self-regulation associated with negative appraisals in social settings appear to be an important aspect of N and related traits.

C. METACOGNITION AND MOOD AWARENESS

Metacognition is a special form of appraisal: a person's appraisals of his or her own cognitive processes, including beliefs about self-control of cognition. The S-REF model (Wells & Matthews, 1994) assigns a key role to metacognitive processing in self-regulation. Metacognitive beliefs influence a person's choice of coping, in that rumination or attempts at palliative thought control are more likely if the person believes that carrying out these mental activities will help with the problem (Wells, 1997). Metacognition of the self as a social agent is an important aspect of social functioning. Cheek and Melchior (1990) attribute shyness to metacognitive processing of self-relevant social cognitions, such that the shy person is preoccupied with his or her social competence and appearance to others. Maladaptive metacognitions, such as beliefs that thoughts are uncontrollable, may block self-transformation through knowledge restructuring.

Cartwright-Hatton and Wells (1997) developed the Meta-Cognitions Questionnaire (MCQ) for assessment of metacognitive style; that is, a person's typical metacognitions. It assesses five dimensions: positive beliefs, uncontrollability of thoughts, (lack of) cognitive confidence, need for control, and cognitive self-consciousness. Scores were highly stable over a 5-week period. Trait anxiety correlated with all five subscales and correlated at .68 with total score ($N = 104$). Hence, trait anxiety (and presumably N) is quite strongly related to (1) the general importance the person places on cognitive self-regulation and (2) various specific beliefs about cognition, which may be maladaptive. Test anxiety relates both to metacognitions, as assessed by the MCQ, and, independently, to a dysfunctional coping style in examination settings (Matthews, Hillyard, & Campbell, in press).

Mood awareness is another form of self-referent appraisal, referring to appraisal of the internal state (see Figure 1). Mayer, Salovey, Gomberg-Kaufman, and Blainey (1991) claim that people have a self-reflective or meta-experience of mood, which includes not only awareness of mood states, but also action to change mood through strategies of thoughts of action—suppression and denial. Another approach (Swinkels & Giuliano, 1995) has distinguished mood monitoring from mood labeling. The former process, referring to frequent evaluation of mood, is associated with N, negative affect, and private and public self-consciousness. Swinkels and Giuliano see mood monitoring as likely to lead to maladaptive rumination, although it also may promote empathy toward others. Mood labeling (i.e., being able to describe and explain one's moods) correlates positively with E, positive affect, and self-esteem, and negatively with N, social anxiety, and alexithymia. Clarity of thought about one's moods may promote evaluation of coping options.

In general, it is often difficult to distinguish (1) direct regulation of states from more general coping efforts and (2) self-regulation of mood from self-regulation of cognition. Nevertheless, there seem to be systematic individual differences in processing information related to the person's own moods, which correlate with personality traits and well-being.

D. WORRY

The concept of worry brings together negative self-appraisal, ruminative coping attempts, and metacognitive beliefs in the utility of worry as a higher-order cognitive syndrome. Wells (1994) developed a trait worry questionnaire, which distinguishes two dimensions of content—social and health worries—and a process dimension of *metaworry*; that is, worry about one's tendencies to worry. Metaworry represents a maladaptive form of self-regulation and seems to be an important component of generalized anxiety disorder (Wells, 1997). It correlates .60 with N and .68 with trait anxiety ($N = 96$). Neuroticism also correlates with social worries ($r = .62$) and, to a lesser degree ($r = .52$), with health worries (Wells, 1994). The magnitude of the correlations reported by Wells (1994, 1997) implies that metaworry, social worry, and metacognition are central to N and trait anxiety.

III. PERSONALITY AND SELF-REGULATION OF REACTIONS TO LIFE STRESS

Thus far, we have described various personality correlates of self-regulative processes. In this section, we review recent work at Dundee (Mohamed, 1996) that aimed to investigate the interrelationships of stress outcomes, cognitive stress process variables, and personality in rather more depth. It focused on neuroticism and dispositional self-consciousness as traits of particular importance to people's reactions to life events. The research addressed three questions concerning individual differences in the appraisals and coping strategies elicited by external demands. It assessed two of the appraisal processes shown in Figure 1: appraisal of external demands (threat, loss, and challenge) and appraisal of coping options, operationalized here as a perceived control. First, how robust are the associations between N, appraisal, and coping across different sources of stress? Second, are associations between N and stress outcome measures mediated by appraisal and coping? Third, how does N compare to measures of dispositional self-consciousness as a predictor of stress process and outcome?

A. NEUROTICISM AS A PREDICTOR OF APPRAISAL AND COPING

Table 2 summarizes data from three studies. In each case, N was assessed with the Eysenck Personality Questionnaire-Revised (EPQ-R) (Eysenck, Eysenck, & Barrett, 1985), and overall stress symptoms were assessed with the General Health Questionnaire (GHQ: Goldberg, 1978). In Study 1 ($N = 218$), subjects were postgraduate students who were asked for single ratings of various dimensions of appraisal and coping across eight stressors. There were consistent individual differences in response across stressors so ratings were averaged to give indices of general style of cognition. In Study 2 ($N = 150$), students were first-year undergraduates

TABLE 2 Correlations between N and Appraisal and Coping Measures
in Three Studies

	1	2	3 (AH)	3 (WK)
Appraisal				
Threat	44**	38**	17**	37**
Loss	−39**	34**	18**	27**
Challenge	−11	06	−08	−14*
Perceived control	−41**	−34**	−17**	−37**
Coping				
Task focus	−21***[a]	20**	−04	−10
Emotion focus	43***[b]	38**	19**	47**
Avoidance	21***[c]	09	10	20**

Note. AH = being away from home; WK = pressure of work. Reproduced from *Stress Processes in British and Overseas Students*, by A. A. R. Mohamed, 1996, unpublished doctoral dissertation, University of Dundee. Used with permission of the author.
[a]Problem focus.
[b]Self-criticism.
[c]Distraction.
*p < .05. **p < .01.

who completed appraisal and coping questionnaires (Endler & Parker, 1990; Ferguson, Matthews, & Cox, in press) for their cognitions of a single stressor, being away from the family home.

Study 3 (N = 207) was conducted in collaboration with Ian Deary. Postgraduate students completed separate sets of questionnaires for two stressors: (1) being away from home and (2) pressure of academic work.

The table shows that, despite differences in sample and the nature of the source of stress, N was consistently related to appraisals of threat, loss, and lack of control, and to emotion-focused coping. The association between N and task focus was somewhat unstable, with one study actually showing a positive correlation, contrary to the general trend in the literature (Costa et al., 1996). As in other studies (e.g., Deary et al., 1996), N was quite strongly correlated with GHQ total score, with *r*s varying from .48 to .62. Morgan, Matthews, and Winton (1995) obtained similar results in a community sample of individuals who suffered property damage as a result of a flood: N predicted negative appraisals, emotion-focused coping, and DSM-III-R trauma symptoms. Table 1 follows the Endler and Parker (1990) model of coping, with emotion focus assessed mostly through items referring to self-blame or self-criticism. Study 1 used rating scales based on the Lazarus and Folkman (1984) coping taxonomy, which distinguishes various aspects of emotion focus. Although N was associated with self-criticism, it was not significantly correlated with reappraisal or detachment. Similarly, N was unrelated to attempts to suppress unpleasant thoughts in the Morgan et al. (1995) study. In terms of the theoretical distinctions made previously, these findings suggest that linking N to emotion focus in the broad sense is misleading. Instead, N relates more to self-criticism than to palliative coping or to self-transformation.

The other broad traits measured in this research were extraversion (E) and psychoticism (P). Introverts resembled neurotics in reporting higher levels of stress symptoms, and a tendency to use emotion focus rather than task focus. However, correlations were smaller in magnitude (none exceeded .3) and rather inconsistent across studies. Correlations between P and the stress-related variables did not exceed chance levels.

A subset of the undergraduate sample of Study 2 ($N = 93$) also completed a measure of generalized self-discrepancy, calculated as the sum of the differences between actual and ideal ratings of 16 areas of life important to students. The measure was internally consistent ($\alpha = .82$). It was correlated with threat appraisal ($r = .29$, $p < .01$), loss appraisal ($r = .26$, $p < .05$), emotion focus ($r = .25$, $p < .05$), N ($r = .28$, $p < .01$), and GHQ total score ($r = .36$, $p < .01$). These data are consistent with the hypothesized role of self-discrepancy as an influence on cognitive stress processes, although appraisal and coping perhaps may be related more strongly to self-knowledge related to the specific stressor concerned (being away from home).

B. MEDIATION OF NEUROTICISM EFFECTS BY COGNITIVE STRESS PROCESSES

Mohamed (1996) also investigated the role of appraisal and coping in mediating associations between N and stress outcome, using multiple regression methods. In each study, mediation was no more than partial. Table 3 shows percentages of variances, explained by various sources, for the data of Table 2. Both N alone and the seven cognitive appraisal and coping variables explain substantial percentages of the variance. The amount of variance uniquely explained by each of the two sources may be

TABLE 3   Percentages of Variance Explained by Various Variable Sets in Three Studies

	1	2	3
N	28 (28)	22 (22)	38 (38)
Appraisal and coping	37 (34)	34 (32)	44 (41)
Appraisal, coping, and N	43 (40)	42 (39)	59 (56)
Var. unique to N	6 (6)	8 (7)	15 (15)
Var. unique to appraisal and coping	15 (12)	20 (17)	19 (16)

Note. Data reanalyzed from *Stress Processes in British and Overseas Students*, by A. A. R. Mohamed, 1996, unpublished doctoral dissertation, University of Dundee.

estimated by subtraction from the total variance explained: For example, the unique contribution of N is the total variance minus the variance explained by the cognitive factors. In all three studies, both N and the cognitive variables added significant independent increments to the total variance. The contribution of N was diminished by control for the cognitive variables, but remained appreciable (6%–15%).

These analyses support a *weak transactional model* of the influence of N. Neuroticism may relate to stress vulnerability in part because of its association with somewhat maladaptive styles of appraisal and coping. That is, N is associated with a style of self-regulative processing oriented toward awareness of threat and self-criticism, which may derive from general and context-linked negative self-beliefs. However, N predicts stress outcome over and above individual differences in appraisal and coping, and so it cannot be reduced solely to these factors. The excess predictive power of N may represent biologically mediated effects (Eysenck, 1994), associations between N and information processing inaccessible to conscious awareness, or consciously reportable cognitions not assessed in the study.

C. DISPOSITIONAL SELF-CONSCIOUSNESS AND COGNITIVE STRESS PROCESSES

The second issue addressed by Mohamed (1996) was the role of dispositional self-consciousness as an influence on the stress process. This trait refers to the tendency to engage in self-focused attention, which we hypothesize derives from the person's generic plans for interrogating and scrutinizing self-relevant information. In Study 1, subjects also completed the Fenigstein, Scheier, and Buss, (1975) questionnaire, which assesses three aspects of self-consciousness: private and public self-consciousness (PR and PU), and social anxiety (SO). PR assesses self-reflection, PU assesses awareness of outwardly observable aspects of the self, and SO assesses reactions to being observed by others. Correlations between these scales and N were .28 for PR ($p < .05$), .40 for PU ($p < .01$), and .48 for SO. Table 4 shows the correlations between dispositional self-consciousness measures and the stress-related variables. The table also gives partial correlations, with N controlled. Self-consciousness was associated with a general increase in primary appraisal, including challenge as well as threat and loss, in the case of private and public self-consciousness. Most of these associations were maintained with N controlled. The three Fenigstein et al. scales also tended to relate to greater emotion focus and avoidance, less task focus, and higher overall stress symptoms. However, with N controlled, only PU and SO predicted coping and GHQ score, with SO the only predictor of reduced task focus and increased avoidance. Thus, like N, self-consciousness traits, especially public self-consciousness and social

TABLE 4   Correlations between Three Dimensions of Self-Consciousness
(Fenigstein et al., 1975) and Appraisal, Coping, and GHQ Total Score: Uncorrected
and Corrected for Neuroticism (Mohamed, 1996)

	PR		PU		SO	
	r	Partial	r	Partial	r	Partial
Appraisal						
Threat	25**	15*	41**	27**	40**	25**
Loss	23**	14	36**	23**	32**	17*
Challenge	25**	23**	21**	18*	−09	04
Perceived control	09	03	−20**	−03	−31**	−15*
Coping						
Task focus	03	10	−14*	−06	−31**	−25**
Emotion focus	23**	13	40**	27**	39**	23**
Avoidance	−05	−11	16*	08	26**	18*
GHQ total score	15*	00	40**	22**	44**	25**

Note. Partial *r*: Correlation corrected for confounding by neuroticism.
*$p < .05$.   **$p < .01$.

anxiety, tend to relate to maladaptive cognitive reactions. Unlike N, PR
and PU seem to relate to a general amplification of appraisal of events.

In further analysis of the data, Matthews, Mohamed, and Lochrie
(1998c) showed that relationships between PR and cognition vary with a
person's appraisal of the changeability of situations. High self-consciousness seems particularly maladaptive when situations are appraised as
changeable. People in general tend to use more task focus in these
circumstances, but high PR subjects do not. Instead, they appraise the
situation as threatening, and favor reappraisal as a coping strategy. That is,
self-conscious individuals fail to take advantage of the affordances for
task-directed action that the situation provides.

In general, the influence of dispositional self-consciousness appears to
be similar but distinct from that of N. It seems that N relates to availability
of negative self-knowledge in various respects, including negative self-
beliefs, high self-discrepancy, and plans for metacognition and coping that
focus attention on negative information. Self-consciousness seems to enhance awareness of self-discrepancy, but also may amplify awareness of
positive features of the situation, such as the challenges it affords. Self-
consciousness may tend to relate to the accessibility rather than the
availability of self-relevant beliefs. Studies in which self-focus is manipulated tend to support similar conclusions (Matthews & Wells, 1996). For
example, self-focus impairs attention and performance in high-test-anxious
subjects, but enhances it in subjects low in test anxiety (Carver, Peterson,
Follansbee, & Scheier, 1983). The more social forms of self-consciousness
appear to be more strongly associated with stress outcomes than private

self-consciousness is, implying that awareness of scrutiny by others is particularly effective in activating self-discrepancy.

IV. PERSONALITY AND SELF-REGULATION IN PERFORMANCE ENVIRONMENTS

Studies that investigate transactions between persons and life stressors deal with temporally protracted sequences of events that differ from person to person. Laboratory studies of stress and performance allow the investigation of self-regulation and stress under more controlled circumstances. Such studies cannot, of course, simulate the anguish that may be attendant on real-life events. Hence, as with life stressors, these studies are concerned with appraisal of external demands and personal coping competence (see Figure 1), but they concern minor hassles (Kohn, 1996) rather than major events. By focusing on a restricted set of external demands, we can investigate self-regulative processing in more detail than is possible in the typical study of life events. We discuss the roles of both broad traits, including neuroticism, and of trait self-efficacy as a self-regulative trait that makes explicit reference to performance.

There is a growing literature on self-regulation and motivation in performance environments (e.g., Kanfer, 1990). Self-regulation may be damaging to performance when it diverts attention from task-related processing, as shown empirically in test anxiety research (Sarason et al., 1995) and in studies of complex cognitive skill acquisition (Kanfer & Ackerman, 1989). In other circumstances, self-regulation may promote effective task-directed effort. Bandura's (e.g., 1986) self-efficacy theory supposes that one's beliefs about personal capacity to achieve performance goals influence motivation and performance. Kluger and DeNisi (1996) distinguish task motivation from "metatask" processes. Task motivation processes are driven by discrepancies between a task standard and performance, whereas metatask processes are initiated by self-discrepancies with respect to goals of maintaining self-esteem and control and presenting a good impression. The effects of these processes on task-directed effort and performance are complex and depend on both person and task factors. In general, self-efficacy, anxiety, and task difficulty tend to promote distracting metatask processing, cognitive interference, and performance impairment.

A. COGNITIVE–ATTENTIONAL MECHANISMS FOR ANXIETY EFFECTS ON PERFORMANCE

As previously discussed, various traits related to negative affectivity, such as anxiety, promote self-focused processing and cognitive interference (e.g., Eysenck, 1992; Sarason et al., 1995). The S-REF theory proposes that demanding tasks often elicit a cognitive–attentional syndrome of self-focus, worry, and distress in vulnerable individuals, that interferes with performance. Developing the self-regulative theory of traits requires us to dissect the components of the syndrome by distinguishing different self-regulative functions and their impact on attention, performance, and well-being (see Matthews & Wells, 1996, for a coping-based analysis).

Activation of the executive system (the S-REF) may have both direct and indirect effects on performance. A person's appraisal of his or her coping options within the task environment may initiate task-focused coping, which directly alters processing of task stimuli. Matthews and Wells (1999) attribute the attentional bias commonly found in distressed individuals to adoption of a strategy for voluntary monitoring for threat stimuli. This interpretation of the bias data is supported by experimental data that show context and expectancy effects (see Matthews & Wells, 1999, for a review), and connectionist modeling (Matthews & Harley, 1996). Test anxiety is often associated with motives to withdraw from the situation and reduction of task-directed effort (Geen, 1987), but anxious subjects may sometimes apply additional effort to compensate for anxiety-driven cognitive interference (Eysenck & Calvo, 1992). Depending on circumstances, the anxious individual may over- or undercompensate for the appraised deficit (Matthews, 1999). Adoption of emotion-focused coping may have indirect effects, to the extent that the processing required interferes with task processing. Protracted rumination and self-evaluation seem to be particularly deleterious to performance: Kanfer and Stevenson (1985) showed experimentally that instructions to self-regulate impair performance.

Hence, traits related to anxiety and negative affectivity should not be seen purely as deficit factors. Conceptualizing anxiety as simply a loss of functional processing capacity is a crude and misleading simplification. Anxiety in performance contexts represents an attempt to adapt to an environment characterized by threats to desired self-representations (Matthews, 1999). The behavioral consequences of anxiety depend on the choice of coping strategy, which in turn depends on the accessibility of plans for coping, on-line appraisal of the likely efficacy of those plans, and the constraints placed upon processing by the attentional demands of the S-REF.

B. SELF-REGULATION AND STRESS PROCESSES IN PERFORMANCE ENVIRONMENTS

Recent work at Dundee has attempted to integrate experimental work on stress and performance with the transactional perspective on individual differences in stress reactions discussed in the previous section. A first step is to distinguish different aspects of stress state, such as the well-known distinctions between worry and emotion (Eysenck, 1992) and tension and tiredness (Thayer, 1996). Matthews et al. (1999) presented psychometric and experimental evidence from performance studies that identifies three dimensions of the subjective stress state: task disengagement (e.g., tiredness, boredom, loss of concentration), distress (negative mood, lack of control), and worry (self-focus, loss of self-esteem, cognitive interference). They suggest that these three dimensions represent three key aspects of person–environment transaction in performance environments: commitment to perform well, overload, and self-evaluation, respectively.

Put slightly differently, the three stress state dimensions may represent different modes of self-regulation. Task engagement indexes an orientation toward achieving personal goals through task-directed attention and effort. Distress represents attempts to minimize the damage caused by demands that a person cannot meet successfully. Worry reflects states in which self-evaluation takes precedence over task demands. The S-REF model emphasizes the dynamic interrelationship of these states, especially in pathological states. Matthews et al. (1999) showed that demanding tasks that evoke distress reactions also may elicit increased task engagement and decrease worry: damage limitation here involves "doing one's best" in difficult circumstances. However, in severe anxiety and depression states, distress and worry appear to be reciprocally linked, leading to perseverative cycles of self-referent cognition and negative affect (Wells & Matthews, 1994).

The analysis just outlined makes predictions about the interrelationships between traits, cognitive stress processes, and stress state response. The causal model here is that appraisal and coping processes (influenced by traits and self-knowledge) generate patterns of cognition, motivation, and affect that are indexed by stress state and represent different modes of self-regulation. Hence, individual differences in appraisal and coping should be correlated with stress states. Challenge appraisal and task-focused coping should promote task engagement, and avoidance should relate to task disengagement. Threat stimuli are threatening only to the extent that self-protective actions are difficult. Hence, threat appraisals should be associated with overload of the processing required to maintain personal security and, consequently, with distress. Depending on its immediacy and other factors, threat may call for either direct action or self-reflection, and so no general relationship with the task engagement or worry was predicted. Emotion-focused coping (in the sense of maladaptive problem solving) might be associated with either attempts to deal with overload through self-criticism of one's efforts to deal with it (leading to distress) or more general attempts to review one's feelings about the task environment (leading to worry). In controlled task environments, avoidance is likely to take the form of withdrawing attention from the task rather than engaging in distracting but unavailable activities such as shopping. Hence, avoidance makes more attentional resources available for self-reflection, and so this coping strategy should tend to increase worry.

Similarly, the biasing effect of N may be predicted from its associations with self-regulation. As previously described, relationships between N and commitment of effort to performance seem to be unstable, and so its correlation with task engagement is difficult to predict. However, given that N seems to relate to threat appraisal and emotion focus, N should predict both distress and worry. Matthews et al. (1999) found that in a large sample ($N = 762$) of subjects performing various tasks, N was unrelated to posttask engagement, but did predict posttask distress ($r = .29, p < .01$) and worry ($r = .21, p < .01$). Extroversion was associated with lower distress ($r = -.19, p < .01$), but not with the other dimensions.

In a recent, unpublished study, two of us (G.M. and S.E.C.) investigated individual differences in self-regulation and stress reactions using a version of the Rapid Information Processing task (Battig & Buzzi, 1986), modified to make it particularly demanding. The subject is required to detect sequences of either three odd or three even digits in a stream of single digits. Several experimental conditions were run, but here we focus on the condition intended to be most generally stressful, in which 108 subjects were tested. Each minute, 150 stimuli were presented, leading to poor performance (mean hit rate was ca. 30%). Subjects also were given periodic negative feedback intended to activate self-discrepancy, indicating that they were failing to reach a performance standard. Personality was measured with short versions of the EPQ-R (Eysenck et al., 1985) and Goldberg's (1992) unipolar adjectival markers for the Big Five. Appraisal was measured with the Ferguson et al. (in press) threat and challenge scales and a perceived control scale developed by Mohamed (1996). A new measure of coping with performance environments was used in this study, the Coping Inventory for Task Stress (CITS: Matthews & Campbell, 1998). The CITS was developed through factor analysis of items specifically referring to performance strategies, including items adapted from existing coping questionnaires (e.g., Endler & Parker, 1990; Carver et al., 1989). Three aspects of coping were measured: task focus, emotion focus (i.e. rumination and self-criticism), and avoidance (i.e., mentally withdrawing from the task). As expected, N was correlated with threat appraisal ($r = .31, p < .01$) and with emotion focus ($r = .35, p < .01$), although its correlation with avoidance ($r = .12$) was nonsignificant.

Table 5 summarizes multiple regression analyses that compared appraisal, coping, and two personality factors (EPQ-R E and N scales) as predictors of the three stress state dimensions. It gives both the initial correlation with stress state for each predictor and the partial correlation that indicates whether the predictor makes a significant unique contribution to the equation. Most of the predictions made from the analysis of self-regulation were confirmed. Low task focus and high avoidance were

TABLE 5   Summary Statistics for Multiple Regressions of Three Subjective State Dimensions on Appraisal, Coping, and Personality Measures

	Disengagement $(r^2 = .64)$		Distress $(r^2 = .51)$		Worry $(r^2 = .51)$	
	r	β	r	β	r	β
Appraisal						
Threat	−01	−08	51**	33**	37**	00
Challenge	−52**	−14	00	−09	04	15
Perceived control	−26**	−11	−32**	−18*	−40**	−09
Coping						
Task focus	−54**	−29**	−19*	−24**	03	13
Emotion focus	02	16	49**	28**	65**	50**
Avoidance	67**	52**	00	−42**	49**	48**
Personality measures						
E	−02	03	−17	−04	−12	−02
N	10	08	41**	21**	29**	06

Note. βs are those for the final regression equations.
*$p < .05$.   **$p < .01$.

related independently to task disengagement; the predicted association between challenge and engagement was significant only for the bivariate analysis. The regression data suggest that appraisals of threat and low perceived control were related more strongly to distress than to worry, as expected. Emotion focus was positively related to both distress and worry, but avoidance was associated with increased worry and, in the multivariate data, with reduced distress. Possibly, avoidance buys relief from negative emotions at the expense of loss of interest in the task and increased self-evaluation.

As in previous studies (Matthews et al., 1999), N was related to both worry and distress. The regression data show that the association between N and worry may be entirely mediated by the cognitive stress process variables, but N adds to the prediction of distress even when individual differences in appraisal and cognition are controlled. The data also indicated the roles of other personality variables. Extroversion was unrelated to the variables listed in Table 5. However, both the Goldberg (1992) conscientiousness (C) and agreeableness (A) scales were associated with higher task engagement and lower worry. These scales also correlated with reduced avoidance, and C also was correlated significantly with higher challenge appraisals. Trait anxiety (Spielberger, Gorsuch, & Lushene, 1970) was highly correlated with N ($r = .72$) and showed a similar pattern of correlations.

Subjects in this study also completed a coping questionnaire referring to their real-life experiences of dealing with mentally demanding tasks. It included items from the Endler and Parker (1990) scales, and the Carver et al. (1989) mental disengagement scale. (Note that Carver et al. use "disengagement" to refer to a coping strategy, whereas Matthews et al., 1999, use the term as a state dimension.) The Wells (1994) worry scales and the Jerusalem and Schwarzer (1989) self-efficacy measure were also administered. Table 6 shows the correlational data (for a total sample of 216). Some of the findings from the performance setting were reproduced, such as the associations between N and emotion focus. However, the data also show the limitations of a specific experimental paradigm as an analog of real-world stressors. In particular, E was a stronger predictor in the real-world data, relating to three out of four coping scales. Possibly, demanding real-world tasks often have a social aspect that extroverts manage more adaptively than introverts. Table 6 also confirms that broad traits relate to self-regulation: E, C, and low N all tended to relate to high self-efficacy and low worry. The data also confirmed that coping and self-regulative dimensions are related. Metaworry was significantly correlated ($p < .01$) with high avoidance ($r = .20$), mental disengagement ($r = .39$), and emotion focus ($r = .42$), and negatively correlated with task focus ($r = -.20$). Conversely, self-efficacy was significantly positively correlated with task focus ($r = .57$) and negatively correlated with emotion focus ($r = -.21$) and mental disengagement ($r = -.32$).

In summary, the data on performance reinforce the picture of N as a self-regulative trait that emerged from studies of appraisal and coping with real-world stressors. High N is associated with both negative self-beliefs, such as low self-efficacy, and with plans for self-regulation through worry-related forms of emotion focus and avoidance coping, which tend to be

TABLE 6   Correlations between Personality Scales and (1) Measures of Coping with Mentally Demanding Real-Life Tasks and (2) Measures of Self-Efficacy and Worry

	Eysenck scales		Goldberg scales				
	E	N	E	N	C	A	I
Measures of coping with mentally demanding real-life tasks							
Task focus	24**	−27**	28**	−24**	32**	12	26**
Emotion focus	−03	41**	−20**	37**	−25**	03	−01
Avoidance	15*	10	07	08	−12	04	−07
Mental disengagement	−19**	30**	−21**	07	−35**	−14	−08
Measures of self-efficacy and worry							
Self-efficacy	30**	−33**	28**	−21**	20**	12	35**
Metaworry	−33**	68**	−42**	43**	−15*	−33**	−01
Social worry	−39**	69**	−50**	37**	−26**	−21**	−04
Health worry	−06	36**	−12	33**	−09	−18*	−07

*$p < .05$.   **$p < .01$.

maladaptive in performance settings. Other traits, such as C, A, and E (in real-world settings) are associated with self-beliefs and plans that promote task engagement and reduce worry.

V. AGGRESSIVE BEHAVIOR

In this section, we discuss the application of the social–cognitive framework to individual differences in aggression, building on the substantial overlap between stress and aggression constructs. In terms of the model presented in Figure 1, this section focuses on appraisals of the intentions of others, which aggression researchers describe as *cognitive distortions*, and in coping through various styles of social problem solving. Inadequacies in implementing this form of coping are described as *cognitive deficiencies*.

Research on individuals at risk for the development of conduct and antisocial disorders has been spurred by the dramatic increase in both adult and childhood violence in recent times (Eron, Gentry, & Schlegel, 1994). Insofar as prevention of these highly disruptive disorders ultimately begins with early identification, emphasis has shifted from the study of adult populations to child populations. Indeed, recent studies demonstrating the significant adaptive and psychological impairments associated with childhood aggression (Offord, Boyle, & Racine, 1991), the relative stability of aggression (Kazdin, 1991, 1995), poor prognostic outcomes, dramatic increases in violent juvenile offenses (Eron et al., 1994), and the tremendous costs to society in terms of legal and mental health services and human suffering have provided the impetus for a flurry of research efforts aimed at identifying effective preventive and treatment techniques (Eron et al., 1994; Offord et al., 1991).

According to Berkowitz (1993), much aggression is elicited by emotional and arousing provocations. Typically aggressive behavior is associated with the emotion of anger, although anger does not instigate aggression directly. Lazarus (1991) offered a somewhat different perspective that relates anger to "a demeaning offense against me and mine"; that is, a slight or injury to self-identity. Anger is associated with a basic action tendency to attack aggressively the perpetrator of the offense, although the behavioral expression of anger depends on self-control and choice of coping strategy. In the study summarized in Table 6, the Spielberger trait anger scale was significantly ($p < .01$) correlated with increased use of emotion focus ($r = .31$) and with metaworry ($r = .38$), but not with self-efficacy or mental disengagement.

Social–cognitive and dispositional approaches to aggression concur in distinguishing two aspects of aggressive personality (Caprara, Barbaranelli, & Zimbardo, 1996; Geen, 1990). The first is described as reactive, affective, or impulsive, and refers to a tendency to respond to provocations with anger and verbal or physical aggression. The second refers to the proactive, instrumental, or planned aspect of aggression, as a deliberate choice of means toward achieving external rewards. Caprara et al. (1996) showed that N was highly correlated with reactive aggression, but not with proactive aggression. Low agreeableness was modestly correlated with both forms of aggression. Hence, reactive aggression is closer to the stress processes previously described than is proactive aggression.

Understanding aggression and its social context is a complex, difficult task, as Bandura (1983) states, "aggression is a multifaceted phenomenon that has many determinants and serves diverse purposes" (p. 1). To date, a number of causal explanatory hypotheses have been proposed, including genetic and biological factors, family interactional patterns, socioeconomic factors, and social learning, among others. Here, we focus on cognitive factors and self-regulation. The two types of aggression may represent particular styles of self-regulation. Lazarus' (1991) analysis of anger suggests that reactive aggression relates especially to sensitivity to threat to self-identity and poor self-control. Caprara et al. (1996) see proactive aggression as a social–cognitive factor associated with internalized norms that promote aggression and violence as acceptable behaviors. It may relate also to positive outcome expectancies for aggressive behavior (Dodge & Crick, 1990). In terms of the conceptual distinctions made previously, the two aspects of aggression may be underpinned by cognitive syndromes related both to negative appraisals of others and to choice of confrontive coping strategies.

A. COGNITIVE PROCESSES IN AGGRESSION

The past decade has hosted considerable research directed toward exploring the role of cognitive processes and products in the genesis and maintenance of aggression. A social information processing model proposed by Dodge, Pettit, McClaskey, and Brown (1986) has played a key role in generating studies designed to clarify the cognitive deficits and biases underlying children's aggression. The Dodge et al. model of social exchange conceptualizes social behavior as a function of the child's processing of a set of social–environmental cues, posited to occur in five separable sequential steps: (1) encoding (perception of environmental cues), (2) representation (interpretation of cues), (3) response search (generation of alternate responses), (4) response decision (selection of response), and (5) enactment (execution of response decision). When deficits or biases occur in any of the five steps, aggressive behavior may result. Dodge (1991) explains his framework in this way:

> When presented with a social cue, such as a provocation by a peer or a group of
> peers engaged in a fun game, a child first encodes this information through sensory

reception and perception. The child then mentally represents those cues as threatening or benign through the application of rules acquired in socialization, and may experience emotions such as fear, anger or a desire for pleasure. The child then engages in a response search, in which one or more behavior responses are accessed from long-term memory. These responses are evaluated as acceptable or unacceptable, and one is selected for enactment. (p. 211)

Cognitive–social theories as articulated by Kendall (1985, 1991) and Mischel (1990) both compliment and elaborate on the Dodge et al. information processing framework. Kendall's (1985, 1991) cognitive–behavioral model of child psychopathology places major emphasis on the learning process and the influence of the contingencies and models in the environment, while underscoring the centrality of mediating/information-processing factors in the development of childhood disorders. Kendall differentiates cognitive distortions from cognitive deficiencies within this framework. Cognitive distortions refer to dysfunctional or biased thinking (Kendall, 1993). Aggressive children evidence distortions in their appraisal and attributional processes, and deficiencies in their cognitive efforts to solve social problems (Lochman & Dodge, 1994). There is a parallel here with the anxiety-related biases previously discussed. As with anxiety, aggression may be associated with biases in the content of self-knowledge, which feed into bias in appraisal and coping. Deficiencies are defined as an absence of thinking—a lack of careful information processing in situations in which thinking would be beneficial. In other words, there is a deficit in the processing that supports self-control and social problem solving.

Mischel's (1990) social–cognitive conceptualizations define aggression as involving a general state of arousal whose meaning and consequences depend on the following mutually interactive psychological variables termed *cognitive–social person variables*:

1. How they encode (i.e., represent, symbolize, and group) information;
2. Their behavioral outcome, self-efficacy, and stimulus–outcome expectancies;
3. Their subjective values;
4. Their self-regulatory systems, responsible for the organization of plans, problem-solving styles, rules, self-standards, and self-motivating strategies that guide goal-directed behavior;
5. Their competencies or abilities to construct particular cognitions and behaviors.

Figure 2 illustrates the complimentary nature of the theories of Dodge et al. (1986), Kendall (1985, 1991), and Mischel (1990). Although the theories differ in detail, there is considerable conceptual overlap between them. In concert, these paradigms present a powerful heuristic for exploring the cognitive underpinnings of aggression in children. They also highlight the role of self-regulation in aggression. Typically, aggressive

---

Cognitive Distortions (Kendall, 1993)
Encoding and Representation (Dodge et al., 1986)
Encoding, Expectancies, and Subjective Values (Mischel, 1993)

Cognitive Deficiencies (Kendall, 1993)
Response Search, Response Decision, and Enactment (Dodge et al., 1986)
Self-regulation and Competencies (Mischel, 1993)

FIGURE 2   Cognitive paradigms for study of childhood aggression.

behavior is not "mindless," but a rational coping option, given the child's distorted beliefs.

B. RESEARCH EXPLORING COGNITIVE DISTORTIONS IN AGGRESSIVE CHILDREN

Substantial research has documented encoding and representational distortions in aggressive children. Hostile attributional biases in ambiguous social situations have been found in varied populations of aggressive children and adolescents and in both hypothetical and live peer interactions (Dodge, Murphy, & Buchsbaum, 1984; Dodge et al., 1986; Dodge & Somberg, 1987; Dodge & Tomlin, 1987; Feldman & Dodge, 1987; Lochman, 1987; Lochman & Dodge, 1994; Nasby, Hayden, & DePaulo, 1980; Steinberg & Dodge, 1983; Van Oostrum & Horvath, 1996; Waas, 1988). Moreover, aggressive children have been shown to attend to fewer cues before arriving at an interpretation and to bias their interpretations selectively by attending to hostile rather than neutral or positive cues. Although they are less accurate than nonaggressive peers at detecting prosocial intentions, they are more accurate at detecting hostile intentions (Dodge & Newman, 1981; Dodge et al., 1986). Such distortions are more characteristic of emotionally reactive than of instrumentally proactive aggressors (Dodge, 1991).

Other studies have clarified the expectancies and values that may underlie aggression in children. Slaby and Guerra (1988) assessed the social beliefs of aggressive and nonaggressive adolescents with regard to the legitimacy of aggression, expected outcomes for the aggressor, and expected outcomes for the victim. Results indicated that aggressive youths were significantly more likely than nonaggressives to believe in the legitimacy of aggression and to endorse the view that aggression begets self-esteem. Aggressive adolescents were also more likely to believe that victims do not suffer. Crick and Dodge (1991) found that proactive–aggressive children were more likely to perceive aggression as an efficacious way to achieve social goals and to favor instrumental rather than relationship-enhancing goals in social interactions than were reactive and nonaggressive peers. The aggressive responses of reactive children were more likely to result from perceiving their peers as cruel and malevolent, as results suggested that these youngsters were significantly more likely than other children to attribute hostile intent to peers in ambiguous, provocative situations. Perry, Perry, and Rasmussen (1986) examined the relationships between the aggression of elementary school children and their self-perceived ability to perform aggression and their beliefs about the consequences of aggression. Results indicated that aggressive children were more confident of their ability to engage in aggressive acts than other children. They were also more likely to assume that their aggression would be successful and would be tangibly rewarded. Furthermore, aggressive children tended to take pride in their aggression and were more likely to believe aggression would prevent future provocation by other children.

C. RESEARCH EXPLORING COGNITIVE DEFICIENCIES IN AGGRESSIVE CHILDREN

In recent years, a proliferation of studies have confirmed cognitive deficiencies in aggressive children at the response search, response decision, and enactment steps of the Dodge et al. model or the self-regulatory and competency stages of Mischel's (1993) framework. Illustrative of this work are studies by Lochman and Lampron (1986), Lochman, Lampron, and Rabiner (1989), Rabiner, Lenhart, and Lochman (1990), and Rubin, Bream, and Rose-Krasnor (1991).

Lochman and Lampron (1986) investigated competence in social problem solving using means–end stories in which a problem situation and successful conclusion were presented to aggressive and nonaggressive boys. The children were required to provide an initial solution followed by as many additional solutions as they could generate. Data demonstrated that aggressive boys produced fewer verbally assertive responses, but significantly more direct action responses than nonaggressive boys, with the number of direct action responses increasing during conflicts with teachers and when situations were perceived as more hostile. Lochman et al. (1989) sought to determine if the problem-solving deficiencies of aggressive children were due to an inability to ascertain appropriate alternate solutions similar to those of their nonaggressive peers or to an idiosyncratic approach to retrieving the ideas that are most easily accessed and activated. When both aggressive and nonaggressive boys chose their solutions from a multiple choice format, a sharp decline in the rates of direct action responses was observed, suggesting that, with the aid of cues, aggressive boys were able to respond in a more reflective way rather than selecting the responses that were most readily activated for them. Even with cues, however, aggressive boys retained an idiosyncratic pattern of responses, electing more help seeking solutions in social situations involving antagonistic intentions.

Rubin et al. (1991) explored the relationships between peer assessments of childhood aggression and social problem-solving behaviors and conditions in elementary school-aged children. Repertoires of social problem-solving strategies were determined by children's responses to an open-ended interview and videotaped observations of pairs of children engaging cooperatively in a simple task. Results revealed that aggressive children were more likely to prefer disruptive and confrontational social goals than their less aggressive peers and to suggest solutions involving physical aggression for hypothetical social problems.

Responses to hypothetical questions immediately after hearing them or with a 20-second delay prior to responding were used by Rabiner et al. (1990) to compare the automatic and reflective social problem-solving skills of average, popular, nonaggressive–rejected, and aggressive–rejected children. Data indicated that the automatic responses of both aggressive– and nonaggressive–rejected boys contained fewer verbal assertion solutions and more conflict-escalating solutions than nonrejected boys. When a response delay was imposed, nonaggressive–rejected and nonrejected boys provided qualitatively similar responses; however, aggressive–rejected boys persisted in furnishing fewer verbal-assertion solutions. The researchers reasoned that nonaggressive and nonrejected boys have an acceptable repertoire of appropriate problem-solving strategies, but tend to respond impulsively in social situations, thus failing to access acceptable responses. In contrast, the problem-solving deficiencies of aggressive-rejected boys were not eliminated when they were required to respond reflectively, likely due to inadequate numbers of verbal-assertion solutions in their problem-solving repertoires. These boys showed a deficit in self-control, even when self-regulation was promoted by the delay prior to response.

D. DEVELOPING THE THEORY OF AGGRESSION AND SELF-REGULATION

Taken together, these various findings suggest that aggression (especially reactive aggression) is characterized by a set of beliefs and response tendencies that distort self-regulation in social settings. The aggressive child is more likely to attribute hostility to others, more likely to evaluate aggressive behavior as a successful coping option, and to access antagonistic responses more readily. Stability in aggressiveness may be an expression of individual differences in the plans for self-regulation described by the S-REF model (Wells & Matthews, 1994). Recent work on aggressive personality in driving contexts suggests a similar perspective on adult drivers. Aggressive drivers are characterized by cognitions of other drivers as hostile, and they prefer to use confrontive coping strategies such as gesturing at other drivers, tailgating, and overtaking (Matthews, Desmond, Joyner, Carcary, & Gilliland, 1997). These strategies are evident in both self-reports and objective studies of risky behaviors during simulated driving (Matthews et al., 1998a).

Other theorists adopt a psychobiological perspective, which attributes the inability of aggressive children to delay gratification to neural disinhibition mechanisms. Gray (1987), in a modification of Eysenck's (1967) personality theory, defined personality in terms of individual differences in conditionability and sensitivity to punishment versus reward, these being regulated primarily by two different, but interacting, conceptual brain systems: the behavioral inhibition system and the behavioral activation system. In an application of this model to childhood aggression, Quay (1988a, 1988b, 1988c) hypothesized that aggression involves a persistently overactive reward system that predominates over the behavioral inhibition system. Although cognitive theorists admit that cognitive processes are adjudicated by biologically determined capabilities, they contend that the expression of these capabilities depends on appropriate stimulation (Bandura, 1983). This latter thesis was borne out in a series of studies conducted by Quay and colleagues (Shapiro, Quay, Hogan, & Schwartz, 1988; Daugherty & Quay, 1991), who found that, although aggressive children are hypersensitive to reward and fail to inhibit responding, they do so only under mixed incentive conditions. Thus, as Shapiro and Hynd (1993) argued, potential links with biological or personality bases (Gray, 1987) should not be viewed as deterministic; rather, they yield insight into those conditions of reinforcement that are most likely to predict aggression and, therefore, hold promise for behavioral interventions.

VI. CONCLUSIONS

Styles of self-regulation are an integral aspect of personality. Reconciling the trait and social–cognitive perspectives on self-regulation requires understanding the underlying cognitive architecture. The three-level architecture proposed by Wells and Matthews (1994) has been applied here to understanding individual differences in adaptation to the challenges posed by everyday life events, by demanding tasks, and potential hostility in other people. In each case, self-regulative processing is prone to "cognitive distortions" such as biases in appraisal of the self and of external demands.

Studies of coping strategies and of self-control show that selection and regulation of response is also subject to bias. Within a given situation, these biases may reflect both somewhat idiosyncratic processing of situation-specific cues (especially social cues) and stable self-knowledge, whose content varies with personality traits. Some of the general characteristics of self-knowledge may be indexed by "self-regulative traits" such as dispositional worry, metacognitive style, and self-efficacy.

Across the research areas surveyed, the single most important trait is neuroticism. It relates to various self-referent processes, including appraisals of threat and loss of control across various contexts, negative appraisals of the self as a social agent associated with shyness, and negative or maladaptive metacognitions. Neuroticism also may relate to attributions of hostility to others, via its association with emotionally reactive aggression. More neurotic subjects also prefer to cope through emotion focus and disengagement, as opposed to task focus. Broadly, N represents the negative content of self-knowledge in representing the person as vulnerable, ineffectual, and lacking self-worth. However, the S-REF model (Wells & Matthews, 1994) emphasizes the dynamic nature of self-knowledge, represented primarily as generic plans for handling particular kinds of situation, as opposed to fixed, context-independent propositions. Neuroticism also indexes the availability of plans for handling external demands through metacognitive routines that generate worry. These plans influence behavior in social and performance settings directly through their effects on task strategy and indirectly through generating cognitive interference. In addition, the cognitive–adaptive perspective on personality, articulated elsewhere (Matthews, 1997, 1999), emphasizes that traits are *distributed* across sets of computationally distinct processing routines subserving common adaptive goals. Neuroticism may then relate independently to plans controling a variety of specific self-regulative functions, supporting adaptation to a world that is represented as threatening, hostile, and difficult to control through task-focused action.

Various traits other than N relate to styles of self-regulation. At the level of broad traits, introversion (low E) relates to stress vulnerability and to aspects of self-regulation such as worry and reduced self-efficacy. Matthews (1997) suggests that E relates especially to confidence in handling cognitively demanding environments, which overlap with threatening environments. Low agreeableness relates to both reactive and proactive aggression, although the cognitive underpinnings of the trait require more investigation. Midlevel or narrow traits may relate to further aspects of self-regulation. Some of the correlates of N, such as social anxiety, may relate to the neurotic mode of adaptation within particular contexts: Endler, Parker, Bagby, and Cox (1991) distinguish various context-linked anxiety traits, for example. Similarly, personality during vehicle driving is better characterized by driving-related traits than by general traits (Matthews et al., 1997). Other traits relate to specific elements of the stress process. Dispositional self-focus of attention appears to amplify awareness of discrepancies in self-knowledge and to predispose states of self-focus that may serve to perpetuate emotional distress (Wells & Matthews, 1994). Optimism–pessimism is another important trait that may relate especially to appraisals of outcomes in stressful situations.

Finally, three areas for further research should be highlighted.

1. Assessment of individual differences in self-regulation could be improved. All the self-regulative trait constructs listed in Table 1 have some validity, but they overlap with one another and with neuroticism.

2. Whereas current research relies strongly on self report measures, more evidence on the relationship of personality and self-regulation to behavioral outcome measures is required. Performance research lends itself naturally to objective measures, and, at least in the case of children, there are now quite sophisticated diagnostic systems for exploring the interrelationships between aggressive behaviors and cognitions (e.g., Schwean, Saklofske, Yackulic & Quinn, 1995). We anticipate further personality-oriented research in these areas. Life stress research perhaps requires greater ingenuity in developing behavioral measures.

3. Further progress in developing self-regulative models of personality traits requires a better understanding of environmental factors. Cognitive–adaptive models of personality (Matthews, 1999) propose that traits map onto environmental qualities that require adaptive choices: N maps onto strategies for dealing with potential threat. Self-regulation is one of several classes of processes that support adaptation (involuntary, "automatic" information processing, and neural processes are others). Although the self-knowledge that supports self-regulation is tuned to environmental contingencies, it is often difficult to specify its contextualization precisely for individual traits. For example, it is unclear how far N governs adaptation, especially to social or ego threats, as opposed to threat in general. Refining the tentative cognitive–social framework sketched out here requires investigation of how the structuring of self-knowledge reflects the structure of the adaptive challenges laid down by the environment.

REFERENCES

Alloy, L. B., & Abramson, L. Y. (1979) Judgement of contingency in depressed and non-depressed students: Sadder but wiser? *Journal of Experimental Psychology, 108,* 441–485.

Anderson, J. R. (1982). Acquisition of cognitive skill. *Psychological Review, 89,* 369–406.

Bandura, A. (1983). Psychological mechanisms of aggression. In R. G. Geen & E. I. Donnerstein (Eds.), *Aggression: Theoretical and empirical reviews* (Vol. 1, pp. 1–40). New York: Academic Press.

Bandura, A. (1986). *Social foundations of thought and action: A social cognitive theory*. Englewood Cliffs, NJ: Prentice-Hall.

Battig, K., & Buzzi, R. (1986). Effect of coffee on the speed of subject-paced information processing. *Neuropsychobiology, 16*, 126−130.

Beck, A. T. (1967). *Depression: Causes and treatment*. Philadelphia: University of Pennsylvania Press.

Berkowitz, L. (1993). *Aggression: Its causes, consequences, and control*. New York: McGraw-Hill.

Bolger, N. (1990) Coping as a personality process: A prospective study. *Journal of Personality and Social Psychology, 59*, 525−537.

Caprara, G. V., Barbaranelli, C., & Zimbardo, P. G. (1996). Understanding the complexity of human aggression: Affective, cognitive, and social dimensions of individual differences in propensity towards aggression. *European Journal of Personality, 10*, 133−155.

Cartwright-Hatton, S., & Wells, A. (1997). Beliefs about worry and intrusions: The Meta-Cognitions Questionnaire and its correlates. *Journal of Anxiety Disorders, 11*, 279−296.

Carver, C. S., Peterson, L. M., Follansbee, D. J., & Scheier, M. F. (1983). Effects of self-directed attention and resistance among persons high and low in test-anxiety. *Cognitive Therapy and Research, 7*, 333−354.

Carver, C. S., & Scheier, M. F. (1981). *Attention and self-regulation: A control-theory approach to human behavior*. Berlin: Springer-Verlag.

Carver, C. S., Scheier, M. F., & Pozo, C. (1992). Conceptualizing the process of coping with health problems. In H. S. Friedman (Ed.), *Hostility, coping, and health* (pp. 167−199). Washington, DC: American Psychological Association.

Carver, R. S., Scheier, M. F., & Weintraub, J. K. (1989). Assessing coping strategies: A theoretically based approach. *Journal of Personality and Social Psychology, 56*, 267−283.

Cheek, J. M., & Melchior, L. A. (1990). Shyness, self-esteem, and self-consciousness. In H. Leitenberg (Ed.), *Handbook of social and evaluation anxiety* (pp. 47−82). New York: Plenum.

Costa, P. T., Jr., Somerfield, M. R., & McCrae, R. R. (1996). Personality and coping: A reconceptualization. In M. Zeidner & N. S. Endler (Eds.), *Handbook of coping: Theory, research, applications*. New York: Wiley.

Crick, N. R., & Dodge, K. A. (1996). Social information-processing mechanisms in reactive and proactive aggression. *Child Development, 67*, 993−1002.

Daugherty, T. K., & Quay, H. C. (1991). Response perseveration and delayed responding in childhood behavior disorders. *Journal of Child Psychology and Psychiatry, 32*, 453−461.

Deary, I. J., Blenkin, H., Agius, R. M., Endler, N. S., Zealley, H., & Wood, R. (1996). Models of job-related stress and personal achievement among consultant doctors. *British Journal of Psychology, 87*, 3−30.

Dodge, K. A. (1991). The structure and function of reactive and proactive aggression. In D. J. Pepler & K. H. Rubin (Eds.), *The development and treatment of childhood aggression* (pp. 201−218). Hillsdale, NJ: Erlbaum.

Dodge, K. A., & Crick, N. R. (1990). Social information-processing bases of aggressive behavior in children. *Personality and Social Psychology Bulletin, 16*, 8−22.

Dodge, K. A., Murphy, R. R., & Buchsbaum, K. C. (1984). The assessment of intention-cue detection skills in children: Implications for developmental psychology. *Child Development, 55*, 163−173.

Dodge, K. A., & Newman, J. P. (1981). Biased decision-making processes in aggressive boys. *Journal of Abnormal Psychology, 90*, 375−379.

Dodge, K. A., Pettit, G. S., McClaskey, C. L., & Brown, M. M. (1986). Social competence in children. *Monographs of the Society for Research in Child Development, 51*, 1−85.

Dodge, K. A., & Somberg, D. R. (1987). Hostile attributional biases among aggressive boys under conditions of threat to the self. *Child Development, 58*, 213−224.

Dodge, K. A., & Tomlin, A. M. (1987). Utilization of self-schemas as a mechanism of interpretational bias in aggressive children. [Special issue: Cognition and action]. *Social Cognition, 5*, 280–300.

Emmons, R. A. (1992). Abstract versus concrete goals—personal striving level, physical illness, and psychological well-being. *Journal of Personality and Social Psychology, 62*, 292–300.

Endler, N. S., & Parker, J. D. A. (1990). Multidimensional assessment of coping: A critical review. *Journal of Personality and Social Psychology, 58*, 844–854.

Endler, N. S., Parker, J. D. A, Bagby, R. M., & Cox, B. J. (1991). The multidimensionality of state and trait anxiety: The factor structure of the Endler Multidimensional Anxiety Scales. *Journal of Personality and Social Psychology, 60*, 919–926.

Eron, L. D., Gentry, J. H., & Schlegel, P. (Eds.). (1994). *Reason to hope: A psychosocial perspective on violence and youth.* Washington, DC: American Psychological Association.

Eysenck, H. J. (1967). *The biological basis of personality.* Springfield, IL: Thomas.

Eysenck, H. J. (1994). Personality: Biological foundations. In P. A. Vernon (Ed.), *The neuropsychology of individual differences* (pp. 151–207). New York: Academic.

Eysenck, M. W. (1992). *Anxiety: The cognitive perspective.* Hillsdale, NJ: Erlbaum.

Eysenck, M. W., & Calvo, M. G. (1992). Anxiety and performance: The processing efficiency theory. *Cognition and Emotion, 6*, 409–434.

Eysenck, S. B. G., Eysenck, H. J., & Barrett, P. (1985). A revised version of the Psychoticism scale. *Personality and Individual Differences, 6*, 21–29.

Feldman, E., & Dodge, K. A. (1987). Social information processing and sociometric status: Sex, age, and situational effects. *Journal of Abnormal Child Psychology, 15*, 211–227.

Fenigstein, A., Scheier, M. F., & Buss, A. H. (1975). Public and private self-consciousness: Assessment and theory. *Journal of Consulting and Clinical Psychology, 43*, 522–527.

Ferguson, E., Matthews, G., & Cox, T. (in press). The Appraisal of Life Events (ALE) scale: Reliability and validity. *British Journal of Health Psychology.*

Gallagher, D. J. (1990). Extraversion, neuroticism and appraisal of stressful academic events. *Personality and Individual Differences, 11*, 1053–1058.

Geen, R. G. (1987). Test anxiety and behavioral avoidance. *Journal of Research in Personality, 21*, 481–488.

Geen, R. G. (1990). *Human aggression.* Pacific Grove, CA: Brooks/Cole.

Gray, J. A. (1987). *The psychology of fear and stress* (2nd ed.). Cambridge, UK: Cambridge University Press.

Goldberg, D. (1978). *The General Health Questionnaire.* Windsor: NFER-Nelson.

Goldberg, L. R. (1992). The development of markers for the Big-Five factor structure. *Psychological Assessment, 4*, 26–42.

Higgins, E. T. (1990). Personality, social psychology, and person-situation relations: Standards and knowledge activation as a common language. In L. A. Pervin (Ed.), *Handbook of personality: Theory and research* (pp. 301–338). New York: Guilford.

Jerusalem, M., & Schwarzer, R. (1989). Anxiety and self-concept as antecedents of stress and coping: A longitudinal study with German and Turkish adolescents. *Personality and Individual Differences, 10*, 785–792.

Jones, W. H., Rose, J., & Russell, D. (1990). Loneliness and social anxiety. In H. Leitenberg (Ed.), *Handbook of social and evaluation anxiety* (pp. 247–266). New York: Plenum.

Kanfer, R. (1990). Motivation and individual differences in learning: An integration of developmental, differential and cognitive perspectives. *Learning and Individual Differences, 2*, 221–239.

Kanfer, R., & Ackerman, P. L. (1989). Motivation and cognitive abilities: An integrative/aptitude–treatment interaction approach to skill acquisition. *Journal of Applied Psychology, 74*, 657–690.

Kanfer, F. H., & Stevenson, M. K. (1985). The effects of self-regulation on concurrent cognitive processing. *Cognitive Therapy and Research, 9,* 667–684.

Kazdin, A. E. (1991). Aggressive behavior and conduct disorder. In T. R. Kratochwill & R. J. Morris (Eds.), *The practice of child therapy* (2nd ed., pp. 174–221). New York: Pergamon.

Kazdin, A. E. (1995). *Conduct disorders in childhood and adolescence* (2nd ed.). Thousand Oaks, CA: Sage.

Kendall, P. C. (1985). Toward a cognitive–behavioral model of child psychopathology and a critique of related interventions. *Journal of Abnormal Child Psychology, 13,* 357–372.

Kendall, P. C. (1991). Guiding theory for treating children and adolescents. In P. C. Kendall (Ed.), *Child and adolescent therapy: Cognitive–behavioral procedures* (pp. 3–24). New York: Guilford.

Kendall, P. C. (1993). Cognitive–behavioral therapies with youth: Guiding theory, current status, and emerging developments. *Journal of Consulting and Clinical Psychology, 61,* 235–247.

Kennedy, R. E., & Craighead, W. E. (1988). Differential effects of depression and anxiety on recall of feedback in a learning task. *Behavior Therapy, 19,* 437–454.

Klass, E. T. (1990). Guilt, shame, and embarrassment: Cognitive–behavioural approaches. In H. Leitenberg (Ed.), *Handbook of social and evaluation anxiety* (pp. 385–414). New York: Plenum.

Kluger, A. N., & DeNisi, A. (1996). The effects of feedback interventions on performance: A historical review, a meta-analysis, and a preliminary feedback intervention theory. *Psychological Bulletin, 119,* 254–284.

Kohn, P. M. (1996). On coping adaptively with daily hassles. In M. Zeidner & N. S. Endler (Eds.), *Handbook of coping: Theory, research, applications* (pp. 181–201) New York: Wiley.

Lavallee, L. E., & Campbell, J. P. (1995). Impact of personal goals on self-regulation processes elicited by daily negative events. *Journal of Personality and Social Psychology, 69,* 341–352.

Lazarus, R. S. (1991). *Emotion and adaptation.* Oxford, UK: Oxford University Press.

Lazarus, R. S., & Folkman, S. (1984). *Stress, appraisal and coping.* New York: Springer.

Lochman, J. E. (1987). Self and peer perceptions and attributional biases of aggressive and nonaggressive boys in dyadic interactions. *Journal of Consulting and Clinical Psychology, 55,* 404–410.

Lochman, J. E., & Dodge, K. A. (1994). Social–cognitive processes of severely violent, moderately aggressive and non-aggressive boys. *Journal of Consulting and Clinical Psychology, 62,* 366–374.

Lochman, J. E., & Lampron, L. B. (1986). Situational social problem-solving skills and self esteem of aggressive and nonaggressive boys. *Journal of Abnormal Child Psychology, 14,* 605–617.

Lochman, J. E., Lampron, L. B., & Rabiner, D. L. (1989). Format differences and salience effects in the social problem-solving assessment of aggressive and nonaggressive boys. *Journal of Clinical Child Psychology, 18,* 230–236.

Markus, H., & Cross, S. (1990). The interpersonal self. In L. A. Pervin (Ed.), *Handbook of personality theory and research* (pp. 301–338). New York: Guilford.

Matthews, G. (1997). Extraversion, emotion and performance: A cognitive–adaptive model. In G. Matthews (Ed.), *Cognitive science perspectives on personality and emotion* (pp. 399–442). Amsterdam: Elsevier.

Matthews, G. (1999). Personality and skill: A cognitive–adaptive framework. In P. L. Ackerman, P. C. Kyllonen, & R. D. Roberts (Eds.), *Learning and individual differences: Process, trait and content determinants* (pp. 251–273). Washington, DC: American Psychological Association.

Matthews, G., & Campbell, S. E. (1998, October). Task-induced stress and individual differences in coping. In proceedings of the 42nd Annual Meeting of the Human Factors and Ergonomics Society, Chicago (pp. 821–825).

Matthews, G., & Deary I. (1998). *Personality traits*. Cambridge, UK: Cambridge University Press.

Matthews, G., Desmond, P. A., Joyner, L. A., Carcary, B., & Gilliland, K. (1997). A comprehensive questionnaire measure of driver stress and affect. In E. Carbonell Vaya & J. A. Rothengatter (Eds.), *Proceedings of the International Conference of Traffic and Transport Psychology* (pp. 317–324). Amsterdam: Elsevier.

Matthews, G., Dorn, L., Hoyes, T. W., Davies, D. R., Glendon, A. I., & Taylor, R. G. (1998). Driver stress and performance on a driving simulator. *Human Factors, 40*, 136–149.

Matthews, G., & Harley, T. A. (1996). Connectionist models of emotional distress and attentional bias. *Cognition and Emotion, 10*, 561–600.

Matthews, G., Hillyard, E. J., & Campbell, S. E. (in press). Metacognition and maladaptive coping as components of test anxiety. *Clinical Psychology and Psychotherapy*

Matthews, G., Joyner, L., Gilliland, K., Campbell, S. E., Huggins, J., & Falconer, S. (1999). Validation of a comprehensive stress state questionnaire: Towards a state "Big Three"? In I. Mervielde, I. J. Deary, F. De Fruyt, & F. Ostendorf (Eds.), *Personality psychology in Europe* (Vol. 7). (pp. 334–350). Tilburg, Netherlands: Tilburg University Press.

Matthews, G., Mohamed, A., & Lochrie, B. (1998c). Dispositional self-focus of attention and individual differences in appraisal and coping. In J. Bermudez, A. M. Perez, A. Sanchez-Elvira, & G. L. van Heck (Eds.), *Personality psychology in Europe* (Vol. 6). (pp. 278–285). Tilburg, Netherlands: Tilburg University Press.

Matthews, G., & Wells, A. (1996). Attentional processes, coping strategies and clinical intervention. In M. Zeidner & N. S. Endler (Eds.), *Handbook of coping: Theory, research, applications* (pp. 573–601) New York: Wiley.

Matthews, G., & Wells, A. (1999). The cognitive science of attention and emotion. In T. Dalgleish & M. Power (Eds.), *Handbook of cognition and emotion.* (pp. 171–192) New York: Wiley.

Matthews, G., Saklofske, D. H., Costa, P. T., Jr., Deary, I. J., & Zeidner, M. (1998b). Dimensional models of personality: A framework for systematic clinical assessment. *European Journal of Psychological Assessment, 14*, 35–48.

Mayer, J. D., Salovey, P., Gomberg-Kaufman, S., & Blainey, K. (1991). A broader conception of mood experience. *Journal of Personality and Social Psychology, 60*, 100–111.

Mischel, W. (1990). Personality dispositions revisited and revised: A view after three decades. In L. A. Pervin (Ed.), *Handbook of personality: Theory and research* (pp. 111–134). New York: Guilford.

Mohamed, A. A. R. (1996). *Stress processes in British and overseas students*. Unpublished doctoral dissertation, University of Dundee.

Morgan, I. A., Matthews, G., & Winton, M. (1995). Coping and personality as predictors of post-traumatic intrusions, numbing, avoidance and general distress: A study of victims of the Perth flood. *Behavioral and Cognitive Psychotherapy, 23*, 251–264.

Nasby, W., Hayden, B., & DePaulo, B. M. (1980). Attributional bias among aggressive boys to interpret unambiguous social stimuli as displays of hostility. *Journal of Abnormal Psychology, 89*, 459–548.

Offord, D. R., Boyle, M. C., & Racine, Y. A. (1991). The epidemiology of antisocial behavior in children and adolescence. In D. J. Pepler & K. H. Rubin (Eds.), *The development and treatment of childhood aggression* (pp. 31–54). Hillsdale, NJ: Erlbaum.

Perry, D. G., Perry, L. C., & Rasmussen, P. (1986). Cognitive social learning mediators of aggression. *Child Development, 57*, 700–711.

Quay, H. C. (1988a). Attention deficit disorder and the behavioral inhibition system: The relevance of the neuropsychological theory of Jeffrey A. Gray. In L. M. Bloomingdale & J. Sergeant (Eds.), *Attention deficit disorder: Criteria, cognition, intervention* (pp. 117–125). Oxford, UK: Pergamon.

Quay, H. C. (1988b). The behavioral reward and inhibition systems in childhood behavior disorders. In L. M. Bloomingdale (Ed.), *Attention deficit disorder* (Vol. 3, pp. 176–186). Oxford, UK: Pergamon.

Quay, H. C. (1988c). Reward, inhibition, and ADDH. *Journal of the American Academy of Child and Adolescent Psychiatry, 27,* 262–263.

Rabiner, D. L., Lenhart, L., & Lochman, J. E. (1990). Automatic versus reflective social problem solving in relation to children's sociometric status. *Developmental Psychology, 26,* 1010–1016.

Roger, D., Jarvis, G., & Najarian, B. (1993). Detachment and coping: The construction of a new scale for measuring coping strategies. *Personality and Individual Differences, 15,* 619–626.

Rubin, K. H., Bream, L. A., & Rose-Krasnor, L. (1991). Social problem solving and aggression in childhood. In D. J. Pepler & K. H. Rubin (Eds.), *The development and treatment of childhood aggression* (pp. 219–248). Hillsdale, NJ: Erlbaum.

Sarason, I. G., Sarason, B. R., & Pierce, G. R. (1995). Cognitive interference: At the intelligence-personality crossroads. In D. H. Saklofske & M. Zeidner (Eds.), *International handbook of personality and intelligence* (pp. 285–296). New York: Plenum.

Schaubroeck, J., & Ganster, D. C. (1991). Associations among stress-related individual differences. In C. L. Cooper & R. Payne (Eds.), *Personality and stress: Individual differences in the stress process.* Chichester, UK: Wiley.

Scheier, M. F., & Carver, C. S. (1992). Effects of optimism on psychological and physiological well-being: Theoretical overview and empirical update. *Cognitive Therapy and Research, 16,* 210–228.

Schwean, V. L., & Saklofske, D. H. (1995). A cognitive-social description of exceptional children. In D. H. Saklofske, & M. Zeidner (Eds.), *International handbook of personality and intelligence* (pp. 185–204). New York: Plenum.

Schwean, V. L., Saklofske, D. H., Yackulic, R. A., & Quinn, D. (1995). Assessment of attention deficit/hyperactivity Disorders [Monograph]. *Journal of Psychoeducational Assessment,* 6–21. Knoxville, TN: Psychoeducational Corporation.

Shapiro, S. K., & Hynd, G. W. (1993). Psychobiological basis of conduct disorder. *School Psychology Review, 22,* 386–402.

Shapiro, S. K., Quay, H. C., Hogan, A. E., & Schwartz, K. P. (1988). Response perseveration and delayed responding in undersocialized conduct disorder. *Journal of Abnormal Psychology, 97,* 371–373.

Slaby, R. G., & Guerra, N. G. (1988). Cognitive mediators of aggression in adolescent offenders: An assessment. *Developmental Psychology, 24,* 580–588.

Smith, M. B. (1950). The phenomenological approach in personality theory: Some critical remarks. *Journal of Abnormal and Social Psychology, 45,* 516–522.

Spielberger, C. D., Gorsuch, R., & Lushene, R. (1970). *The State Trait Anxiety Inventory (STAI) manual.* Palo Alto, CA: Consulting Psychologists Press.

Steinberg, M. E., & Dodge, K. A. (1983). Attributional bias in aggressive adolescent boys and girls. *Journal of Social and Clinical Psychology, 1,* 312–321.

Stokes, J. P. (1985). The relation of social network and individual difference variables to loneliness. *Journal of Personality and Social Psychology, 48,* 981–990.

Summerfeldt, L. J., & Endler, N. S. (1996). Coping with emotion and psychopathology. In M. Zeidner & N. S. Endler (Eds.), *Handbook of coping: Theory, research, applications* (pp. 602–639). New York: Wiley.

Swinkels, A., & Giuliano, T. A. (1995). The measurement and conceptualization of mood awareness: Monitoring and labeling one's mood states. *Personality and Social Psychology Bulletin, 21,* 934–949.

Thayer, R. E. (1996). *The origin of everyday moods.* New York: Oxford University Press.

Van Oostrum, N., & Horvath, P. (1996). The effects of hostile attribution on adolescents' aggressive responses to social situations. *Canadian Journal of School Psychology, 13,* 48–59.

Waas, G. A. (1988). Social attributional biases of peer-rejected and aggressive children. *Child Development, 59*, 969–975.

Wells, A. (1994). A multi-dimensional measure of worry: Development and preliminary validation of the Anxious Thoughts Inventory. *Anxiety, Stress and Coping, 6*, 289–299.

Wells, A. (1997). *Cognitive therapy of anxiety disorders: A practice manual and conceptual guide.* Chichester, UK: Wiley.

Wells, A., & Matthews, G. (1994). *Attention and emotion: A clinical perspective.* Hillsdale, NJ: Erlbaum.

Wells, A., & Matthews, G. (1996). Modelling cognition in emotional disorder: The S-REF model. *Behaviour Research and Therapy, 34*, 881–888.

7

ORGANIZATION AND DEVELOPMENT OF SELF-UNDERSTANDING AND SELF-REGULATION

TOWARD A GENERAL THEORY

ANDREAS DEMETRIOU

University of Cyprus, Nicosia, Cyprus

I. INTRODUCTION

Self-regulation may be defined broadly as those actions directed at modifying a system's present state or activity and which are necessary either because that state (or activity) is diverting from a previously set goal or because the goal itself needs to be changed. Under this broad definition, any system, animate or inanimate, living or artificial, may be considered capable of self-regulation once it satisfies three conditions:

1. It must include a self-monitoring function that provides and updates information related to the system's present state or its ongoing activity.
2. It must also include an organized system of self-representations that describe the system's nature, history, tendencies and preferences, and directions for the future. In short, it involves a self-system.

Copyright © 2000 by Academic Press.
All rights of reproduction in any form reserved.

3. It must contain self-modification skills and strategies that can be applied to the present state or activity to direct toward another state or activity.

Self-regulation cannot occur if any one of these three conditions is lacking, because self-monitoring and self-modification are possible only in relationship to the system's self-representations, which provide criteria for the evaluation of the present activity and cues for possible redirections. Likewise, self-concepts cannot be constructed without self-monitoring and self-modification functions to generate information about the self in its various activities.

These processes are studied in many different areas of psychology and with varying emphases. Specifically, psychology of the self focuses more on self-representations and self-concepts than on self-monitoring and self-regulation. Developmental psychology emphasizes self-monitoring and self-awareness rather than self-concepts or self-regulation per se. Clinical and educational psychology, which are concerned with applications rather than with explications, focus on self-regulation. As a result of this divergence in interests and priorities, there is no generally accepted theory that can delineate the nature and development of these processes adequately. The present chapter is intended to be a contribution in this direction. Specifically, this chapter integrates extant research and theory directly related to the nature and development of certain aspects of self-monitoring, self-representation, and self-regulation, including their interrelationships and their relationships with particular dimensions of cognitive functioning and personality. We focus on studies that were designed especially to cut across different domains—such as cognitive, personality, and self-concept development—in order to uncover how self-understanding and self-regulation are related to different personality predispositions or thinking styles. Our aim is to outline a general model of the organization, dynamics, and development of self-understanding and self-regulation that both accommodates and clarifies the intertwining of cognitive and personality development in everyday functioning. Thus, this chapter answers questions such as the following:

1. What is the minimum mental architecture required for a system to be capable of self-monitoring, self-representation, and self-regulation?
2. How do developing persons represent and regulate themselves with regard to various cognitive and personality domains at successive phases of development?
3. How and why do self-monitoring, self-representation, and self-regulation change with development?

In short, this chapter highlights how individuals understand and represent themselves and how they take charge of their own functioning during critical years of development.

II. THE ARCHITECTURE OF SELF-AWARE AND SELF-REGULATED SYSTEMS

Marsh and Iran-Nejad (1992) equated intelligence with self-regulation. According to their definition, intelligence is "the capacity for self-regulation under external (or stimulus-regulated), dynamic (or micro-system-regulated), and mindful (or person-regulated) control" (p. 330). On the basis of this definition, many creatures other than human beings would be considered highly intelligent because they are capable of extremely complex external and dynamic self-regulation. Migratory fish and birds, for example, travel thousands of miles to find their nests with astonishing accuracy, reflecting complex orientation and navigation skills. Moreover, even very simple creatures, such as bees and ants, exhibit behaviors indicative of elaborate representations of space, communication skills, and constructional capabilities. However, these complex behaviors do not denote self-understanding or mindful self-regulation; at best, they are self-regulated in a dynamic systems sense such that any regulation involved is characteristic of the system rather than of the individual animals themselves. In other words, the individual animal has no representation of the whole situation, of itself, or of the sequence of events to follow after a given moment. Moreover, it has no intervention capabilities that could be actualized to intentionally change the course of events (see Elman et al., 1996).

At present only humans are capable of mindful self-regulation. Evolutionary theorists (Donald, 1991; Mithen, 1996) posit that mindful self-regulation became necessary for two complementary reasons. First, as humans gradually moved from their original, and generally, fixed environment to a more variable and frequently changing one, their ecologically dependent systems of perceiving and interacting with the environment were pushed to their limits. Although these systems are highly efficient in stable environments, they fall short of the demands of variable environments, which require computational and conceptual systems capable of grasping and representing underlying relationships in addition to or in spite of appearances and ecological affordances. Systems able to grasp and represent underlying relationships provide flexibility because they enable the individual to view a given pattern of stimuli from the perspective of other perceived or remembered patterns. This flexibility is bought at the cost of having to make interpretations, choices, and decisions, which may not always be right. Thus, mindful self-regulation is necessary as a means to minimize the likelihood of error.

Second, social life as a defining characteristic of humans occurred concomitantly with this shift from a stable to a changing environment. Social life necessitates that individuals interact with both the physical environment and each other. This double kind of interaction requires that individuals must be able to negotiate with each other about their perceptions, conceptions, representations, and ideas about both the environment per se and themselves. In short, it creates a mental environment in addition to or on top of the actual environments we live in. Having a mental environment necessitates that individuals be able to both discriminate their own mental world from those of other individuals and negotiate their own goals and actions with those of the others they live with. These requirements entail the construction of a sense of personal identity or self as the central engine of self-understanding and self-regulation. In this engine, cognitions and dispositions, that is, mind and personality, coexist in an integral system, which acts adaptively under the guidance and constraints of the understanding and interacting capabilities of the person at a given age in a particular environment. In the subsequent texts, we describe the architecture of this integrated system, focusing first on the mind and then on personality.

This chapter was developed on the general assumption that mind and personality are not only complementary, but also similarly organized. Thus, we assume that mind and personality involve systems directed to the environment and systems directed to knowing and handling these systems. The application of these latter systems on the first is constrained and channeled by available processing and action recourses, and dispositions. A model of the general architecture of the mind and personality is depicted in Figure 1.

A. THE MIND

Intelligent systems capable of self-understanding and mindful self-regulation require a hierarchical organization, such that there are processes to be known and regulated, and active processes that can be applied to them. For living beings, the processes to be known relate to either the identity of the body, such as its appearance and boundaries, or the functioning of the body, such as hunger or breathing, or refer to interaction with the environment. Here we emphasize interaction processes, although it is recognized that bodily identity and processes may be very important for some aspects of self-understanding and self-regulation. Simply defined, perceptual processes that provide access to the environment, concepts that represent the environment, mental operations underlying the interactions with the environment, and actual skills and behaviors that are

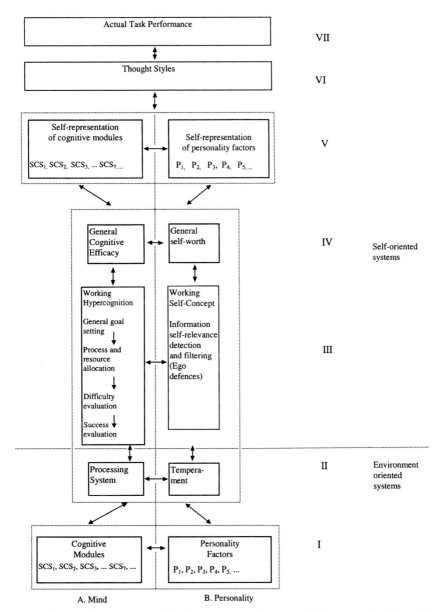

FIGURE 1   The general model of mind, personality, and self. The symbols SCS and P
stand for specialized capacity systems and personality factors, respectively.

applied to the environment are the raw material that can become the object of understanding and regulation.

Self-understanding comprises those processes that enable individuals to register sensations, feelings, conceptions, mental operations, and actions, and represent them as such. Self-regulation involves both individuals' ability to set goals about their own functioning or about the environment and direct their mental and physical functioning so that these goals can be attained. Thus, self-regulation entails the ability to intervene intentionally and systematically in the functioning of the processes that reside at the environment-oriented level of the mind.

The Environment-Oriented Level

It is widely agreed that the level of mind oriented to knowing the environment involves a set of systems, each responsible for representing and processing a particular environmental domain. Currently, there are two dominant approaches to defining environment-oriented systems. The first, which is characteristic of post-Piagetian developmental theory and psychometric tradition, posits that environment-oriented systems of thought are organized according to the specific environmental relationships that they represent and process. The second approach conjectures that thought systems are organized on the basis of ontological criteria; that is, according to the phenomenological characteristics of the objects that need to be known.

The research that my colleagues and I have conducted during the last 20 years aimed to integrate the developmental with the psychometric tradition in the study of intellectual development. This research has identified and delineated seven relationally defined environment-oriented systems:

1. *Qualitative*, which deals with similarity–difference relationships and underlies the construction and use of concepts about the world.
2. *Quantitative*, which deals with quantitative variations and relationships and underlies all aspects of mathematics that humans produce and use.
3. *Causal*, which deals with cause–effect relationships and underlies actions directed to deciphering causal relationships and the explanatory models built to express and explain these relationships.
4. *Spatial*, which deals with orientation in space and the imaginal representation of the environment.
5. *Propositional*, which specializes on the integration of information flowing in verbal interactions and on the evaluation of the validity or invalidity of information provided in these interactions.
6. *Pictographic*, which underlies the representation of the environment or of thoughts themselves through the production of drawings or any other kind of signs.

7. *The Social* system, which concerns interpersonal relationships (Bonoti, 1998; Demetriou & Efklides, 1985, 1989, in preparation; Loizos, 1996; Shayer, Demetriou, & Prevez, 1988).

Gardner (1983) would add somatosensory and musical systems to this list.

It must be noted that some of these domains (that is, the quantitative and the spatial) have been identified for a long time (Thurstone, 1938). Other domains have been mapped as autonomous (the qualitative and the causal) by our research (Demetriou & Efklides, 1985; Demetriou, Efklides, Papadaki, Papantoniou & Economou, 1993a; Shayer et al., 1988). The domain of social understanding is an even more recent addition to the list of autonomous modules. Case et al. (1996) mapped all but the causal and the qualitative system, and proposed a language for specifying the semantic characteristics of each.

Research focused on the different phenomenological aspects of the world has identified three domains: the biological, the physical, and the psychological (Karmiloff-Smith, 1992). Theoretically, these domains are differentiated on the basis of ontological rather than relational and computational characteristics. That is, each domain comprises entities that are unique in important respects, such as appearance and behavior. For instance, animals appear and behave differently than inanimate objects; human behavior is guided by intentions and mental states, which do not exist in the inanimate world. Thus, through evolution, humans evolved mental functions that enable them to deal efficiently with each of these three domains. I have argued that the relationally specified and the ontologically specified domains are, in fact, complementary insofar as relationships involved in the relationally differentiated domains run across the ontological domains. For example, categorical, quantitative, causal, and spatial relations can be found in the biological, physical, and psychological domains (Demetriou, 1998a).

We have postulated that the environment-oriented systems obey certain organizational principles, such that these systems are *domain specific*, *procedurally specific*, and *symbolically biased*. That is, each system (i) specializes in the representation and processing of specific environmental relationships or objects, (ii) involves different types of mental operations and processes that honor the peculiarities of the domain concerned, and (iii) utilizes symbolic systems such as mental images, numerical and mathematical notations, or language, which can facilitate the efficient representation and processing of the relationships in the domain concerned. These structural differences allow the environment-oriented systems to function and develop in relative autonomy (Demetriou & Efklides, 1988; Demetriou, Efklides, & Platsidou, 1993b). Thus, these systems were called specialized capacity systems (SCSs) and they are shown in the bottom left box of Figure 1.

To conclude, the environment-oriented systems are modularized organizations that function as understanding and activity "traps" that can provide advantages under certain conditions and disadvantages under other conditions. That is, if the environmental information is clearly and unambiguously addressed to a given system, a relevant answer or solution can be assembled easily, provided that the necessary mental operations and skills are available. The operation of these systems both reduces the need for control and increases operational efficiency and functional economy. However, if the information does not directly match any one system, and decisions need to be made about the meaning of information or the appropriate course of action, the probability for irrelevant answers or solutions increases. Under these conditions, the appropriate action requires both effort and knowledge so that higher-order operations, residing at the self-oriented level of the mental architecture, become necessary.

The Self-Oriented Level of Knowing

Recently, we coined the term *"hypercognitive system"* to refer to the processes and concepts that reside at the self-oriented level. The adverb "hyper" in Greek means higher than, on top of, or going beyond, and when added to the word "cognitive" it indicates the supervising and coordinating functions of the processes residing at this level (Demetriou et al., 1993b). The input to this system is information coming from the body, the environment-oriented level (see preceding text), and from the general processing system (described subsequently). This information is organized into the maps or models of mental functions that are used to guide the functioning of these systems. Thus, the hypercognitive system involves self-awareness and self-regulation knowledge and strategies, and is conceived as the interface between both the various systems and functions of the mind and the mind and reality. To carry out these interfacing functions, the hypercognitive system comprises working hypercognition and long-term hypercognition.

Working hypercognition refers to a cybernetic cycle of on-line self-monitoring and self-regulation processes that enable the cognitive system to be efficiently and accurately activated according to the requirements of the moment. Working hyper cognition will, therefore, be called upon to make four kinds of decisions:

1. Decisions which underlie goal setting. These include selection of the environment-oriented system to be activated and the most relevant task-specific schemes.
2. Decisions related to the appropriate and efficient use of these schemes, the available processing resources, and other cognitive functions, such as perception. Such decisions refer to procedural aspects of processing a task (i.e., organization of the various steps

and use of general-purpose functions under the particularities of the present occasion) and underlie planning directed to the attainment of the goal set by the first kind of decisions.

3. Evaluations of processing in terms of the effort required or the value of the operation. Obviously, these refer to the level of difficulty imposed by the task. For instance, tasks requiring few and easily assembled processes will be judged as easier than tasks requiring multiple processes. Thus, these decisions influence the motivation to work on a task.

4. Evaluations of the outcomes attained, which compare the solution attained against the initial goal and task-relevant criteria. Thus, these decisions frame how similar problems will be dealt with subsequently.

These four kinds of decisions flow during problem solving in the order presented, with each decision influencing the subsequent ones. For instance, the decision to activate one environment-oriented system instead of another will define the particular procedures to be selected, and these will determine whether the task is considered easy or difficult and thus worth the attempt. Finally, all previous decisions will influence the evaluation of the outcome. A series of studies in our laboratory have provided ample support to this model of working hypercognition (Demetriou & Efklides, 1989; Demetriou et al., 1993b; Kazi, Platsidou, Sirmali, & Kiosseoglou, 1999; Demetriou & Raftopoulos, in press).

The proposed analysis of working hypercognition concurs with general control theory, which postulates that any self-regulated system, from cruise missiles to humans, requires three basic components: (1) a feedforward or directive function that sets the system's goals; (2) a comparator or regulatory function that regularly effects comparisons between the present state of the system and the goal, and (3) a negative feedback control function that registers discrepancies between the present state and the goal, and suggests corrective actions. These three regulatory functions operate under the constraints of an arousal function that defines how the available energy or power is to be used to achieve maximum effects (Ford, 1987). Thus, several recent general theories of self-regulation have integrated variations of this system into their analysis of self-regulation (Brown, 1998; Karoly, 1993; Zimmerman, 2000 this volume).

The Processing Constraints of Working Hypercognition. Cognitive (Baddeley, 1991), psychometric (Jensen, 1980), and developmental psychologists (Case, 1985; Halford, 1993; Pascual-Leone, 1970) concur that humans always operate under conditions of limited resources for representing and processing information about the environment and the self. In an attempt to integrate evidence and theory from all three traditions, we have proposed (Demetriou et al., 1993a) that the available processing potentials may be viewed as a system comprising three dimensions: speed of processing, inhibition, and storage.

Speed of processing refers to the maximum speed at which a given mental act can be executed efficiently. Usually, in tests of speed of processing (Jensen, 1980), the individual is asked to recognize a simple stimulus as quickly as possible, for example, to name a letter or read single words in one's native language.

Inhibition refers to the maximum efficiency with which a decision can be made on the appropriate mental act to be executed according to the moment's requirements. This function usually is tested under conditions that can generate conflicting interpretations, such as the well-known Stroop phenomenon (Stroop, 1935). In this test, words denoting color are written with a different ink color (i.e., the word "red" is written with blue ink) and the individual is asked to name the ink color as quickly as possible. These conditions accurately test inhibition, because the subject is required to inhibit a dominant but irrelevant response (to read the word) in order to select and emit a weaker but relevant response (name the ink color) (Demetriou et al., 1993b; Dempster & Brainerd, 1995; Houghton & Tipper, 1994).

Storage refers to the maximum number of information units and mental acts the mind can efficiently activate simultaneously. A common test of storage is to present the person with a series of numbers, words, sentences, or pictures or combinations of them and ask him or her to recall them after a few seconds.

So defined, the processing system is the locus of self-understanding and self-regulation. That is, at any time, we are aware of the information that is currently active in this system, and our ability to keep processing focused on goal is a function of the inhibition efficiency of this system. Thus, this system may be seen as a dynamic field that intervenes between the environment-oriented and the self-oriented levels of mind and is always occupied by elements of both, in varying proportions. Specifically, the input to this system is environment-relevant information, skills, and processes, which pertain to an environment-oriented system, and management and evaluation processes, which pertain to the hypercognitive system. These latter processes are responsible for effecting the orchestration and the processing of the former and for evaluating the outcome in relationship to the goal. In other words, working hypercognition is the management system that controls the use of the available processing potentials (Demetriou et al., 1993b).

Long-Term Hypercognition.   The products of the functioning of working hypercognition are projected onto and become integrated into long-term hypercognition. Therefore, long-term hypercognition comprises knowledge and rules related to the mind's nature and organization, functions, and uses, which are organized into two distinct but interrelated kinds of structures: a general model of the mind and the cognitive self-image.

The general model of the mind refers to knowledge and beliefs that individuals acquire concerning the general structural and dynamic characteristics of their own mind. These are organized according to the principle of subjective distinctness of cognitive processes and abilities (Demetriou & Efklides, 1988, 1989; Demetriou et al. 1993b). This principle states that cognitive experiences that differ with regard to domain specificity, computational specificity, and symbolic bias are felt or cognized by the thinker as distinct. Otherwise, they are felt or cognized as functionally similar or equivalent. The practical implication of this principle is that the subjective organization of cognitive processes and abilities must, by and large, represent their objective organization. That is, thinkers must recognize that there are both different cognitive functions, such as perception, attention, and memory, and different cognitive structures, such as the environment-oriented systems described previously. Thinkers must also recognize that different tasks (e.g., a mathematical problem, a map-reading problem, or a social interaction problem) entail different mental operations. In our studies of the organization of hypercognitive maps, participants were asked first to solve tasks addressing the different environment-oriented systems. They then were given descriptions of various processes (which, according to the theory, are employed in the processing of each type of tasks) and were asked to specify the processes used to solve each task and to what degree. Overall, participants' responses concurred with the theory. That is, the subjective organization of cognitive processes and functions mirrored its objective organization as described in the preceding text. In Figure 1 this is represented by showing the same SCSs in both the box that stands for the cognitive modules and in the box that stands for their self-representation. Earlier research on metacognition (Brown, 1978; Flavell, 1979) and more recent research on the so-called child's theory of mind (Perner, 1991; Wellman, 1990) and the child's understanding of the organization and functioning of thinking and other cognitive functions (Demetriou et al., 1993a; Fabricius & Schwanenflugel, 1994; Flavell, Green, & Flavell, 1995) provide evidence directly related to this aspect of long-term hypercognition.

Moreover, the individuals' model of the mind specifies how they can use their minds to achieve personal goals without coming into conflict with their particular social or cultural group. For instance, individuals must learn quickly and remember what they learn; they must speak fluently and accurately; they must be socially flexible and considerate; they must control their behavior according to the particularities of the situation. Research on implicit theories of intelligence in our laboratory (Kazi & Makris, 1992) and other laboratories (Sternberg, Conway, Ketron, & Bernstein, 1981) sheds light on this aspect of long-term hypercognition.

The cognitive self-image may be defined as the personalization of an individual's general model of the mind. As such, it comprises the individual's self-representations with regard to the constructs in his or her general model of the mind. Thus, cognitive self-image answers such questions as, Which kinds of problems am I good at solving and which ones am I not so good at solving? How efficient am I in using different cognitive functions such as memory, imagery, and problem solving? How flexible, intelligent, or wise am I? In other words, the cognitive self-image involves all descriptions, implicit or explicit, that individuals attribute to themselves with regard to different mental functions, abilities, strategies, and skills. Research on self-evaluation and self-representation with regard to intellectual functioning is related to this aspect of hypercognition (Demetriou and Kazi, in press; Demetriou, Kazi, & Georgiou, 1999; Harter, 1990; Nicholls, 1990).

Our research on self-image indicates that it involves both constructs that stand for general cognitive abilities, such as one's own speed of processing, working memory, logicality, and learning ability, and also constructs that represent more specific abilities, such as the SCSs. One such study (Demetriou et al., 1999, in press) clearly illustrated how the processing system and the environment-oriented systems together shape the cognitive self-image. Specifically, participants were tested for their performance on tasks measuring speed of processing, and on deductive and inductive reasoning tasks addressed to a particular environment-oriented system, namely, the propositional reasoning system. Based on the participants' performance on these tasks, four groups were formed: (1) slow processors and low reasoners, (2) slow processors and high reasoners, (3) fast processors and low reasoners, and (4) fast processors and high reasoners. The participants' cognitive self-image with regard to logical reasoning and learning ability was probed with a specifically designed inventory. Findings are illustrated in Figure 2, where the states of the processing system and reasoning are taken as the independent variables, and self-representations of reasoning and learning are taken as the dependent variable. It is clear that the faster in processing and the higher on the reasoning tasks the subjects were, the better they considered themselves in reasoning and learning ability. This finding suggests that the hypercognitive system directly registers and represents the condition of the processing system and the environment-oriented reasoning processes. Representations of the processing system underlie the individual's sense of general cognitive efficiency (or self-efficacy in Bandura's, 1989, terms) and representations of domain-specific systems underlie the individual's domain-specific self-perceptions of efficiencies (or self-efficacies).

We believe that long-term hypercognition clearly is related to active self-monitoring and self-regulatory functions involved in working hypercognition. Thus it seems plausible to assume that the individuals' general

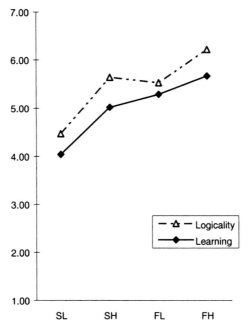

FIGURE 2   Self-attribution of learning and reasoning ability according to the combination of performance on speed of processing and analogical reasoning tasks. The symbols S and F stand for slow and fast speed of processing; the symbols L and H stand for low and high performance on the analogical reasoning tasks. *Note.* From "The Emerging Self: The Convergence of Mind, Personality, and Thinking Styles," by A. Demetriou, S. Kazi, and S. Georgion, 1999, *Developmental Science*, 2. Copyright 1999 by Blackwell Publishers. Reprinted with permission.

knowledge and representations of the organization and functioning of the mind influence how they organize their actions. For instance, if an individual does not recognize that memory implicates an associative function that operates on the basis of spatial and temporal proximity of stimuli, he or she would not capitalize on those properties to maximize memorization of information. A person who does not realize that processing resources are limited would not look for ways to organize information in order to overcome these limitations. Moreover, the cognitive self-image contributes to formation of the individual's short- and long-term goals: for instance, a person who believes that he or she is good at drawing but not in mathematics would prefer drawing activities rather than mathematics. We subsequently present extensive evidence that shows that changes in self-regulation go hand in hand with changes in general understanding of the mind and cognitive self-image.

   Modern neuroscience also conceives of the brain as hierarchically structured. Neuroscientists have shown that there are areas in the brain such as the occipital, temporal, and parietal lobes, that are committed to the understanding of and interacting with different domains in the environment (visual, verbal, and motor information, respectively). These areas report to and are controlled by areas that exert a supervising function, such as the frontal lobes. The functioning and the communication between domain-committed and control-committed structures is constrained by subcortical areas, such as the reticular formation and the hypocampus, which are related to representation of presently needed information (Petrides, 1996; Thatcher, 1994).

B. TEMPERAMENT, PERSONALITY, THINKING STYLES, AND THE SELF

So far, we have focused on the cognitive rather than the dynamic aspects of human understanding, experience, and behavior. However, cognition in general and self-regulation in particular are never entirely cool. Striving to attain a goal generates emotions, which color and influence experience, understanding, and action. Moreover, it is a truism that there are alternative ways to understand, experience, and respond to the same situation. Traditionally, this variation is ascribed to differences in personality and style, which frame emotions and the mind. Personality refers to the individual's more or less stable and decontextualized tendencies and dispositions to interpret and interact with the world in idiosyncratic ways (Caspi, 1998). Thinking styles involve organizing and control mechanisms that orient individuals to particular forms of information processing. These mechanisms originate from both personality dispositions, such as extraversion or openness to experience, and preferred ways to approach and process information, such as abstract conceptualization and reflection as contrasted with doing and experimentation (Sternberg, 1988, Ferrari & Sternberg, 1998). Moreover, there is the self-system itself; that is, "the phenomenological agency that coordinates the demands of the immediate situation with constraints imposed on the individual by dispositions and residues of life experiences" (Graziano, Jensen-Campbell, & Finch, 1997, p. 393).

There is no generally accepted theory on how these systems and functions interrelate or on how they interrelate to the systems and functions of the cognitive aspects of the mind. Our integration of hitherto uncoordinated research on personality and the self suggests that these dimensions of the human personality and the self are organized in the same way as the mind. To substantiate this claim, we compared models of personality, thinking styles, and the self. Panel B of Figure 1 summarizes these models and demonstrates their complementarity and overall similarity with the organization of the mind.

Temperament is considered to be the substrate upon which personality, thinking styles, and the self are constructed. According to Kagan (1994a),

> the word *temperament* is used by some, but not all, scientists to refer to psychological qualities that display considerable variation among infants and young children and, in addition, have a relatively, but not indefinitely, stable physiological basis that derives from the individual's genetic constitution. It is also understood that the inherited physiological processes can mediate different phenotypic displays as the child grows and that experience always influences the form of the behavioral display. The temperamental qualities investigated most often by psychologists, pediatricians, and psychiatrists, which are obvious to parents, include irritability, a happy mood, ease of being soothed, motor activity, sociability, attentiveness, adaptability, approach to or avoidance of novelty, ease as well as intensity of arousal in reaction to stimulation, and regulation of arousal states. (p. 16)

Thus, temperament involves an individual's early tendencies and dispositions, which are then gradually shaped into the dimensions of personality and style. How are these dimensions actualized into patterns of adaptation in the real environment?

Graziano and colleagues (Graziano, Jensen-Campbell, & Finch, 1997; Graziano, Jensen-Campbell, & Sullivan, in press), building on the work of McAdams (1995), proposed that social adaptation is grounded on a three-level hierarchical structure. Level I comprises the so-called Big Five factors of personality, that is, extroversion, agreeableness, conscientiousness, neuroticism, and openness to experience (these factors are symbolized as $P_1 \ldots P_5$ in Figure 1). Individuals high in extroversion are sociable, active, talkative, optimistic, pleasure seeking, self-confident, warm, and uninhibited. Individuals low in extroversion are aloof, withdrawn, shy, and inhibited. Individuals high in agreeableness are soft hearted, generous, kind, forgiving, sympathetic, warm, and trusting. Individuals low in agreeableness are suspicious, headstrong, shrewd, impatient, argumentative, and aggressive. Individuals high in conscientiousness are organized, ambitious, energetic, efficient, determined, precise, industrious, persistent, reliable, and responsible. Individuals low in conscientiousness are distractible, lazy, careless, impulsive, hasty, immature, and defensive. Individuals high in neuroticism are nervous, anxious, moody, tense, self-centered, and self-pitying. Individuals low in neuroticism are confident, self-confident, clear-thinking, alert, and content. Finally, individuals who are open to experience are curious and have wide interests, are inventive, original, imaginative, nontraditional, and artistic. Individuals who are not open to experience are conservative, cautious, and mild.

Level II contains the self-systems, such as global, social, and academic self-esteem: That is, it contains all self-representations, value systems, and general action strategies that translate the Level I dispositions into particular modes of understanding and action.

Finally, Level III involves perceived adaptations to particular task environments, such as academic adjustment, peer relationships, and classroom behavior. According to Graziano and colleagues, the Level II self-systems are differentially related to the Level I personality dispositions and also function as mediators between these dispositions and domain-specific perceived adjustments and related self-narratives. As a result, different types of situation-specific adaptations may originate from the same personality disposition if this is coupled with different kinds of self-representations.

Sternberg's (1988, 1990, 1997; Ferrari & Sternberg, 1998) conception of thinking styles and their relationships to personality and cognitive abilities seems complementary to this outlined model. According to Ferrari and Sternberg, "styles may represent an important missing link integrating intelligence, personality, and real-world performance" (1998, p. 933). Sternberg (1988) called his theory of thinking styles "the theory of mental self-goverment", to stress his view that styles govern the functioning of thinking and self-actualization much as governments govern countries. This theory defines the styles of self-government in terms of several dimensions, such as function and form.

Function refers to what the mind does to cope with the world: Like governments, the mind legislates and plans, implements and executes, judges and evaluates. Thus, there are three styles in the functioning of the mind: the *legislative*, the *executive*, and the *judicial*. "The legislative style characterises individuals who enjoy creating, formulating, and planning for problem solutions." (Sternberg, 1990, p. 140). This style requires high levels of self-awareness and reflectivity and it predisposes people to autonomous, creative, planned, and system-creation activities, such as those that characterize artists, scientists, and policy makers. The executive "style implements rather than plans for execution" (Sternberg, 1988, p. 203) and so requires actual knowledge and problem-solving skills. It predisposes people to rule-following activities, that evolve in well-defined contexts, such as those of the lawyer, police officer, builder, and doctor. Finally, the judicial style involves judgmental activities, such as evaluation of people, systems, ideas, and rules, and it directs to occupations such as judges and admissions officers. Ferrari and Sternberg (1998) claim that "although any complex task typically involves all three functions of self-government, in most individuals, one of the functions tends to be dominant" (p. 927).

Form refers to the preferred ways to approach and handle problems, and Ferrari and Sternberg proposed four forms of self-government: monarchic, hierarchic, oligarchic, and anarchic. "In the monarchic form a single goal or way of doing things predominates. People with a monarchic style tend to focus single-mindedly on one goal or need at a time" (Ferrari & Sternberg, 1998, p. 928). The hierarchic form allows for many goals, of varying priority, so that individuals with a hierarchic style tend to have multiple goals, which are organized hierarchically according to their inter-relationships and importance. The oligarchic form also allows for multiple goals, but considers all goals equally important. Thus, people with an oligarchic style may work toward many goals simultaneously; however, if these goals are not conplementary, none may be achieved. Finally, those with an anarchic style are intolerant of rules and thus avoid organizing and planning goals and activities. Thus, they may shift from one goal or task to another without fully realizing any.

General models of the organization of the self also assume a hierarchi-cal structure, such that there are active processes that produce knowledge about the self, self-representations, and self-descriptions that result from the operation of these processes. In fact, theories positing the self as a hierarchical system are not new: as early as 1890, James (1890) posited that the self involves two hierarchical levels, the "I-self" and the "me-self." The I-self is the knower, in that it comprises all self-observation and self-recording processes. These, in turn, generate the knowledge that we have about ourselves. This constitutes the me-self, which comprises three aspects: a material self, a social self, and spiritual self (James, 1892). The material self subsumes all representations of our bodies and possessions; the social self refers to all characteristics recognized by others; the spiritual self involves our thoughts and dispositions, descriptive and evalua-tive, about ourselves.

James's distinction between a knowing (the I-self) and a known self (the me-self) underlies contemporary theories of the self. Specifically, Markus and Wurf (1987) proposed a model that differentiates the working self-concept from the collection of the individual's self-representations. The working self-concept is directly involved in the formation and control of behavior at both the intra- and the interpersonal level. The model pro-posed that, at the intrapersonal level, the working self-concept influences information processing (e.g., sensitivity to self-relevant stimuli, better processing of self-congruent stimuli, and repulsion or twisting of self-incongruent stimuli), affects motivation (i.e., orientation to choices con-ducive to self-actualization and self-enhancement), and shapes regulation of mental or overt action (by adjustments in the self-concept itself and in the incoming information, but also in overt behavior). At the interpersonal level, the working self-concept is believed to influence social perception (e.g., it is used as a filter for the interpretation and the evaluation of others' behavior), situation and partner choice (e.g., different styles of self-monitoring orient the person to different types of everyday activities), interaction strategies (e.g., the behavior and the signals emitted during interpersonal interactions are intentionally formulated so as to transmit a particular identity to the partner), and reactions to feedback (e.g., self-congruent information is weighted differently as compared to self-incongruent information). Obviously, the similarity between James's I-self and the Markus and Wurf working self-concept, and James's me-self and the Markus and Wurf self-representations is more than apparent.

The preceding organization of self and personality is consistent with the prevailing view on self-esteem, which posits self-esteem as a hierarchical construct, with general self-esteem at the apex, several major domains (that is, academic, social, emotional, and physical self-concept) at a middle level, and several more specific domains within each of these main domains, (e.g., math and science in the academic domain or physical ability and physical appearance in the physical domain) (Bandura, 1989; Bracken, 1996; Byrne, 1995; Harter, 1990, 1998; Hattie, 1992; Marsh, Byrne, & Shavelson, 1992; 1995; Marsh & Hattie, 1996; Oosterwegel & Oppenheimer, 1993; Shavelson & Marsh, 1986).

C. TOWARD AN OVERARCHING MODEL OF MIND, PERSONALITY, AND SELF

The model in Figure 1 shows how the constructs proposed by the various theories are interrelated. We propose that the hierarchical levels of personality and the self-system correspond to the three hierarchical levels of mind depicted by our theory of the cognitive architecture. The model posits that the Big Five factors of personality (that is, Graziano's Level I) correspond to the domain-specific systems that reside at the environment-oriented level of knowing. That is, the domain-specific systems of understanding channel the functioning of the mind, and the Big Five factors channel patterns of action and relationships with the social and cultural environment (see Level I of the model shown in Figure 1). In a similar vein, temperament is considered to be the dynamic aspect of processing potentials, where the processing potentials constrain the complexity and type of information that can be understood at a given age, and temperament constrains how information is received initially and reacted to (see Level II of the model shown in Figure 1). These constructs are controlled by the active processes of self-knowing implicated in James's I-self, the Markus and Wurf working self-concept, or by the monitoring and control processes involved in working hypercognition (see Level III of the model shown in Figure 1). The functioning of these control processes generates feelings and representations of general cognitive efficiency or global self-worth and general self-esteem (see Level IV of the model shown in Figure 1). In parallel to these general self-representations, we have the more localized or specialized self-systems (that is, Graziano's level II, James's me-self, and the Markus and Wurf collection of self-representations). These correspond to the various self-representations that reside in the long-term hypercognitive maps of the organization of the mind (see Level V of the model shown in Figure 1). Thus, the constructs at this level reflect how individuals register and represent themselves with regard to the various dimensions of understanding the world and the various dispositions of interacting with the world. Finally, Sternberg's thinking styles (see Level VI of the model shown in Figure 1) and Graziano's Level III (see Level VII of the model shown in Figure 1) stand on their own as frames that shape perceived or actual adaptations to particular tasks or contexts.

As an integrated representation of the thinking and acting individual, this model captures both the dynamic (that is, the motivational and emotional) and the meaning-making (that is, the representational) components of understanding, experience, and action. Obviously, testing this model in its totality is a gigantic enterprise. However, several studies conducted in our laboratory provided evidence in line with the model. These studies tested various parts of the model and found that self-representations at various levels within the cognitive realm, within the personality realm, and across the two are organized as shown in this model.

One of these studies showed that the Big Five factors of personality are directly related to the cognitive systems. For example, self-representation of cognitive efficiency (i.e., processing and reasoning) and self-monitoring/self-regulation were found to be very closely related to openness to experience. Moreover, four of the five factors of personality were found to intervene, in various combinations with each other, in the formation of thinking styles. Specifically, individuals who were open to experience and neurotic were found to think highly of themselves. In turn, thinking highly of oneself together with being open to experience was found to orient persons to activities requiring originality. Those who were found to think highly of themselves but were not open to experience tended to have a judicial style of thought, which, according to Sternberg, orients to activities requiring evaluation. Interestingly, a combination of neuroticism with extroversion was found to lead to impulsivity; impulsivity itself was negatively related to conscientiousness, which was, however, positively related to systematicity. In turn, systematic personalities tended to have an executive style, which leads to activities with predefined rules. In conclusion, this model suggests how the various dimensions of mind and personality interact to build systems that channel how individuals represent themselves and regulate their relationships with their environment (cf. Demetriou and Kazi, in press; Demetriou et al., 1999b).

III. DEVELOPMENT OF SELF-UNDERSTANDING AND SELF-REGULATION

Recent years have witnessed a proliferation of research on the development of self-understanding and self-regulation, and to conduct an exhaustive review is beyond the scope of this chapter. Our synthesis is designed to illustrate the major landmarks in the development of the individual's (1) understanding of the organization and functioning of the mind, (2) self-representation, and (3) self-regulation. In terms of our theory, the first two subsections discuss the development of long-term hypercognition and the third examines the development of working hypercognition. Table 1 presents an overview of the main developmental trends that will be discussed in these three realms. Finally, we also review research and theory aimed at explaining how and why development in these processes take place.

A. DEVELOPMENT OF THE CHILD'S UNDERSTANDING OF THE ORGANIZATION AND FUNCTIONING OF THE MIND

No substantive evidence exists that prelanguage infants entertain any understanding of the mind. It must be noted, however, that symbolic play, which appears at the end of the second year, such as when an infant uses a banana to pretend he or she is speaking on the phone, indicates implicit metarepresentation. That is, there is an understanding that there are mental states, such as the representation of the telephone, that can be represented by various means not necessarily resembling the initial object (Leslie, 1987). However, an explicit understanding of the mind as a system generating and composed of representations does not appear before 2 to 3 years of age. According to Flavell et al. (1995), preschoolers seem to "have at least a minimal grasp of the bare-bones essentials of thinking: namely that it is some sort of internal, mental activity that people engage in that refers to real or imaginary objects or events" (p. 75). Moreover, they also realize that thinking is different not only from perceiving, but also from other cognitive processes, such as knowing. In one of their experiments, Flavell and colleagues showed that 3-year-olds understand that a person who is blindfolded and has covered ears can neither see nor hear an object, but can think about this object. Another experiment revealed that 3- and 4-year-olds realize that a person is thinking when he or she is in the process of choosing one of several available objects or when he or she is trying to understand how a curious thing happened (such as how a large pear fit into a narrow-necked bottle). Flavell et al. also showed that young preschoolers are aware that a person can have knowledge of things he or she is not currently thinking about. However, there are important aspects of thinking that preschoolers do not understand; specifically, there is compelling evidence that preschoolers do not understand what William James called the "stream of consciousness." That is, they do not realize that thinking is a process that goes on continuously, even during physically inactive periods such as waiting in a doctor's office. For example, in one study by of Flavell et al., preschoolers ignored very clear cues about the

TABLE 1 Development of the Understanding of the Organization and Functioning of the Mind, Self-Representation, and Self-Regulation

Years	Understanding the mind	Self-image	Self-regulation
0–1		Differentiation of the body from the surrounding world	Neurophysiological and sensorimotor modulation
1–2	Implicit metarepresentation (infants use a banana as a telephone)	Self-recognition in the mirror	Means−ends differentiation Sensorimotor schemes are under intentional control
3–5	Understanding that thinking is internal mental activity referring to objects or events Differentiation between perception, knowing, and thinking	Self-concept geared on observable external characteristics	Self-control: awareness and self-initiated notification of action Toddlers can follow requests and commands, but cannot delay gratification
6–8	Understanding the stream of consciousness and inner speech The content of thought can be related with ongoing activity	Taxonomic self-descriptions, generally positive and often inaccurate	Self-regulation through inner speech and other means of attention, motivation, and stimulus control
8–10	Understanding the constructive nature of thought (thought gives meaning). Differentiation between cognitive functions (e.g., attention, memory, and inference)	Trait labels integrating particular self-representations Global self-worth	Short-term goal-selection and planning Mastery over thought, emotional factors, and behavior
11–13	Different kinds of the same cognitive function can be distinguished Differentiation between clearly different thought domains (e.g., mathematical vs. spatial thought)	Higher-order abstractions about the self, although not well integrated	Interest about the future, middle-scale planning, and-systematic regulation of every-day activities
14–16	Awareness of particular cognitive processes and operations Differentiation between similar domains (e.g., causal vs. mathematical thought)	Modularized self-concept involving an accurate global self-concept with accurate domain-specific self-representations	Planning of the future (selection of studies, job selection, etc.)

constant presence of thought activity; the majority denied the statement, "Something is always going on in people's minds, so there must be something going on."

Preschoolers also seem unable to realize that cognitive activities such as looking, listening, reading, and talking necessarily entail thinking and the experience of thought. Although they can at times recognize that mental activity is occurring, they are unable to specify the content of the thinking in spite of very clear signs. For instance, in one experiment by Flavell et al., person A asked person B a thought-provoking question about an object in front of child. Person B said to person A, "That's a hard question. Give me a minute," and she turned to one side giving nonverbal cues that she was trying to find an answer to the question. Preschoolers were not able to indicate that experimenter B was thinking about the object named in the question. Many preschoolers continued to have difficulty with this seemingly simple problem even when experimenter B stared at and touched the object while thinking about it. In fact, preschoolers seem to have difficulty specifying the content of their own thought. For example, when asked about which room in their house they keep their toothbrush, their replies mentioned neither a toothbrush nor a bathroom when they were asked what they had been thinking about.

Preschoolers also are not aware of the associative nature of the mind (Flavell et al. 1995). That is, they do not know that one idea or thought triggers another which triggers another and so on. For example, when preschoolers were told a story about a child who thinks of beautiful flowers while on the beach, they cannot explain why, later the child sees some beautiful flowers, and thinks of the beach. Finally, preschoolers do not seem to understand that thought is only partially controllable; that is, that you can start thinking about something if you decide to but you cannot always stop thinking about something just because you want to.

In another set of studies, Flavell, Green, Flavell, and Grossman (1997) showed that 4-year-olds, in contrast to 6-year-olds, have little knowledge and awareness of inner speech; that is, preschool children did not infer "that a person silently engaged in such intrinsically verbal activities as reading, counting, or recalling items from a shopping list was saying things to herself. They also tended to deny that covert speech is a possible human activity" (p. 39). Moreover, their studies have shown that preschoolers have difficulty noticing their own inner speech. For example, they deny that they engage in inner speech even when they are asked to think silently about the sound of their name.

Finally, we must also note that preschoolers do not conceive of intellectual ability as an internal quality of the mind; rather they seem to associate it with various external characteristics, such as work habits and conduct, and therefore believe that it may be increased by practice and hard work (Flavell et al., 1995). This conception is obviously consistent with their limited understanding of the organizational, functional, and dynamic characteristics of the mind.

These limitations diminish considerably during the early school years, at which age children begin to understand the constructive nature of thought. For example, they understand that it is by thought that one deciphers the meaning of ambivalent expressions (Carpendale & Chandler, 1996). Also, from age 8 to 10 years, children begin to differentiate various cognitive functions, such as memory and inference or attention and thought. However, they cannot discriminate between different aspects of the same cognitive function; for instance, that there are different kinds of memory. Fabricius and Schwanenflugel (1994) reported a series of studies which focused on the awareness of similarities and differences between cognitive functions. In these studies 8- to 10-year-old children and adults were examined. The participants were given simple descriptions of list memory (e.g., getting all the things at the store that your mother requested), prospective memory (e.g., saying happy birthday on the right day to your friend who told you her birthday a long time ago), comprehension (e.g., learning a new board game from the instructions on the box), attention (e.g., listening to what your friend is saying to you in a noisy classroom), and inference (e.g., figuring out what your friend wants when he or she says, "Boy, that cookie looks good!"). The participants were asked to contrast each sentence with all other sentences and indicate the similarity among the processes referred to in each pair of sentences. It was found that from the age of 8 years children can distinguish between memory and inference. Both 10-year-olds and adults (but not the 8-year-olds) realized that the involvement of memory in tasks indicated similar processes. Unlike adults, however, neither 8- or 10-year-olds distinguished between comprehension and attention or between different kinds of memory. By late childhood it seems that children begin to distinguish between different cognitive processes, although this differentiation is very global and limited to processes with clear experiential differences.

Begining in first grade, children understand that each domain involves both a competence component, which refers to the general demands of the domain, and a subjective component, which refers to how they personally value activities within each of the domains. This suggests the first differentiation between a general understanding of the mind and cognitive self-image. However, they do not make finer distinctions between various aspects of competence or subjective value, such as task difficulty, expectations for success, and learning ability within a domain (Eccles, Wigfield, Harold, & Blumenfeld, 1993). In line with these findings, Nicholls (1990) showed that at this age children begin to differentiate the various dimensions of ability and intelligence, recognizing that skill is necessary for successful performance on some tasks and that tasks of different difficulty require different ability. However, children still believe that effort is the primary source of success, and do not recognize that ability may be an underlying system of processes that can be translated into different kinds of performance depending on the particular task.

Awareness of specific cognitive processes and operations develops gradually in adolescence. A series of studies in our laboratory (Demetriou & Efklides, 1989; Demetriou et al., 1993b) has shown that differentiation between problem-solving and reasoning strategies—such as mathematical and spatial problems—is impossible before approximately age 13. At age 14, adolescents begin to differentiate spatial and experimental or mathematical thought, although they cannot differentiate between experimental and mathematical thought. Some differentiation begins at about age 16, culminating during the college years.

The differences and interrelationships between the various dimensions of intellectual competence are constructed during adolescence, when, for example, it is understood that difficulty involves a normative component (i.e., the higher the success rate for a task, the easier the task). At the same time, it is gradually understood that although difficult tasks require more effort, effort compensates for low ability only to a certain degree, and although high ability is an advantage in general, it does not always suffice, because there are tasks where high ability must be complemented by hard and systematic effort. Thus, in adolescence, self-evaluations of intellectual competence and academic achievement become progressively more accurate and modest. Self-evaluation scores and academic self-esteem have been found to decline from late childhood to early adolescence, but beginning in middle adolescence, self-evaluations of performance become more domain-specific, more accurate, and generally more positive (Eccles et al., 1993; Nicholls, 1990; Phillips & Zimmerman, 1990; Stipek & McIver, 1989).

B. DEVELOPMENT OF SELF-REPRESENTATION

For the newborn, recognition of the self centers on the body. Although some evidence suggests that 3-month-old infants can differentiate their body from the surrounding physical environment and other persons (Butterworth, 1995), the first signs of a self-concept do not appear until about age 15 months. At this age, but not earlier, infants begin to recognize themselves in a mirror (Lewis & Brooks-Gunn, 1979). Later, during the early preschool years, more differentiated self-representations begin to be formed, which usually depend on observable characteristics viewed in isolation and which are unrealistically positive (I have blue eyes; I can run fast; I am happy). In early to middle childhood, representations gradually become interconnected, especially if they refer to very obvious or strong characteristics or experiences. This results in taxonomic self-descriptions (I am good, fast, clever, etc.) that indicate a continuity of self-representation over time. Because thought is still unidimensional at this stage (Case et al., 1996), opposites such as good and bad, and happy and sad cannot be truly integrated, and self-representations are still generally positive and, therefore, frequently inaccurate, because the negative side of a dimension is avoided.

At about the age of 2 years, children are aware of the fact that others evaluate them. Stipek, Recchia, & McClintic (1992) showed that at this age (but not earlier) children look to an adult for appraisal after finishing a task. Self-evaluations and others' evaluations are not yet integrated, however, but indications begin to appear at about the age of 3 when children are able to internalize others' performance criteria for tasks. This marks the onset of a more objective and accurate system of self-evaluation and self-representation (Higgins, 1987).

In middle to late childhood, higher order generalizations are possible due to the ability to build bidimensional concepts (Case, 1985, 1992) or representational systems (Fischer, 1980), which allow for a variety of trait labels that integrate self-evaluations and self-representations (for example, I am smart because I do well in different areas, such as English and Social Studies). Moreover, the integration of opposites is possible at this phase (e.g., although I am generally smart, I am not very good at math), so that self-evaluations become more differentiated and accurate. The concept of global self-worth also appears at this phase (Harter, 1990), indicating that the I-self now functions as a general self-monitoring and self-evaluation agent that can integrate the various aspects of the me-self.

In early adolescence thought can conceive of the possible (Inhelder & Piaget, 1958), the suppositional (Demetriou, 1998b), and the abstract (Case, 1985, 1992; Fischer, 1980), because representations can be viewed from the perspective of other representations (Demetriou, 1998b; Demetriou, et al., 1993b). Thus, the traits of the previous phase now can be integrated into higher order abstractions about the self (for instance, I am intelligent because I am smart and creative; I am extroverted because I am rowdy and talkative). Case, Fischer, and Higgins, all concur that abstractions about the self are not yet well integrated at this age. Thus, although both positive and negative abstractions may coexist within the self-system, they are not subsumed under a common self-concept that associates them with different domains, such that one may excel in one domain and fall short in another.

In middle adolescence, abstractions begin to be linked. As a result, adolescents are able to represent themselves as both intelligent and airheaded, extroverted and introverted, and so forth. Thus, at this phase, a more accurate and modularized representation of the self becomes possible, enabling adolescents to pair their various qualities with different types of activities, preferences, and orientations. Self-questioning in terms of "Who am I?" and "What do I want to become in life?" may elicit a generalized self-definition, such as "I want to become a famous person" or a "useful person." At the same time, a specialized answer also can be given when self-questioning focuses on how this general self-definition is to be actualized. For example, when answering the question, "What career is more suitable for the realization of my ambitions given that I am talented in A and not so skilled in B," the adolescent can specify alternative occupations. This indicates that a self-system that is both integrated and differentiated begins to be established at this phase, although command of this system is not fully developed. As a result, in middle adolescence, adolescents may vacillate between extremes and exhibit inaccuracies and distress when the balance shifts to the negative side of dimensions and characteristics.

In late adolescence, the individual becomes able to coordinate abstractions into higher order abstractions and thus develop a coherent self-concept, which was missing in middle adolescence. For instance, the seemingly incompatible poles of a dimension (e.g., extrovert vs. introvert) can now be integrated into a higher order dimensions (e.g., "flexible"; i.e., one can behave as an extrovert in some situations and as an introvert in others). As a result, self-evaluation now can be more accurate, because each of the various dimensions and modules of the self can be approached and evaluated in relation to the specific context.

C. DEVELOPMENT OF SELF-REGULATION

Kopp (1982) proposed that human self-regulation develops along four levels: modulation, control, self-control, and self-regulation. We now suggest that these four levels represent the major hallmarks in the development of working hypercognition and working self-concept (or the I-self).

Specifically, neurophysiological modulation is established from birth to 2 to 3 months of age, and refers to the establishment of control over arousal states and reflexes. Obviously, self-initiated control is totally nonexistent in neurophysiological modulation; arousal states and reflex systems are controlled by the interaction between the condition of the organism and the external stimuli facing the neonate, meaning that control at this phase obeys the laws of dynamic systems. Therefore, working hypercognition proper, that is, a stream of consciousness of which one is aware, is lacking at this phase.

Sensorimotor modulation is attained during the following phase, which lasts until approximately age 1. At this level, self-control refers to coordinated nonreflexive voluntary action that aims at particular goals, such as reaching for an object. Like neurophysiological modulation, sensorimotor modulation "does not involve consciousness, prior intention, or awareness of the meaning of a situation" (Kopp, 1982, p. 203). However, it does enable very flexible mastery of ongoing patterns of activity in response to changes in stimulation. Thus, there seems to be a differentiation in action between the mind and the self, on the one hand, and the environment, on the other.

During the second year, control per se is established. That is, behavior is initiated intentionally, means are differentiated from ends, and there is awareness of social demands and thus compliance with simple orders. In fact, at about the age of 12 months, infants become able to walk. Walking signifies dynamic control over very different and complex body–environment systems, such as walking over different surfaces, stepping on stairs, and so forth. Moreover, it signifies the beginning of self-initiated movement in the environment, which, by definition, requires planning (where to go) and self-regulation (to reach the goal) (Zelazo, 1998). Likewise, imitation of complex behavior is possible during the second year, although it still depends on the presence of a model. Imitation requires control because the attempt to reproduce a sequence of actions necessitates both monitoring the model (or, later, a representation of the model) and regulating one's own actions so that these actions mirror the model's actions. Self-initiated inhibition of an action is also possible at this stage if there have been strong aversive consequences for this action in the past. Even control of emotion may be possible during the second year. Recent studies (e.g., Malatesta, Culver, Tesman, & Sheppard, 1989) have shown that in an attempt to regulate their expression of emotions, one-year-olds compress their lips and knit their eyebrows to control their sadness and anger. The reader is reminded that facial self-recognition appears at this phase, signifying that working hypercognition as the mind's eye and controller now exists, although explicit self-awareness of it is still lacking.

Self-control begins at the end of the second year. In self-control, the balance shifts from the environment as such or from the dynamics of the action in context to the intending person as such. That is, self-control involves awareness and self-initiated modification of action as a result of remembered information (that is, of goals, self-concept, past performance, etc.). The appearance of representation in general and the symbolic functions, such as language, in particular, is clearly related to the change from sensorimotor modulation to self-control. Thus, from this phase onward, children start to behave according to both their will and social expectations in the absence of external monitors. Moreover, children are now able to follow requests and commands (Crockerberg and Lintman, 1990; Schneider-Rosen & Wenz-Gross, 1990), signifying the ability to translate external information about their behavior into all those mental and overt acts necessary to effect a particular request. In other words, this capability implies self-monitoring and self-direction processes that build an internal model of the request and then modulate and regulate the actualization of this model into actual behavior.

Self-control is regarded as distinct from self-regulation (Kopp, 1982). At the level of self-control there is only limited flexibility to adapt to new demands, and there is "a limited capacity for delay and waiting. In contrast, self-regulation is considered to be adaptive to changes. It is a distinctly more mature form of control and presumably implicates the use of reflection and strategies involving introspection, consciousness, or metacognition" (Kopp, 1982, p. 207). Self-regulation as previously defined begins to appear at about the age of 3 to 4 years.

The so-called *delay of gratification* paradigm has produced some very interesting studies about the development of self-regulation. These studies revealed some of the mechanisms that underlie the shift of emphasis in the control of behavior from external to internal sources. In a delay of gratification study, children are usually given two choices: a small reward that is immediately available or a large reward that requires a period of waiting. In an early study (Mischel and Ebbesen, 1970), children 3 to 5 years old were offered the choice of waiting 15-minutes for a very attractive snack or ringing a bell for a smaller treat if the 15-minute period was too long. Very few preschoolers were able to wait the entire 15-minute period. A subsequent study (Vaughn, Kopp, & Krakow, 1984) showed, however, that there are systematic changes in the ability to delay gratification during the preschool years. In this study, 18-, 24-, and 30-month-old toddlers were tested under three conditions: (1) They were asked to refrain from touching a nearby toy telephone; (2) They were instructed not to eat raisins placed under a cup until given permission; (3) They were told not to open a gift until the experimenter had finished working. It was found that the ability to resist these temptations was practically nonexistent at the age of 18 months, because these infants succumbed to the temptation almost immediately; 24-month-olds were able to wait for about a minute; 30-month-olds waited for almost 2 minutes. Other studies have shown that the ability to delay gratification develops considerably throughout the primary school years, so that by the age of 10 to 12 children wait for the larger but delayed incentive instead of choosing the smaller but immediately available one (Mischel, 1986).

With development, self-regulation gradually evolves into planfulness, which is long-term or strategic self-regulation. That is, planfulness integrates, under an overarching plan, the main goals and objectives, subgoals, if needed, the strategies and actions needed to attain goals and subgoals, and a time plan that specifies when strategies and actions are to be applied. So defined, planfulness is not present before the age of about 9 years. In her classic study of the development of visual scanning strategies, Vurpillot (1968) showed that children younger than this age do not formulate a plan that would allow them to compare two houses systematically and exhaustively in order to find out if they are entirely similar or if they differ in some characteristics. In fact, many of Piaget's classic formal operational tasks (Inhelder and Piaget, 1958) may be considered as tests of planfulness. For example, tasks that require designing an experiment to test a hypothesis presuppose that one is able to conceive of the hypothesis and its implications from the beginning and also specify the experimental manipulations that test which of the implications do occur and do not occur. It is well known that these tasks are not solved before the age of 13 to 14 years. It is more than a coincidence that it is only from middle adolescence onward that persons become planful with regard to their short- and long-term goals and thus able to subordinate their thoughts and behavior to the attainment of these goals. For instance, from the age of 13 to 14, adolescents begin to think of what they would like to become in life and follow a long-term plan, such as a particular course of education, to realize their ambitions. Subordinating one's life under multiple long-term plans, such as to have a family, succeed professionally, and have an interesting social life, is an even later attainment, which begins in early adulthood (Erikson, 1963).

Clearly, as it becomes more strategic and planful, self-regulation comes under the control of the person's general theory of mind and self-image, on the one hand, and the person's personality and style, on the other hand. In the next section, we try to explain how these systems interact during development, thereby causing development.

IV. EXPLAINING THE DEVELOPMENT OF SELF-UNDERSTANDING AND SELF-REGULATION

There are two approaches to the explanation of human development in general. One stresses intraindividual dynamics as a source of developmental change and tries to understand how an initial change in any system within the individual causes changes in other systems. The second approach stresses the interindividual dynamics of change and tries to understand how the interaction between individuals causes changes within the interacting individuals. Obviously, the two approaches are complementary. On the one hand, the interaction between two persons may initiate a change in a particular system in each of the two persons, according to the principles underlying interindividual dynamics. Subsequently, however, this change may start to propagate within each individual and affect other systems according to intraindividual dynamics. On the other hand, a change that occurs within an individual according to the principles of intraindividual dynamics may affect the interactions of this individual with other individuals, thereby causing changes according to interindividual dynamics. The following discussion focuses on the intra- and interindividual dynamics of change with regard to self-understanding and self-regulation.

A. INTRAINDIVIDUAL DYNAMICS IN THE DEVELOPMENT
OF SELF-UNDERSTANDING AND SELF-REGULATION

We have argued elsewhere that intraindivual developmental causality is synergic (Demetriou, 1998a, b; Demetriou & Raftopoulos, 1999). This is due to the very nature of the architecture of the mind and personality. That is, the presence of environment-oriented and self-oriented systems in the person suggests that the functioning of any of the environment-oriented systems will, by definition, cause changes in self-understanding. That is, our knowledge of the mind and ourselves increases as we grow older, because the various activities we have to engage in activate different cognitive functions, tendencies, and characteristics, thereby providing the opportunity for us to observe, compare, and contrast them both intra- and interpersonally. For example, the realization that unpleasant thoughts cannot be stopped at will may be the first step in our understanding of the stream of consciousness. Repeated engagement in problem-solving activities in different domains enables the developing person to realize that the mental operations he or she performs in the various domains are not the same.

Moreover, developmental causality is synergic because any change, once it has occurred in any system, will sooner or later affect other systems associated to this system, because it transforms the dynamics of the relationships between the systems. A telling example is that which connects maturational changes in the interconnectivity of different areas of the brain with self-monitoring and self-regulation. Specifically, it is now believed that the brain undergoes a series of maturational cycles in which various parts of the brain are both better interconnected with each other and with the frontal lobes. The frontal lobes are considered to be responsible for the executive control of novel responses and self-awareness with regard to the command of novel responses (Stuss, 1992; Thatcher, 1994). Case (1992) proposed that these cycles in the development of the brain are directly implicated in the development of processing capacity, which, in turn, is implicated in the development of self-regulation. Zelazo (1998) has suggested that many of an infant's achievements during the second year of life (such as means–end coordination, symbolic play, and even walking) are due to the fact that at this phase the infant becomes able to place at least two units of information (sensations, feelings, movements, objects, etc.) in mental focus or working hypercognition. In turn, this is due to the fact that processing has become as fast as needed to bring a new unit into mental focus before the unit previously in focus fades away.

The Rothbart and Bates (1998) theory of temperamental control moves along the same lines. According to this theory, the ability to monitor and inhibit inappropriate impulses and tendencies depends on the development of attentional networks, because they enable the individual to corepresent internal tendencies and external stimuli. This is so because resisting a temptation requires awareness and simultaneous representation of two competing objects (the temptation, such as an immediately available and a more distant, but more valued, reward), the emotional–motivational consequences of each choice, and the mental or actual operations that can be used to direct attention and action from the lesser to the more important goal. Self-regulation is not possible in these situations insofar as this complex of representations cannot be held simultaneously in an active state. This simultaneity occurs at the age of 5 years; that is, at the age at which delay of gratification was found to be possible. Therefore, the development of self-regulation seems to follow the development of both processing potentials and working hypercognition.

Developmental synergy is also obvious in the relationships between the development of self-understanding and self-regulation. That is, preschool children can neither recognize mental processes clearly nor even comprehend that they can use one process to affect the functioning of another. Naturally, then, they do not use these processes as a means of self-regulation. With development in the understanding of the nature and functioning of these processes and in self-representation with regard to each of them, self-regulation of behavior and thought becomes increasingly more efficient.

The mechanisms involved in the development of the ability to delay gratification may be invoked as an example. The studies that investigated the development of this ability revealed that distraction is the primary means by which children attempt to delay gratification. Children try to divert their attention with overt or mental actions that transform or conceal the temptation. Some children cover their eyes so that they cannot see the tempting stimuli; others sing so that they are otherwise engaged during the waiting period; others transform the incentive mentally so that they represent it as being unappealing rather than attractive.

The use of distraction as a means to delay gratification develops systematically in a way that is consistent with the pattern of development outlined above. Preschoolers do not know that distraction can help them resist temptations, and thus they do not use it even when instructed to do so or taught self-instructional strategies; instead, they continue to focus attention on the desirable properties of the incentives, which leads them to succumb to rather than resist the temptation. Efficient use of distraction appears at about the age of 6 to 8 years, when children begin to employ simple strategies, such as covering their eyes or the object itself. Cognitive distractions that result in transformation of the incentives do not appear until early adolescence. Kuhl (1992) posits that although early school-age children are capable of attention control, only later can they use motivation control as a means of self-regulation.

B. INTERINDIVIDUAL DYNAMICS IN THE DEVELOPMENT
OF SELF-UNDERSTANDING AND SELF-REGULATION

Individuals under normal conditions always develop with others. There-fore,

> Individual development is an abstraction which does not actually exist. That is, the changes occurring in an individual are in fact part of overlapping cycles of *codevelopment*. A cycle of codevelopment is the dynamic situation in which the changes which occur in an individual affect and are affected by the changes which occur in other individuals in the cycle. A given individual may be part of a number of cycles of codevelopment, such as the family, the classroom, and the peer group. (Demetriou, 1996, p. 31).

This general conception of development implies that self-understanding and self-regulation develop in the individual as a result of codevelopment. In other words, self-understanding is based on counderstanding and self-regulation is based on coregulation. That is, individuals come to know their own mind and self by observing others functioning and from their interactions with others; moreover, they sharpen their self-regulatory skills and abilities by regulating and being regulated by others.

Counderstanding and coregulation is possible because, according to many infant researchers, the infant is born with built-in intersubjectivity skills (Kougioumoutzakis, 1985; Meltzoff & Moore, 1995; Trevarthen, 1979). According to Trevarthen, *intersubjectivity* is grounded on joint patterns of awareness that enable the interacting individuals to recognize and control each other's intentions and behavior. Thus, intersubjectivity comprises observational, representational imitative, and regulatory (self-regulatory and coregulatory) skills that enable the individual to actively handle interpersonal interactions and continuously strengthen both a sense of self and others. Joint attention is a cognitive–social process that requires intersubjectivity skills. In joint attention, two or more persons can focus their attention on a common object and they are able to monitor changes in the object's and each other's behavior so as to keep the object in focus, such as when one points to a moving object (by gaze and/or by pointing) and the other follows. Research has shown that infants begin as early as 2 to 4 months of age to adjust their gaze when their adult partner changes the direction of his or her sight, although they are not very accurate until the age of about 12 months (Butterworth & Cochran, 1980). In the period between 11 and 15 months, the various aspects of joint attention, such as gaze and point following, become well controlled by the infant (Carpenter, Nagell, & Tomasello, 1998). In fact, from this age onward, interactional synchrony (Fogel, 1993), that is, the ability for concerted interactions and exchange of information, is well established and covers most aspects of interpersonal interactions, including taking turns during verbal interactions and social referencing.

Internalization is the main mechanism that transforms coregulation into self-regulation. Internalization refers to the processes underlying the individual appropriation of shared meaning and interactions. In other words, it refers to the processes that enable individuals who participate in an interaction episode to give personal meaning to the information exchanged during the interaction and reconstruct for themselves the mental or overt actions taking place in the interaction so that they subsequently can use these actions outside the interaction episode and independently of each other.

Vygotsky (1934/1962) proposed that *private speech*, that is, speech directed to the self, is the primary medium of internalization of social rules, social expectations, and self-regulation, because it enables children to monitor their behavior and plan activities. His research showed that private speech develops from an unsophisticated external activity, where children talk to themselves out loud using whole phrases until the age of 4 years, to an abbreviated form at the age of 5 to 6 years when only single words are used, until finally it becomes fully internalized and is thus transformed into inner speech.

Luria's (1961) research on the development of early self-control upholds Vygotsky's theory. In a series of experiments $1\frac{1}{2}$ to 5-year-old children were given a rubber ball that they were told to either squeeze or not squeeze. Children also were asked to give these instructions to themselves. This experiment enabled Luria to examine how children control their behavior following external instructions and using self-directed instructions. It was found that 3- and 4-year-old children were able to follow the positive instruction "press," yet they were unable to inhibit their behavior and follow the instruction "don't press." In fact, the louder the instruction was, the more they pressed. By the age of 5, however, children were able to follow both the experimenter's instructions and their own instructions and refrain from pressing, indicating that they were able to use speech as a means of self-regulation.

Vygotsky's and Luria's theories and findings about the use of private speech as a means of self-regulation are consistent with recent findings on the awareness of private speech. The reader is reminded that, according to Flavell et al. (1997), children are not aware of inner speech before the age of 5 to 6 years. It appears, therefore, that they start to be able to use a given process to influence another when they become aware of the existence of this process. This leads to another interesting conclusion about the interaction between the intra- and interindividual dynamics of the development of self-understanding and self-regulation. Specifically, self-understanding and self-regulation are parts of cycles of counderstanding and coregulation, but counderstanding and coregulation cannot go much further than the individual's current self-understanding and self-regulation potentials. These determine how interindividual interactions and scaffolding will be individually appropriated. Gradually, of course, interindividual interactions and scaffolding enhance the possibilities of individual appropriation by providing models and examples that can help the individual gauge, calibrate, evaluate, and expand, his or her own self-representations and self-regulatory systems.

C. LOOKING TO THE FUTURE: INTEGRATING RESEARCH ON MIND, PERSONALITY, AND SELF

Personality research suggests that the basic structure of personality remains invariant from early childhood. Costa and McCrae (1997), after reviewing a large body of research, concluded that "the five factor model of personality appears to apply equally well to school children, college students, and adults from the full age range" (p. 280). Evidence related to the development of cognitive style is very similar, and suggests that the basic dimensions of cognitive style, such as reflection–impulsivity or field dependence–independence, are in place very early in life. Moreover, research indicates that an individual's position on these dimensions becomes stabilized rather early in development (Kagan, 1965; Witkin, Goodenough, & Karp, 1967), thereafter functioning as a factor of individual differences on measures of intellectual abilities (Zelniker, 1989), cognitive development (Pascual-Leone & Goodman, 1979), and social skills. These findings suggest strongly that personality and style channel how an individual is self-represented and self-regulated.

A longitudinal study presented by Mischel and colleagues fully supported these findings. Parents of children involved in a delay of gratification study were asked in a follow-up study (10 years later) about the competencies and shortcomings of their children. The findings were very clear: Children who were unable to delay gratification in the initial study were characterized as impatient adolescents, unable to postpone gratification. In contrast, those children able to delay gratification were characterized as adolescent who were academically more competent, more socially skilled, better able to cope with stress, and more confident and self-reliant. Moreover, these children obtained higher scores on the Scholastic Aptitude Test (Mischel, Shoda, & Peake, 1990; Shoda, Mischel, & Peake, 1990). These findings on the relationships between the development of self-control and personality fully concur with the model proposed here, which posits direct links between the processing system, self-representation of cognitive efficiency, and personality.

In fact, there is evidence that temperamental characteristics in infancy are related to activity before birth. That is, DiPietro, Hodgson, Costigan, and Johnson (1996) showed that more active fetuses were more difficult, unpredictable, undaptable, and active infants. This suggests that there is a direct relationship between neurobehavioral attributes before birth and later emotional and social dispositions. In line with these findings, Kochanska, Coy, Tjebkes, and Husarek (1997) showed that certain measures of conscience (such as compliance and internalization of and adherence to rules and standards) and moral cognition correspond to various measures of inhibitory control. Based on this evidence, Kochanska et al. (1997) proposed "that early differences in inhibitory control forecast future personality development, and especially adult differences in conscientiousness or constraint, one of the Big Five" (p. 274).

Although promising, this research is only the beginning, because many crucial questions are still unanswered. For example, we know next to nothing about the mechanisms underlying the integration of temperamental qualities with the processes involved in the processing system, such as speed of processing and inhibition, and changes in this integration with development. Kagan (1994b) used a Strooplike experimental design and found that inhibited individuals take longer time to read fearful words (e.g., drown, kill, shy, poison) as compared to words with a pleasant connotation (e.g., love, fond, friend); unhibited individuals were not affected. This finding implies that personality dispositions are directly involved in how information is initially registered and interpreted by the individual. When does this involvement begin and how does it change with development? How does it affect subsequent self-regulatory actions in persons of different temperaments and styles? Moreover, we still do not know how initial differences in the parameters of processing efficiency, such as speed and inhibition, are transformed into feelings of cognitive self-efficacy that may make a person open to experience.

Another set of questions is concerned with self-awareness itself. For example, why are some individuals more self-aware and reflective than others in the first place? According to the model proposed here, this is to be expected because self-awareness is an autonomous component of the mental architecture. However, there is no research on how these initial differences interact with differences in the other levels and systems of the mental architecture and the temperamental dispositions to generate different types or styles of self-representation and self-regulation. Moreover, we still do not understand how initial differences in the functioning of the various domain-specific systems of thought, such as mathematical, causal, or social thought, shape particular attitudes to problem solving that are then formulated into personal strategies, orientations, and choices.

Also, there is little research on the interaction between the developing person's temperamental dispositions and parenting style. Specifically, Kochanska (1995, 1997) showed that different types of temperament require different types of parental discipline if high levels of conscientiousness are to be attained. That is, gentle discipline, which keeps the level of anxious arousal low, promotes conscience in fearful children. However, positive motivation and security of attachment promotes conscience in fearless children. To our knowledge, there is no evidence to suggest how the different types of parenting styles and discipline interact with temperament to shape the other personality types discussed here, such as openness to experience, agreeableness, neuroticism, and extroversion.

Likewise, to date, there is no research on the development of thinking styles as specified by Sternberg and as discussed here. Ferrari and Sternberg (1998) suggest that thinking styles are affected by parenting style (some parents are more encouraging of independence and originality), schooling (certain schools or teachers orient students to legislative occupations as contrasted to others that orient students to executive style activities; see Grigorenko & Sternberg, 1995), and culture (some cultures orient their members to self-autonomy and independence; others stress conformity and reciprocal support; see Triandis, 1989). However, neither Sternberg nor anyone else has empirically traced the development of each of these styles or the possible changes that may take place in their relationships with various dimensions of cognitive abilities, the self-system, or personality (Sternberg, personal communication, 21 October 1997). Ferrari and Sternberg (1998) pointed out that any research focusing on how children develop requires new theories that would integrate the development of mental abilities with the development of thinking styles and personality into a unified framework. Any effort to develop these theories requires evidence on the developmental interpatterning of changes in cognitive processes and abilities, the various aspects of self-evaluation and self-representation sketched herein, and thinking styles.

V. CONCLUSIONS

In this chapter, we proposed a general model of the organization and development of self-understanding and self-regulation. This model integrates research and theories advanced in traditionally separate fields within psychology, mainly cognitive, developmental, personality, and self psychology. According to this model, humans are capable of self-understanding and self-regulation because evolution has provided them with self-oriented processes that specialize on the representation and manipulation of the processes oriented to the understanding of and interaction with the environment. These self-oriented processes provide a huge adaptational advantage to humans as compared to other species because they enable them, as a species, to cope with practically every variation in the world. Practically this is effected because each individual can construct his or her own profile of abilities and skills for interrelating and interacting with the world.

In this profile both the meaning-making and processing (or cognitive), the motivational and emotional (or personality), and the action (or behavior) processes and functions, although distinct, are dynamically inter-twined. As shown in Figure 1, these processes and functions are organized in very complex networks, both horizontally and hierarchically. It is impor-tant to note that in each level, all three kinds of processes are equipoten-tial in principle. At different moments their relative effects may vary as a function of the external situation and the way they are sensed and mapped by the individual. Mapping refers to the processes by which the lower processes in the system are represented, symbolized, and projected onto a higher level. Thus, self-understanding actually refers to the maps con-structed by the projection of processes and functions from lower to higher levels in the hierarchy. In this hierarchical system, one might argue that self-regulation is the dynamic or active aspect of self-understanding. That is, problem-solving failures necessitate reorganizations at the level of the environment-oriented systems. Effecting reorganization enhances and re-fines the mental maps we have of the skills involved, and the self-mapping and self-modification processes and skills themselves.

Thus self-understanding and self-regulation advance in parallel during development. Remember that, with development, self-representations (i) involve more dimensions that are better integrated into increasingly more complex structures, (ii) move along a concrete to abstract continuum so that they become increasingly more abstract and flexible, and (iii) become more accurate with regard to the actual characteristics and abilities to which they refer. The knowledge available at each phase defines the kind of self-regulation that can be effected. Thus, self-regulation becomes increasingly focused, refined, efficient, and strategic. Practically, this im-plies that our information processing capabilities and temperamental dis-positions come under increasing a priori control of our long-term hyper-cognitive maps and our self-definitions. In other words, they come under what Freud (1952) might call ego control. That is, cognitive, motivational, and emotional functioning come under the increasing control of the individual himself or herself rather than of the dynamics of the situations as such.

Development always has three kinds of constraints: the processing potentials available, the condition of each of the domain-specific systems of understanding the world, and temperamental dispositions. These define upper limits and alternative pathways for self-understanding and self-regulation. Moreover, they suggest that an achievement of self-understand-ing and self-regulation in one domain may need to be reconstructed anew, at least to a certain extent, in another domain.

Humans are social creatures: They understand and regulate each other as much as they understand and regulate themselves. Styles of and needs for self-understanding and self-regulation vary, depending on developmen-tal phase, temperamental, and personality predispositions. Meeting indi-vidual needs is facilitated if socialization practices are organized according to the style that is appropriate for the individual. Failures of this kind may result in failures in self-understanding and self-regulation, with negative consequences for both the individual and the group. The clinical and criminological literature abounds with stories about these consequences.

REFERENCES

Baddeley, A. (1991). *Working memory.* UK: Oxford University Press.

Bandura, A. (1989). Regulation of cognitive processes through perceived self-efficacy. *Developmental Psychology, 25,* 729–735.

Bonoti, F. S. (1998). *Pictographic expression of categorical causal, and spatial relations as a function of the developmental condition of the corresponding specialized structural systems and processing capacity.* Unpublished doctoral dissertation. Thessaloniki, Greece: Aristotle University of Thessaloniki.

Bracken, B. (1996). Clinical applications of a context-dependent multi-dimensional model of self-concept. In B. A. Bracken (Ed.), *Handbook of self-concept.* New York: Wiley.

Brown, A. L. (1978). Knowing when, where and how to remember: A problem of metacognition. In R. Glaser (Ed.), *Advances in instructional psychology* (Vol. 1, pp. 77–165). Hillsdale, NJ: Erlbaum.

Brown, J. D. (1998). *The self.* Boston: McGraw-Hill.

Butterworth, G. (1995). An ecological perspective on the origins of self. In J. L. Bermudez, A. Marcel, & N. Eilan (Eds.), *The body and the self* (pp. 87–105). Cambridge, MA: MIT Press.

Butterworth, G., & Cochran, G. (1980). Towards a mechanism of joint visual attention in human infancy. *International Journal of Behavioral Development, 3,* 253–272.

Byrne, B. M. (1995). Academic self-concept: Its structure, measurement, and relation with academic achievement. In B. A. Bracken (Ed.), *Handbook of self-concept.* New York: Wiley.

Carpendale, J. I., & Chandler, M. J. (1996). On the distinction between false belief understanding and subscribing to an interpretive theory of mind. *Child Development, 67,* 1686–1706.

Carpenter, M., Nagell, K., & Tomasello, M. (1998). Social cognition, joint attention, communicative competence from 9 to 15 months of age. *Monographs of the Society for Research in Child Development, 63* (4, Serial No. 255).

Case, R. (1985). *Intellectual development: Birth to adulthood.* New York: Academic Press.

Case, R. (1992). The roles of the frontal lobes in the regulation of cognitive development. *Brain and Cognition, 20,* 51–73.

Case, R., Okamoto, Y., Griffin, S., McKeough, A., Bleiker, C., Henderson, B., & Stephenson, K. M. (1996). The role of central conceptual structures in the development of children's thought. *Monographs of the Society for Research in Child Development, 61* (1–2, Serial No. 246).

Caspi, A. (1998). Personality development across the life course. In W. Damon (Series Ed.), & N. Eisenberg (Vol. Ed.), *Handbook of child psychology: Vol: 3: Social, emotional, and personality development* (5th ed., pp. 311–388). New York: Wiley.

Costa, P. T., Jr., & McCrae, R. R. (1997). Longitudinal stability of adult personality. In R. Hogan, J. Johnson, & S. Briggs (Eds.), *Handbook of personality psychology* (pp. 269–290). San Diego, CA: Academic Press.

Crockerberg, S., & Lintman, C. (1990). Autonomy as competence in 2-year-olds: Maternal correlates of child defiance, compliance, and self-assertion. *Developmental Psychology, 26,* 961–971.

Demetriou, A. (1996). Outline of a general theory of cognitive change: General principles and educational implications. *The School Field*, *7*, 7–42.

Demetriou, A. (1998a). Nooplasis: 10 + 1 postulates about the formation of mind. *Learning and Instruction*, *8*, 271–287.

Demetriou, A. (1998b). Cognitive development. In A. Demetriou, W. Doise, & K. F. M. van Lieashout (Eds.), *Life-span developmental psychology* (pp. 179–269). London: Wiley.

Demetriou, A., & Efklides, A. (1985). Structure and sequence of formal and postformal thought: General patterns and individual differences. *Child Development*, *56*, 1062–1091.

Demetriou, A., & Efklides, A. (1988). Experiential structuralism and neo-Piagetian theories: Toward an integrated model. In A. Demetriou (Ed.), *The neo-Piagetian theories of cognitive development: Toward an integration* (pp. 173–222). Amsterdam: North-Holland.

Demetriou, A., & Efklides, A. (1989). The person's conception of the structures of developing intellect: Early adolescence to middle age. *Genetic, Social, and General Psychology Monographs*, *115*, 371–423.

Demetriou, A., Efklides, E., Papadaki, M., Papantoniou, A., & Economou, A. (1993a). The structure and development of causal-experimental thought. *Developmental Psychology*, *29*, 480–497.

Demetriou, A., Efklides, A., & Platsidou, M. (1993b). The architecture and dynamics of developing mind: Experiential structuralism as a frame for unifying cognitive developmental theories. *Monographs of the Society for Research in Child Development*, *58* (5–6, Serial No. 234).

Demetriou, A., and Kazi, S. (in press). *Self-image and cognitive development structure, functions, and development of self-evaluation and self-representation in adolescence*. London: Routledge.

Demetriou, A., Kazi, S., and Georgion, S. (1999). The emerging self: The convergence of mind, personality, and thinking styles. *Developmental Science*, *2*, (2).

Demetriou, A., & Raftopoulos, A. (1999). Modeling the developing mind: From structure to change. *Developmental Review*, *19*, issue 9.

Dempster, F. N., & Brainerd, C. J. (Eds.), (1995). *Interference and inhibition in cognition*. San Diego, CA: Academic Press.

DiPietro, J. A., Hodgson, D. M., Costigan, K. A., & Johnson, T. R. B. (1996). Fetal antecendents of infant temperament. *Child Development*, *67*, 2568–2583.

Donald, M. (1991). *The origins of the modern mind*. Cambridge, MA: Harvard University Press.

Eccles, J. S., Wigfield, A., Harold, R. D., & Blumenfeld, P. (1993). Age and gender differences in children's self- and task perception during elementary school. *Child Development*, *64*, 830–847.

Elman, J. L., Bates, E., Johnson, M. H., Karmiloff-Smith, A., Parisi, D., & Plunket, K. (1996). *Rethinking innateness: A connectionist perspective on development*. Cambridge, MA: MIT Press.

Erikson, E. H. (1963). *Childhood and society* (2nd ed.). New York: Norton.

Fabricius, W. V., & Schwanenflugel, P. J. (1994). The older child's theory of mind. In A. Demetriou and A. Efklides (Eds.), *Intelligence, mind, and reasoning: Structure and development* (pp. 111–132). Amsterdam: North-Holland.

Ferrari, M., & Sternberg, R. J. (1998). The development of mental abilities and styles. In W. Damon (Series Ed.), & D. Kuhn and R. Siegler (Vol. Eds.), *Handbook of child psychology* Vol. 2: *Cognition, perception and language* (5th ed., pp. 899–946). New York: Wiley.

Fischer, K. W. (1980). A theory of cognitive development: The control and construction of hierarchies of skills. *Psychological Review*, *87*, 477–531.

Flavell, J. H. (1979). Metacognition and cognitive monitoring: A new area of cognitive developmental inquiry. *American Psychologist*, *34*, 906–911.

248   PART I.   GENERAL THEORIES AND MODELS OF SELF-REGULATION

Flavell, J. H., Green, F. L., & Flavell, E. R. (1995).Young children's knowledge about thinking. *Monographs of the Society for Research in Child Development*, *60* (1), Serial No. 243.

Flavell, J. H., Green, F. L., Flavell, E. R., & Grossman, J. B. (1997). The development of children's knowledge about inner speech. *Child Development*, *68*, 39–47.

Fogel, A. (1993). *Developing through relationships: Origins of communication, self, and culture.* New York: Harvester-Wheatsheaf.

Ford, D. H. (1987). *Humans as self-constructing living systems: A developmental perspective on behavior and personality*, Hillsdale, NJ: Erlbaum.

Freud, S. (1952). *A general introduction to psychoanalysis*. New York: Washington Square Press.

Gardner, H. (1983). *Frames of mind: The theory of multiple intelligences*. New York: Basic Books.

Graziano, W. G., Jensen-Campbell, L. A., & Finch, J. F. (1997). The self as a mediator between personality and adjustment. *Journal of Personality and Social Psychology*, *73* (2), 392–404.

Graziano, W., Jensen-Campbell, L. A., & Sullivan, G. (in press). Temperament, activity and expectations for later personality development. *Journal of Personality and Social Psychology*.

Grigorenko, E., and Sternberg, R. J. (1995). Thinking styles. In D. H. Saklofske, and M. Zeidner (Eds.), *International handbook of personality and intelligence* (pp. 205–229). New York: Plenum Press.

Halford, G. (1993). *Children's understanding: The development of mental models*. Hillsdale, NJ: Erlbaum.

Harter, S. (1990). Causes, correlates, and the functional role of global self-worth: A life-span perspective. In R. J. Sternberg and J. Kolligian, Jr. (Eds.), *Competence considered* (pp. 67–97). New Haven, CT: Yale University Press.

Harter, S. (1998). The development of self-representations. In W. Damon (Series Ed.), & N. Eisenberg (Vol. Ed.), *Handbook of child psychology: Vol. 3: Social, emotional, and personality development* (5th ed., pp. 553–617). New York: Wiley.

Hattie, J. (1992). *Self-concept*. Hillsdale, NJ: Erlbaum.

Higgins, E. T. (1987). Self-discrepancy: A theory relating self and affect. *Psychological Review*, *94*, 319–340.

Houghton, G., & Tipper, S. P. (1994). A model of inhibitory mechanisms in selective attention. In D. Gagenbach & T. H. Carr (Eds.), *Inhibitory processes in attention, memory, and language* (pp. 53–112). New York: Academic Press.

Inhelder, B., & Piaget, J. (1958). *The growth of logical thinking from childhood to adolescence*. London: Routledge and Kegan Paul.

James, W. (1890). *Principles of psychology*. Chicago: Encyclopedia Britannica.

James, W. (1892). *Psychology: The briefer course*. New York: Henry Holt.

Jensen, A. R. (1980). *Bias in mental testing*. New York: Free Press.

Kagan, J. (1965). Impulsive and reflective children: Significance of conceptual tempo. In J. D. Krumboltz (Ed.), *Learning and the educational process*. Chicago: Rand McNally.

Kagan, J. (1994a). On the nature of emotion. *Monographs of the Society for Research in Child Development*, *59*, (2–3, Serial No. 240): 7–24.

Kagan, J. (1994b). *Galen's prophesy: Temperament in human nature*. London: Free Association Books.

Kargopoulos, P. V., & Demetriou, A. (1998). Logical and psychological partitioning of mind: Depicting the same picture? *New Ideas in Psychology*, *16*, 125–139.

Karmiloff-Smith, A. (1992). *Beyond modularity: A developmental perspective on cognitive science*. Cambridge, MA: MIT Press.

Karoly, P. (1993). Mechanisms of self-regulation: A systems view. *Annual Review of Psychology, 44*, 23–52.

Kazi, S., & Makris, N. (1992). Laymen's implicit theories about the intelligence of children and adults. *Psychology: The Journal of the Hellenic Psychological Society, 1*, 52–70.

Kochanska, G. (1995). Children's temperament, mothers' discipline, and security attachment: Multiple pathways to emerging internalization. *Child Development, 66*, 597–615.

Kochanska, G. (1997). Multiple pathways to conscience for children with different temperaments: From toddlerhood to age 5. *Developmental Psychology, 33*, 228–240.

Kochanska, G., Coy, K., Tjebkes, T. L., & Husarek, S. J. (1997). Individual differences in emotionality in infancy. *Child Development, 69*, 375–390.

Kohnstamm, G. A., & Mervielde, I. (1998). Personality development. In A. Demetriou, W. Doise, & K. F. M. van Lieashout (Eds.), *Life-span developmental psychology* (pp. 399–445). London: Wiley.

Kopp, C. B. (1982). Antecedents of self-regulation: a developmental perspective. *Developmental Psychology, 18*, 199–214.

Kougioumoutzakis, I. (1985). *The development of imitation during the first six months of life.* (Uppsala Psychological Report No. 377). Uppsala, Sweden: Uppsala University Press.

Kuhl, J. (1992). A theory of self-regulation: Action versus state orientation, self-discimination, and some applications. *Applied Psychology: An International Review, 41*, 97–129.

Leslie, A. M. (1987). Pretence and representation: The origins of theory of mind. *Psychological Review, 94*, 412–426.

Lewis, M., & Brooks-Gunn, J. (1979). *Social cognition and the acquisition of the self.* New York: Plenum.

Loizus, L. N. (1996). Expressing verbal descriptions through drawing. *Psychology: The Journal of the Hellenic Psychological Society, 3*, 71–92.

Luria, A. R. (1961). *The role of speech in the regulation of normal and abnormal behavior.* New York: Liveright.

Malatesta, C. Z., Culver, C., Tesman, J. R., & Sheppard, B. (1989). The development of emotion expression during the first two years of life. *Monographs of the Society for Research in Child Development, 54* (1–2, serial no. 219).

Markus, H., & Wurf, E. (1987). The dynamic self-concept: A social psychological perspective. *Annual Review of Psychology, 38*, 299–337.

Marsh, G. E., & Iran-Nejad, A. (1992). Intelligence: Beyond a monolithic concept. *Bulletin of the Psychonomic Society, 30*, 329–332.

Marsh, H. W., Byrne, B. M., & Shavelson, R. J. (1992). A multi-dimensional, hierarchical self-concept. In T. M. Brinthaupt & R. P. Linka (Eds.), *The self: Definitional and methodological issues* (pp. 44–95). Albany: State University of New York Press.

Marsh, H. W., & Hattie, J. (1996). Theoretical perspectives on the structure of self-concept. In B. A. Bracken (Ed.), *Handbook of self-concept* (pp. 38–90). New York: Wiley.

McAdams, D. P. (1995). What do we know when we know a person? *Journal of Personality, 63*, 365–396.

Meltzoff, A., & Moore, K. (1995). A theory of the role of imitation in the mergence of self. In P. Rochat (Ed.), *The self in early infancy.* (pp. 73–93). New York: Elsevier.

Mischel, W. (1986). *Introduction to personality* (4th ed.). New York: Holt, Rinehart, & Winston.

Mischel, W., & Ebbesen, E. B. (1970). Attention in delay of gratification. *Journal of Personality and Social Psychology, 16*, 329–337.

Mischel, W., Shoda, Y., & Peake, P. K. (1988). The nature of adolescent competencies predicted by preschool delay of gratification. *Personality and Social Psychology, 54*, 687–696.

Mithen, S. (1996). *The prehistory of the mind.* London: Thames & Hudson.

Nicholls, J. G. (1990). What is ability and why are we mindful of it? A developmental perspective. In R. J. Sternberg & J. Kolligian, Jr. (Eds.), *Competence considered* (pp. 11–40). New Haven, CT: Yale University Press.

Oosterwegel, A., & Oppenheimer, L. (1993). *The self-system: Developmental changes between and within self-concepts.* Hillsdale, NJ: Erlbaum.

Pascual-Leone, J. (1970). A mathematical model for the transition rule in Piaget's developmental stages. *Acta Psychologica, 32,* 301–345.

Pascual-Leone, J., & Goodman, D. (1979). Intelligence and experience: A neo-Piagetian approach. *Instructional Science, 8,* 301–367.

Perner, J. (1991). *Understanding the representational mind.* Cambridge, MA: MIT Press.

Petrides, (1996). Fronto-hippocampal interactions in mnemoric processing. In N. Kato (Ed.), *The hippocampus: Functions and clinical relevance* (pp. 289–301). Amsterdam: Elsevier.

Phillips, D. A., & Zimmerman, M. (1990). The developmental course of perceived competence and incompetence among competent children. In R. J. Sternberg and J. Kolligian, Jr. (Eds.), *Competence considered* (pp. 41–66). New Haven, CT: Yale University Press.

Rothbart, M. K., & Bates, J. E. (1998). Temperament. In W. Damon (Series Ed.), & N. Eisenberg (Vol. Ed.), *Handbook of child psychology: Vol. 3. Social, emotional, and personality development* (5th ed., pp. 105–176). New York: Wiley.

Schneider-Rosen, K., & Wenz-Gross, M. (1990). Patterns of compliance from eighteen to thirty months of age. *Child Development, 61,* 104–112.

Shavelson, R. J., & Marsh, H. W. (1986). On the structure of self-concept. In R. Schwarzer (Ed.), *Anxiety and cognition.* Hillsdale, NJ: Erlbaum.

Shayer, M., Demetriou, A., & Pervez, M. (1988). The structure and scaling of concrete operational thought: Three studies in four countries. *Genetic, Social, and General Psychology Monographs, 114,* 307–376.

Shoda, Y., Mischel, W., & Peake, P. K. (1990). Predicting adolescent cognitive and self-regulatory competencies from preschool delay of gratification: Identifying diagnostic conditions. *Developmental Psychology, 26,* 978–986.

Sternberg, R. J. (1988). Mental self-government: A theory of intellectual styles and their development. *Human Development, 31,* 197–224.

Sternberg, R. J., Conway, B. E., Ketron, J. L., & Bernstein, M. (1981). People's conceptions of intelligence. *Journal of Personality and Social Psychology, 41,* 37–55.

Stipek, D., & McIver, D. (1989). Developmental change in children's assessment of intellectual competence. *Child Development, 60,* 521–538.

Stipek, D., Recchia, S., & McClintic, S. (1992). Self-evaluation in young children. *Monographs of the Society for Research in Child Development, 57* (serial no. 226).

Stroop, J. R. (1935). Studies of interference in serial verbal reactions. *Journal of Experimental Psychology, 18,* 643–662.

Stuss, D. T. (1992). Biological and psychological development of executive functions. *Brain and Cognition, 20,* 8–23.

Thatcher, R. W. (1994). Cyclic cortical reorganization: Origins of human cognitive development. In G. Dawson and K. W. Fischer (Eds.), *Human behavior and the developing brain* (pp. 232–266). New York: Guilford.

Thurstone, L. L. (1938). Primary mental abilities. *Psychometric Monographs, 1.*

Trevarthen, C. (1979). Communication and cooperation in early infancy: A description of primary intersubjectivity. In M. Bullowa (Ed.), *Before speech* (pp. 321–347). New York: Cambridge University Press.

Triandis, H. C. (1989). The self and social behavior in differing cultural contexts. *Psychological Review, 96,* 506–520.

Vaughn, B. E., Kopp, C. B., & Krakow, J. B. (1984). The emergence and consolidation of self-control from eighteen to thirty months of age: Normative trends and individual differences. *Child Development, 55,* 990–1004.

Vurpillot, E. (1998). The development of scanning strategies and their relation to visual differentiation. *Journal of Experimental Child Psychology, 6,* 632–650.

Vygotsky, L. S. (1962). *Thought and language.* Cambridge, MA: MIT Press. (Original work published in 1934)

Wellman, H. M. (1990). *The child's theory of mind.* Cambridge, MA: MIT Press.

Witkin, H. A., Goodenough, D. R., & Karp, S. A. (1967). Stability of cognitive style from childhood to young adulthood. *Journal of Personality and Social Psychology, 7,* 291–300.

Zelazo, P. R. (1998). McGraw and the development of unaided walking. *Developmental Review, 18,* 449–471.

Zelniker, T. (1989). Cognitive style and dimensions of information processing. In T. Globerson and T. Zelniker (Eds.), *Cognitive style and cognitive development* (pp. 172–191). Norwood, NJ: Ablex.

Zimmerman, B. J. (2000). Attaining self-regulation: A social cognitive perspective. In M. Boerkaert, P. R. Pintrich, & M. Zeidner (Eds.), *Handbook of self-regulation* (Chap. 2). San Diego, CA: Academic. (This volume)

8

THE ROLE OF

INTENTION IN

SELF-REGULATION

TOWARD INTENTIONAL

SYSTEMIC MINDFULNESS

SHAUNA L. SHAPIRO AND GARY E. SCHWARTZ

University of Arizona, Tucson, Arizona

There have been substantial developments in theory and research on self-regulation over the past four decades. This chapter explores the progression of self-regulation understanding from nonconscious self-regulation (Wiener's cybernetic homeostatic model) to conscious attentional self-regulation (Schwartz, 1977, 1984, 1990) to the nature of conscious attentional self-regulation (e.g., mindfulness; Kabat-Zinn, 1982). Drawing upon insights from Weiner's and Schwartz's models, as well as the work of Kabat-Zinn and colleagues on mindfulness, we posit an expanded model for self-regulation theory. The purpose of this chapter is to introduce intention explicitly into self-regulation theory (i.e., what is the nature of the attention—"mindfulness qualities"—and what is the framework within which the self-regulation system is practiced—"systemic perspectives"). Furthermore, this chapter proposes a model, intentional systemic mindfulness (ISM), that provides both the goal for intention as well as the process for implementing it within self-regulation. ISM examines two critical aspects of intention: mindfulness qualities (how we attend) and systemic perspectives (why we attend).

Self-regulation in biology is an ancient notion captured in proverbs such as "the balance of nature," but it became a modern science with the

Copyright © 2000 by Academic Press.
All rights of reproduction in any form reserved.

introduction of Wiener's (1948) cybernetics. Wiener himself applied this engineering concept to living systems. Self-regulation can be defined as the process by which a system regulates itself to achieve specific goals. In his work on human self-regulation, Schwartz (1977, 1984, 1990) expanded self-regulation to include conscious as well as nonconscious regulation. During the past 20 years, Kabat-Zinn and colleagues have added an extremely effective technique for self-regulation by helping to bring "mindfulness," a form of Buddhist meditation, to mainstream Western medicine. Mindfulness is a conscious, impartial self-regulation, defined as "moment-to-moment awareness" (Kabat-Zinn et al., 1992, p. 937). Mindfulness adds to conscious self-regulation by explicitly infusing "attention" with seven mindfulness qualities: acceptance, nonjudging, nonstriving, patience, trust, openness,[1] and letting go (Kabat-Zinn, 1982; Kabat-Zinn et al., 1992). Systems theory extends the range of applications of mindfulness, enlarging its focus to embed the symptom and self in larger systems (the systemic perspectives). Thus, ISM[2] is a systems theory approach to mindfulness applied to human self-regulation and all self-regulation techniques.

In ISM *intention* is primal, providing the mindfulness qualities and systemic perspectives that should infuse *attention*. However, the majority of current theories of self-regulation, with few exceptions (e.g., Kabat-Zinn, 1982; Kabat-Zinn & Chapman-Waldrop, 1988; Kabat-Zinn et al., 1992), do not explicitly address the multifaceted nature (e.g., physical, emotional, social, spiritual) of restoring or enhancing health and wellness. This chapter discusses an explicit and comprehensive model (ISM) that bridges the theories of East and West and establishes a connected and unifying approach to self-regulation and health. This model provides a contextual perspective for expanding self-regulation theory, as well as a rationale for intention within self-regulation. The core of ISM is intention—the intention to (1) pay attention utilizing the foregoing seven mindfulness qualities as well as five additional affective qualities—generosity, empathy, gratitude, gentleness, and loving kindness—and (2) pay attention within a systems perspective, the simultaneous consciousness of being a whole and being part of a larger whole. The implications of ISM for self-regulation therapies are numerous and suggestions for future research are discussed.

---

[1] Openness refers to the Buddhist quality of the beginner's mind.
[2] We have chosen to call this model *intentional systemic mindfulness* ISM to explicitly emphasize the interrelated systemic components that are a part of Kabat-Zinn's mindfulness work.

I. SYSTEMS THEORY, SELF-REGULATION,
AND MINDFULNESS

Ecologist, Barry Commoner, captured the essence of systems theory in his teaching that everything is connected to everything else (Commoner, 1990). Systems theory argues that fundamental systemic metaprinciples exist in nature and can be applied to systems at all levels. A complex system should be regarded as a "whole" rather than as an aggregate of component parts and local relationships to be studied in isolation. The system as a whole regulates the interaction of its parts or subsystems. To interact, these parts must be connected. The connections enable the parts to affect each other's behavior, but, more importantly, allow the system to control the global operation. This interactive organizational process within systems is termed self-regulation. Living systems maintain inner balance, harmony, and order through their capacity to self-regulate via feedback loops between particular functions and systems (Schwartz, 1977, 1984, 1990).

Out of the interaction between systems, emergent properties evolve. For example, the interaction between hydrogen and oxygen atoms produces a novel emergent property: water. Every system is a whole composed of subsystems and simultaneously is part of a suprasystem. A human being can be thought of as composed of subsystems (organs), part of larger suprasystems (families, communities, cultures), and as a whole system in and of himself or herself. The same rules apply to humans as they do to atoms. The interaction between hydrogen and oxygen can be seen as a metaphor for relationships. For example, just as hydrogen brings out special properties from oxygen and vice versa, when humans interact they bring out emergent properties in each other.

This chapter draws most from the interconnectedness component of systems theory. In discussing the systems concept of interconnectedness, it is important to go beyond the standard reductionist account that explains connectedness purely as relationships between parts, leaving out governance (regulation) by the whole. Systems theory is the effort to study complex systems holistically, recognizing the interconnectedness of all the parts and the large number of nonlinearly interdependent variables involved. The variables are connected through feedback loops and implement the system's self-regulation. This dynamic synergistic interaction can be observed on all levels from subatomic physics and cellular biology to social, political, and global systems. An example at a biological level is ontogeny, where development of the embryo is regulated by a genetic "plan" that is responsive at every stage to environmental influences transmitted somatically. An example within a family system can be seen when parents are loving and respectful to each other they are engaged in feedback loops that promote connection and wholeness. These feedback loops affect their individual relationship, as well as their relationships with their children, which in turn affects the dynamics of the family as a whole.

II. SELF-REGULATION

Self-regulation is a systems concept. Self-regulation is based on positive and negative feedback loops. Positive feedback loops engender heterostasis, leading to change, growth, and development. Negative feedback loops engender homeostasis, which is a stable state that a living organism strives to maintain by keeping vital parameters within viable limits. Both positive and negative feedback loops foster learning and memory (Schwartz and Russek, 1997a). When the homeostatic model is extended from fixed to changing environments, the theory of evolution adds the important parameter of adaptability. Watzlawick, Beavin, and Jackson (1967) described both positive and negative feedback loops:

> ...part of a system's output is reintroduced into the system as information about the output. The difference is that in the case of negative feedback this information is used to decrease the output deviation from a set norm or bias—hence the adjective "negative"—while in the case of positive feedback the same information acts as a measure for amplification of the output deviation, and is thus positive in relation to the already existing trend toward a standstill or disruption. (p. 30)

This definition parallels Carver and Scheier's use of the term "feedback" in social facilitation. For example, they describe the operation of a negative feedback loop in social behavior: "self-directed attention leads to the engagement of a cybernetic feedback loop by which discrepancies between present behavior and a standard of comparison are reduced" (Carver & Scheier, 1981, p. 45). Balance between positive and negative feedback within a system is crucial. If a system has only negative feedback loops, it will remain stagnant; however, if a system contains only positive feedback, then it eventually will explode. Interconnection and wholeness stem from this balance.

One early and foundational model of self-regulation stems from Weiner's (1948) cybernetics. This is based on homeostasis and evolved from his work on antiaircraft guns in World War I. The idea was that the guns would adjust to changing motion of the target aircraft and make a hit. Another example of self-regulation can be seen when you attempt to touch your finger to your nose. If your eyes are open, you receive continual feedback and it is much easier; if your eyes are closed, then this task is much more difficult.

Schwartz (1984, 1990) expanded the notion of self-regulation from automatic response to conscious self-regulation. When system parameters exceed performance limits, the system self-regulates either nonconsciously or consciously. Conscious self-regulation requires that the human being pay attention to the process. Self-regulation automatically (nonconsciously) occurs all the time; however, by bringing conscious attention, the feedback is amplified. This increased feedback leads to greater connection and subsequent self-regulation. For example, if individuals are requested simply to pay attention to their breathing, with no intention to alter their breathing in a particular way (e.g., increase or decrease respiration rate, respiration amplitude, or respiration regularity), typically respiration becomes slower, deeper, and more regular. However, if subjects are instructed to pay attention to their heartbeats, with no intention to alter their heart rate in a particular way, especially with the aid of kinesthetic feedback (feeling one's own pulse), respiration typically becomes shallow and irregular while beat to beat changes in heart rate become more regular (Schwartz, 1984). These selective self-regulation effects with focused attention illustrate the relationship between conscious awareness of organ systems and specific physiological effects.

Schwartz's model of self-regulation involves "attending," which is similar to the Buddhist term mindfulness, and yet, Schwartz's model is goal oriented conscious attention, whereas Kabat-Zinn's model emphasizes conscious (purposeful) attention with no specific goals: "paying attention in a particular way; on purpose, in the present moment, and nonjudmentally" (Kabat-Zinn, 1994, p. 4). Kabat-Zinn's model of mindfulness differs from Langer's (1989) mindfulness in that it extends the focus on attention to include the nature of attention (e.g., mindfulness qualities brought to the attention; reviewed subsequently). Furthermore, Langer focuses on "mindlessness" and does not emphasize self-regulation practices (e.g., meditation) designed to cultivate mindfulness. Finally, Langer (1989, p. 71) does not address the "cosmology" or "moral aspect of mindfulness" that is significant in Kabat-Zinn's model. In teaching mindfulness, focus is on the experiential practice itself. Mindfulness practice involves concentrated moment to moment attention focused inward, attending to thoughts, feelings, and body sensations as they arise. Research has demonstrated that mindfulness may be an effective intervention for anxiety disorders, chronic pain, and psoriasis in its own right (Kabat-Zinn, 1982; Kabat-Zinn et al., 1992; Miller, Fletcher, and Kabat-Zinn 1995), as well as being an effective complement to more traditional medical and psychological therapies (Teasdale, Segal, & Williams, 1995).

III. SELF-REGULATION TECHNIQUES AND POTENTIAL LIMITATIONS

There are several different models of self-regulation and numerous techniques that follow from these models. Techniques that have been used as vehicles to develop self-regulation and mindfulness are meditation, biofeedback, guided imagery, and exercise. These techniques share a goal of health enhancement and disease (symptom) reduction through teaching the individual to simply attend (bare awareness) and thereby connect and self-regulate. However, for many practitioners and patients, the context within which these strategies are implemented is a Western reductionist approach to stress management, focusing on symptom alleviation instead of acknowledging the larger process from a systems perspective (Shapiro, 1982, 1994). These techniques, therefore, share limitations that may prevent the individual from achieving "optimal health," defined by the World Health Organization (1946) as more than the absence of disease, involving mental, physical, and social well-being.

Reductionistic self-regulation theories cannot explicitly address all of the multilevels that create and sustain optimal health. Numerous self-regulation techniques simply intend to return things to normal (e.g., blood pressure) and do not address more systemic intentions. There is nothing wrong in using meditation to lower blood pressure. However self-regulation techniques that explicitly address intention toward ISM may be more effective at promoting healing on a systemic level as well as on a symptom level.

IV. PSYCHOPHYSIOLOGICAL RESEARCH ON SELF-REGULATION — PHYSIOLOGY AND ENERGY

The research on psychophysiological self-regulation is voluminous and documents that different techniques that focus on different components or subsystems have different effects (e.g., progressive muscle relaxation produces greater effects on muscular tension than autogenic training techniques involving images of warmth; reviewed in Lehrer and Woolfolk, 1993).

Many relaxation, meditation, and imagery techniques including Qigong, massage, and noncontact therapeutic touch, implicitly or explicitly involve focused attention to the body. From a dynamical energy systems perspective (the thesis that physical systems interact not only through the sharing of matter, but the sharing of energy and information as well; Schwartz and Russek, 1997a), relaxed self-attention should result in enhanced connectivity between the brain and the body. Enhanced connectivity between the brain and the body may be achieved by at least two mechanisms: (1) physiological mechanisms that employ peripheral negative feedback loops and (2) biophysical mechanisms or loops that involve direct energetic resonance between the peripheral organ and the brain.

A recent study by Song, Schwartz, and Russek (1998) illustrates the potential for selective self-regulation that bridges traditional physiological and modern energetic models of interaction (Schwartz and Russek, 1997a). Nineteen channels of EEG, ECG, and EOG were recorded from 22 subjects during attention to heart versus eye sensation trials, with and without kinesthetic feedback to augment sensory awareness. Analyses of the EEG synchronized with the ECG revealed significant post-R spike EEG effects for heart focused attention (especially with touching), probably reflecting increased baroreceptor and somatosensory feedback, and pre-R spike EEG effects for heart focused attention (independent of touching), possibly reflecting direct energetic interactions between the heart and the brain. These findings suggest that physiological and energetic mechanisms both may be involved in techniques whose goal it is to promote mind–body integration and health.

If simple attention to the body can foster increased synchronization between the brain and the body—not only physiologically, but energetically as well—the potential for ISM is increased accordingly. From a systems perspective, energy circulates within and between organisms, and energy can be directed to achieve specific goals (*energy* is defined by physics as the capacity to do work; see Schwartz and Russek, 1997a, 1997b). Furthermore, the psychology, biology, and physics of self-regulation all point to the suggestion that a key to fostering self-regulation lies in the nature of the intention to direct attention to achieve a desired goal. This insight requires that we expand our current models of self-regulation to include the process of intention.

V. ELABORATION OF AN EXPANDED SELF-REGULATION MODEL: INTENTION

According to Schwartz (1984), self-regulation is the process through which a system maintains stability of functioning as well as flexibility and the capacity for change in novel situations. When a system goes out of balance, the restoration of order requires attention to reestablish connectedness. Because human beings can be thought of as systems, when illness occurs, attention also is needed to reestablish connectedness and subsequently health. This has been described by Schwartz as a pathway model of self-regulation: attention → connection → regulation → order → health. Cultivating conscious attention leads to connection, which leads to self-regulation and ultimately order and health. However, the intention with which this attention is applied may be crucial. An expanded model of self-regulation theory, therefore, includes intention as an initiating antecedent: intention → attention → connection → regulation → order → health. However, the question arises, "Intention toward what?"

VI. INTENTION

Intention is a global property of the entire system (e.g., person). In this context, we are using intention following Webster's (1977) definition that focuses on "purpose" and "direction" as opposed to the definition that focuses on an "ultimate end." Intention can be thought of as toward a means as opposed to a single, ultimate goal (which would imply an end state and does not fit within a systemic model). However, according to Gollwitzer and Brandstatter (1997), both the "goal intention" as well as the "implementation intention" (process) are important. Thus, although the emphasis is on the process (implementation intention), multiple goal intentions are developed simultaneously, but they are derived within a nonlinear, systemic perspective and therefore an "ultimate" end is never completed.

VII. INTENTIONAL SYSTEMIC MINDFULNESS: MINDFULNESS QUALITIES AND SYSTEMIC PERSPECTIVES

In response to the question, "Intention toward what?," we propose, "Toward ISM." ISM (shown in Figure 1) establishes a framework for developing goal intentions (from the micro to the macro; see Figure 2) as well as a process of implementing them (open, nonjudgmental attention to all stimuli) within self-regulation theory. In developing both goal and implementation intentions, ISM integrates two components: systemic perspectives (Figure 2) and mindfulness qualities (Table 1).

For clarity of presentation, mindfulness qualities are discussed first. Consistent with Ajzen's recognition of the importance of the relationship between attitudes and intention to behavior and health (Ajzen, 1996), this model makes explicit a set of attitudinal (mindfulness) qualities to incorporate into self-regulation practice. The term "mindfulness qualities" refers to the intention to incorporate and bring into conscious attention 12 cognitive-affective mindfulness qualities defined by Kabat-Zinn (1990) and elaborated by Shapiro, Schwartz, and Bonner (1998). These 12 mindfulness qualities include nonstriving, nonjudging, acceptance, patience, trust, openness,[3] and letting go (Kabat-Zinn, 1990) as well as gratitude, gentleness, generosity, empathy, and loving kindness (Shapiro, Schwartz, & Bonner, 1998) (see Table 1). The latter qualities were incorporated to explicitly address the affective (heart) qualities of mindfulness. According to Tanahashi, the Japanese characters of mindfulness are composed of two interactive figures: one mind, and the other heart (Santorelli, 1999).

[3] Openness: derived from beginner's mind, "a mind that is willing to see everything as if for the first time" (Kabat-Zinn, 1990, p. 35).

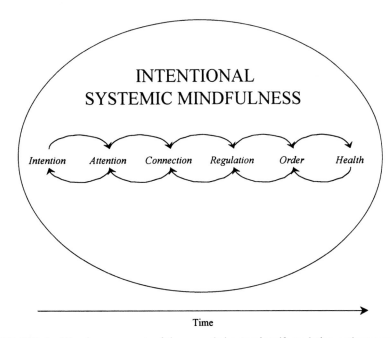

Time

FIGURE 1   The six components of the expanded systemic self-regulation pathways model over time. The arrows indicate how each phase is directly or indirectly connected to all others. Each phase both sends and receives direct or indirect feedback to all other phases as a dynamic systemic process.

Therefore, perhaps a more accurate translation of the Japanese is heart-mindfulness (Shapiro & Schwartz, in preparation).

The mindfulness qualities are involved in a synergistic co-evolution, in that the cultivation of one facilitates the cultivation of others. ISM encourages the cultivation of all qualities simultaneously; however, for each individual, the practice and development of these qualities will be different. A systemic vision recognizes a multiplicity of satisfactory stable equilibiria that continue to evolve to new equilibiria. As a result, the level of activity of each mindfulness quality varies and yet the intention is to cultivate all qualities. The qualities operate as "inputs" during both the intention and attention phase.

Mindfulness qualities specify the way one attends. Attention by itself is not enough. It is crucial to attend in a particular way, with the intention to incorporate the mindfulness qualities as part of the self-regulation technique. It is not simply paying attention, but the intention behind it, that may be important for enhancing health. For example, Schwartz (1984) mentions grooming as a healthy form of attention that leads to self-regulation and improves health. However, it is possible that if individuals groom themselves with the intention to incorporate the qualities of striv-

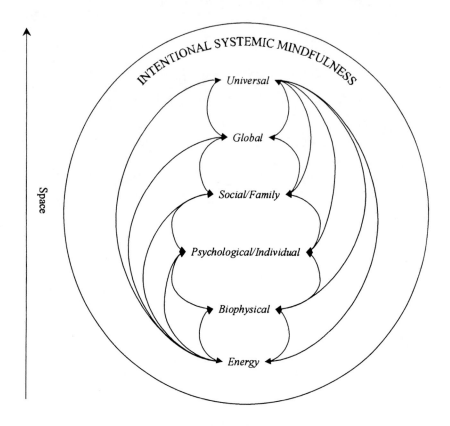

All possible interactions not shown in figure

FIGURE 2   Six systemic levels in space, from the micro (energy) to the macro (universal). The arrows indicate how each level is directly or indirectly connected to all others. Each level both sends and receives direct or indirect feedback to all other levels as a dynamic systemic process. All possible arrows (hence interactions) not are shown.

ing, need for perfection, self-criticism, and frustration, then this attention will not be health promoting and may instead be harmful. This same behavior of grooming, performed with a conscious intention to infuse the attention with mindfulness qualities of acceptance, generosity, nonjudgementalness, may indeed be health promoting.

To consider another example, if people who attend to their blood pressure attend with fear that they will not be able to control it or with anger at themselves for having high blood pressure, this may have deleterious effects on their health or at least impede the potential healing effects of the self-regulation technique. The intention to attend with mindfulness qualities may be health enhancing in itself. Utilizing these qualities, we focus attention on ourselves in a loving and gentle way, open to whatever

TABLE 1   Mindfulness Qualities

Nonstriving: Nongoal oriented, remaining unattached to outcome or achievement
Nonjudging: Impartial witnessing, observing without evaluation and categorization
Acceptance: Open to seeing and acknowledging things as they are
Patience: Allowing things to unfold in their time, bringing patience to both ourselves and to others
Trust: Trusting both oneself and the process of the self-regulation practice itself
Openness: Seeing things as if for the first time, creating possibility by paying attention to all feedback
Letting go: Nonattachment, not holding on to thoughts, feelings, or experiences
Gratitude: The quality of reverence, appreciating and being thankful for the present moment
Gentleness: Characterized by soft, considerate, and tender quality; soothing, however not passive, undisciplined, or indulgent
Generosity: Giving within a context of love and compassion, without attachment to gain or thought of return (the content of giving does not have to be material)
Empathy: The quality of feeling and understanding another person's situation—their perspectives, emotions, actions (reactions)—and communicating this to the person
Loving kindness: A quality embodying benevolence, compassion, and cherishing, a quality filled with forgiveness and unconditional love

---

*Note.*These categories are offered heuristically, reflecting the general idea that there are mindfulness qualities that should be part of the intention phase as well as the attention phase of the pathway model. A commitment (intention phase) is made to bring the qualities to the practice and then the qualities are themselves cultivated throughout the self-regulation practice itself (attention phase). See Kabat-Zinn (1990, pp. 33–40) for detailed definitions of the first seven qualities.

we may find. This attention involves a stance of impartiality, letting go and cultivating patience for whatever is present, and a willingness just to listen to and accept in loving kindness all the parts of our whole.

It is also crucial to discuss the systemic perspectives within which the attending occurs. *Systemic perspectives* refer to the intention to incorporate into the practice of mindfulness the awareness that symptoms themselves exist as part of larger systems (see Figure 2). This aspect of ISM is akin to the term "holon," which was coined by Koestler (1978) and refers to a system that is "both a whole composed of parts and a part composing larger wholes." ISM requires the simultaneous consciousness of being a whole and being part of a larger whole (systemic perspectives) while incorporating the mindfulness qualities.

This context of "wholeness" is created by the intention with which the individual approaches the attention (self-regulation technique). It is necessary to look at intention from a systemic perspective, explicitly acknowledging multiple intentions directed at multiple levels: (1) awareness of interconnection, (2) awareness of dynamic interaction and constant change, (3) awareness of levels (micro–macro), and (4) awareness of wholeness (wholes within larger wholes).

The process of ISM is to develop multiple intentions in an attempt to heal and recognize all levels from the specific symptom (blood pressure) to the largest level (universe.) Thus, approaching self-regulation within systemic perspectives involves seeing and recognizing the interconnection of all things, and intending to acknowledge and heal each piece and simultaneously the larger whole. Practicing a self-regulation technique within the context of ISM leads to a feeling of being supported by and connected with oneself as well as with a larger supportive system. These feelings of support and interconnectedness may have health enhancing properties. The literature supporting this hypothesis will be discussed in Section IX.

Many self-regulation techniques fall short by focusing on a symptom and ignoring the system. For example, a person may practice meditation solely to become aware of blood pressure and thereby lower it. However, if this is done without the proper intention, it may exacerbate the situation as discussed earlier. ISM addresses these shortcomings. A self-regulation technique practiced with intention toward systemic perspectives includes multiple levels of intention, combining the intention to heal blood pressure with an intention to promote the well-being of the entire circulatory system, especially the heart. This in turn leads to enlarging the intention to heal the heart to incorporate the knowledge that the heart is part of the body, conceived of as a psychosomatic self. The self is then recognized as embedded within interpersonal relationships, family, and community, and, therefore, the intention to heal interpersonal relationships is added also. This awareness stimulates recognition that these relationships are part of a larger community (humankind), which creates the intention to acknowledge the connectedness of all beings. Finally, the recognition develops that this greater community is connected to the earth and that humans are interconnected and interdependent with all beings and with the earth itself.

Because of the continual evolving nature of intention, the expanded self-regulation pathway model is not a simple linear sequence. ISM is dynamic, a continual process of expanding and redefining intention (mindfulness qualities and systemic perspectives; see Figure 1). It is a system of many variables that are connected in nonlinear fashion and, thus, it is impossible to separate the pathways—it is the opposite of discrete. Yet, throughout this continual transformation, the intention to attend with the mindfulness qualities (acceptance, loving kindness, etc.) remains constant, as does commitment to eventually acknowledging all systemic perspectives. ISM, therefore, is not only the plan and the execution of the plan, but the modification of the plan based on the feedback of the actual experience (see Figure 1). ISM is change fueled by the intention to incorporate mindfulness qualities and systemic perspectives.

For example, one cannot be expected to immediately embrace (or even grasp) the intention of healing the universe. Because ISM is both nonlinear and dynamic, it provides the opportunity for continual growth and transformation. As one becomes increasingly mindful, through the cultivation of attention, the formulation of one's intentions changes (see Figure 1). Through becoming aware—expanding one's scope of intentionality— deeper levels of previously unrecognized feedback are discovered and amplified. Continuing along the systemic self-regulation pathway model (Figure 1), this constantly increasing feedback guides the movement and allows the process to flow in a dynamic manner as opposed to disjointedly moving from each phase to the next. Thus, as the grounding theory underlying the self-regulation pathway model, ISM opens the potential that, eventually, multiple intentions will be adopted. As one continues the process, one moves through concern for the specific symptom to concern for the larger context of one's symptoms.

ISM is both the theory and the practice, exercising guidance throughout the entire self-regulation pathway model. It pervades the whole system (self-regulation pathway model), providing the overarching principles that cause the flow as well as the means to sustain this flow. One has to be mindful continually of the increasing levels of feedback in order to deepen one's mindfulness qualities, expand one's systemic perspectives, and sustain the flow.

VIII. APPLICATIONS OF INTENTIONAL SYSTEMIC MINDFULNESS TO SELF-REGULATION TECHNIQUES

We suggest that optimal health enhancement and disease prevention and resolution stem from systemically mindful self-regulation techniques more so than from nonsystemically mindful self-regulation techniques. "Optimal health enhancement" can be translated and measured using outcome variables that span the immunological level (e.g., NK cells) and the physiological level (e.g., blood pressure) to the psychological (e.g., depression, anxiety), the social (quality of life), and the spiritual (spirituality measure) levels. ISM teaches the individual to adopt the intention to heal from a qualitative and contextual level that may promote healing on all levels (symptom, self, family, political, universal). Systems heal both downward and upward, smaller to larger and larger to smaller. Thus, the person (a system) heals on multiple levels, creating a greater opportunity to reach optimal health (physical, emotional, social, spiritual well-being). ISM is both a means (the technique used to achieve this whole) and an end (a way of living, being, and interacting in the world).

The healing effects of "consciously paying attention" may depend upon the mindfulness qualities and systemic perspectives in which this self-regulation is practiced. Through self-regulating techniques (meditation, biofeedback, hypnosis, imagery, yoga), the individual attends and connects to his or her "self," and is often able to regulate blood pressure and body temperature, and achieve a state of physiological hypoarousal—the "relaxation response" (Benson, 1975). The literature demonstrates that no technique is inherently better than another in terms of self-regulation for a specific clinical problem (Shapiro, 1994). We suggest that a self-regulation technique practiced with the intention toward ISM is qualitatively and quantitatively "better" than one practiced with no intention.

IX. CONNECTEDNESS AND INTERCONNECTEDNESS

It is commonly recognized at the molecular biochemical level that connection is crucial for regulating physical health. However, if connectedness is fundamental to the functioning of our body, it seems plausible that it is important on social and psychological levels as well. As Schwartz and Russek (1997b) remind us, the words "health" and "heal" come from the Anglo-Saxon "hal," which means whole (Webster, 1977). Perhaps feeling whole and connected is primal to cultivating physical and emotional health. ISM, by fostering interconnnectedness and wholeness (during both the intention and attention phases of the pathway model), may be health enhancing.

It can be argued that in the past scientific research literature, positive association between social support and health was really tapping into the healing effects of connectedness and wholeness. The effects of social support are well documented. As Berkman, (1995, p. 245), a pioneering researcher in the field states, "there is now a substantial body of evidence that indicates that the extent to which social relationships are strong and supportive is related to the health of individuals who live within such social contexts." In the past 20 years, numerous studies have concluded that people who feel isolated and disconnected have a greater risk of death from all causes. The converse has been found also: People who feel loved and connected are healthier and live longer.

One of the first prospective longitudinal community-based studies that documented the relationship between health and social support was the Alameda County study. This study found that men and women who did not have a strong social network were 1.9 and 3.1 times more likely to die in a 9-year followup (Berkman & Syme, 1979). There have been at least eight community-based prospective studies since, all indicating a relationship between social support and mortality rates independent of socioeconomic status, self-reported physical health status, and health practices such as smoking, diet, alcohol consumption, exercise, and utilization of preventive health services (Berkman & Syme, 1979; Blazer, 1982; House, Robbins, & Metzner, 1982; Kaplan et al., 1988; Orth-Gomer & Johnson, 1987, Orth-

Gomer, Unden, & Edwards, 1988; Ruberman et al., 1984; Schoenbach et al., 1986; Seeman et al., 1993; Welin et al., 1985; Williams et al., 1992).

The literature also demonstrates that facilitating feelings of support and connection through group intervention is health enhancing. Spiegel, & Bloom, Kraemer, & Gottheil (1989) conducted a prospective intervention focusing on group cohesion, support, sharing, and trust for patients with metastatic breast cancer. A 10-year followup showed that women in the intervention group survived 36.3 months compared to 18.9 months in the control group (Spiegel et al., 1989). In a similar study, Fawzy et al. (1993) found a three times greater chance of survival in patients with malignant melanoma who received a group support intervention.

In the Lifestyle Heart Trial, 41 patients with angiographically documented coronary artery disease were assigned randomly to an intervention group or a "usual-care" control group. The intervention consisted of a low-fat vegetarian diet, moderate exercise, smoking cessation, stress management, and support groups. The usual-care group received standard traditional medical care. At a 1-year followup, 82% of the intervention group showed significant regression of severe coronary atherosclerosis, whereas the control group continued to worsen (Ornish et al., 1990). The stress management (imagery, meditation, yoga) and social support components of the intervention were designed intentionally to help participants enhance connectedness with self, others, and a higher power (Ornish, 1991).

Even more recent studies consistently document the relationship between love, spirituality, and health. In a study exploring the relationship between the perception of parental care and health, Russek and Schwartz (1997) found that feelings of warmth and closeness with parents predicted health status for 35 years. Another study examined the effects of social support and religion on men and women who had undergone open heart surgery 6 months previously. The study revealed a four times greater risk of mortality 6 months after surgery in men and women who lacked participation in organized social groups, and a three times greater risk for those who did not draw strength and comfort from their religion (Oxman et al., 1995).

Reductionistic self-regulation techniques, practiced without intention (mindfulness qualities and systemic perspectives) may never access this resource of interconnectedness associated with healing. However, practicing self-regulation with the intention toward ISM (developing the mindfulness qualities and systemic perspectives) may help facilitate greater health enhancing feelings of support and connection (interconnection). For example, the systemic perspectives may enable the individual to connect to a larger self and, thereby, become more whole. As Kabat-Zinn (1994, p. 226) describes, "When we are in touch with being whole, we feel at one with everything. When we feel at one with everything we feel whole." Self-regulation techniques facilitated with the intention toward systemic perspectives aim to foster this healing sense of "ultimate belonging" which the Benedictine monk Steindal-Rast (1989) refers to as "God."

The mindfulness qualities also may facilitate feelings of love, connection, and support. The systemic pathway model (Figure 1) can be applied to all levels, from the individual to the global, suggesting that the theory attention (embodying the mindfulness qualities) leads to greater connection and greater health is not limited to an individual or biological process. An example can be seen when applying this model to interpersonal relationships. Bringing a compassionately open attention to relationships may lead to greater connection, love, and health. We can develop our capacity to feel (accept) and express love through attention, but only through an attention couched in trust, acceptance, and generosity (mindfulness qualities). As the foregoing research suggests, when we feel loved and cared for unconditionally, or in theologian Paul Tillich's (1952) words "accepted," we have improved health and well-being. Thus, a self-regulation technique (attention) practiced with the intention toward ISM (mindfulness qualities and systemic perspectives) may facilitate the health enhancing feelings of interconnection and love.

X. GENERAL PRINCIPLES OF INTENTIONAL SYSTEMIC MINDFULNESS INTERVENTIONS

General principles of ISM that could transfer across intervention settings include (1) an emphasis on the intention of the selfregulation intervention, (2) cultivating a compassionate, nonjudgmental (mindfulness qualities) attention throughout the intervention, (3) viewing the intervention as a continual process as opposed to an end in itself, and (4) adopting systemic perspectives that acknowledge and address interconnectedness and wholeness.

XI. FACILITATING INTENTION SYSTEMIC MINDFULNESS

An effective way to facilitate interconnectedness is probably to practice self-regulation with others (groups, couples, and student and teacher). A community (sangha) provides an organizing context, facilitating direct experience of greater connection. One example can be seen in Kabat-Zinn's work with mindfulness meditation groups (Kabat-Zinn, 1982; Kabat-Zinn et al., 1992; Miller et al., 1995). Further examples are the Lifestyle Heart Trial intervention (Ornish, 1991) and historical teacher and disciple practices of the ancient traditions (Buddhism, Hinduism, Judaism).

XII. DIRECTIONS FOR FUTURE RESEARCH

There are multiple directions for future research. First and most importantly, self-regulation interventions with an intention toward ISM need to be compared to self-regulation interventions without any explicit intentions. An example of this would be to measure the psychological and physiological effects of diaphragmatic breathing with the intention toward ISM versus diaphragmatic breathing with no explicit intention. We hypothesize that the systemic mindful intervention would benefit the individual on multiple levels of health. Furthermore, future research should focus on creating reliable and valid self-report measures to assess ISM (e.g., one's intentions, the degree to which one understands and is able to integrate ISM into the self-regulation) as well as measures to assess systemic health (an assessment sensitive to the multiple levels of health). Because ISM is an overarching approach to self-regulation, it can be studied and applied to various specific techniques such as biofeedback and relaxation.

XIII. IMPLICATIONS FOR HEALTH AND MEDICINE

In discussing the implications of ISM, it is crucial to emphasize again that ISM is not simply another self-regulation technique (although it can be applied to self-regulation techniques). ISM can be viewed as a way of living, a "way of being" (Kabat-Zinn, 1992). Thus, the implications of ISM span multiple levels from the micro to the macro, each interacting with and stimulating the others.

On an individual level, intention toward ISM will amplify feedback and thus should deepen connections and self-regulatory processes within the body. Furthermore, ISM provides a compassionate contextual perspective for self-exploration, potentially leading to greater insight and psychological well-being, and allowing greater reception of more accurate and complete information that can be processed without attaching judgment. One's intention to embody the mindfulness qualities within a systems context of interconnectedness should affect not only one's relationship with self, but all interpersonal relationships, bringing greater compassion and insight to family, friends, colleagues, and even casual acquaintances and strangers.

A natural outgrowth of practicing self-regulation techniques with the intention toward ISM is that the cultivation of feelings of compassion, impartiality, and interconnectedness often translate into action (e.g., greater service to community). This is because the practice frequently results in feelings of interconnectedness and the realization that there is no separation between self and other. ISM cultivates the capacity to understand another person's point of view and the ability to acquire information nonjudgmentally. Social psychology has demonstrated the phenomena of cognitive filtering and schema: In all spheres of life, people often attend to stimuli that support their beliefs and filter out those which do not. This process usually occurs at a nonconscious level, and people are, therefore, unaware that they have lost crucial information that could be applied to health and well-being.

XIV. SUMMARY

This chapter addressed the possible implications of making intention explicit in self-regulation theory. It responds to the question, "Intention toward what?," by developing a model of ISM. ISM provides a comprehensive and integrative approach to self-regulation and health. Through directing intention toward the two components of the model, mindfulness qualities and systemic perspectives, a more accepting, compassionate, and systemic approach is brought to self-regulation practices and techniques. A challenge for future research is to develop instruments that measure intentionality and health systemically (e.g., biopsychosocial–spiritually) and determine whether ISM techniques lead to more systemic improvements in overall health and well-being. The evolution of self-regulation theory toward ISM will expand the simple stress management and symptom reduction intention of self-regulation techniques toward a more comprehensive approach to human intention.

ACKNOWLEDGMENTS

We thank the editors Monique Boekaerts, Paul Pintrich, and Moshe Zeidner for the care and constructive feedback they provided. Their editing skill greatly contributed to the evolution of this chapter. The first author acknowledges Jon Kabat-Zinn, whose writings first interested her in this field. Finally, we deeply thank Benedict and Nancy Freedman for their invaluable suggestions and support.

REFERENCES

Ajzen, I. (1996). The directive influence of attitudes on behavior. In P. M. Gollwitzer & J. A. Bargh (Eds.), *The psychology of action: Linking cognition and motivation to behavior.* (pp. 385–403).
Benson, H. (1975). *The relaxation response.* New York: Morrow.
Berkman, L. (1995). The role of social relations in health promotion. *Psychosomatic Medicine, 57,* 245–254.

Berkman, L. F., & Syme, S. L. (1979). Social networks, host resistance and mortality: A nine year follow-up study of Alameda County residents. *American Journal of Epidemiology, 109,* 186–204.

Blazer, D. (1982). Social support and mortality in an elderly community population. *American Journal of Epidemiology, 115,* 684–694.

Carver, C., & Scheier, M. (1981). The self-attention-induced feedback loop and social facilitation. *Journal of Experimental Social Psychology, 17*(6), 545–568.

Commoner, B. (1990). *Making peace with the planet.* New York: Pantheon.

Fawzy, F., Fawzy, N., Hyun, C., Elashoff, R., Guthrie, D., Fahey, F., & Morton, D. (1993). Malignant melanoma: Effects of an early structured psychiatric intervention, coping, and affective state on recurrence and survival 6 years later. *Archives of General Psychiatry, 50,* 681–689.

Gollwitzer, P. & Brandstatter, V. (1997). Implementation intentions and effective goal pursuit. *Journal of Personality and Social Psychology, 73*(1), 186–199.

House, J. S., Robbins, C., & Metzner, H. L. (1982). The association of social relationships and activities with mortality: Prospective evidence from the Tecumseh community health study. *American Journal of Epidemiology, 116,* 123–140.

Kabat-Zinn, J. (1982). An outpatient program in behavioral medicine for chronic pain patients based on the practice of mindfulness mediation: Theoretical considerations and preliminary results. *General Hospital Psychiatry, 4,* 33–47.

Kabat-Zinn, J. (1990). *Full catastrophe living.* New York: Bantam Doubleday Dell Publishing Group.

Kabat-Zinn, J. (1994). *Wherever you go there you are.* New York: Hyperion.

Kabat-Zinn, J., Massion, A. O., Kristeller, J., Peterson, L. G., Fletcher, K. E., Pert, L., Lenderking, W. R., & Santorelli, S. (1992). Effectiveness of a meditation based stress reduction program in the treatment of anxiety disorders. *American Journal of Psychiatry, 149,* 936–943.

Kabat-Zinn, J., & Chapman-Waldrop (1988). Compliance with an outpatient stress reduction program: rates and predictors of program completion. *Journal of Behavioral Medicine 11*(4), 333–352.

Kaplan, G. A., Salonen, J. T., Cohen, R. D., Brand, R. J., Syme, S. L., & Puska, P. (1988). Social connections and mortality from all causes and cardiovascular disease: Prospective evidence from eastern Finland. *American Journal of Epidemiology, 128,* 370–380.

Koestler, A. (1978). *Janus: A summing up.* London, UK: Hutchinson.

Langer, E. (1989). *Mindfulness.* Reading MA: Addison-Wesley.

Lehrer, P., & Wolfolk, R. (Eds.). (1993). *Principles and practice of stress management.* New York: Guilford.

Miller, J., Fletcher, K., & Kabat-Zinn, J.(1995). Three-year follow-up and clinical implications of a mindfulness meditation-based stress reduction intervention in the treatment of anxiety disorders. *General Hospital Psychiatry, 17,* 192–200.

Ornish, D. M. (1991). *Dr. Dean Ornish's program for reversing heart disease.* New York: Random House.

Ornish, D. M., Brown, S. E., Scherwitz, L. W., Billings J. H., Armstrong, W. T., Ports, T. A., McLanahan, S. M., Kierkeide, R. L., Brand, R. J., & Gould, L. (1990). Can lifestyle changes reverse coronary atherosclerosis? The lifestyle heart trial. *The Lancet, 336,* 129–133.

Orth-Gomer, K., & Johnson, J. (1987). Social network interaction and mortality: A six year follow-up of a random sample of the Swedish population. *Journal of Chronic Disorders, 40,* 949–957.

Orth-Gomer, K., Unden, A. L., & Edwards, M. E. (1988). Social isolation and mortality in ischemic heart disease. *Acta Medica Scandinavia, 224,* 205–215.

Oxman T. E., Freeman, D. H., Manheimer E. D. (1995). Lack of social participation or religious strength and comfort as risk factors for death after cardiac surgery in the elderly. *Psychosomatic Medicine, 57*, 5–15.

Ruberman, W., Weinblatt, E., Goldberg, J. D., & Chaudhary, B. S. (1984). Psychosocial influences on mortality after myocardial infarction. *New England Journal of Medicine, 311*, 552–559.

Russek, L., & Schwartz, G. E. (1997). Feelings of parental caring predict health status in mid-life: A 35-year follow-up of the Harvard Mastery of Stress Study. *Behavioral Medicine, 20*, 1–13.

Santarelli, S. (1999) *Heal Thy Self*. New York: Bell Tower.

Schoenbach, V. J., Kaplan, B. G., Freedman, L, Kleinbaum, D. G. (1986). Social ties and mortality in Evans County, Georgia. *American Journal of Epidemiology, 123*, 577–591.

Schwartz, G. E. (1977). Psychosomatic disorders and biofeedback: A psychobiological model of disregulation. In J. D. Maser and M. E. P. Seligman (Eds.), *Psychopathology: Experimental models*. San Francisco: W. H. Freeman.

Schwartz, G. E. (1984). Psychobiology of health: A new synthesis. In B. L. Hammonds and C. J. Scheirer (Eds.), *Psychology and health: Master lecture series* Vol. 3 (pp. 145–195). Washington, DC: American Psychological Association.

Schwartz, G. E. (1990). Psychobiology of repression and health: A systems approach In J. Singer (Ed), *Repression and dissociation: Implications for personality theory, psychopathology and health*, (pp. 337–387). Chicago: University of Chicago Press.

Schwartz, G. E., & Russek, L. (1997a). Dynamical energy systems and modern physics: fostering the science and spirit of complementary and alternative medicine. *Alternative Therapies, 3*(3), 46–56.

Schwartz, G. E., & Russek, L. (1997b). The challenge of one medicine: Theories of health and eight "world hypotheses." *Advances: The Journal of Mind-Body Health, 13* (3), 7–23.

Seeman, T. E., Berkman, L. F., Kohout F., Lacroix, A., Glynn, R., & Blazer, D. (1993). Intercommunity variations in the association between social ties and mortality in the elderly: A comparative analysis of three communities. *Annual Epidemiology, 3*, 325–335.

Shapiro, D. H. (1982). Overview: Clinical and physiological comparisons of meditation with other self-control strategies. *American Journal of Psychiatry, 139*, 267–274.

Shapiro, D. H. (1994). Examining the content and context of meditation: A challenge for psychology in the areas of stress-management, psychotherapy, and religion/values. *Journal of Humanistic Psychology, 34*, (4), 101–135.

Shapiro, S., Schwartz, G. E., & Bonner, G. (1998). The effects of mindfulness-based stress reduction on medical and premedical students. *Journal of Behavioral Medicine. 21*, 581–599.

Shapiro, S. & Schwartz, G. E. (in preparation) *Heart-Mindfulness*.

Song, L. Z. Y. X., Schwartz, G. E. R., & Russek, L. G. R. (1998). Heart-focused attention and heart-brain synchronization: Energetic and physiological mechanisms. *Alternative Therapies in Health and Medicine, 4*(5), 44–63.

Spiegel, D., Bloom, J. R., Kraemer, H. C., & Gottheil, E. (1989). Effect of psychosocial treatment on survival of patients with metastatic breast cancer. *The Lancet, 2*, 888–891.

Stiendal-Rast, D. (1989). The mystical core of organized religion. *ReVision, 12*(1), 11–14.

Teasdale, J. D., Segal, Z., & Williams, M. (1995). How does cognitive therapy prevent depressive relapse and why should attentional control (mindfulness) training help? *Behavioral Research and Theory, 33*, (1), 25–39.

Tillich, P. (1952) *Courage to be*. New Haven, CT: Yale University Press.

Watzlawick, P., Beavin, J. H., & Jackson, D. D. (1967). *Pragmatic of human communication: A study of interactional patterns, pathologies and paradoxes*. New York: Norton.

Webster, N. (1977). *Webster's new twentieth century dictionary of the English language*. Unabridged, 2nd ed. New York: Collins World.

Welin, L., Tibblin, G., Svardsudd, K., Tibblin, B., Ander-Peciva, S., Larsson, B., Wilhelmsen, L. (1984). Prospective study of social influences on mortality: The study of men born in 1913 and 1923. *Lancet, 1*, 915–918.

Wiener, N. (1948). *Cybernetics; Control and communication in the animal and the machine.* New York: Wiley.

Williams, R. B., Barefoot, J. C., Califf, R. M., Haney, T. L., Saunders, W. B., Pryof, D. B., Hlatky, M. A., Siegler, I. C., & Mark, D. B. (1992). Prognostic importance of social and economic resources among medically treated patients with angiographically documented coronary artery disease. *Journal of the American Medical Association, 267*, 520–524.

World Health Organization. (1946). Constitution. Geneva, Switzerland.

9

COMMUNAL ASPECTS OF SELF-REGULATION

TAMARA JACKSON, JEAN MACKENZIE, AND
STEVAN E. HOBFOLL

Kent State University, Kent, Ohio

I. INTRODUCTION

Self-regulation is typically viewed as a systematic process of human behavior that provides individuals with the capacity to adjust their actions and goals to achieve desired results (Carver & Scheier, 1982). Self-regulation models have implied that personal, internal processes are the primary determinants of behavior. These attributes include self-esteem (Baumeister, Heatherton, & Tice, 1993), self-attention (Carver, Blaney, & Scheier, 1979), and cognitive resources such as intelligence and coping skills (Sternberg, 1988; Thayer, Newman, & McClain, 1994). By placing emphasis on these personal resources, traditional theories of self-regulation confer onto self-control, independence, and self-reliance the pivotal role in this process (e.g., Carver & Scheier, 1982). Focus on the self is primarily derived from a Western, European male-dominant culture that encourages individuals to be "autonomous, self-directing, unique, and assertive, and to value privacy and freedom of choice" (Kim, Triandis, Kagitcibasi, Choi, & Yoon, 1994, p. 7). Although individualism is heavily emphasized and valued in the concept of self-regulation, people do not, of course, always function in isolation from each other.

Traditional models of self-regulation assume that behavior is determined by individual goals and needs with limited influence from others or the environmental context. Based on individualism, self-regulation concepts assume that the social structure is based on "equality, equity, noninterference, and detachability" (Kim et al., 1994, p. 7), and the

Copyright © 2000 by Academic Press.
All rights of reproduction in any form reserved.

questionable assumption that every person can exercise free will. Relatedly, self-regulation implies that individual behavior is predominantly regulated by internal forces, therefore negating the impact of external factors. Consequently, many of these models fall short of recognizing that people, in general, and certain groups of people, in particular, may both operate in a more socially mediated fashion and lack the social and economic resources needed to independently control their lives. Thus, they may neither choose nor be free to SELF-regulate their behavior.

In this chapter, we review existing theories of self-regulation, discuss the limitations of these models, and offer alternative theories that address the communal components that influence behavior. We also discuss a subset of social factors, specifically coping, social support, and power, and how they are associated with the self-regulation process. Because necessary social and economic resources are not distributed evenly, some individuals are at a disadvantage in their self-regulatory abilities. Acknowledging the multiple determinants of self-regulation, we highlight the argument that self-regulation is not a process that is based on free will and individual abilities alone.

A. COMMUNAL REGULATION

In an effort to expand the purview of self-regulation theories that focus predominantly on individual attributes and behaviors, we emphasize the communal context in which self-regulation occurs. Seen from more of a collectivist perspective, communal regulation recognizes that individuals self-regulate and monitor their actions within a network of socially mediated factors, such as family, organizational, and group-based needs, goals, and desires. Kagitcibasi (1994) argued that autonomy and relatedness to others are dual human needs, and self-regulation theory must recognize the interaction and the need to synthesize the two characteristics to promote optimal human functioning. Indeed, we wish to move from self-regulation to a more communal *self-in-social-setting regulation* in which individual behaviors are recognized as nested within a wider collectivist context.

B. EMBEDDED SOCIAL COMPONENTS OF SELF-REGULATION MODELS

Much interest has emerged in understanding self-regulatory behavior. Research on behavioral self-regulation has predominantly focused on processes such as controlling thoughts and emotions (Mayer & Gaschke, 1988) and attention management (Mikulincer, 1989) to explain goal-oriented action and adaptive functioning. The common factor among concepts of self-regulation is the significant emphasis on the self and how attending to it is a necessary component to success and adaptive functioning. Self-attention and self-management, and their impact on determining individual behavior are primary areas of interest in the process of self-regulatory actions.

Self-Attention and Self-Regulation

Self-focus or attention influences self-regulatory behavior by activating a control process that compares individuals' actual behavior to their ideal standard and increases personal awareness of how the two components may differ (Duval, Duval, & Mulilis, 1992). Essentially, self-regulatory behavior serves as a feedback loop to decrease the amount of discrepancy between ideal and desired behaviors. Carver and Scheier (1982) argued that the primary function of a feedback system during self-regulation "is not to create 'behavior.' Its purpose is instead to create and maintain the perception of a specific desired condition; that is, whatever condition constitutes its reference value or standard of comparison" (p.113). In other words, self-directed attention promotes the regulation of personal actions by altering perceived actual behaviors to conform to a valued point of reference and portray a desired personal image (Carver & Scheier, 1990). Such regulatory responding is thought to be adaptive because it alters behavior in order to avoid future misfortune and to compensate for previous losses when situations of failure are encountered. Factors such as amount of positive and negative expectancies also influence behavioral changes that are enacted to decrease self-standard discrepancies and maintain a valuable self-image. For example, favorable outcome expectancies are associated with increased personal attempts to conform to standards, whereas expectancies of negative outcome are associated with overall avoidance of the situation (Carver, Blaney, & Scheier, 1979).

The tendency to self-regulate to decrease levels of discrepancy between the actual self and a valued behavioral standard is associated with the differentiation between ideal self-guides, such as individuals' hopes, and ought self-guides, such as the sense of duty, obligation, and commitment (Higgins, Roney, Crowe, & Hymes, 1994). The ideal self-regulatory system emphasizes achieving positive outcomes by decreasing discrepancy to a reference point, whereas the ought belief system strives to avoid negative outcomes by magnifying incompatibility to an undesired end state. In either condition, people are presented as being principally responsible for determining their pattern of behavior.

Although the theory of self-standard discrepancy sounds individualistic because the focus is on self-attention and personal attempts to alter behavior, it is heavily laden with social influences from external factors. Many of the concepts on which self-discrepancy theories are based (e.g., standards, points of reference, concepts of ideal and ought selves, and expectancies) derive from culturally based notions of acceptable behavior that are rooted in socially based roles. Because people do not function in a social vacuum, "the behavior of one person influences the behavioral options of another in ways that are not random. ... Self-regulation simply proceeds with regard to the group as a system concept rather than to the self image" (Carver & Scheier, 1982, p. 131). For example, Eisenberger, Mitchell, and Masterson (1985) found that the provision of external rewards increased self-control behavior and personal effort because it served to represent a standard for acceptable social responding. It is apparent that behavioral standards typically are not individually derived. Instead, they are susceptible to environmental influences and are based on the feedback and behavior of others within people's social network.

Additionally, self-standard discrepancy theories appear individually bound because the primary theme is that people are independently comparing themselves to each other and striving to reduce discrepancies. Because such research is typically conducted among individuals who are not directly connected with each other, the concept of communal comparison is overlooked. For example, family members may avoid comparing themselves with each other in efforts to reduce intrafamilial strife. Instead, they may communally compare themselves with a particular standard to enhance a joint sense of well-being and satisfaction. Similarly, social comparison with the intention of reducing discrepancy among those who are socially intertwined (e.g., marital partners) may not be desirable because individual differences within close interpersonal relationships may complement each other and promote healthy interactions. Throughout self-standard discrepancy theories, individual differences are presented as interfering variables that need to be reduced as much as possible. However, an alternative is to view the differences as a source of diversity and as a beneficial opportunity to learn from each other in a reciprocal and communal manner.

Self-Management and Self-Regulation

Self-management may be viewed as an application of self-regulation. Its function is to initiate plans and actions to achieve desired goals. Self-management consists of the ability to effectively integrate three components of self-regulation: (1) appropriately identify the problem, formulate an accurate mental representation of the event, and plan behavior according to relevant information, (2) implement cognitive activity in a manner that will promote personal success and satisfaction, and (3) monitor and evaluate internal and external feedback to execute behavior to meet obligations and duties (Sternberg, 1988). The inability to direct behavior in response to these components is typically associated with poor self-management and falling short of attaining desired results. For example, Baumeister, Heatherton, and Tice (1993) argued that although elevated self-esteem is frequently viewed as being desirable, it may interfere with effective self-regulatory processes that are essential for adaptive self-management. They found that individuals with high self-esteem tended to poorly self-manage their behavior during times of perceived high ego threat as compared to situations of low ego threat because they were more likely to make commitments and execute behaviors that were incommensurate with their personal abilities. Environmental realities (e.g., level of personal control and personal reinforcement) appear to play a significant role in people's ability to self-manage. Therefore, the negation of such objective factors usually is accompanied by maladaptive behavioral responses.

Self-management also occurs in response to self-regulation of emotion. Thayer (1978, 1989) argued that mood is closely connected with states of bodily arousal and impacts internal feelings of energy and tension. Self-regulation of mood may serve as an important foundation for effective self-management because it "involves behaviors that modulate energy and tension to optimal levels" (Thayer, Newman, & McClain, 1994); therefore, an individual may seek to change either or both dimensions to promote adaptive functioning. Likewise, the inability to regulate and maintain an emotional equilibrium is thought to be a source of diminished self-management and psychological functioning. Bromberger and Matthews (1996) found that low instrumentality or the inability to seek out and engage in behaviors indicative of decreased emotional distress was associated with higher prevalence of depressive symptoms and poorer mood regulation.

Although concepts of self-management emphasize processes within the individual (i.e., self-regulation), the importance of social influences, such as feedback loops, social roles, and standards in human behavior, are also highlighted. For example, concepts such as behavioral expectations focus on how social standards and roles impact personal functioning. External factors, such as environmental opportunities and positive reinforcement from others, are also strong determinants of individual behavior. Individuals often look toward others within their social network for behavioral guidance, confirmation of appropriate display of actions or emotions, and as a source of modeling for adaptive and acceptable functioning. Many times, stress-relieving behaviors rely on social aspects, such as seeking support from others, to provide guidance and meaning during a distress-provoking situation. The impact of these social influences in the self-management process further elucidates the idea that individual behavior is ultimately a product of external, culturally based cues.

Health Appraisals Are a Component of Self-Regulation

Health appraisals serve as an illustration of how the processes of self-regulation and self-management are influenced by external social factors. Health appraisals develop in response to self-regulatory actions, such as personal perceptions and emotional reactions to health threat, and they influence the planning and initiation of behaviors that are appropriate to these perceptions and reactions (Leventhal, Nerenz, & Steele, 1984). Croyle and Hunt (1991) highlighted the importance of socially mediated actions such as social comparison on determining the emotional, cognitive, and behavioral responses during the stages of health appraisal. For example, eliciting opinions from others and evaluating personal well-being relative to a known social standard have a strong impact on coping responses and levels of behavioral adjustment to health-related stress.

As acknowledged, some theories of self-regulation, in particular social cognitive models (e.g., Bandura, 1986; Clark, 1987; Zimmerman, 1989), do recognize social context as a component of self-directed behavior. However, the impact of socially mediated factors often assumes a status that is far inferior to individually based components. To use a Gestalt figure–ground analogy, theories that emphasize self-regulation place the individual as the figure and social context as the ground. In other words, although the social setting is included in the portrait of self-regulation, it clearly falls out of focus and its level of contribution or importance to the overall figure diminishes.

In contrast, the notion of *self-in-social-setting regulation* places social context as the figure and individual factors (e.g., goals) as the ground. In so saying, the focus shifts to concepts of communality and interpersonal relatedness, emphasizes the role of social influence, and promotes a collectivist manner of responding to environmental demands and conforming to external standards. Communal perspectives directly acknowledge that individual behavior does not occur in isolation and that behavioral standards and expectations are not developed in an idiosyncratic manner. Instead, people look toward others to make sense of personal situations and execute individual responses. Even the concept of pain is imbued with sociocultural meaning. Whether pain is purely physical, spiritual, the product of guilt, or possession by demons reflects cultural concepts that define for the self pain's existence and its purpose. Pain for one culture may be something to be endured, for another something to be avoided, and for still another something to be accepted as part of spiritual healing. Self-regulation would have pain as internal, mentally mediated, and personally controllable, at least in part. However, these very conceptions are products of a Protestant view of pain and its purpose.

C. INDIVIDUALISTIC TERMS OF TRADITIONAL MODELS OF SELF-REGULATION

Concept of Individualism

Traditional theories of self-regulation present people as an entity separate from the social context in which they function. They are also heavily rooted in the concept of self-contained individualism that emphasizes self-control and the perception of a distinct boundary between oneself and others (Sampson, 1988). Individualism is based on the belief that the concept of the self does not extend beyond personal physical being and that a person's functioning and destiny are separate from others (Spence, 1985). Personal goals and needs take precedence over group or communal goals (Han & Shavitt, 1994), and personal fate and a sense of internal control are highly emphasized (Triandis, 1990).

Although individualistic traits may appear callous and promote a sense of isolation, they are often viewed as the foundation to being self-reliant and productive (Perloff, 1987). The sharp delineation between the self and others often has been viewed by individual theorists (e.g., Perloff, 1987; Spence, 1985) as a sign of good mental health and effective social functioning. Being more communal comes to be seen as a sign of weakness, social unsophistication, and lowered potential and productivity. As a result, the concept of individualism has been presented as the necessary component for success, achievement, and personal happiness.

Myth of Individualism

The premise of individualism assumes that self-regulation and, subsequently, self-management are predominantly within individuals' control and the main purpose is to exercise personal will even if it means exhibiting little consideration for others. Ironically, the individualistic approach to self-regulation and coping misrepresents the actual male behavior after which these theories are presumably modeled. In reality, the individual as an independent agent is stereotypic even when applied to Western men, most of whom tend to be deeply embedded in complex social networks. Although the role of caretaker and meeting others' needs has been presented as a feminine phenomenon and thus negated, many mainstream theories do not recognize that "feminine" behaviors allow men the luxury of maintaining an illusory sense of self-regulation and personal control (Eagly, 1987).

Miller (1986) presented a scenario of a woman whose main consideration for accepting a job was whether she could make special arrangements to have equal time to devote to her job and perform the duties needed to care for her family. On the other hand, her husband's main considerations were salary, career development, and self-improvement. Although both the husband and wife were self-regulating and adapting their behavior to pursue their desired goals, traditional theories of individualism and self-regulation would more than likely view the husband's form of self-regulation as more adaptive because his behavior was driven predominantly by personal goals and needs that promote a sense of individual control while conceptualizing the wife's behavior as being less than optimal because her goals were intertwined with and predominantly based in the needs of others (e.g., her family). Hence, she may be perceived as failing to develop as a self-sufficient, independent person from an individual perspective (Eagly, 1987). Although it is clear from this description that the woman is regulating her individual behavior based on external circumstances, the husband's dependence on external resources (e.g., the wife's behavior), as related to his ability to self-regulate is less obvious. Whereas the husband's self-regulatory practices are readily apparent and rewarded for being geared toward individual productivity, the wife's behavior, which is influenced by *self-in-social-setting regulation* (e.g., considering the overall well-being, needs, and desires of family members), may be overlooked and even negated because the emphasis is not predominantly on personal empowerment. This illustration contradicts the belief that self-reliance and individualism are the primary routes to personal success and fulfillment. Instead, it provides support for the concept that self-directed behavior is embedded within the context of a social setting either directly (e.g., assisting others in meeting their needs and goals) or indirectly (e.g., benefiting from the actions of others in achieving individual goals).

D. CONCEPT OF INTERRELIANCE

The preceding scenario highlights the point that self-reliance and communal behavior do not exist in isolation from each other. Although social stereotypes that label men as self-reliant and women as communal are frequently perpetuated in Western society, the point is that both genders practice a combination of both behaviors. The concept of interreliance may be the key to optimal functioning within a social context and communally working together for the well-being of a collective group, such as a family. Unlike individualism, interreliance acknowledges that people do not act in isolation from each other or have complete control over their own actions (see Hobfoll, 1998).

In this fashion, social support can be conceptualized as a system of interreliance characterized by a "dynamic process of transactions between people and their social networks that takes place in an ecological context" (Hobfoll & Vaux, 1993, p. 688). Individuals may actively seek out support and maintain relationships as a way to maximize their own personal resources and increase adaptive functioning. In so doing, relationships derived from social support can provide beneficial resources for individuals, such as affection, advice, and money, that may enhance their ability to self-regulate. People depend upon and use others within their social network to accomplish goals, and cannot readily isolate themselves from their environment. Hence, self-regulation is an interdependent, social process. Moreover, unless individuals provide feedback, connectedness, or exchange value for the support they receive, their access to social support will be curtailed (Kelley, 1979; Clark, Mills, & Powell, 1986).

In accordance with the concept of interreliance, a more accurate conceptualization is that self-regulation is a social process, rather than principally a self-reliant process. People do not act independently because their individual needs typically are weighed against the needs of others who will be impacted by their decisions and actions. Individual goals are intertwined with social goals and are accomplished through interpersonal interaction. We may imagine the self as reliant, and this is certainly one layer of the regulation process, but it is a layer always embedded in a broader social context.

E. THE IMPACT OF CULTURE ON SELF-REGULATORY BEHAVIORS

Collectivism and Culture

Traditional models of self-regulation overlook and even negate the foundations on which the value systems for women and certain ethnic minority groups are based. In opposition to the perception of being self-contained, many women and ethnic minority groups tend to employ a sense of ensembled individualism or collectivism that characterizes a less demarcated boundary between self and others. Contrary to self-contained individualism, the goal of collectivism is to achieve harmony and work toward the well-being of oneself and others by operating within the surrounding social context (Sampson, 1988; Yamaguchi, 1994). It is apparent that self-regulation and personal control are strongly impacted by communal influences. In addition, interpersonal relationships within certain cultures consist of communal efforts such as exchange and reciprocity (Clark et al., 1986; Mills & Clark, 1982) which, although they exist in Western culture, are more centrally defining in other cultures (Gao, 1996). These relational postures further require more cautiousness, communication, and consideration of the needs of other. This translates to an even greater need for interdetermined acts and shared reliance of means and consequences.

Many cultures recognize individuals as agents for communal welfare (Triandis, 1990). In many African cultures, the welfare of the general community is placed above individual members. Individual needs and goals are pursued in the interest of communal needs and not personal benefit. African culture emphasizes an interdependence between the community and the individual. When people work for the overall well-being of the community, they directly benefit from individual actions as a whole (Moemeka, 1996). Similarly, Chinese culture is strongly rooted in the ideas of Confucianism. Within Confucian philosophy, the self is defined by the surrounding social context and seen as an extension of relational networks and thus cannot be separated from the existence of others (Gao, 1996).

The emphasis is on the social context and the need to consider the goals and needs of others in order to define and care for the self.

Related to a collectivist perspective, many ethnic minority groups in the United States and Northern Europe, especially recent non-Western immigrants who have not yet assimilated into European–American philosophies, experience difficulty adapting to the individualistic ideal of self-regulation that is promoted in the United States and Western Europe. The sense of connectedness and viewing oneself in relation to others is a vital part of survival for many ethnic minority individuals. Familial ties and social relationships are considered a priority for many individuals within the Asian- (Gao, 1996), Hispanic- (Rogler, Malgady, & Rodriguez, 1989; Shkondriani & Gibbons, 1995), and African (Moemeka, 1996) American communities. Thus, the people in these communities may view the mainstream, individualistic culture as callous, removed, and nonconducive to personal growth (Keefe & Casas, 1980). Among Hispanic and Southeast Asian immigrants, it is thought that the psychological stress caused by disrupted social ties or cultural traditions during the process of acculturation may be a risk factor for physical illness and maladjustment (Ying & Akutsu, 1997; Vargas-Willis & Cervantes, 1987). Communal lifestyles promote reciprocity and working together for the wellness and regulation of the community as a whole.

Although theories of self-regulation argue that behavior is determined by internal, personal factors, collectivist perspectives view individual behavior as a product of communal expectations. For example, Islam argues that individuals are not free to make their own choices; instead, they must follow in the direction that has been determined by others (Harre, 1981). Similarly, the Chinese and African cultures view the self as embedded within a social context and defined by external norms and expectations from the community. As a result, individuals are defined and their behaviors are influenced according to the role they occupy in society. In addition, the role expectations of the individual extend to protecting the welfare of fellow community members (Gao, 1996; Moemeka, 1996). It appears that some cultures gain strength by intertwining themselves with others, not by isolating themselves and relying predominantly on internal resources.

Gender Socialization

Similar to many ethnic minority cultures, some women have views of interpersonal relations that conflict with the traditional perspective of self-regulation. Although it is a part of human nature to serve each other's needs to survive, individualistic societies tend to view such collectivist behavior as a sign of subordination and social inferiority. Women are socialized to believe that their individual happiness and self-identity is derived from nurturing and meeting the needs, wishes, and desires of others, specifically men and children (Katz, Boggiano, & Silvern, 1993; Miller, 1986). A traditional, individualistic approach overlooks the purpose and benefits of exhibiting nurturing behavior and concern for others because it lacks self-reliance and self-regulation abilities (Katz et al., 1993). However, this behavior may more appropriately be viewed as an indicator of strength, good health, and a strong sense of self gained through interactions with others (Triandis, Bontempo, Villareal, Asai, & Lucci, 1988). In addition, such communal behavior contributes to women's ability to be responsive to others' needs while simultaneously benefiting from these social exchanges and maintaining an integrated sense of self (Miller, 1986; Lykes, 1985).

Issues of Power Inequality

Self-regulation is a process that assumes individuals have equal control over their external environment. This assumption is, of course, inaccurate because society consists of people who possess differing degrees of economic, political, and social power. Individuals with little power may be capable of self-regulation, but are prevented because of external circumstances outside of their immediate control to exercise personal choice. Additionally, traditional models of self-regulation make the assumption that people have many resources (e.g., power, money, and support) to assist in the coping process. However, when such models are applied to groups of individuals who are frequently subjected to conditions of discrimination or considered to be of inferior social status (e.g., women, ethnic minorities, or impoverished individuals), such populations may appear flawed (Hobfoll, Cameron, Chapman, & Gallagher, 1996; David & Collins, 1991; Moritsugu & Sue, 1983). The context of individuals' situations, including access to resources, must be considered in order to understand barriers that prevent action (Banyard & Graham-Bermann, 1993; Hobfoll, 1988, 1989).

Role entrapment, for example, is an external condition that hinders personal control and serves as an obstacle to self-regulation for many women and ethnic minority individuals. Role entrapment refers to mainstream society's feelings of prejudice and negative stereotypes toward members of certain groups. These feelings manifest themselves in conditions of inequality and subservience for select populations (Royce, 1982). As a result, members of underprivileged populations may experience many external barriers (e.g., difficulty securing a stable well-paying job, ongoing conditions of poverty, low economic and political power) to their ability to self-regulate. It may be difficult to self-regulate when encountering a system that creates numerous economic and social restraints.

Although environmentally based conditions may be factors that are external to the individual, the lack of adequate external resources can significantly impact internally driven processes and behaviors (i.e., self-regulation). Hence, socially based conditions resulting in diminished personal control over external factors (e.g., unemployment, economic disadvantage) may impact on internal conditions, such as feelings of compromised self-efficacy (Belle, 1990). Based on theoretical notions, self-efficacy is a personal factor that promotes the ability to direct behavior to achieve desired outcomes (Bandura, 1997). However, individuals with limited power over their external environment may encounter numerous obstacles to their goals, independent of levels of individual efforts, and experience decreased perceptions of personal control. In contrast, individuals of privileged social status tend to have a higher sense of personal efficacy because they have more power over their environment and possess more resources to execute behaviors to achieve desired goals. Therefore, it appears that external conditions can facilitate or hinder individuals' ability or desire to optimally self-regulate their behavior.

Communal Power

Empowerment may be defined as a connection with others. Unlike traditional meanings of power that focus on having control over others, communal power promotes interacting and connecting through relationships with others (Amaro, 1995; Surrey, 1991). For women who tend to be more collective than males, collective empowerment may be especially beneficial. According to Surrey (1991), "the sense of powerlessness of the individual is supplanted by the experience of relational power" (p. 176). The same holds true for ethnic minorities, such as African–Americans, Asians, and Latinos, who often are more collective in orientation than the dominant, Western culture. Many minorities derive empowerment through group achievement and cohesiveness, rather than individual accomplishments and self-reliance (Triandis, McClusker, & Hui, 1990). Empowerment is a long and complicated process that necessitates continued support. Although personal power is necessary to encourage individual action, the causal social conditions that contribute to disempowerment must be confronted in order to understand self-regulatory behavior from a universal perspective.

When discussing ethnic and gender differences in communal ideology, it is, however, important not to stereotype all women and members of various ethnic minority groups (e.g., African–Americans, Hispanics) as being collectivist in their approach. Intra-ethnic and -gender differences should be taken into consideration also. Although there is a large body of theoretical literature that supports collective ideology as a central belief among women and ethnic minority cultures, empirical evidence supporting this perspective is limited. Similarly, minimal research of self-regulatory behavior has been conducted among ethnic minorities, thus, hindering the possibility of ethnic comparisons. Future research is needed to elucidate the relationship between collectivism and ethnic minority status and how that relationship may qualify practices of self-regulation.

II. COPING AS SELF-REGULATION

The coping literature has recognized that individuals may respond to stressful situations in various ways, which are partly based on personal and psychological resources (Pearlin & Schooler, 1978). Coping styles generally have been dichotomized into two major divisions: problem focused and emotion focused (Folkman & Lazarus, 1980). The problem focused approach is represented as an active, task-oriented response activated to problem solve by changing the source of the stress or its aftermath. Emotion-focused coping, on the other hand, has been described as an emotional response, such as self-preoccupation and fantasizing, that serve as a passive way to withstand a stressful event (Endler & Parker, 1990; Folkman & Lazarus, 1980).

The characteristics and health outcomes related to these two coping styles have been examined extensively. Problem-focused, or instrumental, coping has been associated with healthier mental and physical functioning (Aspinwall & Taylor, 1992; Bromberger & Matthews, 1996; Endler & Parker, 1990), less depression (Billings and Moos, 1984), greater self-esteem (Swindle, Cronkite, & Moos, 1989), better illness management (Kvam & Lyons, 1991), and healthier sexual behaviors (Folkman, Chesney, Pollack, & Phillips, 1992). Emotion-focused coping, in contrast, has been associated with poorer psychological and physical health outcomes. Research also indicates that women are more likely than men to practice emotion-focused coping and thus are more susceptible to experiencing psychological distress as a result (Aneshensel & Pearlin, 1987; Billings & Moos, 1984; Solomon & Rothblum, 1986). Although a large body of literature supports the idea that problem-focused coping is related to better psychological and physical functioning, there is also an indication that emotion-focused techniques may have superior effects in certain situations. For example, emotion-focused coping has been associated with decreased feelings of pain and threat during ongoing life stressors, such as chronic physical illnesses (Kessler, Price, & Wortman, 1985).

In addition to being presented as the superior coping behavior, problem-focused coping is associated with personal characteristics that promote self-control, determination, and power. For example, a sense of hardiness has been identified as a necessary component of successful coping. Individuals with a hardy coping style are thought to have self-efficacious beliefs of their ability to exert control over their environment and maximally utilize resources available to them. Additionally, hardiness represents the ability to "...find opportunities for the exercise of decision-making, the confirmation of life's priorities, the setting of new goals, and other complex activities [appreciated] as important human capabilities" (Kobasa & Puccetti, 1983 p. 840). Similar to previous findings on emotion-focused styles of coping, Kobasa and Puccetti also argued that a high degree of hardiness is associated with better coping, more effective problem-solving skills, and more adaptive responses to stress, whereas low hardiness is associated with an ineffective method of emotional coping characterized by distraction and self-pity. Although hardiness is just one view of coping, this perspective is representative of the built-in biases of coping theories in general, with their emphasis on "rugged individualism" as an ideal.

A. SOCIAL CONTEXT OF COPING

Consistent with the championing of "rugged individualism," when socially based coping techniques such as seeking social support have been studied in the traditional literature, they typically have been equated with the less effective forms of coping (e.g., Endler & Parker, 1990; Thayer et al., 1994). However, because the problem- versus emotion-focused dichotomy of coping styles clearly favors concepts of independence, self-reliance, and personal control characterized by an orientation that idealizes hardiness and problem-focused coping, support seeking may become negatively embedded in comparison. When questionnaires cue for self-reliance, as the *sin quo non* of well-being, seemingly open questions about social coping may be responded to negatively in this context. Likewise, alternative views of coping are often viewed with greater skepticism (Kabayashi, 1989). By so doing, the fact that coping behavior tends to be more characteristically influenced by the social context in which individuals live is negated (Hobfoll, Dunahoo, Ben-Porath, & Monnier, 1994; Lyons, Mickelson, Sullivan, & Coyne, 1998).

Most life stressors are usually socially bound and intertwined with others from the surrounding environment (Lyons et al., 1998). Pearlin (1993) argued that stress is "the consequence of engagement in social institutions, whose very structure and functioning can engender and sustain patterns of conflict, confusion, and distress" (p. 311). Difficulties associated with certain social roles, such as spouse, parent, and co-worker, often serve as primary sources of stress (Cronkite & Moos, 1995) because of the limitations and demands imposed upon individuals' positions in society (Pearlin, 1993). Therefore, the adoption of more socially embedded strategies for coping and self-regulation that consider the needs, values, standards, and rules of involved others may enhance efficacy in achieving desired results.

Individual coping efforts have social consequences and often consist of interactions with others (Coyne & Smith, 1991; Pearlin, 1991). Consequently, adopting a social perspective in coping is important because behavior simultaneously affects the well-being of individuals who are socially intertwined (Wethington & Kessler, 1991). The ability to cope and regulate individual behavior optimally, particularly during times of stress, must correspond to the ability to function and cause change within an interpersonal context. It follows that socially based theories of coping represent a more comprehensive, holistic depiction of behavior when confronting stressful events.

Unlike traditional approaches to coping that focused predominantly on the efforts of the individual, models that consider the social context of coping tend to bring new interpretations to this arena as new patterns of coping effectiveness begin to emerge. For example, prosocial coping styles are related to better emotional health as compared to antisocial approaches (Dunahoo, Hobfoll, Monnier, Hulsizer, & Johnson, 1998). In addition, prosocial behaviors such as seeking social support are identified as predictors of active coping behaviors (Zea, Jarama, & Bianchi, 1995) as opposed to passive, ineffectual methods.

B. MULTIAXIAL MODEL OF COPING

To address the culture, gender, and individual biases inherent in traditional coping theories, social and communal influences need to be incorporated. In attempts to represent the interrelatedness of both individualistic and communal orientations of coping, Hobfoll et al. (1994) developed the multiaxial model of coping. This model highlights the idea that individuals' coping styles are determined by situational importance, a cycle of resource loss and gain, and their relationship to others. This theory also underscores the idea that coping action varies according to people's consideration of others around them. The multiaxial model consists of three dimensions of coping that include (1) active–passive, (2) prosocial–antisocial, and (3) directness–indirectness. Coping behavior is thought to occur along these continuous dimensions simultaneously. This model is presented in Figure 1.

Active versus Passive Coping

The active–passive dimension of multiaxial models reflects the level of coping activity. This axis represents how active individuals are in confronting stressful situations. Active coping is characterized as behaviors that are enacted to access resources in preparation against a potential stressor, to offset the negative impact of confronted stressors, or to restore depleted resources. In contrast, passive coping reflects inactivity and is recognized as strategies that consist of avoidance of a stressor. The model also recognizes that reactions to stressful events may be characterized by inaction and avoidance in order to conserve resources for later mobilization when they might be more effective or better amassed to meet the challenge.

Prosocial versus Antisocial Coping

The multiaxial model posits that coping can be further demarcated on a continuum between prosocial and antisocial endpoints. The prosocial–antisocial axis of the multiaxial model emphasizes that coping action differs

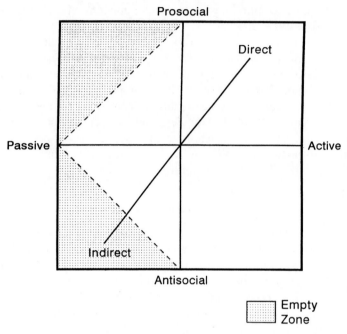

FIGURE 1   The multiaxial model of coping.

in the degree to which it considers the social environment and incorporates concern for other individuals. Antisocial coping includes behaviors that are intentionally antagonistic toward others or that display an overall disregard for others' well-being. In addition, antisocial strategies are implemented to achieve individual goals by exploiting and overpowering others. Antisocial coping, such as aggression, may facilitate goal achievement, but it may be detrimental to physical and emotional well-being (Johnson, 1990) and may deplete other resources beneficial to the coping process (e.g., social support; Lane & Hobfoll, 1992).

In contrast to the antisocial approach, an active, prosocial style of coping emphasizes building coalitions, seeking social support from others, and considering the well-being of others when contemplating an action plan to attain goals (Triandis et al., 1990). Prosocial strategies tend to be particularly effective in situations that require mutual cooperation. Relational issues, such as condom negotiation and monogamy, may serve as illustrations of this point. For women, condom negotiation with partners is not within their individual control; instead, it is an act that requires the cooperation of both partners (Amaro, 1995). The negotiation process could be collective and prosocial in that both partners compliment each other and reach a mutual agreement. On the other hand, this situation could create a state of competitiveness if partners cannot compromise and reach consensus. Similarly, the decision as to whether to maintain a monogamous relationship is also a communal act that could result in either mutual agreement and intimate bonding or divergent and competing plans for relationship commitment.

Indirect versus Direct Coping

The third dimension of the multiaxial model addresses the pattern of coping directness and how it translates into prosocial and antisocial forms of coping. By promoting individualism, Western philosophy emphasizes directness. Being direct is equated with honesty, forthrightness, and manliness. Indirect actions are perceived, in contrast, as manipulative or dishonest means to satisfying needs. However, in communal terms, indirectness connotes a more positive style of interacting that represents a sign of respect for others, sophistication, and an interest in maintaining amicable relations (Triandis, 1990). For example, individualist cultures are more likely to resort to competition to resolve conflicts, whereas collectivists are more prone to engage in indirect, face-saving strategies, such as mediation and bargaining (Leung, 1987).

In addition to influencing interactional styles, indirectness also highlights the importance of achieving goals through stage setting or altering the collective environment. To illustrate this point, Western corporations are increasingly adopting a teamwork approach in the realization that working together promotes increased productivity. To optimize team efforts, it is necessary for members to be familiar with each other and learn to communicate. Collective social interactions in the workplace contribute to an increased ability to develop mutual goals and plans, and promote understanding and knowledge sharing among team members. To encourage such interactions, corporations are increasingly adopting techniques to facilitate a communal atmosphere, such as a nonhierarchical organizational structure and joint financial incentive programs for employees, where individual rewards are based on group efforts (Erez & Somech, 1996). Creating opportunities to increase collaborative efforts among colleagues is an indirect, yet effective method of increasing work productivity.

C. COMMUNAL MASTERY

Our most recent research may serve as one further illustration of the distinction between self-regulation and communal regulation. In particular, we move here to how individuals perceive the self *vis-a-vis* others in terms of regulating their behavior. As we have asserted throughout this chapter, self-regulation considers the self as the *primum mobile* that generates coping behavior and eventuates successful outcomes. It assumes that the self is the conduit through which behavior is regulated. A communal orientation implies that the self is inextricably tied with others in an interwoven fashion. The self and the other are ensembled (Sampson, 1988); that is, a unit or group of complementary parts that contribute to a single effect.

These distinct conceptualizations result in very different research questions and approaches. For example, in examining Self-mastery and Self-efficacy, questionnaires ask for responses to items such as, "I have a great deal of control over things that happen to me." A more communal mastery orientation would change such an item to reflect the self nested in relationships with others, such as "By joining with friends and family, I have a great deal of control over the things that happen to me." Those people who have a more individualized mastery orientation would answer in the affirmative to the former item. However, they might respond in a neutral or even a negative manner to the latter item to the extent that they see themselves as the authors of their fate, or might even see others as interfering with them in achieving their goals. More communally oriented individuals would likely see their self-reliance as interconnected with their relationships.

We designed a new measure of Communal Mastery based on this notion (see Table 1). *Communal Mastery* is defined as the tendency to see oneself as having the potential for success through behavior that is an interwoven process of the self in relation to others. When compared to Self-Mastery, we found Communal Mastery to be more closely related than Self-Mastery to receipt of social support, quality of support received, team leadership style, prosocial coping, and less antisocial coping. Women were also more likely to score higher on Communal Mastery than men. Contrary to seeing interdependence as a weakness, those people high in Communal Mastery were no less likely to utilize assertive action in their coping responses. Moreover, communal mastery was not related to a more external locus of control, but rather to a shared control.

Consistent with the findings of others (Kessler et al., 1985), Communal Mastery did seem to come at a price. Specifically, Self-Mastery was more highly negatively correlated with anger and depression than was Communal Mastery, suggesting that Communal Mastery may sacrifice the self to some extent. Those people high in Communal Mastery worried more, especially about their relationships, and were more likely to consider the needs of others. However, those high in Communal Mastery were lower in depression and anger than those low in Communal Mastery, indicating that it was nonetheless an emotional resource. It appears though that Self-Mastery is more "efficient" at preserving the well-being of the self. Perhaps, in part, because people high in Communal Mastery do worry about their social relationships, Communal Mastery was more strongly related to relationship success than was Self-Mastery.

Hence, in contrast to self-regulation models, communal regulation theory again in this instance yields a different kind of questionnaire, with

TABLE 1   Communal Mastery Scale

Directions: Below are some statements people make about themselves. Tell me how much you agree or disagree with the statements. The choice may be difficult on some of them: just tell me how you GENERALLY FEEL. Please remember to fill in the appropriate circles on the answer sheet.

1 = Strongly Disagree
2 = Somewhat Disagree
3 = Somewhat Agree
4 = Strongly Agree

I Generally Feel	Strongly Disagree	Somewhat Disagree	Somewhat Agree	Strongly Agree
1. By joining with friends and family, I have a great deal of control over the things that happen to me	1	2	3	4
2. Working together with friends and family I can solve many of the problems I have	1	2	3	4
3. There is little I can do to change many of the important things in my life, even with the help of my family and friends	1	2	3	4
4. Working together with people close to me I can overcome most of the problems I have	1	2	3	4
5. What happens to me in the future mostly depends on my ability to work well with others	1	2	3	4
6. I can do just about anything I set my mind to do because I have the support of those close to me	1	2	3	4
7. With the help of those close to me I have more control over my life	1	2	3	4
8. What happens to me in the future mostly depends on my being supported by friends, family, or colleagues......................	1	2	3	4
9. I can meet my goals by helping others meet their goals	1	2	3	4
10. Friends, family, and colleagues mainly get in the way of my accomplishing goals	1	2	3	4

Note. Used by permission of S.E. Hobfoll, Kent State University

qualitatively different results as to the strengths of socially interdependent individuals. Although we are just embarking on this new line of research, the results are promising and indicate that when research adopts a communal model, social behavior is not related to weakness, but strength and particular success in social context, contrary to what has been shown when agenic models are adopted (Endler & Parker, 1990).

D. DIRECTIONS FOR FUTURE RESEARCH

The potential limitations posed by emphasizing individualism, self-reliance, and personal control over and beyond the influence of social context and relatedness were consistently highlighted throughout the chapter. To address these concerns, future research examining the processes of self-regulation should incorporate themes derived from a communally based model of self-directed behavior. There are some models of self-regulation that have directly acknowledged the role of social context and conceptualized individual behavior as being intertwined with larger interpersonal functioning (e.g., social cognitive models). However, it appears that their focus remains principally on individuals and how social context plays a role in their pursuit of personal goals. Although this perspective extends beyond traditional theories that tend to heavily emphasize individualism and discount socially mediated factors, the recognition of engaging in individual efforts to address group-based needs and goals seem to be overlooked.

In addition to focusing on how social context interacts with personal factors (e.g., cognitive processes) to direct behavior toward individual goals, models of communal regulation emphasize how social context calls upon individuals also to gear their behavior toward group-oriented goals and desires. Specifically, individuals direct their behavior to achieve goals that are beneficial to their social network affiliations (e.g., organizations, families) as well as for their individual gain. Future research incorporating a communal perspective should further investigate what strategies individuals use to establish a balance between achieving goals that are mutually beneficial for themselves as well as for other members in their social environment. Similarly, it is important also to examine how these strategies may differ according to social status, resource availability, and level of orientation to a collectivist or communal perspective.

Communal regulation recognizes social context as a prominent feature as opposed to a background of self-directed behavior. This approach may allow the concept of self-regulation to expand and increase its universal applicability. Furthermore, unlike traditional models of self-regulation rooted in individualism, the idea of *self-in-social-setting regulation* may provide a more comprehensive definition of what constitutes and determines self-regulatory behavior. This challenges, in particular, the assumption of free will presupposed by self-regulatory models.

When incorporating models of communal regulation, it is important not to fall prey to conceptualizing communal regulation as being a form of collectivism that exists as a polar opposite to individually based self-regulation. Instead, the focus should incorporate a balance between communal and individualistic self-regulation for optimal functioning. Just as collectivist perspectives view individualism as being contrary to interpersonal functioning and serving as a hindrance to personal satisfaction, concepts of individualism view social enmeshment as a sign of personal weakness. It is apparent that both concepts are extreme in their views and may harbor their own limitations. In efforts to circumvent this dilemma, research incorporating a model of communal regulation should be aware of this potential downfall and recognize that individual- and social-based efforts do not exist in isolation.

III. SUMMARY AND CONCLUSION

In this chapter, we attempted to highlight major biases that exist in traditional theories of psychology. Because such theories typically have been operationalized and developed according to the values and standards of a Western, European philosophy, they have reflected a rather narrow band of human behavior. They either have isolated competing explanations of behavior or have presented them in a less favorable light. For example, within traditional theories, individualism connotes strength and adaptability, whereas communal or collectivist patterns of behavior are indicative of submissiveness and a less influential status in society. Because of this underlying bias, alternative concepts of human behavior previously have received minimal attention in the mainstream study of psychology.

Reflecting the bias toward individualism, self-reliance and self-regulation typically have represented notions that are highly valued in our society, such as self-control, personal freedom, and accountability. On an individual level, processes that focus on the self and are geared primarily toward personal advancement are viewed as prerequisites for productivity and adaptive functioning. As a result, the shortcomings of an individualistic philosophy often are overlooked. For example, perspectives primarily focusing on self-focus, in reality, are not optimally adaptive and even can be counterproductive when practiced to an extreme. In contrast, a more societal perspective recognizes the shortcomings of a purely individualistic approach and highlights the notion that behaviors do not occur in a social vacuum. Therefore, the focus shifts to viewing environmental factors, such as standards, norms, and interpersonal interactions within people's social environment, as predominant determinants of behavior.

Although individualistic and collectivist approaches differ in their conceptualization of sources of human behavior, it is important to realize that they do not exist in isolation. They should be seen as processes that coexist to produce optimal levels of functioning and adaptability within the environment. For example, concepts that focus on self-focus and management should incorporate social comparison and expectations as a major component. Similarly, communalism needs to recognize that self-reflection and a certain degree of self-control and personal responsibility are essential processes in behavioral monitoring and motivation. By acknowledging the existing strengths and weaknesses of each perspective, it becomes clear that both communalism and individualism complement and build upon each other in order to fully understand human behavior within a social context.

ACKNOWLEDGMENT

Work on this chapter was made possible, in part through the support of the NIMH Office of AIDS Research (Grant 1RO MH45669) and the Applied Psychology Center, which was founded through a grant from the Ohio Board of Regents to support psychological research on applied issues in psychology.

REFERENCES

Amaro, H. (1995). Love, sex, and power: Considering women's realities in HIV prevention. *American Psychologist, 50*, 437–447.

Aneshensel, C. S., & Pearlin, L. I. (1987). Structural contexts of sex differences in stress. In R. C. Barnett, L. Biener, & G. K. Baruch (Eds.), *Gender and stress*. New York: Free Press.

Aspinwall, L. G., & Taylor, S. E. (1992). Modeling cognitive adaptation: A longitudinal investigation of the impact of individual differences and coping on college adjustment and performance. *Journal of Personality and Social Psychology, 6*, 989–1003.

Bandura, A. (1986). *Social foundations of thought and action: A social cognitive theory.* Englewood Cliffs, NJ: Prentice-Hall.

Bandura, A. (1997). Self-efficacy: *The exercise of control*. New York, N.Y.: W. H. Freeman.

Banyard, V. L., & Graham-Bermann, S. A. (1993). Can women cope? A gender analysis of theories of coping with stress. *Psychology of Women Quarterly, 17*, 303–318.

Baumeister, R. F., Heatherton, T. F., & Tice, D. M. (1993). When ego threats lead to self-regulation failure: Negative consequences of high self-esteem. *Journal of Personality and Social Psychology, 64*, 141–156.

Belle, D. (1990). Poverty and women's mental health. *American Psychologist, 45*, 385–389.

Billings, A. G., & Moos, R. H. (1984). Coping, stress, and social resources among adults with unipolar depression. *Journal of Personality and Social Psychology, 46*, 877–891.

Bromberger, J. T., & Matthews, K. A. (1996). A "feminine" model of vulnerability to depressive symptoms: A longitudinal investigation of middle-aged women. *Journal of Personality and Social Psychology, 70*, 591–598.

Carver, C. S., Blaney, P. H., & Scheier, M. F. (1979). Reassertion and giving up: The interactive role of self-directed attention and outcome expectancy. *Journal of Personality and Social Psychology, 37*, 1859–1870.

Carver, C. S. & Scheier, M. F. (1982). Control theory: A useful conceptual framework for personality-social, clinical, and health psychology. *Psychological Bulletin, 92*, 111–135.

Carver, C. S. & Scheier, M. F. (1990). Principles of self-regulation: Action and emotion. In E. T. Higgins & R. M. Sorrentino (Eds.), *Handbook of motivation and cognition:Foundation of social behaviors*, (Vol. 2, pp. 3–52). New York: Guilford Press.

Clark, N. M. (1987). Social learning theory in current health education practices. *Advances in Health Education and Promotion, 2*, 251–275.

Clark, M. S., Mills, J., & Powell, M. C. (1986). Keeping track of needs in communal and exchange relationships. *Journal of Personality and Social Psychology, 51*, 333–338.

Coyne, J. C., & Smith, D. A. (1991). Couples coping with a myocardial infarction: A contextual perspective on wive's distress. *Journal of Personality and Social Psychology, 61,* 404–412.

Cronkite, R. C., & Moos, R. H. (1995). Life context, coping processes, and depression. In E. E. Beckman & W. R. Leber (Eds.). *Handbook of depression, second edition* (pp. 569–590). New York: Guilford Press.

Croyle, R. T., & Hunt, J. R. (1991). Coping with health threat: Social influence processes in reactions to medical test results. *Journal of Personality and Social Psychology, 60,* 382–389.

David, R. J., & Collins, J. W. (1991). Bad outcomes in black babies: Race or racism? *Ethnicity and Disease, 1,* 236–244.

Dunahoo, C. L., Hobfoll, S. E., Monnier, J., Hulsizer, M. R., & Johnson, R. (1998). Even the Lone Ranger had Tonto: There's more than rugged individualism in coping, *Anxiety, Stress, and Coping, 11,* 137–165.

Duval, T. S., Duval, V. H., & Mulilis, J. P. (1992). Effects of self-focus, discrepancy between self and standard, and outcome expectancy favorability on the tendency to match self to standard or to withdraw. *Journal of Personality and Social Psychology, 62,* 340–348.

Eagly, A. H. (1987). *Sex differences in social behavior: A social role interpretation.* Hillsdale, NJ: Erlbaum.

Eisenberger, R., Mitchell, M., & Masterson, F. A. (1985). Effort training increases generalized self-control. *Journal of Personality and Social Psychology, 49,* 1294–1301.

Endler, N. S., & Parker, J. D. A. (1990). Multidimensional assessment of coping: A critical evaluation. *Journal of Personality and Social Psychology, 58,* 844–854.

Erez, M., & Somech, A. (1996). Is group productivity loss the rule or the exception? Effects of culture and group-based motivation. *Academy of Management Journal, 39,* 1513–1537.

Folkman, S., Chesney, M. A., Pollack, L., & Phillips, C. (1992). Stress, coping, and high-risk sexual behavior. *Health Psychology, 11,* 218–222.

Folkman, S., & Lazarus, R. S. (1980). An analysis of coping in a middle-aged community sample. *Journal of Health and Social Behavior, 21,* 219–239.

Gao, G. (1996). Self and other: A Chinese perspective on interpersonal relationships. In W. B. Gudykunst, S. Ting-Toomey, & T. Nishida (Eds.), *Communication in personal relationships across cultures* (pp. 81–101). London: Sage.

Han, S., & Shavitt, S. (1994). Persuasion and culture: Advertising appeals in individualistic and collectivistic societies. *Journal of Experimental Social Psychology, 30,* 326–350.

Harre, R. (1981). Psychological variety. In P. Heelas & A. Lock (Eds.), *Indigenous psychologies: The anthropology of the self* (pp. 79–103). New York: Academic Press.

Higgins, E. T., Roney, C. J., Crowe, E., & Hymes, C. (1994). Ideal versus ought predilections for approach and avoidance: Distinct self-regulatory systems. *Journal of Personality and Social Psychology, 66,* 276–286.

Hobfoll, S. E. (1988). *The ecology of stress.* New York: Hemisphere.

Hobfoll, S. E. (1989). Conservation of resources: A new stress theory. *American Psychologist, 44,* 513–524.

Hobfoll, S. E. (1998). *Stress, culture, and community: The psychology and philosophy of stress.* New York: Plenum.

Hobfoll, S. E., Cameron, R. P., Chapman, H. A., & Gallagher, R. W. (1996). Social support and social coping in couples. In G. R. Pierce, B. R. Sarason, & I. G. Sarason (Eds.), *Handbook of social support and the family* (pp. 413–433). New York: Plenum.

Hobfoll, S. E., Dunahoo, C. L., Ben-Porath, Y., & Monnier, J. (1994). Gender and coping: The dual-axis model of coping. *American Journal of Community Psychology, 22,* 49–82.

Hobfoll, S. E., & Vaux, A. (1993). Social support: Social resources and social context. In L. Goldberger, & S. Breznitz (Eds.), *Handbook of stress: Theoretical and clinical aspects* (2nd ed., pp. 685–705). New York: Free Press.

Johnson, E. H. (1990). *The deadly emotions: The role of anger, hostility, and aggression in health and emotional well-being*. New York: Praeger.

Kabayashi, J. S. (1989). Depathologizing dependency: Two perspectives. *Psychiatric Annals, 19,* 653–658.

Kagitcibasi, C. (1994). A critical appraisal of individualism and collectivism: Toward a new formulation. In U. Kim, H. C. Triandis, C. Kagitcibasi, S. Choi, & G. Yoon (1994). *Individualism and collectivism: Theory, method, and applications* (pp. 52–65). Thousand Oaks, CA: Sage.

Katz, P. A., Boggiano, A., & Silvern, L. (1993). Theories of female personality. In F. L. Denmark & M. A. Paludi (Eds.), *Psychology of women: A handbook of issues and theories* (pp. 247–280). Westport, CT: Greenwood Press.

Keefe, S. E., & Casas, J. M. (1980). Mexican Americans and mental health: A selected review and recommendations for mental health service delivery. *American Journal of Community Psychology, 8,* 303–326.

Kelley, H. H. (1979). *Personal relationships: Their structure and processes*. Hillsdale, NJ: Erlbaum.

Kessler, R. C., Price, R. H., & Wortman, C. B. (1985). Social factors in psychopathology: Stress, social support, and coping processes. *Annual Review of Psychology, 36,* 531–572.

Kim, U., Triandis, H. C., Kagitcibasi, C., Choi, S., & Yoon, G. (1994). *Individualism and collectivism: Theory, method, and applications* (pp. 1–11). Thousand Oaks, CA: Sage.

Kobasa, S. C., & Pucetti, M. C. (1983). Personality and social resources in stress resistance. *Journal of Personality and Social Psychology, 45,* 839–850.

Kvam, S. H., & Lyons, J. S. (1991). Assessment of coping strategies, social support, and general health status in individuals with diabetes mellitus. *Psychological Reports, 68,* 623–632.

Lane, C., & Hobfoll, S. E. (1992). How loss affects anger and alienates potential supporters. *Journal of Consulting and Clinical Psychology, 60,* 935–942.

Leung, K. (1987). Some determinants of reactions to procedural models for conflict resolution: A cross-national study. *Journal of Personality and Social Psychology, 53,* 898–908.

Leventhal, H., Nerenz, D. R., & Steele, D. J. (1984). Illness representations and coping with health threats. In A. Baum, S. E. Taylor & J. E. Singer (Eds.), *Handbook of psychology and health* (Vol. 4, pp. 219–252). Hillsdale, NJ: Erlbaum.

Lykes, M. B. (1985). Gender and individualistic vs. collectivist bases for notions about the self. Special issue: Conceptualizing gender in personality theory and research. *Journal of Personality, 53,* 356–383.

Lyons, R. F., Mickelson, K. D., Sullivan, M. J. L., & Coyne, J. C. (1998). Coping as a communal process. *Journal of Social and Personal Relationships, 15,* 579–605.

Mayer, J. D., & Gaschke, Y. N. (1988). The experience and meta-experience of mood. *Journal of Personality and Social Psychology, 55,* 102–111.

Mikulincer, M. (1989). Cognitive interference and learned helplessness: The effects of off-task cognitions on performance following unsolvable problems. *Journal of Personality and Social Psychology, 57,* 129–135.

Miller, J. B. (1986). *Toward a new psychology of women*. (2nd ed.). Boston: Beacon Press.

Mills, J., & Clark, M. S. (1982). Communal and exchange relationships. In L. Wheeler, (Ed.), *Review of personality and social psychology*. (Vol. 3). Beverly Hills: Sage.

Moemeka, A. (1996). Interpersonal communication in communalistic societies in Africa. In W. B. Gudykunst, S. Ting-Toomey, & T. Nishida (Eds.), *Communication in personal relationships across cultures* (pp. 197–216). London: Sage.

Moritsugu, J., & Sue, S. (1983). Minority status as a stressor. In R. D. Felner, L. A. Jason, J. N. Moritsugu, & S. S. Farber (Eds.), *Preventive psychology: Theory, research, and practice* (pp. 162–174). New York: Pergamon.

Pearlin, L. I. (1991). The study of coping: An overview of problems and directions. In J. Eckenrode (Ed.), *The social context of coping* (pp. 261–276). New York: Plenum.

Pearlin, L. I. (1993). The social contexts of stress. In L. Goldberger & S. Breznitz (Eds.), *Handbook of stress: Theoretical and clinical aspects* (2nd ed., pp. 303–315). New York: Free Press.

Pearlin, L. I., & Schooler, C. (1978). The structure of coping. *Journal of Health and Social Behavior, 19,* 2–21.

Perloff, R. (1987). Self-interest and personal responsibility redux. *American Psychologist, 42,* 3–11.

Rogler, L. H., Malgady, R. G., & Rodriguez, O. (1989). *Hispanics and mental health: A framework for research.* Malabar, FL: Krieger.

Royce, A. P. (1982). *Ethnic identity: Strategies for diversity.* Bloomington: Indiana University Press.

Sampson, E. E. (1988). The debate on individualism: Indigenous psychologies of the individual and their role in personal and societal functioning. *American Psychologist, 43,* 15–22.

Shkodriani, G. M., & Gibbons, J. L. (1995). Individualism and collectivism among university students in Mexico and the United States. *Journal of Social Psychology, 135,* 765–772.

Solomon, I. J., & Rothblum, E. D. (1986). Stress, coping, and social support in women. *Behavior Therapist, 9,* 199–204.

Spence, J. T. (1985). Achievement American style: The rewards and costs of individualism. *American Psychologist, 40,* 1285–1295.

Sternberg, R. J. (1988). Mental self-government: A theory of intellectual styles and their development. *Human Development, 31,* 197–224.

Surrey, J. L. (1991). The "self-in-relation": A theory of women's development. In J. D. Jordan, A. G. Kaplan, J. B. Miller, I. P. Stiver & J. L. Surrey (Eds.), *Women's growth in connection* (pp. 162–180). New York: Guilford Press.

Swindle, R. W., Cronkite, R. C., & Moos, R. H. (1989). Life stressors, social resources, coping, and the 4-year course of unipolar depression. *Journal of Abnormal Psychology, 98,* 468–477.

Thayer, R. E. (1978). Toward a psychological theory of multidimensional activation (arousal). *Motivation and Emotion, 2,* 1–34.

Thayer, R. E. (1989). *The biopsychology of mood and arousal.* New York: Oxford University Press.

Thayer, R. E., Newman, J. R., & McClain, T. M. (1994). Self-regulation of mood: Strategies for changing a bad mood, raising energy, and reducing tension. *Journal of Personality and Social Psychology, 67,* 910–925.

Triandis, H. C. (1990). Cross-cultural studies of individualism and collectivism. In G. Jahoda, H. C. Triandis, C. Kagitcibasi, J. Berry, J. G. Draguns, & M. Cole (Eds.), *Nebraska Symposium on Motivation: Vol. 37 Cross-cultural perspectives* (pp. 41–134). Lincoln: University of Nebraska Press.

Triandis, H. C., Bontempo, R., Villareal, M., Asai, M., & Lucca, N. (1988). Individualism–collectivism: Cross-cultural perspectives on self-ingroup relationships. *Journal of Personality and Social Psychology, 54,* 323–338.

Triandis, H. C., McCusker, C., & Hui, C. H. (1990). Multimethod probes of individualism and collectivism. *Journal of Personality and Social Psychology, 59,* 1006–1020.

Vargas-Willis, G., & Cervantes, R. G. (1987). Consideration of psychosocial stress in treatment of the Latina immigrant. Special issue: Mexican immigrant women. *Hispanic Journal of Behavorial Sciences, 9,* 315–329.

Wethington, E., & Kessler, R. C. (1991). Situations and processes of coping. In J. Eckenrode (Ed.), *The social context of coping* (pp. 13–30). New York: Plenum.

Yamaguchi, S. (1994). Collectivism among the Chinese: A perspective from the self. In U. Kim, H. C. Triandis, C. Kagitcibasi, S. Choi, & G. Yoon, *Individualism and collectivism: Theory, method, and applications* (pp. 175–188). Thousand Oaks, CA: Sage.

Ying, Y. W., & Akutsu, P. D. (1997). Psychosocial adjustment of Southeast Asian refugees: The contribution of sense of coherence. *Journal of Community Psychology, 25,* 125–139.

Zea, M. C., Jarama, S. L., & Bianchi, F. T. (1995). Social support and psychosocial competence: Explaining the adaptation to college of ethnically diverse students. *American Journal of Community Psychology, 23,* 509–531.

Zimmerman, B. J. (1989). A social cognitive view of self-regulated learning. *Journal of Educational Psychology, 82,* 297–306.

DOMAIN-SPECIFIC MODELS AND RESEARCH ON SELF-REGULATION

10

SELF-REGULATION IN ORGANIZATIONAL SETTINGS

A TALE OF TWO PARADIGMS

JEFFREY B. VANCOUVER

Ohio University, Athens, Ohio

I. INTRODUCTION

It was the best of times, it was the worst of times, it was the age of wisdom, it was the age of foolishness, it was the epoch of belief, it was the epoch of incredulity. (Dickens, 1859, p. 1)

Dicken's novel portrays the very different approaches two cities took to adapt to the paradoxical issues of their day. This chapter describes two approaches industrial/organizational (I/O) psychologists have taken to understanding the complexity of human behavior in organizational settings. One approach focuses on individual decision making; the other on the structure of interrelated parts. The first arises from a long history of the study of cognitive processes in individuals; the other arises from an equally long history of the study of communication within and between systems. Both of these approaches have been joined, if somewhat tenuously, in theories of self-regulation. This chapter reviews these two paradigms and their role in understanding self-regulation in organizational settings. Meanwhile, the union of these approaches is less than complete and portends the casualties that characterize a revolution. Preferring a more peaceful evolution, I represent some of the underlying issues that have arisen from the histories of the paradigms and present a model that more fully completes the merger begun in the self-regulation literature.

Copyright © 2000 by Academic Press.
All rights of reproduction in any form reserved.

Given the breadth of the backgrounds possible for readers of this chapter, a brief description of I/O psychology is in order. I/O psychologists' domain ranges from the description and measurement of individual differences for purposes of selection and performance appraisal to the creation of interventions designed to increase performance or satisfaction among workers. In recent times we have observed that organizations have become more complex, jobs more dynamic, and workers more autonomous (Katzell, 1994). This has led to an increased appreciation of the individual in determining individual and organizational outcomes. Thus, to develop interventions, redesign environments, and choose people to participate in these organizations in ways that maximize performance, satisfaction, and prosocial and health-oriented behaviors requires a deep understanding of how individuals conduct themselves in these fluid contexts. Several self-regulation models have emerged in I/O psychology to help provide that understanding. The underlying elements of these theories will be described in more detail later, but first definitions of self-regulation (SR) and self-regulated learning (SRL) are presented to ground the reader in the approach to SR taken in this chapter.

II. DEFINITIONS

Defining SR and SRL in a domain of science is difficult. Researchers each tend to take their own approach and the number of definitions cumulate as a function of the number of researchers. In the case of SR and SRL, most definitions emphasize the cognitive decision-making paradigm (e.g., Kanfer, 1990; Karoly, 1993). In this chapter, a more generic approach is taken.

A. SELF-REGULATION

In general, regulation refers to keeping something regular; to maintaining a variable at some value despite disturbances to the variable. The value at which the variable is maintained is called the desired state. For a system to regulate a variable itself (i.e., self-regulation), the desired state must be internally represented within the system. In psychology, internally represented desired states are often called goals (Austin & Vancouver, 1996). The goal construct is perhaps the most common and central component in self-regulation theories (Kanfer, 1990).

In I/O psychology, humans, groups, and organizations are systems of interest (Vancouver, 1996), but it is the former that has received the most attention in terms of SR. For example, I/O psychologists are interested in the role of individuals in regulating their level of performance (e.g., Vancouver, 1997). Indeed, performance long has been a critical topic in I/O psychology (Katzell & Austin, 1992), but earlier conceptions of the worker focused on either the properties of organizations (e.g., reward systems) or the *passive* properties of individuals (e.g., intelligence) on performance. SR models emphasize the active role of individuals in the process of determining their levels of performance. This new focus began with the humanist movement in psychology in the 1950s and 1960s (Katzell & Austin, 1992), but reached a more mature level in the 1980s after the articulation of SR in theories of organizational behavior (e.g., Ashford & Cummings, 1983).

Simultaneously, the importance of goals in increasing performance was receiving substantial empirical support (Locke, Shaw, Saari, & Latham, 1981). The research was driven inductively (Locke & Latham, 1990), but SR theories have arisen to provide a theoretical base (Locke, 1991a). Interestingly, the goals common to the goal-setting literature are usually attainment goals, as opposed to maintenance goals more common to regulation descriptions (Austin & Vancouver, 1996). The difference is subtle, so an example is useful.

Consider a "widget" maker. Widgets are a generic, fictional product that is useful for exposition. In the maintenance context, a widget maker might monitor the state of the shelves in his or her store. He or she might have a goal related to keeping the shelves full. As customers purchase widgets, the widget maker must make more, but only enough, to fill the shelves. That is, as the customers disturb the variable (i.e., state of shelves), the widget maker acts to return the state of the shelves to the desired state for them (i.e., full). Specifically, maintenance implies keeping the perception of the state of a variable regular; actions occur *when* disturbances move a variable from the desired state or the desired state changes. In the attainment context, the widget maker might have a goal for the number of widget to produce in a day. Actions occur *until* a desired state is reached. Once that desired state is reached, the phenomenon of interest ends. Each workday begins anew with zero widgets made and ends when the goal is reached.

To achieve or maintain a goal, the system must be able to act to affect its environment (i.e., goal-directed behavior). Often SR refers not to the actions per se, but to the processes that mediate or support the actions. For example, Karoly (1993) defined SR as processes "that enable an individual to guide his/her goal-directed activities over time and across changing circumstances (contexts). Regulation implies modulation of thought, affect, behavior, or attention …" (p. 25). For example, our widget maker might remove an object from his or her line of sight that tends to distract him or her from making widgets. The behavior, removing the object, affects attention that can be applied to the behavior of widget making, for which the individual has a goal. However, this conception of SR simply may be a special case of general SR. That is, the removal of distracting objects implies a desired state of no distractions. Hence, the removal of the object is a means to accomplish the goal of no distractions, which happens to facilitate the making of widgets. Indeed, this description of self-regulating self-regulation foreshadows later descriptions of a fundamental model in one of the paradigms.

Another key feature in the broader definition of SR requires that the system have the capacity to assess the current state of the variable. To compensate for disturbances to a variable being maintained or to know when a goal is attained, the system must know (i.e., internally represent) the current state of the variable. A system's actions accord with the difference between the current state as perceived by the system and the desired state as internally represented by the system. Without the ability to perceive the variable's current state, the effect of actions on variables must be calculated by the system. Several models of SR describe human behavior as calculative, and more will be said about this in the last section of this chapter.

As with the means feature, some conceptualizations of SR focus on the assessment feature. For example, SR can refer to processes that bring the current state of a goal to conscious attention (see Karoly's definition in the preceding text or Carver & Scheier's, 1981, description of self-focus). Likewise, for many, SR refers to the behaviors required to monitor and improve the quality and quantity of information on goal progress. For example, when individuals ask someone else to tell them how they are doing on a task, they may be responding to a sense of inadequate information regarding performance, such that they must do something (e.g., ask) to get that information. This conceptualization parallels the focus on goal-directed behavior described previously. A system that is "responding to a sense of inadequate information regarding performance" implies a desired level of information. Hence, the content of the goal has changed, not the process of self-regulation. It is merely a special case of a more generic description.

B. SELF-REGULATED LEARNING

Self-regulated learning (SRL) is a much smaller topic in I/O psychology because learning is a much smaller topic (Weiss, 1990). To understand SRL, we must first define learning. The common definition is that learning is a relatively permanent change in knowledge or skill produced by experience (Weiss, 1990). Self-regulated learning can be tied to the three key features of self-regulation: goals, actions, and assessment. Hence, in this chapter SRL refers to (a) the creation of new goals, (b) the creation of new means to maintain or attain goals, or (c) changing ways to assess (i.e., perceive) current states. As with SR, SRL has been defined more narrowly to refer to behaviors and mechanisms that improve the creating, affecting and assessing features. That is, SRL often refers only to learning general mechanisms for improving self-regulation as opposed to learning general or specific mechanisms for regulating variables.

A general SRL mechanisms of interest to I/O psychologists includes learning to set specific, measurable goals when creating new goals. This general mechanism is likely to improve the regulation of any variable for which specific, measurable goals are set. Hence, salespersons who specify the number of new client calls, the number of follow-up calls, and the number of sale closes to be attained in a day will be able to regulate those factors better than salespersons who do not quantify these aspects of their performance. This is the point behind budgeting. Setting budget goals might not assure one can meet them, but it goes a long way toward improving money management. For I/O psychologists, general mechanisms, because of their application in a variety of settings, tend to be of more interest than specific mechanisms. However, a single mechanism may underlie both general and specific learning. The nature of this mechanism is the topic of the final section of this chapter.

C. SUMMARY

Given the breadth of the definition of SR and SRL used in this chapter, the number of I/O theories related to the concept is overwhelming. Austin and Vancouver (1996) listed 31 theories featuring goals or goallike concepts in psychology since 1905. I/O psychologists have used most if not all of these theories in their work. Vancouver (1996) listed 49 recent theoretical contributions to the study of organizational behavior that comply with the definition of SR given herein, and more have been published since the lists were compiled (e.g., Kluger & DeNisi, 1996).

In addition, several of the contributions are integrations of the past work of others. For example, Ford (1992) attempted to integrate 31 theories from psychology, a list that only partially overlaps Austin and Vancouver's, into a single self-regulation theory of motivation. Likewise Edwards (1992) integrated the stress literature as it pertains to organizational settings using a self-regulation heuristic. Kanfer and Heggestad (1997) reviewed and integrated much of the individual differences literature pertaining to self-regulation. Kanfer (1990) also reviewed self-regulation models as part of her review chapter on motivation theories in I/O psychology. She included three theories: goal-setting (Locke & Latham, 1990), social cognitive theory (Bandura, 1986), and control theory (Carver & Scheier, 1981). Finally, Locke (1991a) edited a special edition of *Organizational Behavior and Human Decision Processes* on cognitive self-regulation models. His criteria reduced the number of theories to just three as well: goal setting, social cognitive theory (SCT), and the theory of planned behavior (Ajzen, 1991).

Rather than review all of these theories in detail, I review the two core paradigms that have contributed to most, if not all, of these theories. In addition, the fundamental issue that drives this chapter relates to the conflicts between these paradigms. In particular, the explicit exclusion of control theory from Locke's list of SR theories is indicative of a rift among SR theorists that requires an examination of the core ideas in the two paradigms.

III. TWO PARADIGMS

Naming the paradigms is difficult because so many people have contributed to them, so many variations exist, and so many connotations (both good and bad) have been placed on the various labels that any label will not do them justice. Keeping that caveat in mind, I label the first paradigm "cybernetic systems." Systems theories and cybernetics arose almost simultaneously, and they influenced each other to such an extent that they now can be considered one (Richardson, 1991). In I/O psychology, the theory that most exemplifies the cybernetic-systems paradigm is control theory (Carver & Scheier, 1981; Lord & Hanges, 1987).

The second paradigm is the "decision-making" paradigm, which includes problem-solving models. Unlike the cybernetic–systems paradigm, which reaches well beyond psychology, the decision-making paradigm stems from the cognitive science field, which broaches only a few fields besides psychology (Gardner, 1985). In I/O psychology, the exemplar decision-making theory is expectancy theory (Vroom, 1964), which as Locke (1991a) notes, has been incorporated into all of the theories in his list.

With an eye on the end product, the more complete union of these two paradigms, the review highlights some fundamental gaps and misdirections that have impeded the union. Specifically, problems have emerged that relate to point of view and type of processing (i.e., parallel versus serial). The point-of-view problem relates to understanding who is regulating what in autonomous, agential models of systems. The type of processing problem refers to the tendency for theories to model either parallel or serial processes, but not both, a current problem for cognitive psychology (Baddeley, 1994).

To address these issues, I take the dynamic quality of system interaction and the cybernetic structure seriously, not simply as a heuristic to help integrate several theories (e.g., Edwards, 1992; McKenna & Wright, 1992). According to Richardson (1991), the casual attitude is one of the roadblocks to the adoption of feedback thinking in the social sciences:

> Some social scientists view the use of the feedback concept in social science as "borrowing an idea from engineering."... Perception of feedback as an analogy represent a weak intellectual commitment to the idea as an explanatory tool. Weak commitment, as Kuhn (1962/1970) suggests, means rapid abandonment in the face of minor anomalies. The perception of feedback as an analogy rather than as a fact of life in living system weakens efforts to understand the role of feedback and circular causality in social systems. (p. 327)

Meanwhile, some cybernetic–systems models have not acknowledged the attentional bottleneck so fundamental to the decision-making paradigm (Simon, 1994). The attentional bottleneck has been used to account for the serial processing indicative of thinking, planning, and decision making. The task, then, is to describe how a system composed of cybernetic structures can think, plan, and make decisions over time. This task is reserved for the end of the chapter. The result is a structural model of decision making and a cybernetics systems theory that can handle both parallel and serial processing.

A. CYBERNETIC–SYSTEMS PARADIGM

The review of the cybernetic–systems paradigm begins with general systems theory. Richardson (1991) speculated that general systems theory began with a philosophy seminar given by Ludwig von Bertalanffy at the University of Chicago in 1937. General systems theory describes a basic, but not necessarily intuitive, observation witnessed across several disciplines of science (e.g., von Bertalanffy was a biologist). The observation was that properties of systems and/or their environments remained stable despite instability in their environments. One interesting example of this can be found in ecological systems and led to Lovelock's Gaia hypothesis that the earth is a living system. The specific observation is that despite the constant rise in the temperature of the sun, the temperature of the earth has remained relatively stable over the course of millions of years. Based on these observations and some mathematics to describe them, von Bertalanffy (1950) launched a substantial intellectual movement to integrate theories and domains of study across chasms previously considered unassailable. This movement was to be joined by several other grand theories on the nature of systems.

Primary among these other grand theories was cybernetics (Rosenblueth, Wiener, & Bigelow, 1943; Wiener, 1948). Cybernetics drew upon an idea that was proving useful in engineering, the negative feedback loop (see Figure 1). In Wiener's (1948) model, the input to the system is some reference signal determined by an engineer or user from which is subtracted any feedback of the output of the system. Depending on the difference of the feedback from the reference signal, an error is magnified

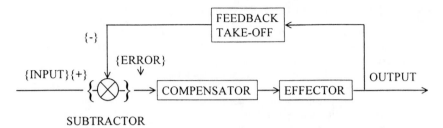

FIGURE 1   Powers's (1978) adaptation of Wiener's (1948) control system diagram. Copyright © 1978 by the American Psychological Association. Reprinted with permission.

(or not) in a compensator, which engages an effector, which causes the output, which is fed back, and so on. Thus, by monitoring the results of its own output, the system can regulate that output.

The feedback and goal-striving mechanisms articulated in cybernetic models were quickly seen as one key explanation for von Bertalanffy's stability-despite-instability observation (Richardson, 1991). It is important to note that not all stability-despite-instability observations can be explained with cybernetic principles. Marbles will roll to the bottom of bowls regardless of initial placement of the marble or movements of the bowl; water in a glass will return to level regardless of the amount of jousting to the glass; and the earth will maintain a fairly constant temperature despite the sun's constantly increasing temperature. All of these examples involve stability-despite-instability (i.e., regularity), and all can be modeled with feedback mathematics, but none involves an internally represented desired state (i.e., a goal) with the cybernetic mechanisms needed to maintain that state. Hence, to be consistent with the definition of SR, only cybernetic processes are considered here.

Additional theories and theorists informed and built on cybernetic–systems thinking over the years (e.g., Ashby, 1956), but in I/O psychology, Katz and Kahn's (1978) *The Social Psychology of Organizations* has been the most influential. Like the other theorists, they emphasized that systems are composed of interrelated parts and that the parts themselves are composed of less complex systems and structures. For example, organizations are composed of humans, which are composed of cybernetic structures, which are composed of still smaller and simpler structures. Because of this configuration, they advised that when thinking about any particular system, the component systems and the higher-order systems of which the focal system is a member need to be thought about as well. The point of view all too often taken in science, systems theorists argue, is that of attempting to isolate the focal system without realizing that the system acts in a constellation of other systems (Lazlo, 1976). To this day, a systems view is endorsed by nearly everyone in the field of I/O psychology, management science, and organizational theory. Yet, several people have argued that it has been so diluted and the various renditions made so narrow in scope as to misrepresent the concept (e.g., Ashmos & Huber, 1987; Colarelli, 1996; Vancouver, 1994, 1996).

1. Perceptual Control Theory

Meanwhile in the cybernetic subcomponent, 1978 also saw an important attempt to communicate a variant on cybernetic thinking, perceptual control theory (PCT), to the psychological community (Powers, 1978). Unlike living systems, PCT is primarily a theory of human systems. However, the model is grand in the sense that Powers and his colleagues (Powers, Clark, & McFarland, 1960a, 1960b; Powers, 1973) attempted to articulate a theory of human psychology that explained all behavior.

Grand theories of psychology are looked upon with great suspicion in American psychology (Frese & Zapf, 1993), and Powers's theory is no exception (Locke, 1994). Eventually, Powers's model was taken up by two social psychologists, Carver and Scheier (1981, 1982a, 1982b), whose book and papers were cited by I/O psychologists (e.g., Campion & Lord, 1982; Lord & Hanges, 1987; Taylor, Fisher, & Ilgen, 1984). From there, the cybernetic–systems model has made its way into still narrower theories of motivation and self-regulation. However, those theories have omitted much of Powers's ideas. Thus, it is important to go back to some of the original work to reexamine the fundamental concepts, because these concepts speak to the central difficulties involved in merging the two paradigms that form my tale.

First, Powers made some important changes to Wiener's original conceptualization of the negative feedback loop. These changes correct two of the point-of-view errors in cybernetic–systems theories recently criticized (cf., Locke, 1991b, 1994).

The first point-of-view error, or "objectification blunder" as Powers (1978) called it, relates to some simplifications in Wiener's original model. Powers's (1978) depiction of the control system (see Figure 2) added two elements missing from Wiener's model: the input function and disturbances. Figure 2 should be familiar to the student of SR. Like Wiener's model, it is structural. The lines represent where signals can pass and the boxes represent functions that transform the values or nature of signals. In particular, the input function translates information about the current state of the variable into a signal the system can compare with the internally represented desired state. Wiener provided no mechanism to accomplish this, yet it is arguably the most central function. Without it the thermostat could not detect the temperature of the room and our widget maker could not detect the state of his or her shelves or how many widgets he or she has produced.

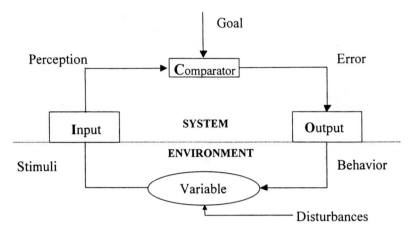

FIGURE 2 Cybernetic–control systems diagram that is similar to Powers (1973) and Carver and Scheier (1981). "Stimuli" is used where "feedback" was the label used in the earlier diagrams. This was renamed because feedback refers only to the effect of behavior on the variable, not disturbances, which also act on the variable. Also "goal" is used where Powers (1973) used the term "reference signal" and Carver and Scheier (1981) use the term "standard."

The omission of the input function assumes the point of view does not matter when assessing the state of the variable. For psychology, where it is well known that the perception of an object is not necessarily the same for all observers, this omission is very problematic. It assumes objectivity where none exists. Indeed, the input function determines the variable. Walter B. Cannon's (see Mook, 1996) theory of homeostasis was incorrect, not because the processes described were incorrect (it was a control process), but because his guess regarding what about glucose was being monitored (and hence, controlled) was wrong.

The second omission was the disturbance term (see Figure 2). Without disturbances, system outputs completely determine the state of the variable. Hence, it is reasonable to see why Wiener described his model as one of the control of output. Without an input function and any influences on the variable beyond the output of the system, the value that is compared to the desired state (i.e., the goal) could be output. However, drafts affect the temperature of a room and customers influence the number of widgets on the shelves. The specific nature of these effects on the variable are unimportant (i.e., no functions need to be described for these effects on the variable) because the input function assesses the variable, not the antecedents on the variable. This is an extremely important attribute of control systems. Systems need not "understand" the world to regulate their variables, they merely need a means to assess it, a goal for it, and a means to affect it.

Interestingly, it appears that our widget maker can be described as controlling output (i.e., behavior), in the attainment goal context because there is no disturbance effect. The number of widgets produced, (the variable) is completely a function of the number of widgets assembled. However, if the widget maker is placed in an employment context with a quality control inspector who periodically rejects a widget that has been made, we would see that the widget maker can handle disturbances: He or she will replace rejected widgets with new ones. This mistaking of the control of perceptions with the control of behavior is referred to as the behavioral illusion (Marken, 1997).

Figure 2 also exposes a second point-of-view error, the "input blunder" (Powers, 1978). Wiener labeled the goal "input" (see Figure 1). Technically, it is correct to say that these signals are input into the feedback loop. However, the implication of the word "input" is that the signal comes from outside the system (it is input into the system, not into the loop). This was often true for the types of systems that Wiener described, but not for agential systems like humans. Thus, Powers's drawing of the cybernetic unit shows more clearly the boundary between the system and its environment (see Figure 2).

Although the diagram shows that input into the system comes in the form of stimuli to the input function, the source of the goal is more mysterious. Another of Powers's major contributions to psychology and self-regulation was to place the functioning of any particular loop within a constellation of hierarchically arranged loops (Powers et al., 1960a). In this configuration, the goals for one loop, or cybernetic unit, were outputs from higher-order units (see Figure 3). Thus, goals were not determined by entities outside the system, but from inside—from the self.

One less than generous way to categorize this contribution is to say that the mystery was elaborated. What Powers did was to place a stacked set of additional cybernetic units (10 by last count) between the unspecified source of the topmost reference signal and the boundary-spanning cybernetic units (Powers, 1988). The mystery remains, but one possible answer is that the signal was there since the control structure emerged during an early period in evolutionary development (Gallistel, 1985).

The persistence of the mystery is clearly a key factor in psychology not embracing PCT, but the power of the elaboration of the hierarchical structure has played a very important role in understanding self-regulation in complex systems (Austin & Vancouver, 1996; Carver & Scheier, 1981; Cropanzano, James, & Citera, 1992; Ford, 1987; Karoly, 1993; Lord & Levy, 1994; Nelson, 1993). It makes complex perceptions understandable as a combination of molecular perceptions rising up the hierarchy. It provides an explanation of complex behavior as a function of goals and subgoals. Indeed, given this depiction, it makes more sense to say that one is not choosing behaviors to accomplish desired tasks, but that one is

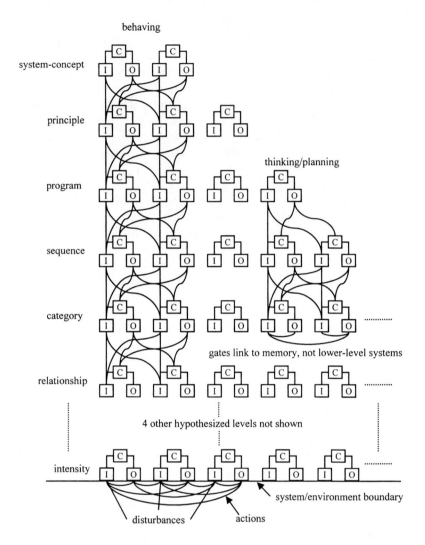

FIGURE 3   Adaptation of Powers's (1988) model of the hierarchy of control. Information flows up from input functions (I) to comparator functions (C) and to other input functions. Information flows down from output functions (O) to comparator functions or to input functions.

choosing subgoals (Austin & Vancouver, 1996). The goal levels for the last set of subgoals determine muscle tensions, which is where the system acts on the environment. Hence, it is the bottom-most cybernetic units that bridge the gap between thought and action (cf. Guthrie, 1935).

Powers (1988) provided a pictorial representation of the hierarchy (see Figure 3). Although it looks complex, begin by understanding that each set of three boxes labeled "I," "C," and "O" represent the input, comparator, and output function of the simple cybernetic unit (see Figure 2). Thus, the model is parsimonious. Second, the lines between the units show the lines of communication between the functions. Input lines pass signals up the hierarchy from the input functions of lower-level units to the input functions of higher-level units. Output lines pass signals from the output functions of higher-level units to the comparators of lower-level units.

A significant difference between this representation and that of others (e.g., Carver & Scheier, 1981; Lord & Levy, 1994) is the multiple connections shown between the units. This is important because it captures the parallel processing of these units. Signals are passed up the input function lines and down the output function lines simultaneously and across numerous units. A second difference between this representation and those of others is the depiction of thinking/planning on the right-hand side of Figure 3. I will hold off talking about that aspect until later in the chapter.

In the meantime, an example using the widget maker is useful. Recall that his or her goal is shelves full of widgets. To maintain this goal he or she makes widgets. Making widgets requires subgoals (e.g., obtain parts, have part A connected to part B, etc.). Over time, these subgoals produce all the actions required to complete a widget. Thus, as customers purchase widgets, an error is created between the goal and the widget maker's perception of the state of the shelves. This is not a problem; it simply changes the levels of the subgoals required to make widgets.

This changing of subgoals need not be a conscious process. Indeed, because the widget maker knows what to do to make widgets, he or she need not think about it (thinking is described later). Instead, the output function translates the error into subgoal signals for specific lower-level units. Those subgoals in turn creates errors (i.e., discrepancies between the subgoal and the perception for that unit) in the cybernetic units involved. For example, to make a widget, the first subgoal may be "have raw materials." This signal is not a behavior (e.g., get raw materials), because the process of getting the materials requires another host of subgoals (e.g., perceive yourself walking toward the raw materials). To meet the goal of walking in a particular direction requires a host of muscles operating in a coordinated, yet parallel manner. Fortunately, that coordination developed when our widget maker was a young child; he or she need not think about that either.

This description of subgoals of perceptions can be awkward, but it is important to be theoretically consistent. It clearly highlights the role of goals in behavior and, therefore, the role of self-regulation. Note, however, that this description does not match everyone's description of self-regulation because conscious processes are not necessarily involved (cf. Locke, 1991a; Kanfer, 1990).

Before leaving PCT, it is important to note that the more formal (i.e., mathematical) version of Powers's model includes a gain factor and a lag factor. Gain is analogous to Wiener's compensator. It has been equated with importance (Austin & Vancouver, 1996) and the level of arousal associated with a discrepancy from the goal (Ford, 1987). In an operating control unit, gain determines the precision of the unit (Powers, 1978). Units with higher gain maintain their variables at their reference level more precisely than units with lower gain because they amplify error (i.e., discrepancies). In living systems, gain reflects the state of the energy–matter subsystem (Miller, 1978), but for Powers's model this is only likely to be true for the lowest-level units because they use the muscles to act on the environment. Powers incorporated gain into the output function; hence, it does not appear as its own function in Figure 2.

To understand the impact of gain, let us return to the widget maker. Suppose that our widget maker makes both widgets and gadgets. For both, the goal is to keep the shelves stocked, but for widgets the gain is higher. Over time we would see much less variance in the state of the widget shelves than the state of the gadget shelves. Widgets have priority. One could speculate that this is likely the case if widgets represent a greater profit margin for our widget maker. That is, gains are determined by a control unit seeking to maximize profit. Gains are not controlled; they are part of the output function that regulates the maximization of profit.

The other factor, lag, reflects the speed at which the cybernetic unit reduces discrepancies. Lags occur in the environmental side and the system side of control systems. On the environment side, things can take different times for information to flow (e.g., departments that submit monthly versus daily reports). On the system side, lag is determined by the time scale over which the state of the variable is averaged (Powers, 1973). If a cybernetic unit responds more quickly than the lower-level units to which it has sent goals, the system will oscillate. In hierarchical control systems, higher-level units can adjust the gain of rapidly responsive lower-level units to prevent oscillation and smooth out responses (Powers, 1973).

Meanwhile, Ashby (1956) argued that complex systems are able to anticipate disturbances and hence prepare or act before the perception of the current state deviates from the desired state. This is particularly important when lags in the environment preclude the ability of the system to maintain a variable on-line (i.e., in real time). For example, our widget maker might develop a clever advertising scheme. Expecting that the advertising will lead to a run on widgets, the widget maker builds an extra supply of widgets so that the stock does not run out before more can be made.

Ashby's description of control systems acting on anticipated discrepancies differs somewhat dramatically from PCT. In PCT, compensations for lags can occur as the system develops experience with the variable of interest. Hence, initially our widget maker will not anticipate the effect of advertising on the state of the shelves in the store. However, with experience, the widget maker will develop a control system that monitors the level of supplies. That control system normally has a goal of zero. Yet, when a higher-level control system perceives a new ad campaign, it will change the goal from zero to some number that is a function of the amount of error in the higher-level control system. The higher-level control system may be monitoring profit. Whenever our widget maker perceives that profits are lower than desired, he or she sets a goal of developing an advertising campaign and creating a supply of widgets.

2. Plans and Cybernetics

Before leaving the cybernetic–systems paradigm, one additional theory needs to be described. When Powers began his work (Powers et al., 1960a, 1960b), psychology was reacting to behaviorism's limited description of human behavior as purposeless and environmentally driven. Indeed, along with Powers (who was originally trained as a physicist), several prominent psychologists were articulating a revolution in thought and method. Noteworthy among them were Miller from Harvard, Galanter from the University of Pennsylvania, and Pribram from Stanford, who published their efforts in a book titled *Plans and the Structure of Behavior* (Miller, Galanter, and Pribram 1960). *Plans* used the cybernetic structure in a significant way to describe a possible theory of human behavior. Specifically, Miller et al. described a cybernetic feedback unit, the TOTE (test, operate, test, exit), as the primary unit of analysis.

The PCT and TOTE models are very similar (Austin & Vancouver, 1996). Not only are both based on the negative feedback loop, but both describe a hierarchical structure of these units to explain complex behavior. Both try to incorporate the power of the cybernetic unit and the complex system-level phenomena that can be explained when multiple units are connected in hierarchical structures. Both use the cybernetic unit to move beyond the behaviorist architecture of the reflex arc, and both describe the circular causality of the loop. Yet, each focuses on different problems, and thus emphasizes different properties available to hierarchically arranged units. In an attempt to develop a general model of behavior, Powers highlighted the central role of behavior as a means of keeping a perception in line with a fixed or varying goal. Hence, perception is the focus of perceptual control theory.

Meanwhile, Miller et al. (1960) were trying to close the gap between thought and action. They were interested in the behaviors exhibited and, particularly, the sequential pattern of those behaviors. Specifically, they were interested in how humans form and implement plans, where plans are sequences of behaviors conceived to achieve goals. Thus, where Powers was more concerned with the input side of the loop, Miller et al. (1960) were more concerned with the output side. Fortunately for Miller et al., they had an analogy for understanding plans. The analogy was the computer program, with its hierarchical structure, digital (on/off) units, and serial operation.

The TOTE model adopts these computer program properties. That is, a TOTE unit is either on or off (i.e., it is digital), and only one unit is on at a time (i.e., they operate in series). This description is substantially different from Powers's description of units operating in parallel. The TOTE description corresponds to the phenomonological experience of serial thinking and, I should add, a great deal of empirical evidence once the concept of chunking could be applied to the data (Miller, 1956). It was only more recently that the power of the parallel distributive processing (PDP) models and their description of analog processing that psychologists could realize that the PCT model might correspond better than the TOTE model to the biological constraints of the mind.

The source of this fundamental difference between the TOTE model and PCT is what the authors claim passes over the arrows in their models. For PCT, what passes is information, not in the information theory sense of reduced uncertainty, but in the electrical sense of current or a signal (Powers, 1973). In TOTE, what passes across includes three elements: energy, information, and control.

In TOTE, the concept of energy is the medium of the signal. It is probably closest to Powers's thinking because the amount of "energy" indicates the level of the signal. On the other hand, for Miller et al., information relates to information theory in that what is passed (i.e., the signal or energy) can degrade as it passes over the channel. This understanding fueled the move to digital computers, because if the signal could be interpreted as only one of two values, the receiver is less likely to err in determining the value of the signal than if a continuous signal needed to be interpreted. More recently, many engineers have come to realize that digital signals truncate information (e.g., Kosko, 1993). The third element that passes according to TOTE is control. For Miller et al., this was the most important notion of what passes, and the most unfortunate, because it dramatically changes the way a system can operate. In TOTE, control refers to the sequencing of activities. The analogy used was the running of code in a computer program. For example, in a batch file (a type of computer program), each line executes one at a time because each line represents a set of signals that need to pass through the central processing unit (CPU) or instructions regarding which signals are passed through. The CPU is a bottleneck. Only a single set of instructions and values can pass at one time. Thus values are operated on according to the instructions and pass the results on (in the form of other instructions or values), usually to be used by other lines of code.

For the purposes of this chapter, the difference in the two conceptualizations of the cybernetic unit comes down to the issue of parallel versus serial processing. TOTE runs in series. The test (or comparison) determines whether the unit operates or exits. If it exits, control is passed to another unit. The structure of the units (that is, which unit is next engaged when one is exited or what subunits are engaged when a unit is operating) determines the sequential nature of behavior for the system. On the other hand, PCT runs in parallel. All the units are comparing (testing) their perceptions with their goals and outputting signals to lower-level units depending on the results of the comparison. The structure determines the speed they test (e.g., higher-level units test at slower speeds), which units pass signals to which other units, and the nature of that signal (e.g., an output for determining a goal or gain, or an input for determining a perception). The sequencing of behavior is the job of one particular level in the hierarchy, appropriately referred to as the sequence level (Powers, 1988).

Of these two conceptualizations, the serial has clearly dominated. So pervasive is the serial description that many theories heavily influenced by PCT (e.g., Carver & Scheier, 1981; Klein, 1989) implicitly or explicitly incorporate it. Not only did it correspond to the computer analogy, so important at the time for defeating one of the behaviorists' main arguments,[1] but it also corresponded to psychology's general understanding of cognitive functioning. We seem to think in series. With the rejection of behaviorism, phenomenal experience was again a legitimate source of observation, and the work of Simon, Newell and others legitimatized the observation with working models. Miller et al. were influenced heavily by the work of Newell, Simon, and Shaw, to which they had direct access (Miller et al., 1960). Interestingly, the work of these other researchers stemmed primarily from the decision-making paradigm. TOTE was the first model to bring these two paradigms together, but the effort was flawed. To this day we are attempting to correct that flaw.

3. Summary

This section reviewed the cybernetic–systems paradigm and two specific theories within the paradigm, PCT and TOTE. In general, the cybernetic–systems paradigm describes a model of nested systems interacting in parallel that provide stability where there is instability. More complex systems are described by the integration of simpler systems, with the relatively simple cybernetic system receiving the most attention. The PCT model drops the role of systems greater in complexity than the human system from this description. The TOTE model not only drops higher-order systems, but also the parallel processing of the component systems. For understanding how a self-regulating system operates in an environment of other self-regulating systems, both simplifications are problematic. Yet, a large number of systematic observations support a model of limited cognitive capacity and serial decision making. Perhaps these observations indi-

---

[1]The behaviorists argued that systems like those described by cognitive psychologists could not work. The computer showed that they could.

cate that serial decision-making models are more appropriate for under-standing human systems. I review that paradigm next.

B. THE DECISION-MAKING PARADIGM

Like the cybernetic–systems paradigm, this part of the tale begins in the 1930s, with the contributions of Tolman (1932) and Lewin (1936). Like Miller et al. (1960) in the previous paradigm, Tolman and Lewin were largely reacting to behaviorism. Specifically, Tolman's reaction was to articulate two internal, latent constructs—expectancy and valence—as mediators between stimuli and response. These mediators later were related to subjective expected utility models used to predict various courses of action (Edwards, 1954). Lewin also articulated these intervening vari-ables as the highly measurable constructs of expectancies, instrumentali-ties, and valences (Lewin, 1951; Lewin, Dembo, Festinger, & Sears, 1944). These constructs became the basis of several models of decision making, even though they were relabeled often along the way (Austin & Vancou-ver, 1996; Kanfer, 1990).

Most decision-making models use a variant of the subjective expected utility (SEU) notion. In these models, "utility" is described hedonistically (i.e., to maximize pleasure and minimize pain). Utility is generally opera-tionalized as the degree to which an option is seen as rewarding or punishing (Stevenson, Busemeyer, & Naylor, 1990). The "subjective" ele-ment focuses on our limitations in cognitive processing (e.g., Miller, 1956; Simon, 1955), and the self-biases and heuristics we employ to get beyond our limitations (e.g., Kahneman, Slovic, & Tversky, 1982). The "expected" element requires that we carry models of the world in our heads (i.e., mental models) and use them to predict the consequences of our actions (e.g., Bandura, 1986; Stevenson et al., 1990).

For these mental models to be of any use, a somewhat predictable world is required. Returning to the widget maker illustrates this point. Recall the advertising scheme that the widget maker anticipates will lead to an increase in sales of widgets. Predicting the level of sales requires sufficient data from past experience with similar conditions to calculate contingen-cies. However, the effect of a particular, new advertising campaign is an unknown. It may work well or work poorly. The widget maker easily could overproduce, which could be a major problem if widgets are a perishable good, or underproduce, which would result in the loss of sales and possibly customers. The cybernetic–systems approach to this problem would be to seek to decrease the lag in widget making (Lord & Maher, 1990; Senge, 1990). This would allow the widget maker to respond to the effect of the campaign instead of guess at its effect. Perhaps the question for this chapter is whether nature selected for the decision-making approach, the cybernetic-systems approach, or some combination.

According to decision-making theories, the models in our heads reflect our beliefs about contingencies and the value of consequences (Austin & Vancouver, 1996). The contingencies include beliefs about one's own capacities to affect the environment (i.e., self-efficacy, capacity beliefs) or the probabilities that effort will lead to results (i.e., expectancy), and beliefs about the relationships between objects in the environment (i.e., instrumentalities, outcome expectancies, context beliefs). Beliefs about consequences include the anticipated value of the outcomes from the person's perspective (e.g., valence). The SEU theories attempt to articulate mathematical combinations of these constructs that parallel the way they are combined in our minds prior to making choices. The hope is that the mathematics can generalize to all individuals, whereas the levels of the constructs will differ for different individuals. Hence, SEU theories are nomothetic models that explain, or account for, individual differences. Nonetheless, they describe a limited aspect of human behavior in that they apply only to the prediction of choices among options (Stevenson et al., 1990). Furthermore, the usefulness of predictions regarding the effects of the choices on future states works only when (a) the world is predictable, (b) the person can reasonably accurately model that predictability in their minds, and (c) the cues necessary for the prediction are somewhat accurately knowable (Lord & Maher, 1990).

Despite these inherent limitations in the phenomenon to which they might reasonably apply, decision-making theories have had such a strong impact on psychology and the study of motivation in I/O psychology that some people consider all aspects of motivation to be a choice (Campbell & Pritchard, 1976). Until recently, the primary theory of motivation in I/O psychology was expectancy theory (Vroom, 1964), and the aspect of social cognitive theory (SCT; Bandura, 1986, 1991) that has received the most attention in I/O is the self-efficacy component. Indeed, the more dynamic potential of SCT and decision-making models has been ignored mostly. The reason for this lack of dynamic conceptualizing and studies may be traceable to the original contributors, Lewin and Tolman.

Lewin, because he perceived difficulties in testing and modeling dynamic processes in humans, emphasized the immediate prediction of behavior (preferably a molar prediction) based on the current state of the system. Ironically, Wiener had the exact same reservation about testing cybernetics with human, particularly social phenomena (Richardson, 1991). Lewin also preferred general statistical laws to specific idiographic prediction because of the difficulty of assessing all the parameters within an individual. His development of practical methods for assessing a few key states and his relatively successful prediction with those variables also contributed substantially to its adoption. Indeed, earlier, more complex versions of his topographic theorizing have seen less success (Hill, 1985).

Likewise, Tolman was not only molar, but also did not tend to take himself too seriously (Hill, 1985). The molarity stance left his rats buried in thought (Guthrie, 1935). He never tried to get to the molecular level of the muscles. According to Hill (1985), Tolman's whimsical stance made it difficult for anyone to take his theoretical work seriously, even if his empirical work was stellar.

These attitudes, with some exceptions, heavily influenced decision-making models in the ensuing years. Specifically, decision-making models tend to share several features in common. First, they tend to be nondynamic (cf. Kleinmuntz, 1993), referring to the choices given a static situation. Hence, they cannot account for changing environments (Kanfer, 1990) or changing internal states. This feature is reflected in the role of goals in decision-making models, which is that they are all but ignored, even though both Tolman and Lewin used the goal construct as a major component of their theorizing. This omission is possible because when using a static model of decision making, the goal properties of expectancies and valences can be conceived of as static. There is no need to account for the possibility that as individuals accomplish their goals, valences and expectancies can change. The second common feature is that they are serial. Decisions are made one at a time, owing by most accounts, to the attentional bottleneck (Simon, 1994).

Although the serial and static qualities are indicative of much of the research in this area, there are exceptions. Problem solving is an aspect of the decision-making paradigm that incorporates goals and change. Stevenson et al. (1990) noted that "the terms problem solving and decision making are often used interchangeably" (p. 285). Yet, they argue that the problem-solving branch is much more dynamic in that it refers more to the "construction" of alternatives, whereas decision making is about the "selection" of alternatives. While maintaining a distinction, a more detailed look at the problem-solving aspect of the decision-making paradigm is required.

1. Problem Solving

Once dynamics enters back into the picture, the goal reemerges as key. According to Proctor and Dutta (1995), "most contemporary research on problem solving originates from the work of Newell and Simon (1972) ..." (p. 204). Newell and Simon speak of the understanding and searching processes of a problem space determined by the problem task. Different understandings can lead to different representations of the problem space, but it is the processes of searching that most interests us here. Again, to quote Proctor and Dutta (1995),

> If human information processing capacity were unlimited, it would be possible to consider simultaneously the entire set of problem states and relations between the problem states. However, processing capacity is limited such that only one problem space operator can be applied and only a limited number of states considered at a

time (Newell, 1980). Consequently, strategies for searching the problem space are an important part of problem solving. To accomplish the problem solution requires a search through the problem space in which operators are applied and new states are considered. Search proceeds by selecting a state and then an operator; applying the operator to the present state, thereby producing a new state; and deciding whether to move into the new state and whether the goal state has been achieved. If the goal state has not been achieved, this general procedure is repeated. For all but the most trivial problems, successful search will depend on some strategy for evaluating progress toward the goal and selecting the next move within the problem space. (p. 206)

Two interesting points are made in this paragraph. First, the search process is described as serial because of the limited capacity of the central information processor (again, the computer analogy is strong in this work). Second, the role of goal states and anticipated possible states (i.e., constructed new states) is key to describing the processes. Specifically, the model compares the newly constructed state with the goal state and operates differently based on that comparison. This description is exactly analogous to the TOTE model. This not a coincidence. Recall that Miller et al. were heavily influenced by the (then preliminary) work of Newell, Simon, and colleagues. Subsequently, Newell and Simon read and incorporated the TOTE model.

Although problem solving and decision making are generally conceptualized as serial, the long-term behavioral implications of these processes are not. For instance, Anderson's (1983) adaptive control of thought (ACT) theory attempts to deal with the observation that problem solving appears to heavily tax cognitive processing, but that over time that demand relaxes. In other words, problem solving begins as a serial process, but it does not end that way. Not that the problem-solving behaviors disappear; instead, they can be executed rapidly and while other cognitively taxing processing is also occurring. These are indicative qualities of "automatic" processing (Schneider & Shiffrin, 1977; Shiffrin & Schneider, 1977). Ironically, these types of processes needed to be considered seriously after Miller's (1956) description of the limits of cognitive processing because of his use of the concept of chunking. Chunks, which formed after practice, allowed the system to group what had been several pieces of information into one. Thus, the system could objectively handle greater amounts of information because it was subjectively reducing that information into fewer pieces.

2. In Sum

In this section I review the general decision-making paradigm. In this case, the general model is more limited than the first paradigm in that it attempts to describe the processes involved in the selection of choices. In line with the more practical side of its founders, the decision-making paradigm has tended to be molar, static, and serial. However, returning to the more conceptual work of its founders, dynamic, goal-centered processes have been reintroduced in Newell and Simon's (1972) description of problem solving. Owing to the relatively more recent work in automatic and parallel processing, attempts have been made to describe the process of movement from serial to parallel processing. This is a process addressed again after a description of the conflicts that emerged between the paradigms and among SR theories in I/O psychology.

IV. THE PARADIGMS IN INDUSTRIAL–ORGANIZATIONAL PSYCHOLOGICAL THEORIES OF SELF-REGULATION

Prior to reviewing the paradigms, two short lists of I/O-specific theories were presented (Kanfer, 1990; Locke, 1991a). The two theories that overlapped the lists, goal-setting theory and SCT, incorporate parts of both paradigms. Each is discussed subsequently. In addition, action theory, which is a popular self-regulation theory in European occupational psychology (Frese & Zapf, 1993) incorporates both paradigms and also is described subsequently.

A. GOAL-SETTING THEORY

Goal-setting theory was inductively derived from the application of various manipulations (Locke, 1968; Locke & Latham, 1990). For much of its history it was atheoretical. It describes the generally positive impact of specific, challenging goals and feedback on performance. Control theory has been used to explain these findings (Campion & Lord, 1982), but Locke has adamantly rejected that explanation (Locke, 1991b, 1994; Locke & Latham, 1990). Generally, much more attention is given to the decision-making aspects of goal-setting theory (Naylor & Ilgen, 1984). Much research and conceptualizing focuses on the antecedents of accepting or choosing difficult goals, and goal commitment (Kanfer, 1990). Most of these antecedents relate to the expectancies and values placed on the accomplishment of the goal. Indeed, once Garland (1984) resolved the instrumentality paradox by showing that the contradictory predictions of goal-setting theory and expectancy theory could be resolved by distinguishing between relationships found within experimental groups from those found between groups, the marriage of goal-setting and expectancy theory was complete (Locke, 1991a). In addition, Locke embraced several concepts from SCT and incorporated them into his theory (Kanfer, 1990).

B. SOCIAL COGNITIVE THEORY

In I/O psychology, Latham and his colleagues (Frayne & Latham, 1987; Latham & Frayne, 1989; Latham & Locke, 1991) adopted SCT as a guiding framework for constructing work behavior interventions in SR. The reader is encouraged to look at this work directly. SCT incorporates several classes of goals (e.g., performance, social, self) and cognitive evaluations of contingencies, capabilities, and outcomes. The cognitive evaluations parallel the expectancy–value models, particularly of Lewin (Bandura, 1991). Indeed, perhaps the central construct of SCT is self-efficacy, which is a judgment of one's capacity to perform at a given level. Self-efficacy presumably improves on expectancy because it includes not only the notion of the contingency between the person and action, but also links to attributions and goals of competency (e.g., Deci & Ryan, 1985). Another concept, forethought, allows humans to anticipate the consequences of their actions and judge the value of those consequences. Together these elements are housed in an "executive control system" that Bandura claims may be superimposed onto the negative feedback operation of cybernetic systems (Bandura, 1991). Likewise, he claims that the hierarchical goal structure is inadequate for explaining the discrepancy creation that occurs as individuals strive for higher levels of performance after successful performance. He claims his theory reflects an open loop, whereas PCT reflects a closed loop. Because of the role of this distinction in the conflict, the difference between an open and closed loop conceptualization needs further elucidation.

Open and closed have been used as adjectives to describe both loops and systems. Part of the conflict may arise from confusing these concepts (Vancouver, 1998). Specifically, any system that interacts with its environment is open. It is a requirement of living systems (Richardson, 1991). Powers (1988) noted that his theory refers to open systems, which can be seen in the crossing of the environment–system border in Figure 2. Meanwhile, Powers described a closed negative feedback loop. Powers uses closed to emphasize the circular causality of the loop: The actions of the system affect subsequent actions. Our widget maker makes widgets until the number of widgets he or she has made meets his or her goals. This is the fundamental contribution of Rosenblueth, Wiener, and Bigelow (1943). It is very different from the behaviorist's reflex arc architecture, which posits that behavior is solely a function of environmental stimuli. The arc ends with behavior. The loop never ends; it is closed.

On the other hand, Bandura (1991) calls the loop open because goals and other elements in the loop can change. In particular, Bandura emphasizes the system's influence on the loop. At first, Bandura's description seems perfectly compatible with the PCT description of the hierarchical goal structure, because goal signals impact the loop (i.e., determine goal levels) from higher-level units within the system, but outside the focal loop. Also, disturbances to the environmental variables are outside the loop and impact behavior because the system compensates for the disturbances. Hence, the loop as described by Powers always has been "exposed," if not open.

Yet neither the disturbance nor the hierarchical structural influences capture Bandura's problem with the closed loop concept. He claims additional, internal influences. In general, the name given to these internal influences is volition (Locke, 1991a). Volition, which is often a central concept in SR, may be a causality or a hero in the conflict that underlies the tale of the two paradigms. However, at this point, it is so difficult to get agreement regarding its meaning, much less its existence, and evidence from SCT and PCT has been used to validate it (Sappington, 1990), so that it is likely to provide little help. More specifically, Bandura (1991) evokes self-system concepts, like self-motivation and self-satisfaction, to explain the tendency for humans to seek challenging goals, to persist when they accomplish no (hypothesized) higher-level goal, and even to derive pleasure from the pursuit, regardless of the consequences.

For Powers, these concepts (e.g., volition, self-satisfaction, etc.) fly in the face of science (Powers, 1991). They do not describe the mechanisms by which they work. For Locke (1991a), that is the point. Mechanisms imply determinism. Instead, Locke prefers to adopt the soft determinism commonly found in the decision-making paradigm (i.e., one can measure expectancy–value concepts to predict behavior, but one can never ultimately identify the source of the values).

Attempts to combine control theory and decision-making theories have emerged (Hyland, 1988; Klein, 1989; Lord & Hanges, 1987). However, these are similar to SCT and goal-setting theory in that they describe the predictive advantage of using expectancy–value concepts with control theory concepts, not the structure mechanisms involved. Another theory, action theory, does this and more. It is discussed next.

C. ACTION THEORY

Action theory perhaps best exemplifies the combination of the cybernetic–systems and decision-making paradigms. Its central advocates tend to be German (Frese & Zapf, 1993; Hacker, 1985), and they have developed a very rich and comprehensive theory. Action theory derives from Tolman and Lewin (Frese & Sabini, 1985a), but unlike decision-making theories in American psychology, it kept the goal concept. The TOTE model was highly influential as well (Frese & Sabini, 1985b; Frese & Zapf, 1993). Thus, cybernetic principles underlie much of the work.

The similarities between action theory and PCT are dramatic (see Table 1). Action theory has attended to the goal hierarchy and considers both serial and parallel (i.e., automatic) processing. However, according to Frese and Zapf (1993), an explanation for parallel processing has not been incorporated into the theory. Hence, it is considered a major theoretical gap for action theory. The opposite problem exists for PCT. What is

TABLE 1   Comparing Action Theory with Perceptual Control Theory

	Action theory	Perceptual control theory
Focus	Purposeful behavior	Purposeful behavior
Working principles	Objective reality; internal constructs	Objective reality; internal constructs
Basic construct	Goal (conscious)	Goal (conscious or unconscious)
Basic building block	Cybernetic unit	Cybernetic unit
Controlled construct	Action	Perception
Basic structure	Hierarchical (4 or 5 levels)	Hierarchical (11 levels)
Operation	Serial (controlled) & parallel (automatic)	Parallel & serial
Related theoretical problem	How does system handle multiple goals simultaneously?	Why is serial necessary at all?
Feedback	All information relating to current state	Aspect of current state caused by actions
Knowledge	Representation of condition–action–result interrelations (operative image system)	Representation of source weights and operations of perceptions: goals for lower level systems and source of goals (functions)
Error	Potentially avoidable goal nonattainment	Discrepancy of perception from goal

unaccounted for is serial processing. This is an interesting difference, which I will address subsequently.

Finally, three vocabulary terms—feedback, knowledge, and error—differ (but overlap) between the two theories. These are not all just semantic differences. By calling all the input into the system "feedback," the theory implies that all the variance to the environmental variable is a function of the output of the system (which is fed back) and not a combination of the system's output and disturbances. This harks back to the objectification blunder discussed earlier. Indeed, several control theorists call input "feedback," but conceptually this adds ambiguity to the term.

A second difference is the understanding of the nature of knowledge. For action theory, knowledge is the representation of contingencies between conditions, actions, and outcomes. For PCT, knowledge is represented in the functions. It may be that each function is a series of weighted connections that transform the signals passing between the functions, but it is unclear whether the weighted connections might include representations of contingencies.

The differences between the meaning of the term error does appear to be semantic. For the purposes of this chapter, I use error in the PCT sense. Error in the action theory sense is what I later call out-of-tolerance error. Nevertheless, I/O psychologists are well served by reading the research by action theorists regarding their concept of error (see, for example, Reason & Zapf, 1994).

D. SUMMARY

In I/O psychology the combination of cybernetic and decision-making concepts is common, yet their marriage is a tenuous one due to conflicts between the adherents (e.g., Bandura, 1989; Powers, 1991). New theories that incorporate both are populating management (e.g., Tsui & Ashford, 1994) and psychology journals (e.g., Kluger & DeNisi, 1996). For example, Kluger and DeNisi (1996) conducted a meta-analysis of the feedback intervention literature and found a great deal of variation in the results. Their approach to filling the gap between the evidence of the effectiveness of a prominent I/O intervention and the desired level of effectiveness was to detail the theory of the phenomenon better. Labeled feedback intervention theory (FIT), Kluger and DeNisi essentially detailed the implications of feedback if control theory accurately described humans. Likewise, Tsui and Ashford's (1994) theory of the adaptive self-regulation quality of managers utilizes both decision-making and cybernetic principles. Yet, the conflict between the decision-making and cybernetic–systems approaches is not likely to abate without addressing some fundamentals. In the next section, I describe an aspect of Powers's theory that has received little attention, especially from Powers himself, but might provide the architecture that joins the paradigms.

V. MERGING THE PARADIGMS

The juncture of cybernetics and decision making describes another source of exposure for the closed loop. Specifically, it addresses the question of changes in the functions. Given that changes to the functions provide a relatively permanent change to the system, this particular mechanism also relates to self-regulated learning.

A. LEARNING IN THE ACTION HIERARCHY

Few people in psychology appear aware of the explanation of learning within PCT (e.g., Hill, 1985). Instead, the theory is usually presented as describing how someone currently regulates, not how that regulation came about (e.g., Carver & Scheier, 1981). To describe learning in self-regulation requires describing how the input functions, output functions, and comparator functions come into existence or change. Describing the processes of change is much less daunting then describing creation; hence, only the former is discussed here. To circumscribe the task even more, I describe only changes to the output functions. These are the functions that determine the goal levels for lower-level units and, ultimately, action. It is here that the union of decision making and cybernetics is likely to be found.

Like Kuhl's (1994) homunculi or Minsky's (1986) minds, the model involves agents operating on agents. In this case, the agents are individual cybernetic units. Figure 4 illustrates the mechanism. The agent acted upon is the perceptual unit. Acting on this perceptual unit is an internal unit (cf, intrinsic unit, Powers, 1973), which monitors the error coming from the perceptual unit's comparator. It has a desired level of error, or goal'. The prime symbol distinguishes the internal unit components and values from the perceptual unit's. Further, the internal unit has an output function (e.g., O') that acts on, at a minimum, the output function of the perceptual unit. The action of the internal unit's output function is to change the perceptual unit's output function. Powers (1973) calls change to a function the "reorganization" of that function. Thus, if a discrepancy arises between the internal unit's perception and its goal, its output function reorganizes the output function of the perceptual unit.

The exact mechanism of reorganization is less clear. In 1973 Powers wrote, "The effects of the outputs of the reorganizing system must be such as to change the properties of behavioral systems. ... Several mechanisms are known to have such effects: synaptic thresholds can be altered chemically or by neural signals; new synaptic connections can grow even in the adult brain, and presumably can wither away, too" (p. 185). The exact nature of these neurological processes are important, but are beyond the tale presented here. Suffice it to say, if learning occurs and that learning

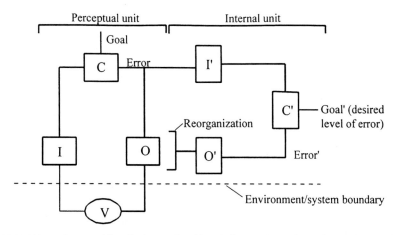

FIGURE 4   Reorganizing the internal unit's relation to the action unit. I = input function; C = comparator function; O = output function; V = variable.

changes the brain in some way, the processes that control that learning need to be specified. That is what the reorganization model provides.

Specifically, reorganization changes the way errors are handled in the perceptual unit. However, not just any perceptual unit error will lead to reorganization. A well-functioning control system might experience a great deal of error during normal operation (e.g., the thermostat in your home). Instead, the input function for this internal unit may be one of three types. One type might assess the magnitude of error, where goal prime defines the boundary value. Anything beyond that level is out of bounds. The second type of input function might assess the length of error. For example, chronic error indicates a problem for the perceptual unit. Error that rises and falls within normal bounds does not indicate a problem for that unit. Whereas error that plateaus and remains, even though within bounds in magnitude, might usefully trigger reorganization. The third type of input function might assess rate of progress. Again, error is allowed and expected, but if it is not reduced rapidly enough, given the lag indicative of units at the particular level of the hierarchy in question, it might indicate a time for a change in tactics. The three types of errors all indicate errors that are out of tolerance. If they are sufficiently large (i.e., greater than goal prime), they create error prime. As mentioned earlier, these comprise the subset of errors action theorists call errors (e.g., Frese & Zapf, 1993).

Error in the internal unit results in changes to the perceptual unit's output function because the internal unit's output function is engaged. The changes effect the error in the perceptual unit, which the internal unit is monitoring. When that error begins dropping, error prime drops to zero and reorganization stops. The perceptual unit's output function is now organized in a way that reduces the errors it experiences. That is, the negative feedback loop is functioning again.

To take this description out of the abstract, let us return to our hard working widget maker. Recall that his or her goal is to keep the widget shelves full. When a customer purchases a widget, the state of the shelves deviates from full, thus creating an error in his or her cybernetic unit. This error is simply handled by setting the subgoals levels necessary to make widgets. Suppose, however, that after a successful advertising campaign, the widget maker has trouble keeping enough widgets on the shelves. This creates a chronic error in the keep-shelves-full control unit. This chronic error may prompt the widget maker to change the way he or she makes widgets until a more efficient method is found. Failing that, the widget maker might decide to hire another worker to keep up with the demand. The result is that the goal remains the same, "keep the shelves full," but the subgoals (i.e., output function) change.

Were these changes simple, the preceding description of reorganization might be adequate. However, the neurological mechanisms require a trial-and-error approach to problem solving (i.e., out-of-tolerance error correction). Although this description might sometimes apply (e.g., when guessing), individuals often change behavior more smoothly and more effectively than simply trial and error. Fortunately, owing to the hierarchical nature of control systems hypothesized to exist within the individual, a more effective reorganization process can be articulated: A process that is very consistent with the decision-making and problem-solving processes described earlier. To do this requires memory and one more architectural component.

B. GATES AND MODES OF OPERATION

The architectural component is a gate that switches the flow of information between the environment and memory. Placing a gate at the foot of the input function and another at the foot of the output function provides four modes of operation for any given control unit (Powers, 1973; Vancouver, 1996). Table 2 lists the four modes and the condition of each gate that uniquely describes each mode. Note that one might be uncomfortable with the dichotomous nature of this description, preferring instead to conceive of a mechanism that determines the relative weight of the information that comes from these sources. However, the dichotomous mechanism is easier to describe and may be correct. The exact form of the mechanisms can be the source of future theory building and empirical testing.

Within the cybernetic–systems paradigm, the mode that I have been describing up to this point is the behaving mode. Information about the current state of the environmental variable comes from the environment. Information about subgoals needed to determine muscle tensions that cause action on the environment are sent down the hierarchy to the muscles and, thus, to the environment.

The next mode, observing, takes in information from the environment, but simply stores it in memory. No actual behaviors regarding the particular control unit are attempted. This mode is most analogous to Bandura's modeling concept. Representations of environmental variable states that can reduce discrepancies (i.e., control perceptions) can be stored in memory for later use. For this to work, we must connect the representations (or

TABLE 2   Modes of Operation

	Input gate	Output gate
Behaving	Environment	Environment
Observing	Environment	Memory
Thinking	Memory	Memory
Assuming	Memory	Environment

symbols, to use Bandura's term) to output functions. This is not straight-forward, but the thinking mode provides the vehicle.

In the thinking mode, both the input gate and output gate are set to memory. This may be the serial decision-making and problem-solving mode that allows relatively effective behavioral choice in response to out-of-tolerance error. Figure 3 is needed to understand how this might work. Under the label "thinking/planning" are several control units with connections between the levels. However, unlike their neighbors to the left, the units do not connect all the way down to the environment/system boundary. Instead, gates controlled by the internal cybernetic units switch the outputs of certain perceptual units to the inputs of their own and other units. Phenomenologically, this would be like thinking to yourself, "If I did this, that would happen," and it likely involves attentional processes (Powers, 1973). The process creates a guess regarding the likely percep-tions following the setting of subgoals at certain levels. These guesses are based on the past perceptions that resulted when the subgoals where set at those levels. That is, the thinking mode allows a system to test its potential subgoal specifications prior to engaging with the environment.

At least two assumptions are required to connect this architectural model with the decision-making paradigm. First, the subgoal patterns must be tied to specific, potential perceptions. Hence, when a subgoal configu-ration is "tested," it retrieves the perceptions that arose in the past when that configuration was used. Valence (e.g., anticipated value) is then the reduction in errors (e.g., discrepancies of perceptions from goals) produced by the subgoal configuration. This seems a reasonable assumption when the configuration and the perceptions are within the same system. How-ever, if observation mode (e.g., behavioral modeling) is to work, the subgoal configuration that created the perceptions observed must be knowable by the observing system. This requires a symbolic processing system (e.g., Newell, 1990).

The second assumption is that the probabilities that a subgoal configu-ration will lead to a perception (or set of perceptions) can be retrieved or generated during the thinking process. These probabilities are the ex-pectancies and instrumentalities associated with subgoal configurations. They and the valences become relevant when multiple alternative subgoal configurations might work to reduce errors. Then the alternatives can be tested for the highest probability of the most error reduction. Of course, the tests are only as good as the predictability of the environment, the memory stores used to form the hypothesized state of the variable, and the probabilities. Given these limitations, it is perhaps not surprising that we find that extensive planning procedures do not work and do not tend to be descriptive of behaviors of individuals working on complex tasks (e.g., Carroll, 1997).

So when our widget maker contemplates the dire state of his or her shelves, he or she might think about the perception of full shelves. To accomplish this goal, the widget maker sees in his or her mind's eye that it requires making widgets as rapidly as they are bought. The widget maker might think about past actions that have led to perceptions of rapid widget making, where these actions are represented as subgoal configurations in his or her memory, or might remember that when a larger supply of raw materials was purchased, he or she could work more rapidly at making widgets. Alternatively, the widget maker might use higher-level goal configurations and their perceptions (e.g., stored universal plans; Earley & Shalley, 1991) to "see" this connection at a more abstract level. Hence, a subgoal configuration that increases the desired level of raw materials on hand is adopted. To accomplish this, the widget maker also changes the desired level of raw materials bought from each supplier. The widget maker might envision giving cash to a supplier and realize the need to get more cash from the bank before visiting suppliers or he or she will run out in the middle of the transaction. Thinking about all the subgoals more, the widget maker might wonder about the ability of his or her car to hold all the raw materials. If the widget maker does not think about all the subgoals, has no past experience, or is met with an unexpected disturbance, he or she might be unable to accomplish the new subgoals without modifications.

Thus, I am suggesting that the reorganization of a higher-level output function involves two processes: it changes the output function and it puts lower-level units in thinking mode, so that the reorganized function can be tested. Powers (1991) pointed out that because the memories used for testing are so likely to be flawed and that parallel processing is much more efficient, the system can much more effectively interact on-line in parallel with real-time data. Indeed, in the lower levels, it is very difficult to see much merit in using thinking to predict environmental states, or in operating in series. The system can receive information and act very rapidly, simply, and simultaneously to disturbances to the variables (Marken, 1992). There is no need to anticipate those disturbances or to extrapolate the likely effects on the perceptions of environmental variables when setting subgoals at certain levels. However, at higher levels this is less likely to be true and the model proposed nicely conforms to a great deal of research in psychology (Austin & Vancouver, 1996), especially on decision making (Beach, 1990; Newell, 1990).

C. SOME DATA

One line of research seems especially relevant to the role of attentional processes in control systems. Vallacher and Wegner (1987), under the rubric "action identification theory," described a series of studies on out-of-tolerance error. One particularly simple, but clever, study illustrates the principle. This experiment had two conditions. In both conditions participants were to drink a cup of coffee. However, in one of the conditions they used a regular cup; in the other they used a dribble cup (i.e., a trick cup that makes it very difficult to get the liquid out without spilling on yourself). After some time with the coffee, the experimenter asked the participants what they were doing. The participants in the regular cup condition reported getting a good drink, getting a caffeine buzz, or other goals associated with drinking coffee. The participants in the dribble cup condition reported that they were trying to get the liquid into their mouths. Actually, the students in the regular cup condition were trying to get the liquid into their mouths, but the subgoals (i.e., output functions) required to do that were well practiced and nothing in the environment caused the discrepancies in any of the subsystems to go out of tolerance. On the other hand, in the dribble cup condition, perceptions relating to the flow of the liquid into one's mouth, and not one's lap, were so far from the normal, that errors were out of bounds. This resulted in the system trying (and thinking) about ways to get to the perception (liquid in mouth) desired.

This description conforms to Powers's (1973) speculation that conscious attention indicates what unit is reorganizing. Another speculation of Powers that was written for the 1973 book, but not published until recently, relates to the role of emotions (Powers, 1992). Carver and Scheier (1990) looked into similar ideas, focusing on the rate-of-progress type internal system. Specifically, they reviewed a large amount of research demonstrating the relationship between rate of progress toward goal attainment and emotional reactions: Too slow and the person has a negative reaction and brings attentional resources to bear on the problem; faster than expected and more favorable emotions arise.

In I/O psychology, Beach (1990) and Mitchell and Beach (1990) described a theory of decision making in which comparisons are made between anticipated or current perceptions and desired perceptions. They use the TOTE term "image" instead of perception, which inspired their theory's title, image theory. According to image theory and the evidence they are collecting (e.g., Beach, 1993), the system engages in more systematic search and serial decision making only when comparisons are too far off tolerance. Otherwise, it hums along automatically regulating the variables in its environment, without the need for conscious decision making.

Other researchers in I/O psychology have described the connection of cybernetic and decision-making models and the role of automatic processes in goal-directed behavior (e.g., Klein, 1989). Also, research studies have supported the combined role of cybernetic and decision-making principles (e.g., Kernan & Lord, 1990; Klein, 1991; Tubbs, Boehne, &

Dahl, 1993). However, no one has attempted to describe the cybernetic architecture required to account for both approaches.

VI. CONCLUSION

A book chapter is insufficient for communicating the specifies of self-regulation theories in I/O psychology. Instead, I have tried to give the reader a review of the two general paradigms that have informed those theories and some of the conflicts that have arisen between the paradigms. Nonetheless, specifics are important, so I have tried also to detail a specific model at the point where the two paradigms merge.

Throughout this chapter the difference between serial and parallel processing has been emphasized. I have argued that cybernetic–systems theory tends to describe humans as a system operating in parallel (TOTE is the exception). Meanwhile, the decision-making paradigm tends to describe humans as serial. Yet systems act both ways. Specifically, it appears that when in the thinking and observation mode, the cybernetic units process in series. Why this is the case is not exactly clear. Nonetheless, hypotheses can be generated with the architecture described. For example, consistent with much of cognitive psychology, one might speculate that when the output gate is set to memory, short-term memory (STM) is used. Thus, although units can be operating in parallel, units in thinking and observation mode must share this limited resource, which forces serial processing (the attentional bottleneck). Other hypotheses should be entertained, like the limitations in physical systems (e.g., time is serial, sight is unidirectional). Nonetheless, the key issue is that a description of learning can integrate the two types of processing into a single model.

Three suggestions come to mind regarding the focus of future work for self-regulation. First, much work can continue to examine a relatively narrow class of systems (e.g., the manager) and how those systems affect and are affected by the constellation of systems surrounding them (e.g., Tsui & Ashford, 1994). Second, close examination of the similarities and differences in the variants of cybernetic–systems and decision-making models is necessary. This examination not only simplifies the scientist's work by eliminating redundancy of concepts and theory, but also exposes key gaps in understanding to which empirical and theoretical work can be focused. We should try to resolve those places where highly overlapping theories like control theory and action theory disagree. This research is often basic in nature, but will ultimately prove more useful than micro problem solving.

A third approach for self-regulation would be to focus on methodological issues (Marken, 1997). The methodological implications of cybernetic systems are a major stumbling block to validating the model. It is likely that one reason decision-making research proceeded down the static, snapshot path was because of the difficulties in conducting research in dynamic environments and estimating parameters in dynamic models. Fortunately, researchers are beginning to create dynamic environments (e.g., Dörner & Schaub, 1994; Kleinmuntz, 1993; Rasmussen, Brehmer, & Leplat, 1990), and systems dynamic researchers (Levine & Fitzgerald, 1992; Richardson, 1991) have been creating dynamic models. However, short of qualitative analysis and action research (Runkel, 1990), applied psychologists have had little help in testing the more dynamic aspects of their theories. A firm grasp of the breadth of the cybernetic–systems paradigm is likely to be most useful because many people have grappled with the problem for a long time (Richardson, 1991). For I/O psychologists, simply reading the other chapters in this book is likely to lead to relevant and novel study designs.

To return to my allusion of Dicken's novel, many psychologists fear the creation of a single paradigm for psychology for the reasons that prompted Dicken's to write his novel of the French revolution. They fear that the numerous old dictators of the past will be slain, only to have a few new dictators emerge. However, no revolution is necessary. The fundamentals for merging the two paradigms are already well established. The transition from the feudal serfdom of individual theories to the ordered yet democratic rule of law of a few paradigms can be nonviolent. We should not fear that the paradigms will rule to their idiosyncratic whims, because they have been with us all along. Instead, and especially for the applied psychologist, it means a deeper understanding of the nature of complex systems operating in complex environments is developing. With that understanding comes more accuracy in prediction and more hope in the effectiveness of inventions. This seems to be a far, far better thing.

REFERENCES

Ajzen, I. (1991). The theory of planned behavior. *Organizational Behavior and Human Decision Processes, 50,* 179–211.

Anderson, J. R. (1983). *The architecture of cognition.* Cambridge, MA: Harvard University Press.

Ashby, W. R. (1956). *An introduction to cybernetics.* London: Methuen.

Ashford, S. J., & Cummings, L. L. (1983). Feedback as an individual resource: Personal strategies for creating information. *Organizational Behavior and Human Performance, 32,* 370–398.

Ashmos, D. P., & Huber, G. P. (1987). The systems paradigm in organization theory: Correcting the record and suggesting the future. *Academy of Management Review, 12,* 607–621.

Austin, J. T., & Vancouver, J. B. (1996). Goal constructs in psychology: Structure, process, and content. *Psychological Bulletin, 120*(3), 338–375.

Baddeley, A. (1994). The magical number seven: Still magic after all these years? *Psychological Review, 101*, 353–356.

Bandura, A. (1986). *Social foundations of thought and action.* Englewood Cliffs, NJ: Prentice-Hall.

Bandura, A. (1989). The concept of agency in social–cognitive theory. *American Psychologist, 44*, 1175–1184.

Bandura, A. (1991). Social cognitive theory of self-regulation. *Organizational Behavior and Human Decision Processes, 50*, 248–287.

Beach, L. R. (1990). *Image theory: Decision making in personal and organizational contexts.* New York: Wiley.

Beach, R. L. (1993). Broadening the definition of decision making: The role of prechoice screening of options. *Psychological Science, 4*, 215–220.

Campbell, J. P., & Pritchard, R. D. (1976). Motivation theory in industrial and organizational psychology. In M. D. Dunnette (Ed.), *Handbook of industrial and organizational psychology* (pp. 63–130). Chicago: Rand McNally.

Campion, M. A., & Lord, R. G. (1982). A control systems conceptualization of the goal-setting and changing processes. *Organizational Behavior and Human Performance, 30*, 265–287.

Carroll, M. (1997). Human-computer interaction: Psychology as a science of design. *Annual Review of Psychology, 43*, 61–83.

Carver, C. S., & Scheier, M. F. (1981). *Attention and self-regulation: A control theory approach to human behavior.* New York: Springer-Verlag.

Carver, C. S., & Scheier, W. F. (1982a). An information processing perspective on self-management. In P. Karoly & F. H. Kanfer (Eds.), *Self-management and behavior change* (pp. 93–128). New York: Pergamon.

Carver, C. S., & Scheier, M. F. (1982b). Control theory: A useful conceptual framework for personality-social, clinical, and health psychology. *Psychological Bulletin, 92*, 111–135.

Carver, C. S., & Scheier, M. F. (1990). Origins and functions of positive and negative affect: A control-process view. *Psychological Review, 97*, 19–35.

Colarelli, S. M. (1996). Establishment and job context influences on the use of hiring practices. *Applied Psychology: An International Review, 45*, 153–176.

Cropanzano, R., James, K., & Citera, M. (1992). A goal hierarchy model of personality, motivation, and leadership. In L. L. Cummings & B. M. Staw (Eds.), *Research in organizational behavior* (Vol. 15, pp. 267–322). Greenwich, CT: JAI Press.

Deci, E. L., & Ryan, R. M. (1985). *Intrinsic motivation and self-determination in human behavior.* New York: Plenum.

Dickens, C. (1859). *A tale of two cities.* New York: Sheldon.

Dörner, D., & Schaub, H. (1994). Errors in planning and decision-making and the nature of human information processing. *Applied Psychology: An International Review, 43*, 433–453.

Earley, P. C., & Shalley, C. E. (1991). New perspectives on goals and performance: Merging motivation and cognition. In G. Ferris & K. Rowland (Eds.), *Research in personnel and human resources management* (Vol. 9, pp. 121–157). Greenwich, CT: JAI Press.

Edwards, J. R. (1992). A cybernetic theory of stress, coping, and well-being in organizations. *Academy of Management Review, 17*, 238–274.

Edwards, W. (1954). The theory of decision making. *Psychological Bulletin, 51*, 380–418.

Ford, D. H. (1987). *Humans as self-constructing living systems: A developmental perspective on behavior and personality.* Hillsdale, NJ: Erlbaum.

Ford, M. E. (1992). *Motivating humans: Goals, emotions, and personal agency beliefs.* Hillsdale, NJ: Erlbaum.

Frayne, C. A., & Latham, G. P. (1987). Application of social learning theory to employee self-management of attendance. *Journal of Applied Psychology, 72*, 387–392.

Frese, M., & Sabini, J. (Eds.). (1985a). *Goal directed behavior: The concept of action in psychology.* Hillsdale, NJ: Erlbaum.

Frese, M., & Sabini, J. (1985b). Action theory: An introduction. In M. Frese and J. Sabini (Eds.), *Goal-directed behavior* (pp. xvii–xxv). Hillsdale, NJ: Erlbaum.

Frese, M., & Zapf, D. (1993). Action as the core of work psychology: A German approach. In H. C. Triandis, M. D. Dunnette, & L. M. Hough (Eds.), *Handbook of industrial and organizational psychology* (2nd ed., Vol 4, pp. 271–340). Palo Alto, CA: Consulting Psychologists' Press.

Gallistel, C. R. (1985). Motivation, intention, and emotion: Goal directed behavior from a cognitive–neuroethological perspective. In M. Frese and J. Sabini (Eds.), *Goal-directed behavior* (pp. 48–66). Hillsdale, NJ: Erlbaum.

Gardner, H. (1985). *The mind's new science*. New York: Basic Books.

Garland, H. (1984). Relation of effort–performance expectancy to performance in goal setting experiments. *Journal of Applied Psychology, 69*, 79–84.

Guthrie, E. R. (1935). *The psychology of learning*. New York: Harper & Row.

Hacker, W. (1985). Activity: A fruitful concept in industrial psychology. In M. Frese & J. Sabini (Eds.), *Goal-directed behavior* (pp. 262–283). Hillsdale, NJ: Erlbaum.

Hill, W. F. (1985). *Learning: A survey of psychological interpretations* (4th ed.). New York: Harper & Row.

Hyland, M. B. (1988). Motivational Control Theory: In integrative framework. *Journal of personality and social psychology, 55* 642–651.

Kahneman, D., Slovic, P., & Tversky, A. (1982). *Judgment under uncertainty: Heuristics and biases*. Cambridge, UK: Cambridge University Press.

Kanfer, R. (1990). Motivation theory in I/O psychology. In M. D. Dunnette & L. M. Hough (Eds.), *The handbook of industrial/organizational psychology* (2nd ed., pp. 75–170). Palo Alto, CA: Consulting Psychologists Press.

Kanfer, R., & Heggestad, E. D. (1997). Motivational traits and skills: A person-centered approach to work motivation. *Research in Organizational Behavior, 19*, 1–56.

Karoly, P. (1993). Mechanisms of self-regulation: A systems view. *Annual Review of Psychology, 44*, 23–52.

Katz, D., & Kahn, R. L. (1978). *The social psychology of organizations* (2nd ed.). New York: Wiley.

Katzell, R. A. (1994). Contempory meta-trends in industrial and organizational psychology. In M. D. Dunnette & L. M. Hough (Eds.), *Handbook of industrial and organizational psychology* (Vol. 4, 2nd ed.). Palo Alto, CA: Consulting Psychologists Press.

Katzell, R. A., & Austin, J. T. (1992). From then to now: The development of industrial–organizational psychology in the United States. *Journal of Applied Psychology, 77*, 803–835.

Kernan, M. C., & Lord, R. G. (1990). The effect of valence in single and multiple goal environments. *Journal of Applied Psychology, 75*, 194–202.

Klein, H. J. (1989). An integrated control theory model of work motivation. *Academy of Management Review, 14*, 150–172.

Klein, H. J. (1991). Further evidence on the relationship between goal setting and expectancy theories. *Organizational Behavior and Human Decision Processes, 49*, 230–257.

Kleinmuntz, D. N. (1993). Information processing and misperceptions of the implications of feedback in dynamic decision making. *System Dynamics Review, 9*, 223–237.

Kluger, A. N., & DeNisi, A. (1996). The effects of feedback interventions on performance: A historical review, a meta-analysis and a preliminary feedback intervention theory. *Psychological Bulletin, 119*, 254–284.

Kosko, B. (1993). *Fuzzy thinking: The new science of fuzzy logic*. New York: Hyperion.

Kuhl, J. (1994). *Motivation and volition*. In G. d'Ydewalle, P. Eelen, & P. Bertelson (Eds.), *International perspectives on psychological science* (Vol. 2, pp. 311–340). Hove, UK: Erlbaum.

Kuhn, T. S. (1962/1970). *The structure of scientific revolutions*. Chicago: University of Chicago Press.

Latham, G. P., & Frayne, C. A. (1989). Self-management training for increasing job attendance: A follow-up and a replication. *Journal of Applied Psychology*, *74*(3), 411–416.

Latham, G. P., & Locke, E. A. (1991). Self-regulation through goal setting. *Organizational Behavior and Human Decision Processes*, *50*, 212–247.

Lazlo, E. (1976). Nonempirical criteria in the development of science. In E. Lazlo & E. B. Sellon (Eds.), *Vistas in physical reality* (pp. 107–121). New York: Plenum.

Levine, R. L., & Fitzgerald, H. E. (Eds.) (1992). *Analysis of dynamic psychological systems*. New York: Plenum.

Lewin, K. (1936). *Principles of topological psychology*. New York: McGraw-Hill.

Lewin, K. (1951). *Field theory in social science*. New York: Harper.

Lewin, K., Dembo, T., Festinger, L., & Sears, P. S. (1944). Level of aspiration. In J. M. Hunt (Ed.), *Personality and the behavior disorders* (pp. 333–378). New York: Ronald.

Locke, E. A. (1968). Toward a theory of task motivation and incentives. *Organizational Behavior and Human Performance*, *3*, 157–189.

Locke, E. A. (1991a). Introduction to Special Issue. *Organizational Behavior and Human Decision Processes*, *50*, 151–153.

Locke, E. A. (1991b). Goal theory vs. control theory: Contrasting approaches to understanding work motivation. *Motivation and Emotion*, *15*, 9–28.

Locke, E. A. (1994). The emperor is naked. *Applied Psychology: An International Review*, *43*, 367–370.

Locke, E. A., & Latham, G. P. (1990). *A theory of goal-setting and task performance*. Englewood Cliffs, NJ: Prentice-Hall.

Locke, E. A., Shaw, K. N., Saari, L. M., & Latham, G. P. (1981). Goal-setting and task performance: 1969–1980. *Psychological Bulletin*, *90*, 125–152.

Lord, R. G., & Hanges, P. J. (1987). A control system model of organizational motivation: Theoretical development and applied implications. *Behavioral Science*, *32*, 161–178.

Lord, R. G., & Levy, P. E. (1994). Moving from cognition to action: A control theory perspective. *Applied Psychology: An International Review*, *43*, 335–398.

Lord, R. G., & Maher, K. J. (1990). Alternative information-processing models and the implications for theory, research, and practice. *Academy of Management Review*, *15*, 9–28.

Marken, R. S. (1992). *Mind readings: Experimental studies of purpose*. Gravel Switch, KY: Control Systems Group.

Marken, R. S. (1997). The dancer and the dance: Methods in the study of living control systems. *Psychological Methods*, *2*, 436–446.

McKenna, D. D. & Wright, P. M. (1992). Alternative metaphors for organization design. In M. D. Dunnette & L. M. Hough (Eds.) *Handbook of industrial and organizational psychology* (Vol. 3, 2nd ed., pp. 901–960). Palo Alto, CA: Consulting Psychologists Press.

Miller, G. A. (1956). The magical number seven, plus or minus two: Some limits on our capacity for processing information. *Psychological Review*, *63*, 81–97.

Miller, G. A., Galanter, E., & Pribram, K. H. (1960). *Plans and the structure of behavior*. New York: Holt.

Miller, J. G. (1978). *Living systems*. New York: McGraw-Hill.

Minsky, M. (1986), *The society of mind*. New York: Touchstone.

Mitchell, T. R., & Beach, L. R. (1990). "...Do I love thee? Let me count..." Toward an understanding of intuitive and automatic decision making, *Organizational Behavior and Human Decision Processes*, *47*, 1–20.

Mook, D. G. (1996). *Motivation: The organization of action* (2nd ed.). New York: Norton.

Naylor, J. C., & Ilgen, D. R. (1984). Goal-setting: A theoretical analysis of a motivation technology. In B. M. Staw & L. L. Cummings (Eds.), *Research in organizational behavior* (Vol. 6, pp. 95–140). Greenwich, CT: JAI Press.

Nelson, T. D. (1993). The hierarchical organization of behavior: A useful feedback model of self-regulation. *Current Directions in Psychological Science*, *2*, 121–126.

Newell, A. (1980). Reasoning, problem solving, and decision processes: The problem space as a fundamental category. In R. S. Nickerson (Ed.), *Attention and performance* (Vol. 8, pp. 693–718). Hillsdale, NJ: Erlbaum.

Newell, A. (1990). *Unified theories of cognition.* Cambridge, MA: Harvard University Press.

Newell, A., & Simon, H. A. (1972). *Human problem solving.* Englewood Cliffs, NJ: Prentice-Hall.

Powers, W. T. (1973). *Behavior: The control of perception.* Chicago: Aldine.

Powers, W. T. (1978). Quantitative analysis of purposive systems: Some spadework at the foundations of scientific psychology. *Psychological Review, 85,* 417–435.

Powers, W. T. (1988). An outline of control theory. Conference Workbook for *Tests in Cybernetic Theory,* American Society for Cybernetics Conference, Felton, CA.

Powers, W. T. (1991). Commentary on Bandura's "Human agency." *American Psychologist, 46,* 151–153.

Powers, W. T. (1992). On emotions. *Living control systems* (Vol. 2, pp. 31–40). Gravel Switch, KY: Control Systems Group.

Powers, W. T., Clark, R. K., & McFarland, R. I. (1960a). A general feedback theory of human behavior: Part 1. *Perceptual and Motors Skills Monograph, 11,* 71–88.

Powers, W. T., Clark, R. K., & McFarland, R. I. (1960b). A general feedback theory of human behavior: Part 2. *Perceptual and Motor Skills Monograph, 11,* 309–323.

Proctor, R. W., & Dutta, A. (1995). *Skill acquisition and human performance.* Thousand Oaks, CA: Sage.

Rasmussen, J., Brehmer, B., & Leplat, J. (Eds.) (1990). *Distributed decision making: Cognitive models of cooperative work.* Chichester: Wiley.

Reason J. T., & Zapf, D. (1994). Errors, error detection, and error recovery [Special issue]. *Applied Psychology: An International Review, 43,* 427–584.

Richardson, G. P. (1991). *Feedback thought: In social science and systems theory.* Philadelphia: University of Pennsylvania Press.

Rosenblueth, A., Wiener, N., & Bigelow, J. (1943). Behavior, purpose, and teleology. *Philosophy of Science, 10,* 18–24.

Runkel, P. J. (1990). *Casting nets and testing specimens: Two grand methods of psychology.* New York: Praeger.

Sappington, A. A. (1990). Recent psychological approaches to the free will versus determinism issue. *Psychological Bulletin, 108,* 19–29.

Schneider, W., & Shiffrin, R. M. (1977). Controlled and automatic human information processing: I. Detection, search, and attention. *Psychological Review, 84,* 1–66.

Senge, P. M. (1990). *The fifth discipline.* New York: Doubleday.

Shiffrin, R. M., & Schneider, W. (1977). Controlled and automatic human information processing: II. Perceptual learning, automatic attending, and a general theory. *Psychological Review, 84,* 127–190.

Simon, H. A. (1955). A Behavioral model of rational choice. *Quarterly Journal of Economics, 69,* 99–118.

Simon, H. A. (1994). The bottleneck of attention: Connecting thought with motivation. *Nebraska Symposium on Motivation, 41,* 1–21.

Stevenson, M. K., Busemeyer, J. R., & Naylor, J. C. (1990). Judgment and decision-making theory. In M. D. Dunnette & L. M. Hough (Eds.) *Handbook of Industrial and Organizational Psychology* (Vol. 1, 2nd ed., pp. 283–374). Palto Alto, CA: Consulting Psychologists Press.

Taylor, M. S., Fisher, C. D., & Ilgen, D. R. (1984). Individuals' reactions to performance feedback in organizations: A control theory perspective. In K. Rowland & G. Ferris (Eds.), *Research in personnel and human resources management* (Vol. 2, pp. 81–124). Greenwich, CT: JAI Press.

Tolman, E. C. (1932). *Purposive behavior in animals and men.* New York: Appleton-Century-Crofts.

Tsui, A. S., & Ashford, S. J. (1994). Adaptive self-regulation: A process view of managerial effectiveness. *Journal of Management, 20,* 93–121.

Tubbs, M. E., Boehne, D. M., & Dahl, J. G. (1993). Expectancy, valence, and motivational force functions in goal-setting research: An empirical test. *Journal of Applied Psychology, 78,* 361–373.

Vallacher, R. R., & Wegner, D. M. (1987). What do people think they're doing? Action identification and human behavior. *Psychological Review, 94,* 3–15.

Vancouver, J. B. (1994, August). Individual and organizational systems fit. In T. Welchan (Chair), *New Directions in Fit.* Presented at the Academy of Management Annual Conference, Dallas.

Vancouver, J. B. (1996). Living systems theory as a paradigm for organizational behavior: Understanding humans, organizations, and social processes. *Behavioral Science, 41*(3), 165–204.

Vancouver, J. B. (1997). The application of HLM to the analysis of the dynamic interaction of environment, person and behavior. *Journal of Management, 23*(6), 723–746.

Vancouver, J. B. (1998). *Clarifying Semantic Misunderstandings in the Control Theory Debate.* Paper presented at the meeting of the American Psychological Association, San Francisco, CA.

von Bertalanffy, L. (1950). An outline of general system theory. *British Journal of the Philosophy of Science, 1,* 139–164.

Vroom, V. H. (1964). *Work and motivation.* New York: Wiley.

Weiss, H. M. (1990). Learning theory in industrial and organizational psychology. In M. D. Dunnette & L. M. Hough (Eds.) *Handbook of industrial and organizational psychology.* (Vol. 1, pp. 171–222). Palo Alto, CA: Consulting Psychologists Press.

Wiener, N. (1948). *Cybernetics: Or control and communication in the animal and the machine.* Cambridge, MA: MIT Press.

11

SELF-REGULATION AND HEALTH BEHAVIOR

THE HEALTH BEHAVIOR GOAL MODEL

STAN MAES AND WINIFRED GEBHARDT

Leiden University, Leiden, Netherlands

I. INTRODUCTION

The interest of psychologists in health behavior undoubtedly has increased as a consequence of the dramatic change in causes of death in Western countries over the past century. Around 1900 the most important killers in Western countries were communicable diseases such as influenza, pneumonia, tuberculosis, and diphtheria. After the Second World War, accidents and chronic illnesses such as cardiovascular diseases, cancer, and chronic obstructive pulmonary diseases became the most important killers in Western countries. Whereas microorganisms play a causal role in communicable diseases, the causes of most chronic diseases and accidents are to a large extent behavioral or behavior related. As much as half of mortality is currently due to unhealthy behavior (Maes & Van Elderen, 1998). For example, smoking is a proven risk factor for cardiovascular diseases, cancer and chronic obstructive pulmonary diseases. People who maintain regular physical activity are less likely to fall victim to heart diseases, stroke, chronic obstructive pulmonary diseases, diabetes, and osteoporosis. Unhealthy diet has been shown to be associated with cancer, cardiovascular diseases, and diabetes. Excessive body weight increases the risk of cardiovascular diseases, especially if other risk factors are present. Use of alcohol is related to various types of accidents and cirrhosis of the liver, and drug use is related to accidents and crime.

Copyright © 2000 by Academic Press.
All rights of reproduction in any form reserved.

Experiencing stress is associated with chronic conditions such as high blood pressure, gastrointestinal diseases, and infectious diseases, as well as suicide (World Health Organization, 1988).

Because most of these unhealthy behaviors are habitual, they are not easy to change. Early models, which implied that the mere provision of information, incitement of fear, or use of social power could influence these behaviors, have proved to be unsuccessful (Maes, 1990). In reaction to these early models, health behavior models have become more sophisticated over time. For example, Edwards's (1961) subjective expected utility theory was applied to health behavior. According to this theory, a person who is confronted with two or more possible actions will choose the one with the greatest subjective expected utility. Subjective expected utility is a function of the subjective probability that an action will lead to particular outcomes and the expected utility of these outcomes. For example, according to this theory, a communication on exercising to prevent heart disease will lead to a change in behavior if the person becomes convinced that (a) heart disease is a bad thing and (b) exercising will prevent him or her from developing it. Models that have been applied widely to health behavior, such as the health belief model (Rosenstock, 1974) and the protection motivation theory (Rogers, 1975), were influenced by subjective expected utility theory. For example, in the health belief model, it is assumed that the health threat as perceived by the individual is dependent on the beliefs about one's personal susceptibility to a specific illness (= outcome) and the beliefs about the anticipated severity (= utility) of the consequences of this illness. In addition to the perceived health threat, the anticipated effectiveness of a specific health measure determines whether a person will adopt the health behavior. The anticipated effectiveness is based on beliefs that the specific measure will reduce risk and beliefs that the benefits of the health measure exceed the costs. In short, in the health belief model four conditions are expected to determine whether or not an individual will engage in preventive health behaviors: (1) whether one regards oneself as susceptible to the condition, (2) whether one believes that the condition has potentially serious consequences, (3) whether one believes that the proposed behavior will lead to a reduction in one's susceptibility to the condition or to its severity, and (4) whether one expects the benefits of the behavior to outweigh its costs.

Models like these can be regarded as rudimentary self-regulation models, because personal beliefs, values, and expectations are essential features of these models. However, because self-regulation can be defined as a sequence of actions and/or steering processes intended to attain a personal goal, one can question whether the principles of self-regulation are adequately represented in these models.

In this chapter, after a brief discussion of the above-mentioned models, we will introduce basic issues of self-regulation, including goal setting, goal hierarchy, goal conflict, and regulatory processes. Ford's motivational system theory forms the basis for this introduction. Subsequently, the health behavior goal model is introduced. This model, which was developed by us, incorporates both self-regulation constructs and predictors from the already mentioned health behavior models. Following the introduction of the health behavior goal model, empirical evidence in the domain of exercise behavior and smoking is reported. Finally, conclusions and directions for future research are presented.

II. CURRENT HEALTH BEHAVIOR MODELS AND SELF-REGULATION

As previously mentioned, self-regulation can be defined as a sequence of actions and/or steering processes intended to attain a personal goal. In other words, self-regulation consists of the individual's attempt to control his or her own behavior over time and across contexts to achieve self-chosen goals. Any model of self-directed behavior should, therefore, include an adequate representation of the concept of personal goals and of the process of approximation toward personal goals. Existing models of health behavior do not fully meet these criteria.

A number of models, for example, the health belief model (Rosenstock, 1974), Rotter's (1982) social learning theory, the theory of reasoned action (Fishbein & Ajzen, 1975), the theory of planned behavior (Ajzen, 1985), Bandura's social learning theory (Bandura, 1977) and the protection motivation theory (Rogers, 1975), frequently have been applied to the study of health behavior. Table 1 summarizes the main concepts of these theories. In each of the rows of the table, constructs of the various theories that are conceptually similar are presented. In the column at the far left, a general term is given for the concepts within each row.

The role of personal characteristics, such as age and gender, on the process of decision making is mentioned explicitly in the health belief model, but not in the other theories. Environmental characteristics, such as reminders from the external environment that one should change one's behavior (e.g., by means of leaflets), are taken up by both the health belief model and Rotter's social learning theory. In both the health belief model and the protection motivation theory, the importance of "threat appraisal" on the decision to change behavior is stressed. Threat appraisal is assumed to be a combination of perceived susceptibility to a certain disease (e.g., lung cancer) when continuing the current, unhealthy, behavior (e.g., smoking) and the perceived severity of that particular disease. All of the theories include perceived benefits of the new health behavior as important factors that influence behavioral change, although the exact term used for the concept varies between theories. The opposite factors (i.e., per-

TABLE 1 Main Concepts of the Prominent Theories of Health Behavior (Change)

	Health belief model	Rotter's social learning theory	Theory of reasoned action/theory of planned behaviour (TPB)	Bandura's social learning theory	Protection motivation theory
Personal characteristics	Demographic- and socio-psychological factors internal cues to action				
Environmental characteristics	External cues to actions	Situation/social context			
Threat appraisal	Health threat • Perceived susceptibility • Perceived severity				• Perceived susceptibility • Perceived severity Response–efficacy
Perceived benefits	Perceived benefits of action	• Reinforcement (overall expectancy)	Attitude to behavior • Probability of (positive) outcome • Value of outcome	Outcome–expectancy	
Perceived costs	Perceived barriers to action	• Reinforcement value	Attitude to behavior • Probability of (negative) outcome • Value of outcome		• Costs (or perceived barriers) • Internal rewards of current behavior • External rewards of current behavior
Social influence			Subjective norms • Normative beliefs • Motivation to comply		
Perceived competence		Locus of control	Perceived behavioral control (only in TPB) • Probability of control factor • Power of control factor	Self-efficacy	Self-efficacy
Mediating processes	Likelihood of taking health action	Behavior potential	Behavioral intention	Probability of behavior	Protection motivation

ceived costs of change) are explicitly incorporated in the health belief model, the theory of reasoned action, the theory of planned behavior, and the protection motivation theory. Furthermore, the theory of reasoned action and the theory of planned behavior emphasize the influence of the direct social environment on the individual's behavior by incorporating subjective norms. Subjective norms involve beliefs concerning what important others think that one should do (e.g., the belief that my parents would want me to quit smoking; a normative belief), as well as the inclination to conform with this perceived wish (i.e., the motivation to comply). Other health behavior theories do not include such a concept. Expectancies regarding one's capabilities of performing behavior (e.g., self-efficacy or perceived behavioral control) are considered a major determinant of behavior change, particularly in the theory of planned behavior, and the protection motivation theory. These expectancies refer to the expected likelihood that a certain type of behavior would be easy or difficult to perform (e.g., the belief that if I wanted to, I could easily quit smoking). In Table 1 these type of expectancies are summarized by the more general term "perceived competence."

Finally, it is assumed that the individual weighs all of the various factors described within the theory to enable himself or herself to come to a conclusion whether to change behavior. Thus, the person deliberates on all the expected advantages and disadvantages of changing behavior, and the end of this process is characterized by the formation of an intention or a decision either to adopt the new behavior or to continue with the existing behavior. This is assumed to be the primary factor of whether the new behavior will be acquired. The other factors are expected to influence behavior indirectly only (i.e., via the decision or intention to change).

In conclusion, in all of these described theories, a person is regarded as making decisions on a rational basis, and cognitions in the form of expectancies are assumed to be the most important determinants of the decision (or intention) to change behavior. As such, these theories are concerned with the first phase of self-regulation, that is, goal setting. The main question that they address is then, "Which factors influence whether a person will adopt a new behavioral goal" (i.e., changing unhealthy behavior and replace it with a healthy behavior). The processes following this decision are not part of the theory focus. We will elaborate on this issue later on.

It should be noted that the theories, which have been discussed only briefly here, all have been shown to be successful in explaining part of the variance in the attitude toward a new behavior or the intention to adopt this new behavior. Relationships between the theoretical concepts specified in these models and actual behavior or—in the rare cases that it is measured—an actual change in behavior, are much weaker, however. Two principal remarks, which may at least in part explain these findings, can be made concerning the models.

First, although the above-mentioned theories refer to some extent to the importance of goals as determinants of health behavior, the goals in question are set for and not by the individual. In other words, a target health behavior such as weight loss, quitting smoking, or engaging in physical exercise, is defined in an external way and is not related adequately to existing personal goals. As such, these approaches neglect the fact that human beings have to adopt the target as a goal. In addition, people typically pursue multiple goals simultaneously and some of these goals may conflict with the target health behavior. Being physically inactive at a certain moment in time cannot be predicted by beliefs or expectancies alone. At least of equal importance is the fact that physical exercise may interfere with other important personal goals, such as building a relationship, caring for children, studying for an exam, or doing one's job. People do not fail to adopt health behaviors merely because they do not want to quit smoking, engage in physical exercise, or lose weight, but also because they prefer to pursue other goals that are cognitively or behaviorally incompatible with the target health behavior. Thus, the problem with the existing models is that they concentrate on the attainment of an isolated external target and they ignore the fact that goals are by definition internally set.

Second, the above-mentioned models cast goal attainment as an event rather than a process or fail to provide an adequate description of the process of approximation toward health behavior goals. Accounts of the processes linking beliefs or perceptions and acquisition of the target behavior typically are restricted to one mediating construct such as the likelihood of taking action, behavior potential, behavioral intention, probability of behavior, or protection motivation. In contrast, many authors in the self-regulation literature draw a distinction between goal setting, planning, and goal striving, on the one hand, and monitoring, attainment, revision, and persistence, on the other (Austin & Vancouver 1996). The importance of identifying distinct steps in the process of change or approximation toward a goal also has been stressed by various other models that have been used in the study of health behavior change. Examples are Janis and Mann's (1968) theory of conflict, Prochaska and DiClemente's (1986) transtheoretical model, Weinstein's (1988) precaution adoption process, and Schwarzer's (1992) health action process approach. Table 2 shows the various stages as discerned by these four theories.

The theories differ somewhat in the nature of the stages that are differentiated in the process of changing toward a new behavior. The transtheoretical theory describes a global process of behavior change, regardless of the motives for change. The three other theories, on the other hand, refer explicitly to a factor that is assumed to lead to behavior

TABLE 2   Main Concepts of the Prominent Stage Theories of Health Behavior Change

Theory of Conflict	Transtheoretical model	Precaution adoption process	Health action process approach
	Precontemplation (stage 1)	No knowledge of hazard (stage 0) Learn about hazard (stage 1)	
Appraisal of new challenge (stage 1)	Contemplation (stage 2)	Believe in significant likelihood for others (Stage 2)	Health threat (begin. of stage 1; i.e., motivation phase): • Threat severity
	Contemplation (stage 2)	Acknowledgment of personal susceptibility (stage 3)	• Threat vulnerability
Evaluation of behavioral alternatives (stage 2)	Contemplation (stage 2)		• Self-efficacy expectancies • Outcome–expectancies
Selection of best alternative (stage 3)	Contemplation (stage 2)	Decide to take precaution (stage 4)	Behavioral intention (end of stage 1)
Commitment to selected behavior (stage 4)	Preparation (stage 3)		Action plans (begin. of stage 2; i.e., volition phase)
	Action (stage 4)	Take precaution (stage 5)	Action
Adherence to new behavior (stage 5)	Maintenance (stage 5)		Action control, e.g., delay of gratification (end of stage 2)

change; that is, a perceived threat (precaution adoption theory and the health action process approach) or, more positively stated, a new challenge (theory of conflict).

Both the transtheoretical theory and the precaution adoption process incorporate a precontemplation phase, during which the person is not yet contemplating a change of behavior. In the precaution adoption process, a further division is made between a phase during which one has no knowledge of the negative health consequences of his or her current behavior, and a later phase during which one does have this information but still is undecided whether to alter his or her behavior.

The contemplation phase is characterized by appraisal of the new challenge, which may involve an estimation of the severity of the threat and of the personal vulnerability to this threat. Furthermore, the person makes a selection of the best behavioral alternative to handle the threat (coping appraisal) during this phase (theory of conflict and health action process approach). In the health action process approach, it is assumed that one estimates (1) the extent to which he or she believes that the behavior will be effective in reaching the goal (outcome expectancies) and (2) the extent to which he or she is capable of executing the behavior (self-efficacy expectancies).

In the transtheoretical model and the health action process approach, the preparation phase is the period during which a person has decided to change and is making plans of action. This phase is included in the theory of conflict as a commitment to a new policy. The next phase, that is, initiation of actual behavior change (action stage), is the final stage of the precaution adoption process approach. In the theory of conflict as well as in the health action process approach, on the other hand, the end of the process is defined by a state of adherence to the new behavior even in the face of difficulties. Control processes will induce the person to persevere by commitment to perform the new behavior, and by delaying gratification until the goal is reached. This final state of goal achievement coincides with the maintenance stage in the transtheoretical model. Thus, generally, a precontemplative, a contemplative, a preparative, and an active and/or a maintenance stage are distinguished, although the exact definition of each of these stages may be different in kind. Clearly, from this perspective, approximation toward a goal is a complex decisional and actional process. Each stage is in itself part of the process of self-regulation.

III. SELF-REGULATION AND THE PERSONAL GOAL STRUCTURE

A basic tenet of self-regulation theory is that motivation to change behavior exists when the individual wishes to reduce a perceived discrepancy between his or her actual state and a desired state (Scheier & Carver, 1988). The desired state is, however, broadly defined and may involve various goals. To perceive a discrepancy between actual and desired states, the person has to be self-focused and action oriented (Kuhl, 1981).

The desired state can be influenced by three different types of factors: (1) expectations, (2) affective factors, and (3) desired self-conceptions (Markus & Wurf, 1987). Expectations concern the anticipated consequences of various behaviors in terms of costs and benefits, as well as the perceived ability of the person to perform these behaviors. The affective factors include the innate needs of the individual, and learned and more specific motives and values, which all can lead to another, preferred state of being. Desired self-conceptions are influential because people do not act only to accomplish specific achievements, but also choose those activities that support their own definitions of the self.

Changes in external as well as internal conditions may result in alterations in each of these factors and, consequently, lead to other desired states. For example, an individual may be motivated to start engaging in physical exercise because exercise facilities have been provided at work and many colleagues encourage him or her to participate, and/or because he or she is confronted with lower back pain symptoms. In each of these circumstances, the expectations concerning the behavior (e.g., it will not be a great effort to go to a gymnasium), the individual's values (e.g., if others think that physical activity is that important, then maybe it is) and even self-conceptions (e.g., if my very unhealthy looking boss can do physical activity, then I can do it as well, even though I always thought that I was not the sporty type) may change.

Goals can thus be defined as thoughts about desired states or outcomes. Personal goals represent a variety of (un)desired states or outcomes and also direct the person to achieve (or avoid) these states. These properties of goals are, respectively, the content and the process aspects of goals (Ford, 1992). Whereas many models concentrate on the process aspect, the content aspect has been largely neglected in the literature. Most health or illness behavior models deal with the content aspect by focusing on one single specific target (e.g., losing weight, stopping smoking, or taking prescribed medication) at a time. Even if the person adopts these specific targets as a desired state, they do not exist in isolation. Specific goals form part of a more complex goal structure, characterized by various levels. At the highest level, goals represent personal meaning or the optimization of self-concept. They include other goals concerning health (e.g., being safe and healthy), well-being (e.g., enjoying life as much as possible), personal growth (e.g., developing one's talents to the maximum), and social goals (e.g., being a good mother or partner). These higher-order goals are pursued via subgoals at different levels of specificity, including behavioral goals (e.g., exercising, watching TV, spending time on a hobby, or doing the household chores). Lower-order goals are more concrete and are instrumental in attaining more abstract, higher-order goals. As such, they are subgoals or means to an end. Whereas they are more specific, it is easier for the individual to verify whether lower-order goals have been attained, and for that reason lower-order goals function as a target, which facilitates approximation toward higher-order goals. On the other hand, higher-order goals give meaning and organization to behavioral goals, which means that they function as a purpose (Ford, 1992).

Exploring the relationships between a specific health goal and the larger personal goal structure implies that the personal goal structure of a person can be assessed. A basic requirement for assessment is a taxonomy of human goals as provided by Ford and Nichols (1991), Ford (1992), and Austin & Vancouver (1996). The Ford and Nichols 24-category taxonomy distinguishes between desired within-person consequences (affective goals, cognitive goals, and subjective organization goals) and desired person–environment consequences (self-assertive social relationship goals, integrative social relationship goals and task goals). Maes, Sweeney, and Gebhardt (1998) developed a 52-item goal facilitation scale on the basis of this taxonomy. In a yet unpublished study, the scale was administered to a little over 1,000 health care workers. They were asked how important the prescribed goals were to them and to what extent their work allowed them to fulfill these goals. Items included goals such as doing creative things, experiencing bodily pleasure, feeling like they belonged, not being controlled by others, not being ill, and not being like everyone else. Multiple regression analyses showed that perceived nonfulfillment of goals is a strong predictor of health-related outcomes including somatic complaints, burnout, anxiety, depression, and hostility. The results illustrate that purpose or, in other words, the extent to which activities are related to important and different kinds of higher-order goals, is a highly relevant issue in the area of health and illness (behavior).

IV. GOAL ALIGNMENT, GOAL CONFLICT, AND GOAL BALANCE

The hierarchical organization of goals implies that, within a specific behavior episode, approximation toward a specific goal is more likely if this goal is in line with (and less likely if it is in conflict with) higher-order goals. Approximation toward many health behaviors can create important conflicts at a higher-order level. Losing weight, reducing alcohol consumption, quitting smoking, starting a vigorous program of physical exercise, or avoiding snacks between meals are all examples of behavioral health goals that undoubtedly serve higher-order health goals, but that are frequently in conflict with higher-order well-being goals.

Within a specific behavior episode, there are also important interactions between goals at the same level. At the behavioral level, conflicts also may occur because of energy or time scarcity. In other words, there are different things that one might want to do at a certain moment in time, but one cannot do them all at once. Therefore, the occurrence of a behavior may limit the occurrence of a whole sequence of other behaviors because of the limited capacity or energy of the system. For these reasons, quitting smoking may interfere with studying for an exam, and engaging in physical exercise three times a week may conflict with spending time with a new romantic partner.

Even if there is goal alignment with other behavioral and higher-order goals within a specific behavioral episode, maintaining a specific goal (e.g., following a restrictive diet or doing strenuous physical exercise daily) across time and situations may lead to undesirable consequences in certain situations or in the long run. In other words, one cannot always concentrate on or fulfill one single central goal: There has to be goal balance between behavior episodes (Ford, 1992). For example, focusing only on affective goals may have undesirable consequences for health goals, and concentrating exclusively on task goals may have undesirable consequences for social goals. This highlights another important limitation of existing health behavior models: They concentrate on determinants of a target health behavior within a specific behavior episode, but overlook forces that occur across episodes. Although the stage models do consider change over time, they do not include determinants of change, which are related to the personal organization of goals or, in other words, the self (Csikszentmihalyi, 1990), and they disregard environmental influences, which occur over time. As such, they make content (the personal goal structure) and context abstract.

V. GOAL SETTING AND GOAL ORIENTATION

Apart from the content of a goal, people use cognitive strategies to achieve goals at a behavior episode level. These processes are called goal setting processes. Goal setting is influenced by various goal characteristics. Austin and Vancouver (1996) discerned the following dimensions: (a) importance–commitment, (b) difficulty–level, (c) temporal level, and (d) level of consciousness. Quite some evidence exists that goals are more likely to be fulfilled if (1) they are highly important to the individual, (2) they are not too difficult or too easy to achieve, and (3) they can be reached within a restricted time frame.

The level of consciousness of a goal refers to the fact that individuals may be more or less aware of a goal and that the attainment of a goal may be more or less intentional. Individuals tend to be more aware of achievement-oriented goals than of emotion-oriented goals. In addition, goals that the individual was very aware of at the early stages of attainment may become less conscious as regulation processes become more automatic at later stages. This suggests that fully integrated goals require less mental capacity. Engaging in physical exercise three times a week may become a habit after 1 year, even though it required a lot of monitoring during the first months.

Across episodes, consistencies in styles of goal pursuit, which are called goal orientations (Ford, 1992) can be discerned. Among the many dimensions of goal orientation, a distinction can be made between approach versus avoidance orientation. Approach goals, which involve movement toward a desired outcome, have been studied frequently. Avoidance goals, which are characterized by movement away from an undesired outcome, have received less research attention, yet are at least as important from a health point of view (Coats, Janoff-Bulman & Alpert, 1996). Some behaviors are indeed protective from a health point of view and can be defined as approach goals, whereas others are potentially damaging and should be avoided. Engaging in physical exercise, having regular medical checkups, getting rest and relaxation, sleeping 7 to 8 hours a day, wearing seat belts, and eating healthy food are examples of approach goals. Quitting smoking, reducing alcohol intake, avoiding snacks between meals, reducing intake of animal fat, salt, or sugar, and avoiding stressful or unsafe situations are examples of possible avoidance goals. A higher-order goal such as staying healthy thus can be attained by means of approach or avoidance subgoals and it is important to realize that individuals differ in this orientation. It should be noted that this is true not only for achievement goals, but also for emotional goals.

Another important dimension refers to the fact that goal directed activity can be induced by the person (active orientation) or by external events (reactive orientation). Although many health behavior models assume that approximation toward a health target is induced by the person, many illness behavior models assume that important health targets are achieved by coping with external events. Both models neglect individual differences in goal approximation. Maes, Leventhal, and De Ridder (1996) pointed at the fact that one of the limitations of the Lazarus and Folkman (1984) stress-coping model is the assumption that individuals cope in a reactive way with disease-related events. By focusing exclusively on the way the stressor shapes coping behavior, this and other models indeed have overlooked the effects of the individual's life goals on the meaning and representation of the disease and the selection of coping procedures. For example, a coronary heart patient who is perfectly able to return to work may stop working because it is personally more important to spend more time with his or her spouse, or the patient may violate diet regulations because it is more important to please his or her host. Lazarus (1993) agreed with this point of view.

A comparable criticism may be formulated toward health behavior models. Many of these models disregard the fact that health behavior change frequently occurs because of reactive coping with stressful events or restrictive environments. For example, many people stop smoking after a myocardial infarction and other people may start smoking again to cope with loss of a family member.

Ford (1992) mentioned a third dimension of goal orientation: the maintenance–change dimension. This dimension refers to a tendency to maintain stability or to seek change and self-improvement. In terms of resource theory (Hobfoll, 1988), one could see the tendency to maintain stability as a tendency to conserve existing resources and see the tendency to change as a tendency to gain or develop resources.

Although many other dimensions can be distinguished, such as Kuhl's distinction between state and action orientation, many authors concentrate on (combinations of) the foregoing three dimensions. For example, as Ford (1992) mentions, Kobasa's (1979) hardiness concept, a personal characteristic that proved to be related to favorable health outcomes in executives, can be defined as an active, positive, self-improving orientation.

VI. GOALS, BELIEFS, AND EMOTIONS

Having a goal, the right environment, and the necessary skills are not enough to attain the goal. People also must believe that they have the personal qualities and opportunities to reach the goal. Ford (1992) makes a distinction between context and capability beliefs. Context beliefs refer to whether one has the responsive environment needed to support goal attainment ("Will I have the time to exercise daily?", "Will my spouse support this?", and "Will I find a sports club that will accept me?"). Capability beliefs refer to whether one has the personal skill needed to function effectively ("Will I be able to sport daily?", "Do I have the mental strength?", and "Are my old sports injuries allowing me to do this?"). It should be noted that this distinction approximates Bandura's (1977) concepts of outcome and efficacy expectancies, and that many other health behavior models also incorporate (part of) these concepts.

Even if one believes that an important goal can be reached, one needs to have the energy to do it. Emotions can be seen as the regulatory and the energizing components of behavior. Events that satisfy goals yield positive emotions; events that harm or threaten goals give rise to negative emotions (Frijda, 1988). In other words, pursuing a goal inevitably is accompanied by emotions, which are important determinants of action. They provide us with evaluative information about our interactions with the environment (i.e., the regulatory function of emotions) and facilitate actions toward desired consequences or away from undesired consequences (i.e., the energizing function of emotions; Ford, 1992). As such, it is surprising that in contrast to stress-coping models, where emotions are thought to play a crucial role, emotions are not a main factor in the existing health behavior models. Most of these models can be characterized as social cognition models, which make abstraction from the regulatory and energizing force of emotions.

VII. THE SELF-REGULATION PROCESS

Many of the existing health behavior models describe determinants of a target health behavior or, in the case of the stage models, discern stages of change, but the underlying psychological processes are implicit. In other words, the regulatory principles and mechanism are not explained.

One can distinguish bodily and psychological regulatory processes. All of the existing health behavior models do not include bodily processes. However, bodily processes play an important role in the development and maintenance of many health behaviors, such as physical exercise or relaxation, and especially in the reduction of addictive behaviors, such as smoking, alcohol abuse, or excessive food intake. As a consequence, psychological models should be complemented by biological models, which one can, however, argue are beyond the scope of psychology; therefore we will concentrate here on psychological regulatory mechanisms, which involve cognitive and affective processes.

Emotions or affective states regulate behavior by facilitating (continuation of) behavior that is associated with positive affects and inhibiting behavior that is associated with negative affects. In addition, negative affect motivates the person to change the conditions that lead to negative affect states (Ford & Nichols, 1991).

In terms of cognitive processes, Ford and Nichols (1991) distinguish three kind of mechanisms: (a) feedback mechanisms, which involve monitoring and evaluation of progress toward a goal on the basis of a standard; (b) feedforward mechanisms, which are guided by personal capabilities and context expectancies, and (c) activation of control processes, which are involved in adequate planning and action control to ensure continuation of progress despite competing goals and obstacles.

It is clear that affective states influence all three processes or mechanisms because they can be seen as a standard, and they are associated with outcomes and with competing goals and obstacles. As a consequence, regulatory actions, which are induced by these states, may or may not be congruent with regulatory actions directed at the achievement of a specific health target such as losing weight. This suggests the need for a model, characterized by dual processing such as Leventhal's self-regulation model (Leventhal, 1970, see also Chapter 12). A distinction thus can be made between achievement-directed regulation (e.g., losing weight to stay healthy) and emotion-oriented regulation (e.g., eating to feel good or experience pleasure). There is considerable evidence that the two must be in balance if self-regulation (i.e., the achievement of higher-order goals) is to succeed (Kuhl, 1992). This suggests that salient achievement-oriented goals (e.g., acquisition of a health behavior) will depend on affect states related to goal attainment and persistence, and vice versa. Thus, although health has been shown repeatedly to be one of the most important higher-order goals for human beings, it undoubtably competes with happiness for first place. Some authors even contend that the "pleasure principle" is the main self-regulatory principle of all behavior (Smith, 1977).

Although the health behavior models, that were discussed in the first paragraphs leave these regulatory mechanisms largely implicit, it should be noted that even self-regulation models emphasize some processes more than others. For example, Carver and Scheier (1982) concentrated more on feedback processes, Bandura (1977) and Schwarzer (1992) on feedforward processes, and Kuhl (1992) on activation of control processes.

In summary, in the domain of health behaviors, a theory incorporating self-regulatory principles should differentiate between (1) higher- and lower-order goals, (2) achievement-oriented and emotion-oriented goals, (3) various goal characteristics, (4) goal orientations, and (5) regulatory processes. Furthermore, it should describe the process of goal attainment in terms of subgoals or stages, and the degree of movement toward a specific goal should be conceptualized in terms of the goal's compatibility with the existing personal goal structure.

VIII. THE HEALTH BEHAVIOR GOAL MODEL

Based on all of these considerations, we have developed the health behavior goal (HBG) model. The HBG model (1) assumes that goal approximation is influenced at all stages by the personal goal structure of the individual, (2) includes predictors from the health behavior change models that traditionally have been used to study health behavior, (3) differentiates between health- and affect-related cognitions, and (4) represents a process of change. As such, the HBG model integrates aspects of expectancy–value, stage, and goal theories (see Figure 1). The model has been developed to describe and predict the process of health behavior change.

In the HBG model, change of behavior is assumed to be influenced by various factors. First of all, progression toward the target health behavior will be more likely to occur if the target behavior is consistent with the personal goal structure. This concept, which is at the core of the model, involves all that is of importance to the person; that is, the things a person wants to do in or with one's life. As mentioned before, a distinction should be made between higher-order and lower-order goals. The more a target health behavior conflicts with higher-order goals such as always supporting others, or avoiding pain and discomfort, the smaller the chance that the individual will move toward this target behavior. However, conflicts at the same level, for example, between the target health behavior and other behavioral goals, such as studying or watching TV, also may impede attainment of the target health behavior. If other valued behavioral goals are incompatible with the target health behavior, progress toward the target behavior will be unlikely. Such potential conflicts do not necessarily have important emotional consequences for the individual. It is only when

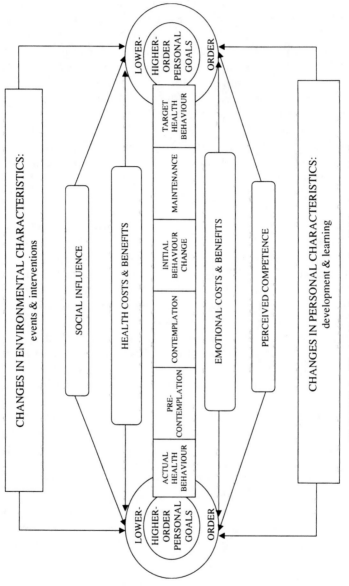

FIGURE 1   The health behavior goal model (main concepts).

the target health behavior has been adopted as a goal that conflict with other salient goals is likely to result in emotional distress. Such distress is especially likely if goal conflict continues over time.

Furthermore, when a target health behavior involves adoption of a new behavior (e.g., physical exercise), the chances of attainment of the target are higher than when the target involves cessation of an existing behavior (e.g., quitting smoking). The probability of adoption of a target health behavior is also higher when it is specific, seen as important, and relatively easy to attain within a reasonable period of time.

In addition to the personal goal structure, the expected consequences of the target health behavior also are assumed to influence the process of behavior change, as in the more traditional theories of health behavior (see Table 1). In the HBG model, these expectancies are divided into the following four categories: (1) perceived health costs and benefits, (2) perceived emotional costs and benefits, (3) social influence, and (4) perceived competence.

Perceived health costs and benefits include all expected health outcomes of executing the target health behavior. For example, one might expect that more exercise, would lead to increased cardiovascular fitness; at the same time, however, one might expect that injury might occur while doing so. Similarly, perceived emotional costs and benefits refer to the expected emotional outcomes of the target health behavior. All anticipated consequences related to the well-being of the person are embodied in this concept. An example is the belief that exercising will lead to improvements in one's psychological state.

Clearly, these expectations representing health or emotional costs and benefits considerations resemble various concepts of the traditional theories of health behavior (e.g., perceived benefits and barriers to action or attitude to behavior; see Table 1). The distinction between health and emotional costs and benefits is based on a distinction between achievement and affect-related cognitions.

The concept of social influence represents a person's appraisal of how the social environment would react to adoption of the target health behavior. For example, a husband might expect his partner to support his efforts to commence and maintain an active life style. It should be noted that in the theory of reasoned action and the theory of planned behavior (see Table 1), the influence of the social environment is limited to social pressure, whereas in the HBG model the concept also incorporates the support of the social network, which can be seen as context beliefs or cognitions.

Finally, perceived competence refers to a person's assessment of his or her capacity to execute the behavior, for example, appraisal of the amount of effort needed to exercise three times or more a week for at least 20 minutes. Perceived competence also includes the individual's estimate of his or her own self-regulatory mechanisms, which may be employed to overcome internal or external constraints. As such, the concept is related to the concept of behavioral control and Bandura's concept of self-efficacy (see Table 1). In other words, perceived competence refers to capability beliefs or cognitions.

Naturally, the concepts are interrelated. For example, each of the four types of expected consequences of the target health behavior is to some extent associated with the personal goal structure. It is plausible to assume that health costs and benefits are related to higher-order goals referring to health issues, and emotional costs and benefits are related to higher-order goals referring to well-being. Social influence will be particularly important for behavior change when it is integrated with higher-order social goals such as being a good partner or lower-order social goals such as spending time with my partner. Likewise, the influence of perceived competence in behavior change may be related to higher-order goals concerning personal growth, such as developing my skills, and becoming better at what I am doing, or lower-order goals, such as spending time on a hobby.

The four types of expectancies of the behavior may also interrelate. For example, social influence may lead to the arousal of certain emotional costs or benefits. When a significant other person such as one's partner conveys that he or she would be extremely appreciative if smoking were banned in the home, an emotional benefit of quitting smoking may involve the gratitude of the partner (in whatever form this may be translated into concrete behavior; for example, doing the dishes or staying at home more often). Another example is that personal competence may influence the expected health costs or benefits. The more one is convinced that he or she is able to perform a specific behavior and maintain it at a certain level, for example, on the basis of previous experience, the more one is likely to expect that the perceived benefits of the new behavior will occur.

Changes in the personal goal structure can occur through changes in environmental and personal characteristics. Environmental characteristics are aspects of the environment that may facilitate or impede adoption of the health behavior (e.g., interventions). Environmental characteristics can be a powerful source of health behavior change. The chances of adoption of a health behavior will be minimal as long as environmental characteristics complicate or impede the initiation of the target health behavior. Also, environmental changes may have a profound influence on all the four types of expected consequences of the advocated behavior. For example, the introduction of an exercise program at the worksite may lead to an increase in (1) social support and pressure, because supervisors and colleagues all participate in the program, (2) the expected emotional benefits, because one assumes that exercising during the break will result in an energy boost afterwards, (3) expected health benefits, because the program will be under professional guidance, and (4) perceived competence, because all colleagues are able to participate in the program and, therefore, it cannot be too difficult.

Personal characteristics include sociodemographic variables such as gender, age, and educational level, as well as various other attributes such as basic goal orientations or styles, including approach–avoidance, active–reactive, maintenance–change, or state–action orientations. Some of these personal attributes may develop or change through learning processes over time and, as such, influence the chances of occurrence of the target health behavior. Again, like the changes in environmental characteristics, changes in personal characteristics also may lead to changes in the expected consequences of the new behavior.

Thus, changes in personal and environmental characteristics may serve, respectively, as internal and external cues to action such as symptoms (internal) or messages and certain events (external). Such cues may lead to the perception of (1) new challenges (I would like to learn a new behavior to achieve a new goal) or (2) a threat (I have to change my behavior to prevent a negative event from happening). If the new goal is highly valued or if the threat is perceived as serious, this may lead to alteration of the relative priority of the goals included in the personal goal structure. In addition, perception of the consequences of certain behaviors (e.g., in terms of health and emotional outcomes) may change. This may, in turn, initiate a process of change.

As can be derived from the figure, the process of change is assumed to occur through certain distinct stages. The starting point of this process is initial health behavior; that is, the actual behavior of the individual that can be observed or otherwise determined. It should be defined in specific terms; for example, the amount of weekly exercise in minutes or the number of cigarettes smoked each day. The target health behavior is the behavior that, if practiced, may benefit the individual's health, either in the short or in the long term. This target health behavior is set outside the individual and applies generally to an entire population or a subset of a population. Examples of target health behavior include exercising three times a week for 20 minutes at a time or quitting smoking. In case the initial health behavior is not in accordance with the target health behavior, the process of change entails at least four stages: the precontemplation stage, the contemplation stage, the initial behavior change stage, and the maintenance stage. The stages are assumed to be sequential, and each stage constitutes an important step in the process of behavior change.

In the precontemplation stage, the individual does not wish to change his or her behavior. In the contemplation stage, actual behavior is still unchanged, but the individual is now motivated to progress toward the target health behavior. During the stage of initial behavior change, the individual starts to change his or her behavior in the direction of the target health behavior. In the final, maintenance stage the health promotive behavior is sustained for a long period. During each of these phases, relapse is possible. These stages of the health behavior goal model are comparable to the general phases described in stage models (see Table 2).

At each stage of behavior change, the individual evaluates whether it is worthwhile to continue to move toward the target behavior, and adjusts his or her behavior accordingly. This process of evaluation and adjustment ends when the goal is either reached or abandoned because goal attainment seems unlikely (Carver & Scheier, 1982) or because other goals have become more important. These evaluations are based on (1) the extent of compatibility between the target health behavior and the personal goal structure, and (2) the perceived immediate consequences of performing the target health behavior. Three distinct regulatory processes can be distinguished in this respect: (1) feedback mechanisms, which imply that progress toward the target is evaluated against an achievement or emotional standard, (2) feedforward mechanisms, which are guided by context and capability expectations regarding the consequences or outcomes of behavior, and (3) action control processes, which guide the person through different stages of progress toward the target by controlling behavioral, cognitive, or emotional obstacles to progression. The relative importance of each of the factors specified in the health behavior goal model is considered to be stage dependent. Changes in personal or environmental characteristics may initiate a process of behavior change, beginning with alteration of the goal hierarchy and eventually leading to the incorporation of the target health behavior in the personal goal structure.

In short, the model's main features are that it (1) incorporates the personal goal structure of the individual, (2) encompasses phases of change, (3) focuses on individual emotional and health costs as well as benefits of changing the behavior, (4) takes into account an individual's perception of his or her own capacities, as well as perceived influence of the direct social environment, and (5) recognizes personal, as well as environmental sources of change.

To test central hypotheses derived from the model, a study was conducted with 526 employees responsible for residential care in seven Dutch nursing homes (Gebhardt, 1997). The employees filled out questionnaires twice, with a 12-month interval between measurements. In this questionnaire, the respondents were asked, among other things, about their current exercise behavior, the anticipated consequences (health and emotional costs or benefits, social influence, and perceived competence) of exercising at least three times a week, and possible conflicting behavioral goals. Results of this prospective study revealed that the five core variables of the model, including the variable for competing goals, were adequate predictors of either progression toward the target health behavior or of relapse to a previous stage. Competing personal goals seem to be particularly important predictors for starting to exercise regularly and for maintaining regular exercise. Moreover, the predictive power of the variables differed over the stage transitions, indicating that the core constructs differ in their relative importance depending on the stage transition.

There is evidence that the model also may be successful in predicting health-compromising behaviors. McKeeman and Karoly (1991) studied the role of interpersonal and intrapsychic goal-related conflict in cigarette smokers ($n = 38$), successful self-initiated quitters ($n = 40$), and recent relapsers ($n = 36$). The three groups, which were matched in terms of age, gender, and smoking background, completed questionnaires retrospectively assessing (a) the degree of conflict among important personal goals and the goal of smoking cessation and (b) perceived social hindrance vis-à-vis their efforts to quit smoking. Results indicated that quitters, in contrast to current smokers and relapsers, recalled significantly less goal-related interpersonal interference and significantly lower levels of goal conflict.

IX. CONCLUSION AND DIRECTIONS FOR FUTURE RESEARCH

Many of the existing health behavior models, including the health belief model, the theory of planned behavior, Bandura's social learning theory, and the protection motivation theory, can be regarded as rudimentary self-regulation models. However, because self-regulation can be defined as a sequence of actions and/or steering processes intended to attain a personal goal, one can question whether essential principles of self-regulation are represented adequately in these models.

First, the target health behavior is defined in these models in an external way; that is, it is set for the individual without relating it to existing personal goals. Most health behavior models focus on one specific goal or target at a time, without linking this goal to higher-order or other behavioral goals. That integration in the personal goal structure gives both meaning and direction to movement toward a specific health target is neglected.

Second, the fact that some models concentrate on one isolated target at a time implies that they focus on the acquisition of a health behavior within a specific behavioral episode. As such, they ignore personal and environmental forces that occur across episodes; that is, over time and across different situations. Although the so-called stage models do consider change over time, they do not include determinants of change that are related to the personal organization of goals and they also disregard environmental influences that occur over time. In other words, unlike the more traditional health behavior models, they concentrate on process, but equally fail to define purpose, content, and context.

Third, the existing health behavior models disregard personal preferences or styles in goal pursuit as tendencies to approach or avoid, to be active or reactive, to be conservative or change-oriented, or to focus on states or actions. Some models within the area of health behavior focus exclusively on one aspect of these dimensions. This is a critique that not only applies to many of the health behavior models mentioned in this chapter, but to many other models of health and illness behavior. For example, traditional stress-coping models are based on the assumption that people tend to cope in a reactive way with stressful events, whereas there is a lot of evidence that individuals also cope with these events in an active, goal-oriented way. Other models do not even take these personal goal orientations into account, although they may prove to be more relevant for the prediction of approximation toward health-enhancing behaviors or, in contrast, the avoidance of health-compromising behaviors.

This brings us to a fourth remark, which is that the nature of the health targets did not get enough attention in the existing models. It is important to note that in addition to the distinction between health-enhancing and health-compromising behaviors, health behaviors also may differ in many other dimensions. This can be illustrated by comparing exercise behavior and smoking behavior on each of the following dimensions:

1. *Time*: To be effective, physical activity should be executed for at least 20 minutes at a time, whereas smoking involves a different time span altogether.
2. *Space*: Adopting physical activity requires a special environment that permits this behavior to take place (safely), whereas quitting smoking does not.
3. *Financial consequences*: Adopting physical activity in many instances costs money, whereas quitting smoking will (eventually) save money.
4. *Frequency of behavior*: Adopting physical activity requires recurrent action, whereas quitting smoking does not, once the subject has reached the maintenance stage of smoking cessation.
5. *Physiological consequences*: Adopting physical activity may lead to increased production of endorphines, whereas quitting smoking may lead to withdrawal symptoms such as those caused by a lack of nicotine.
6. *Dependency on others*: Adopting physical exercise is often related to having a partner in sporting activities or practicing a team sport, whereas quitting smoking is relatively independent of others, although social support and pressure may be essential.
7. *Reward and positive reinforcement*: Adopting physical activity is generally regarded as a very positive behavior, whereas quitting smoking may initially generate a positive response from the environment, but easily may be taken for granted after a longer period of time,

because smoking may have been regarded as unacceptable behavior in the first place.

These criteria can form the basis for a taxonomy of health behaviors that can be used to compare research outcomes. We are convinced that the nature of the target health behavior has been overlooked too frequently as a powerful source of unequivocal research results. Likewise, more subjective characteristics of the health behavior target, such as importance–commitment, difficulty level, temporal level, and level of consciousness, should be assessed, because they may account for important interindividual differences.

Fifth, most of the existing health behavior models are cognitive models; that is, the most important determinants are defined in terms of context and capability beliefs or outcome expectancies. As such, one can question whether other regulatory processes such as bodily and affective regulatory processes received the attention they deserve. Although it can be argued that bodily processes are beyond the scope of psychological models, they do play a very important role in the acquisition and maintenance of health behaviors such as regular physical exercise or in the reduction of addictive behaviors such as smoking, alcohol abuse, or various forms of excessive food intake. However, affective processes always should be integrated into health behavior models by at least differentiating between achievement or health target-related cognitions, on the one hand, and affect-related cognitions, on the other hand. These cognitions do not necessarily require different regulatory mechanisms (such as feedback, feedforward, or action control mechanisms). They are, however, different in nature and are linked to different and possibly conflicting personal health and well-being goals, and, as such, they are an important source of interindividual differences in the pursuit of health behaviors.

Based on all these considerations, we developed the health behavior goal model (HBG), which integrates aspects of expectancy–value, stage, and goal theories. In short, the model's features are that it (1) incorporates the personal goal structure of the individual, (2) encompasses phases of change, (3) focuses on individual emotional and health costs as well as benefits of changing the behavior, (4) takes into account an individual's perception of his or her own capacities, as well as the perceived influence of the direct environment, and (5) recognizes personal as well as environmental sources of change. There is evidence from two studies—one on physical exercise and one on smoking—that competing personal goals do predict (in addition to more traditional determinants) stage transitions toward or away from target health behaviors.

However, more research is needed on other health behavior targets. Additionally, the relationship between health behaviors and higher-order goals should be studied, because both studies concentrated on competing goals at a behavioral level only. This is an important issue for further research, because higher-order goals give purpose to specific health goals. We are currently carrying out research in this direction on exercise behavior, smoking, and use of alcohol in adolescents and cardiac patients. In these two ongoing studies, goal importance and fulfillment scales are applied, that are constructed on the basis of the Ford and Nichols (1991) taxonomy of higher-order goals.

In addition, the ultimate test of a health behavior change model should not be restricted to prospective studies, but also should include intervention studies. Ultimately, only quasi-experimental studies can ascertain which variables favor transition from one stage to another and for which (subset of) subjects. As such, it will be important to determine whether the effectiveness of particular interventions is stage and subject dependent. Much of the existing knowledge concerning health behavior change is derived from models based on expectancy–value theory and cannot be applied satisfactorily to interventions. The more traditional models do not adequately represent the process of change and therefore aim to discover determinants of health behavior for whole populations, rather than to identify subgroups on the basis of process characteristics. Intervention studies also will provide insight into the role of environmental characteristics with respect to the process of change, which is often underestimated in health behavior models. Many changes in health behavior are dependent on the existence of opportunities for contemplation, initiation, change, and maintenance. Self-regulation is possible only if environmental conditions for change are present. As a consequence, social engineering is frequently a necessary precondition for self-regulation, especially in healthy populations, where internal cues (e.g., symptoms) are absent. Although illness and health behaviors are closely related, internal and external pressures for change are more frequently absent in healthy populations; hence, changing health behaviors in healthy populations is more difficult.

Finally, the role of demographic and personal factors, such as goal orientations related to health behavior and health behavior change, should be studied. Like environmental factors, they may be important determinants of the core construct emphasized in the health behavior goal model, and thus of health behavior change.

Although much more research is needed, we hope to have convinced the reader that goal theory can form the cornerstone for an important extension of the more traditional social cognitive models and the stage models, which frequently have been applied to the area of health behavior change.

ACKNOWLEDGMENT

We are indebted to Laura Sweeney for reviewing the English.

REFERENCES

Ajzen, I. (1985). From intentions to actions: A theory of planned behavior. In J. Kuhl & J. Beckman (Eds.), *Action-control: From cognition to behavior*. Heidelberg, Germany: Springer-Verlag.

Austin, J. T., & Vancouver, J. B. (1996). Goal constructs in psychology: Structure, process and content. *Psychological Bulletin,120*(3), 338–375.

Bandura, A. (1977). *Social learning theory*. Englewood Cliffs, NJ: Prentice-Hall.

Carver, C. S., & Scheier, M. F. (1982). Control theory: A useful conceptual framework for personality-social, clinical, and health psychology. *Psychological Bulletin, 92*, 111–135.

Coats, E. J., Janoff-Bulman, R., & Alpert, N. (1996). Approach versus avoidance goals: Differences in self-evaluation and well-being. *Personality and Social Psychology Bulletin, 22*(10), 1057–1067.

Csikszentmihalyi, M. (1990). *Flow: The psychology of optimal experience*. New York: Harper & Row.

Edwards, W. (1961). Behavioral decision theory. *Annual Review of Psychology, 12*, 473–498.

Fishbein, M., & Ajzen, I. (1975). *Belief, attitude, intention, and behavior: An introduction to theory and research*. Reading, MA: Addison-Wesley.

Ford, M. E. (1992). *Motivating humans: Goals, emotions and personal agency beliefs*. Newbury Park, CA: Sage.

Ford, M. E., & Nichols, C. W. (1991). Using goal assessments to identify motivational patterns and facilitate behavioral regulation and achievement. In M. L. Maehr & P. R. Pintrich (Eds.), *Advances in motivation and achievement* (Vol. 7, pp. 51–84). Greenwich, CT: JAI Press Inc.

Frijda, N. H. (1988). The laws of emotion. *American Psychologist, 43*, 349–358.

Gebhardt, W. A. (1997). *The health behaviuor goal model: Towards a theoretical framework for health behavior change*. (Health Psychology Series No. 2). Leiden, Netherlands: Leiden University.

Hobfoll, S. E. (1988). *The ecology of stress*. Washington, DC: Hemisphere.

Janis, I. L., & Mann, L. (1968). A conflict-theory approach to attitude change and decision making. In A. G. Greenwald, T. C. Brock, & T. M. Ostrom (Eds.). *Psychological foundations of attitudes*. New York: Academic Press.

Kobasa, S. (1979). Stressful life events, personality and health: An inquiry into hardiness. *Journal of Personality and Social Psychology, 37*, 1–11.

Kuhl, J. (1981). Motivational and functional helplessness: The moderating effect of state versus action orientation. *Journal of Personality and Social Psychology, 40*, 155–170.

Kuhl, J. (1992). A theory of self-regulation: Action versus state orientation, self-discrimination and some applications. *Applied Psychology: An International Review, 41*, 97–129.

Lazarus, R. S. (1993). Coping theory and research: Past, present and future. *Psychosomatic Medicine, 55*, 234–247,

Lazarus, R. S., & Folkman, S. (1984). *Stress, appraisal, and coping*. New York: Springer-Verlag.

Leventhal, H. (1970). Findings and theory in the study of fear communications. In L. Berkowitz (Ed.). *Advances in experimental social psychology*, Vol. 5, pp. 119–185. New York: Academic Press.

Maes, S. (1990). Theories and principles of health behavior change. In P. Drenth, J. Sergeant, & R. Takens (Eds.). *European perspectives in psychology*, (Vol. 21, pp. 193–208). Chichester, UK: Wiley.

Maes, S., Leventhal, H., & De Ridder, D. (1996). Coping with chronic disease. In N. Endler & M. Zeidner (Eds.). *Handbook of coping*. New York: Wiley.

Maes, S., Sweeney, L., & Gebhardt, W. (1998). *The goal importance/facilitation scale*. Leiden, Netherlands: Leiden University.

Maes, S., & Van Elderen, T. (1998). Health psychology and stress. In M. Eysenck (Ed.). *Psychology: A European text*. London: Addison-Wesley Longman.

Markus, H., & Wurf, E. (1987). The dynamic self-concept: A social psychological perspective. *Annual Review of Psychology, 38,* 299–337.

McKeeman, D., & Karoly, P. (1991). Interpersonal and intrapsychic goal-related conflict reported by cigarette smokers, unaided quitters, and relapsers. *Addictive Behaviors, 16,* 543–548.

Prochaska, J. O., & DiClemente, C. C. (1986). Toward a comprehensive model of change. In W. R. Miller & N. Heather (Eds.). *Treating addictive behaviors.* New York: Plenum.

Rogers, R. W. (1975). A protection motivation theory of fear appeals and attitude change. *Journal of Psychology, 91,* 93–114.

Rosenstock, I. M. (1974). The health belief model and preventive health behavior. *Health Education Monographs, 2,* 354–386.

Rotter, J. B. (1982). Social learning theory. In N. T. Feather (Ed.). *Expectations and actions: Expectancy–value models in psychology.* Hillsdale, NJ: Erlbaum.

Scheier, M. F., & Carver, C. S. (1988). a model of behavioral self-regulation: Translating intention into action. *Advances in Experimental Social Psychology, 21,* 303–346.

Schwarzer, R. (1992). Self-efficacy in the adoption and maintenance of health behaviours: Theoretical approaches and a new model. In R. Schwarzer (Ed.). *Self-efficacy: Thought control of action.* Washington: Hemisphere.

Smith, J. H. (1977). The pleasure principle. *International Journal of Psychoanalysis, 58*(1), 1–10.

Weinstein, N. D. (1988). The precaution adoption process. *Health Psychology, 7,* 355–386.

World Health Organization (WHO). (1988). *Health promotion for working populations* (Technical Report Series, No. 765). Geneva, Switzerland: WHO.

12

REGULATION, SELF-REGULATION, AND CONSTRUCTION OF THE SELF IN THE MAINTENANCE OF PHYSICAL HEALTH

SUSAN BROWNLEE,* HOWARD LEVENTHAL,*
AND ELAINE A. LEVENTHAL[†]

*Rutgers University, New Brunswick, New Jersey
[†]Robert Wood Johnson School of Medicine, New Brunswick, New Jersey

I. THE SELF-REGULATION THEME

The major objective of this chapter is to provide our perspective on the nature of self-regulation as it has been applied to health-relevant behaviors. What distinguishes our approach from that of other, similar approaches is attention to content. Specifically, we define substantive domains in which specific variables that govern self-regulation can be assessed. We also define these variables as complex, bilevel structures, that is, as both abstractions (labels and propositions) and experienced perceptions, something done in few other models (for an exception, see

Copyright © 2000 by Academic Press.
All rights of reproduction in any form reserved.

Epstein, 1973, 1993a). We reject the assumption that the strongest, most useful models are content-free, for example, models with variables such as attitudes, perceived probabilities, and utilities. Although open models are reasonable starting points or frameworks, frameworks become theory only when they define specific, content variables within substantive domains. We know of no scientific theories that have advanced our understanding of natural processes in the absence of substantive content.

A second and related goal is to describe the growth of our theoretical view on the self-regulation process and how it borrowed from and contrasted with the theoretical position of other investigators. Although we refer to empirical data where it is relevant and available, we do not attempt an exhaustive summary of empirical literature. Readers searching for integrative summaries are advised to look elsewhere (e.g., Bishop, 1994; Carver & Scheier, 1981, 1982, in press; Croyle & Barger, 1993; Leventhal, Leventhal, & Cameron, in press b; Ory & DeFries, 1998; Petrie & Weinman, 1997; Skelton & Croyle, 1991; Stoller, 1998). Whereas our perspective informs the text, it draws to a substantial degree on material from our laboratory.

The third of our objectives is to attempt to distinguish among three perspectives on self-regulation: (1) self-regulation as problem solving, (2) self-regulation as self versus other generated goals, and (3) self-construction, or the reorganization and modification of features of the self, and strategies and procedures for problem solving. Although the boundaries between these perspectives are fuzzy rather than sharp, we articulate the defining characteristics of each in the section that follows. With that task completed, we present an overview of the Common-Sense Model (CSM) of self-regulation. We describe the model's origin and compare and contrast it with other models used to understand self-regulative processes relevant to health. Following our treatment of problem solving and goal selection, we turn to the self system and the modification of the content and structure of the self (i.e., self-construction).

II. PROBLEM SOLVING, SELF-REGULATION, AND REGULATION OF THE SELF

An intense, week-long conference with colleagues at Leiden University led us to question what we meant when we used the phrase "self-regulation." Does it point to new insights or is it mere jargon? The absence of any logic for the appearance and disappearance of the phrase from the titles of our integrative and summary papers suggested that either it is an inherently shy pair of words or that we were uncertain of its meaning and utility.[1] It seemed of value, therefore, to address this issue up front.

A. DIMENSIONS ALONG WHICH PROBLEM SOLVING SHADES INTO SELF-REGULATION AND REGULATION OF THE SELF

How do we decide when a process involves self-regulation? Everyday activities such as going to work, preparing meals, and integrating food shopping into daily schedules require problem solving behavior that involves self-regulation only in the sense that the self is the source of action (see Greenwald, 1981). Do these daily tasks differ in a fundamental way from behavior such as taking two aspirins to control or eliminate the headache and feverish feeling of a cold? Does the latter become self-regulation because its targets (i.e., the symptoms) are manifest in the self? Of course, the cues and actions of going to work are also in the self: The meaning of the 7:00 a.m. alarm is in the auditory and interpretive systems of the mind, as is the perception of the road while one is driving. If we assume that a person trying to get rid of a headache and feverish feeling is acting as a commonsense medical scientist (Leventhal, & Diefenbach, 1991; Leventhal, Leventhal, & Contrada, 1998b; Leventhal, Meyer, & Nerenz, 1980), diagnosing the condition as a cold and taking procedures appropriate for its control, then these actions are no less problem solving than those involved in going to work. Although the targets are in the somatic self, they are little different from other external targets (see Table 1). It is unlikely that the headache and feverish feeling were of the actor's choosing or that the actions taken require any change in self-identity or the acquisition of new skills.

It appears more reasonable to view problem solving as self-regulation when the target for problem solving is set by the problem solver and/or when the problem solving focuses on the "machinery" of the self and/or subjective feelings of the self. Managing self-machinery could include activities as narrow as focusing more intently on one's hand while removing an embedded splinter or as broad as varying eating and sleep patterns to minimize jet lag prior to an overseas flight. Self-regulation is also an intimate part of problem solving when an individual makes choices among

[1] Self-regulation appeared in titles in the mid 1980s (Leventhal, Zimmerman, & Gutmann, 1984; Nerenz & Leventhal, 1983) and disappeared and reappeared in the 1990s (Leventhal, Leventhal, & Contrada, 1998). It was not mentioned in our integration of the studies on fear communications (Leventhal, 1970) and it was not salient in our presentations of the Common-Sense Model of Illness Cognition (Leventhal, Meyer, & Nerenz, 1980; Leventhal et al., 1984; Nerenz & Leventhal, 1983). Until our more recent publications, it seemed that we were more likely to use the expression when applying the CSM model to specific health problems such as compliance with treatment (e.g., Leventhal et al., 1984).

alternative outcomes, such as the trade-off between experiencing pain and distress from treatment to avoid the pain and distress of advancing disease (Chapman, 1998). It also seems appropriate to describe problem solving as self-regulation when it is necessary to acquire new procedural knowledge specific for goal attainment.

Finally, "self-construction" may be the most appropriate label when the focus of attention and the goals for problem solving shift to altering self-identities (e.g., who and what one is) and the acquisition of procedural skills for maintaining existent roles and personal function. For example, the construction of new identities and procedures for self-maintenance are involved when a woman newly diagnosed with breast cancer adopts the role of a cancer patient when in treatment and vigorously retains the role of wife and mother when at home (Nerenz & Leventhal, 1983). The patient role is a new identity and the reorganization required to sustain old identities in the face of new circumstances demands the use of both existent and new higher-order strategies. Taking on the single new identity of "cancer patient" is likely to be simpler because it requires only the adoption of new role-relevant coping procedures; the acquisition of procedures for maintaining distinctions among roles is unnecessary (Leventhal, Idler, & Leventhal, 1999).

Although problem solving, self-regulation, and self-construction appear as discrete categories as defined by the Yes entries in the rows of Table 1, the rows should be treated as dimensions without boundaries. Thus, problem solving, self-regulation, and construction of the self, the columns in Table 1, represent idealized definitions of categories that lack distinct boundaries and shade into one another. The dimensions (i.e., rows of the table) can be used to characterize specific health actions: Those with more Yes entries toward the leftmost column are defined as problem solving; those with more entries toward the right side are defined as self-constructions. The pattern of Yes entries depends, however, on the preexistent knowledge and skills of the individual performing the behavior. Thus, the same action may be characterized differently at different points in time for the same person. For example, if a healthy middle-aged male adopts a low fat diet, takes vitamin E supplements, and drinks green tea to reduce the risk of colon cancer, he is best conceptualized as problem solving if these actions require neither new skills or changes in how he goes about his daily activities. The view of these behaviors as simple problem solving will be strengthened if there is no change in self-identity; that is, the behaviors are adopted to reduce existent, perceived familial risk and do not change the actor's views of vulnerability to cancer. Indeed, if the behaviors are correctly characterized as problem solving activities, we can expect them to change in response to new information; for example, all of the behaviors would be cast aside if credible information indicates that they are ineffective or if new information is received about the cause of death of the

TABLE 1   Factors That Are Common to and That Differentiate Problem Solving, Self-Regulation, and Construction of the Self: The Three Types of Activity Emerge as One Moves from the Low to the High End of a Dimension

Dimensions	Problem solving	Self-regulation	Construction of the self
Goal Dimensions			
Goals set by self	—	Yes	Yes?
Modifying current affect level ($-$ & $+$) is goal	Yes	Yes	—
Adding new self-identities	—	—	Yes
Modifying existent self-identities (e.g., adding features to existent roles)	—	—	Yes
Procedural dimensions (i.e., actions taken)			
Monitor & regulate goals	Yes	Yes	Yes
Focus attention: Concentrate on relevant cues and shut out irrelevant cues	—	Yes	—
Control energy level: Rest, clear vision, steady hands, etc.	—	Yes	—
Regulate affect states	—	Yes	—
1) Using automatic tactics	—	—	—
2) With volitional tactics	Yes	Yes	—
Invoke higher-order strategies: Use existent strategies when other tactics fail	—	Yes	Yes?
Create new forms for controlling each of above (i.e., attention, energy level, affect, & strategies)	—	—	Yes

uncle, that is, that he died of untreated appendicitis rather than colon cancer. On the other hand, if the behavioral changes involve the acquisition of new self-identities (i.e., that one is intrinsically (genetically) at risk), the individual may be less willing to change specific preventive behaviors and very unwilling to give up the role of cancer prevention. The question remaining is whether the same "self-regulation" model, (i.e., with common substantive domains and variables similarly structured) can represent these three processes and be an effective guide to empirical research.

III. MODELING PROBLEM SOLVING, SELF-REGULATION, AND SELF-CONSTRUCTION

Table 2 provides an overview of the models that have guided descriptive studies and interventions examining both health behaviors (e.g., preventive actions) and illness behaviors (e.g., diagnostic and treatment activities (Kasl & Cobb, 1966)). A comparison of the models suggests that their commonalities outstrip their differences. The nature of these similarities

TABLE 2 Overview and Rough Chronology of Theoretical Models Guiding Self-Regulation Research on Health and Illness Behavior

Model	Key assumptions	Early references
I. Drive Models	Classically conditioned fear motivates instrumental action; fear reduction reinforces instrumental actions	Miller (1951); Dollard & Miller (1950)
II. Attitude models	Favorableness toward a behavior is a function of its links to more basic attitudes and values	Peake (1958); Rosenberg et al. (1960)
Reasoned action	Probability action will achieve values and perceived favorableness of valued others	Fishbein & Ajzen (1974); Ajzen & Fishbein (1972, 1977)
Planned behavior	Self-efficacy in addition to intention	Ajzen (1991)
III. Models based on utility framework	Perceived path to goal = F (Probability of goal attainment × value)	Lewin (1935); Tolman (1938)
Health Belief Model	Motivation = F [perception of severity & perceived vulnerability] Action = F [motivation & benefits − costs] Action = F [Motivation/benefits − costs/symptoms/self-efficacy]	Hochbaum (1958) Rosenstock (1966) Becker & Maiman (1975)
IV. Parallel response model	Separate paths for danger and fear control Action = F [threat & act plan]; fear effects short lived; fear lowers self-efficacy and blocks action Representations abstract and concrete	Leventhal et al. (1965) Leventhal (1970) Johnson (1975)

Model	Description	References
V. Stress and coping model	Perceptual control of emotion Separate problem and emotion coping	Lazarus (1966) Lazarus & Launier (1978)
VI. Social learning model	Cognitive–behavioral and social learning Perceptual representations and modeling Self-efficacy and performance	Bandura (1969, 1977a, 1977b)
VII. Protection motivation	Separate paths for danger and fear control Adds utility component Motivation = F [perceived Severity × perceived vulnerability] Motivation = F [perceived Severity × preceived vulnerability × self-efficacy]	Rogers (1983)
VIII. Common Sense Model of Illness	Action = F [representation & procedures] Illness representations defined by (A) Abstract and concrete domains (B) Five empirically defined domains Procedures shaped by representation Five domains describe procedures Representations and procedures are context dependent (context = culture; roles; self system)	Leventhal et al. (1980) Leventhal & Diefenbach (1991); Lau et al. (1989) Leventhal & Diefenbach (1991) Leventhal et al. (1998b) Leventhal et al. (in press b)

and differences, and their reason for being can be appreciated best by reviewing them in relation to the development of the Common-Sense Model (CSM) for the analysis of health and illness behavior. The material will familiarize the reader with the theoretical approaches used in health research and show how we borrowed from and modified existent models to make sense of empirical evidence.

The CSM has five properties that distinguish it from other self-regulation models:

1. It specifies that health and illness behaviors are the product of the combined action of the representation of specific illness threats and of the action plans (i.e., procedures) called into play by these representations.
2. It defines five specific, substantive domains for the representation of threat.
3. It postulates that the variables within the five domains for representing threat are bilevel; that is, they are represented both as words (e.g., abstract disease labels) and by concrete, experiential processes (i.e., perceptions of symptoms, sense of time passed, images of danger, etc.).
4. It postulates separate cognitive and affective systems that interact in affecting behavior.
5. It assumes that contextual factors (e.g., social roles, personality) influence behavior by affecting disease representations and procedures for action.

Thus, we expect an individual confronting a disease threat such as cancer will have thoughts and concrete ideas about the identity (label cancer, perceived symptoms of cancer), time frame (expected longevity and feelings or images of events until time of death), cause (thoughts about diet, smoking, and recall of specific events where one succumbed to the temptation of cigarettes or high-cholesterol foods), consequences (pain, and physical and psychological dysfunction), and control of cancer (breast cancer treatable by surgery and chemotherapy; lung cancer perceived as not treatable by any known method), and have emotional reactions to these representations. We also would expect the individual to plan and act (or not act) to prevent, detect, or treat cancer in ways consistent with the representation of the disease, and each of the representations, action plans, and emotional reactions will be affected by contextual factors. We are confronting a complex, dynamic system that is difficult to examine as a totality.

A. THE ORIGINS OF THE COMMON-SENSE MODEL

The CSM developed from a fusion of two lines of research: studies of preventive health behavior that were guided by the Health Belief Model

(HBM: Rosenstock, 1974; Rosenstock, Hochbaum, & Leventhal, 1960) and studies of the effects of fear communications on preventive health practices, which were guided initially by the Fear-Drive Model (Dollard & Miller, 1950).

Health Belief Model: A Utility Approach

The Health Belief Model (HBM) is typical of the utility models that were and still are popular in economic analyses. It posited that health behaviors are motivated by the product of the perception of the severity of a health threat times perceptions of vulnerability to or probability of the threat (Becker, 1974; Becker & Maiman, 1975; Rosenstock, 1974). The specific response selected to avoid threat was that with the greatest number of perceived benefits and the smallest number of perceived losses (see Table 2).

The HBM did not arrive on the scene de novo; it was similar to models of attitudes that proposed that attitudes toward specific actions and objects are the product of the perceived probability of their satisfying a person's values or "utilities" (Peak, 1958; Rosenberg, Hovland, McGuire, Abelson, & Brehm, 1960). The theory of reasoned action (TRA: Fishbein & Ajzen, 1974) and its later version, the theory of planned behavior (TPB: Ajzen, 1991; Ajzen & Fishbein, 1980; Hecker & Ajzen, 1983), are widely used models that fall within the utility framework. Both TRA and TPB propose that favorableness toward specific health actions and intentions to engage in actions, such as quitting smoking or obtaining a mammogram to detect breast cancer, are products of the perceived probability that the act will satisfy more basic attitudes and values (e.g., the likelihood that quitting smoking will achieve values such as increased longevity, monetary savings, etc.). The theory of reasoned action (TRA) added two constructs missing from the HBM: intention and perceived norms. *Perceived norms* involve the actor's perception that valued others (assessed) were favorable toward the proposed action (e.g., approved of quitting smoking). *Intention to act* was seen as a necessary step that mediated (i.e., connected) attitudes and perceived norms to actual behavior (Ajzen & Fishbein, 1972).

The Health Belief Model (HBM) differs from TRA and TPB in three ways: it does not presume that intentions are necessary for action, it overlooks social influence, and it makes a significant step toward providing substantive definitions of its probability and value components (i.e., vulnerability and severity). By contrast, the TRA and other attitude models failed to specify the content of the beliefs and values relevant to specific actions to protect health and manage disease. Whereas our Common-Sense Model defines specific, substantive domains, it continues in the tradition of the HBM and rejects the open approach of the TRA and TPB. CSM departs, however, from both the HBM and the TRA by postulating that the mechanisms underlying the variables comprising the representation of disease threats involve both abstract and experiential or concrete components. Finally, the role of the social context in the CSM is far more complex than that postulated in either the TRA or TRB.

The Fear-Drive Model

The Fear-Drive Model, the second, important source of the CSM, emerged from research in the animal laboratory (Miller, 1951) and was applied relatively unchanged to humans. In its human guise, it was viewed as an operational or behavioral version of the psychodynamics of fear (Dollard & Miller, 1950). The model assumed that fear that was classically conditioned (Pavlovian conditioning) to external cues (lights, sounds, thoughts, and messages about cancer) was a source of motivation and that instrumental responses that reduced these fear states (e.g., the rat's escape from the shock compartment of a shuttle box and the human's quitting smoking or taking a medicine to kill bacteria) were rewarded and learned because they reduced and/or eliminated fear. This combination of classical and instrumental conditioning was presumed to account for the wide range of motivated actions in animals and humans that could not be accounted for by primary drives such as hunger, thirst, and sexuality.

Experimental Studies of Fear Communications

The Fear-Drive Model's contribution to the Common-Sense Model (CSM) came by way of our studies on the effects of threat (fear-arousing) messages on attitudes and behaviors. The studies of response to fear communications were experimental and many were prospective; that is, attitudinal and behavioral outcomes were assessed hours, days, weeks, and months after exposure to the threat messages. Threat level or fear was the major factor varied in these studies (Janis, 1969; Leventhal, 1970), and it typically was orthogonal to other variables (e.g., action plans), the order of presentation of fear material, self-esteem, and delay between message receipt and time for action (Kornzweig, 1967). The presence or absence of specific action instructions (i.e., action plans) was the most important of these other factors (Leventhal, Singer, & Jones, 1965; Leventhal, Watts, & Pagano, 1969). The studies were designed to test a basic assumption of the Fear-Drive Model, which is that high levels of fear would increase acceptance of recommended health actions only when they were accompanied by action plans that facilitated fear reduction. It was the reduction of fear by action plans or by any other factor orthogonal to fear level (e.g., the immediate availability of action; forced rehearsal of action plans after rather than before exposure to the threat message, etc.) that was seen as critical for the acceptance rather than the rejection of a recommended health action. Unfortunately for the Fear-Drive Model, not one of these expectations was supported by data.

The Parallel Response Model: Fear and Cognition
Are Processed in Parallel

The results of the fear communication studies forced an alternative paradigm for understanding how information about health threats was processed en route to overt action. The data that required the shift were as follows. First, no studies confirmed the earlier findings (Janis & Feshbach, 1953) that compliance to recommended health actions was diminished by presenting recommendations as part of high fear in contrast to low fear messages, presumably because high fear stimulated defensive reactions.[2] Rather, in study after study, strong threat messages aroused higher levels of fear and more favorable attitudes toward recommended health practices than did low threat messages. However, the more favorable attitudes and behavioral intentions generated by the high threat messages declined to precommunication baseline as fear subsided; this usually took place within 24 to 48 hours postexposure (Leventhal, 1970). Most importantly, high threat messages rarely if ever produced more overt action than did low threat messages (Leventhal, 1970).

The lack of support for the fear-drive hypothesis does not mean that threat messages were irrelevant for action. There was no action in the absence of either a high or a low threat message: action required exposure to a threat message, high or low, and to an action plan: the combination was essential for action (see Figure 1). The likelihood of action was identical for action plans combined with a high threat message and action plans combined with a low threat message; the level of fear had no effect on the behavioral outcome. Thus, identical numbers of participants were inoculated against tetanus after exposure to either a high or a low threat message as long as the threat messages were combined with an action plan, but neither the plan alone nor the threat messages alone led to action (Leventhal et al., 1965). Likewise, a similar number of participants quit or reduced smoking after exposure to a strong or weak threat message about smoking and lung cancer when the threat messages were combined with action plans (Leventhal et al., 1967).

Finally, data also showed that fear could inhibit actions that moved the individual toward a danger and increased his or her sense of threat (e.g., taking chest X-rays; see Millar & Millar, 1995, 1996, for more recent evidence). There were no signs of inhibition for actions to avoid threat

[2]There is little or no evidence for the assumption that the levels of fear reported in studies of fear-arousing communications stimulates defensive responding. The data show fear effects are short lived and that high fear may disrupt the recipient's sense of competence at executing responses, but does so only for brief periods of time (Leventhal, 1970). It is not entirely clear that there was a main effect in the original Janis and Feshbach study, because the main effect does not seem to be present in a later report that included all subjects and showed an interaction of fear level with individual differences in neuroticism (see Janis & Feshbach, 1954).

such as quitting smoking, although on occasion there were signs that fear facilitated such behaviors (Leventhal et al., 1967). In those cases where fear facilitated or inhibited action, it did so for relatively brief periods of time. A major conclusion drawn from these data was that there are two pathways for processing information about health threats: One is a relatively "cold" cognitive path that generates a representation of the perceived threat and plans for coping; the other is a "hot" path that creates active states of fear and procedures for fear management (see Figure 1).

The results of these studies raised at least three critical questions:

1. What in the specific action plans was critical for generating action?
2. What aspect of the threat message was critical for sustaining overt action for days and weeks well after the decline of fear (see also Lazarus, 1966; Lazarus, Speisman, Mordkoff, & Davison, 1962)?
3. Do the processes involved in fear remain separate from those involved in the perceptual representation of the danger or do they in some way interact with it, and if so, how (see also Lazarus & Launier, 1978)?

In this chapter we focus on the first two of these questions.

Action Plans Are Concrete

The action plans used in the fear studies went well beyond simple recommendations such as get an inoculation or quit smoking: (1) they were specific and concrete, and (2) they embedded the recommended action

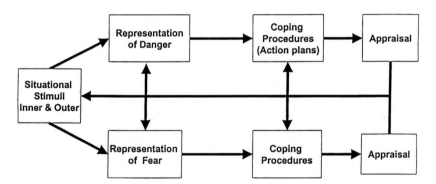

FIGURE 1   The early version of the parallel response model proposed that somatic stimuli and information about disease threats from external sources are processed in two, largely independent routes: As objectively perceived representations of danger (i.e., health threats) and as emotional experience. Action plans or coping procedures are generated to reach goals set by the representations and appraisals of procedural efficacy feedback into the system, revising the procedures, altering the representation, eliminating the eliciting stimulus, and/or arousing or minimizing affective reactions. A similar sequence is involved in coping with fear.

within the individual's daily behavior pattern. The series of steps needed to begin and complete an action such as getting a tetanus shot or reducing smoking were described in detail, and the behaviors were linked to cues and action sequences in the participants' daily lives. For example, the student participants in the tetanus studies were given examples of class changes that would bring them near the student health center and were asked to review their daily class schedules and identify such class changes in their own schedules: The plan laid out the steps to connect the action to the individual's daily behavior. Similar links were created to daily life situations for the procedures to quit smoking.

Are Threat Messages Concrete?

The concrete nature of action plans (i.e., their connecting of specific actions to concrete (visible and palpable) cues) suggested that the representations of illnesses that provide the goals for self-protective behaviors and the cues for starting and directing these behaviors also have an important, concrete component. Whereas high and low threat messages covered the same points in more (high threat) and less vivid (low threat) language, we suspected that elements common to both elicited concrete mental contents from the recipients' existent knowledge base. This hypothesis also was suggested by the findings of the two earliest studies testing the Health Belief Model: Hochbaum's (1958) study of factors that affect people's desire to take chest X-rays to detect lung cancer and Leventhal, Rosenstock, Hochbaum and Carriger's (1960) study on factors that affect taking flu inoculations during the 1957 influenza epidemic. Both of these studies showed that beliefs in vulnerability to disease (lung cancer and flu) predicted behavior if these beliefs were measured at an experiential level rather than by direct questioning. For example, when confronted with a picture of a man walking past an X-ray booth, Hochbaum's (1958) subjects who did not themselves get X-rays explained the behavior by saying, "He did not need an X-ray because he looks healthy."

The hypothesis that concrete cues played a critical role in guiding coping behaviors was supported also by a series of studies on the preparation of patients to cope with noxious medical procedures (Johnson, 1975; Leventhal, Leventhal, Shacham, & Easterling, 1989). For example, patients prepared with concrete information (i.e., the sensations they would experience during endoscopy) and procedures for coping (i.e., how to breathe and swallow the endoscopy tube) gagged less and controlled the rate at which the tube was inserted through the trachea (Johnson, 1975; Johnson & Leventhal, 1974). In summary, the findings from each of these lines of research pointed to the critical role of concrete, perceptual information as a guide to performance. We proposed, therefore, that representations of health threats are both abstract and concrete (Figure 2).

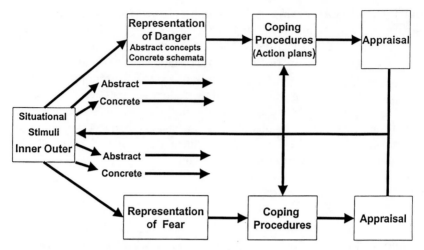

FIGURE 2   The early elaboration of the parallel response model proposed that somatic stimuli and information about disease threats from external sources are processed by abstract, propositional structures and by implicit, concrete structures or schemata. Concrete schemata give preverbal meanings to stimuli (Leventhal, 1984). Concrete schemata are also multi-level, combining organized perceptual information (Leventhal, 1984) with less detailed schemas or images of less structured, early experience such as the rapid movement of objects toward or away from the self (J. Mandler, 1992), events capable of eliciting emotional reactions.

Our confidence was strengthened in the importance of the perceptual features of representations for generating and sustaining motivation for action by theoretical and empirical work in social learning theory (SLT: Bandura, 1969, 1977a). Studies of social modeling clearly emphasized the importance of observation of others as a source of motivation and the acquisition of procedures for action. Similarly, the construct of self-efficacy (Bandura, 1977b), which emphasized the importance of the individual's sense of his or her ability to perform the actions needed to achieve a particular outcome, was similar to our earlier suggestion that signs of the inhibition of overt action by fear were due to fear undermining self-competence for executing plans rather than due to fear stimulating denial (Leventhal, 1970).

IV. ILLNESS COGNITION AND CONTROL THEORY

The version of the Common-Sense Model (CSM) that emerged at the end of the decade of the 1960s (Leventhal et al., 1965; Leventhal, 1970) and the coping stress model that developed at about the same time (Lazarus, 1966; Lazarus & Launier, 1978) provided investigators with a control system framework that was useful for describing problem solving and affect regulation. The pictures used to represent the CSM (Figures 1 and 2; e.g., Leventhal, 1970; Leventhal et al., 1980; Leventhal & Nerenz, 1983) differed, however, from the figures used to represent self-regulation processes in models developed by control theorists such as Carver & Scheier (1981, 1982, in press), Miller, Galanter, & Pribram (1960), and Powers (1973). The figures generated by the latter theorists were built around a simple TOTE (test, operate, test, exit) unit (see Figure 3), and did not have the boxes for representations, procedures, and appraisals present in the figures used to represent the CSM (see Figures 4 and 5).

The boxes in the CSM have a particular purpose: they provide space in which to elaborate the content of the control process. Attention to content is a distinguishing feature of the CSM, and the representation box was to be filled with the attributes that defined illness representations, the procedural box with the cognitive heuristics, strategies, and actions useful for diagnosing the presence of threat and its control, and the appraisal box for spelling out the criteria against which actions are appraised. In short, the picture of the CSM was designed to include domain-specific contents. The TOTE, by contrast (e.g., Carver & Scheier, 1981, 1982, in press; Scheier & Carver, 1992), shows an input function (i.e., the feedback from a response designed to alter an environmental disturbance) that is compared to a

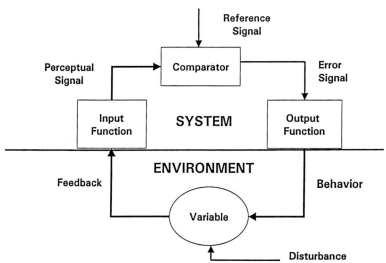

FIGURE 3 The TOTE represents a content-free regulatory device that responds by detecting and evaluating disturbances (comparing the input to a reference signal) and generating an output function and behavior designed to reduce the discrepancy detected in the comparison of input to reference signal. System action repeats until the discrepancy is removed. TOTEs of different types can be organized in hierarchical and parallel arrangements. Adapted from C. S. Carver & M. F. Scheier, in press.

standard or reference value (Figure 3). The picture is content-free and is equally fine as a description of the thermostat controlling the temperature of a house or as the behavior of a person taking a medication to treat a cold.

A. THE SUBSTANCE OF COMMON-SENSE MODELING

The development of substantive domains and specific content variables was the first, major point of departure of common-sense modeling from that of other self-regulation models and other theories used for the analysis of health-relevant behaviors. The identification of these domains and their bilevel structure was critical, therefore, to the development of the CSM. The content of these representations defines the goals or reference values for the regulation process. Once goals and procedures for goal attainment are specified, their sources can be defined and we can evaluate whether the processes identified in the CSM can be applied to self-regulation and self-construction as defined in the second part of this chapter.

The Attributes of Illness Representations

A variety of approaches were taken to identify the content of illness representations. One was to use open-ended interviews to explore the representation and management of everyday illnesses such as the common cold (Lau, Bernard, & Hartmann, 1989; Lau & Hartmann, 1983), chronic asymptomatic illnesses such as hypertension (Baumann & Leventhal, 1985; Meyer, Leventhal, & Gutmann, 1985), and chronic symptomatic illnesses such as respiratory problems (Lacroix, Martin, Avendano, & Goldstein, 1991). A substantial number of these studies were reviewed by Scharloo and Kaptein (1997). A second approach was the use of multidimensional scaling with disease labels and symptoms as stimuli (Bishop, 1991; Bishop & Converse, 1986; D'Andrade, Quinn, Nerlove, & Romney, 1972; Linz, Penrod, Leventhal, & Siverhus, 1981). In both cases, the objective was to identify the content or attributes of representations as seen by study participants (see Lacroix, 1991; Lacroix et al., 1991). Recent studies have used closed items and factor analysis to identify dimensions of diseases such as arthritis (Hampson, Glasgow, & Zeiss, 1994; Schiaffino & Cea, 1995; Schiaffino & Revenson, 1992) and chronic fatigue syndrome (Moss-Morris, Petrie, & Weinman (1996). The dimensions are not always consistent across studies, in part because investigators used different item sets, but mainly because diseases differ from one another (Hampson et al., 1994; Heijmans, & deRidder, in press b). The disease-specific nature of illness representations makes clear that they reflect reality: They are grounded in concrete experience with specific symptoms, the rate of appearance and fluctuation of these symptoms, and the perceived contingencies of symptom fluctuation with environmental and behavioral factors.

Substantive Domains Defining Existent Illness At least five domains have emerged from studies of illness representations (see Figure 4): identity, or the labels and indicators (visible signs, functional declines, and subjective symptoms) that identify the presence of a disease; time lines, or the rates of onset, duration, and recovery associated with each illness; consequences, the functional, economic, social, and psychological consequences of the disease; causes, the environmental pathogens and internal factors generating the disease; and control, or the belief that the disease can be controlled by the self and/or expert intervention (Scharloo & Kaptein, 1997). The content and values of attributes such as time line and control differ by disease and by individual. For example, the symptoms perceived to be associated with elevations of blood glucose vary across diabetics (see Gonder-Frederick & Cox, 1991). Conditions such as coro-

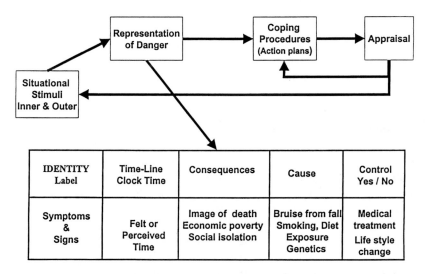

FIGURE 4 Five, substantive domains or attributes of illness representations were defined in later elaborations of the parallel response model: identity, time line, cause, consequences, and control (beliefs about the controllability of the disease). Specific variables can be defined within each domain and the variables within these domains are multilevel, that is, they derive their meaning from both abstract and concrete (perceptual and image-schema) structures. A similar set of attributes applies to action plans or procedures. Thus, procedures are appraised with respect to their impact on the identity (disease label and symptoms), time line (time to symptom relief), cause, and consequences of the threat, and affect the perception of its controllability. Abstract and concrete representations within the five domains may set different and conflicting goals for procedural action and result in different appraisals of action outcomes. This system can be viewed as a mental model for solving health and illness problems.

nary disease, osteoarthritis, and early onset or type 1 diabetes may be seen as similar with regard to chronicity, control, and cure (incurable), but vastly different as to consequences. Colon and breast cancer may be seen as curable if they have not spread, but once they are metastatic, they are more likely to be seen as incurable and uncontrollable. It is extremely important to note, however, that medical models and CSM representations are not the same! For example, in one study the majority of breast cancer patients with metastatic disease believed their disease was acute, that is, that it could be treated and cured just like the measles (Leventhal, Easterling, Coons, Luchterhand, & Love, 1986). Similarly, in her sample of 79 cancer patients, Silverman (1999) found only a weak association between physicians' ratings of poor prognosis and patients' beliefs that their disease was chronic.

Finally, a feature of illness representations that is useful for understanding individual differences in behavior for most diseases may be of no value for understanding individual differences in response for others. For example, virtually all Addison's disease patients agree their illness is genetic in origin; thus, this variable as measured is useless to explain individual differences in adaptation (Heijmans & deRidder, in press b). Reviews of studies of specific diseases can be found in Petrie and Weinman (1997) and Skelton and Croyle (1991).

Domains Defining Risk of Future Illness   Although we assume that the domains in which variables are defined for representing ongoing illness are also applicable to anticipated risks, less empirical work has been done to determine the fit of the domains and their attributes to health in contrast to illness behaviors (Kasl & Cobb, 1966). The transition to prevention and health behaviors will require some restatements and refinements of the variables within domains if not of the domains themselves. For example, higher levels of non-cancer-specific somatic symptoms are related to greater worry about cancer in women who are cancer-free, but this increase in worry occurs only for women who report feeling some degree of vulnerability to cancer (Cunningham et al., 1998; Easterling & Leventhal, 1989). Thus, the labels and indicators (subjective symptoms) that would define the presence or identity of cancer also generate worry about anticipated risk of cancer. However, the impact of symptoms operates within the framework of vulnerability beliefs, a factor that was not stipulated as a variable within the identity domain when examining how the representation of cancer affects illness behavior. Belief in vulnerability may be an important factor when examining how the representation of cancer affects behavior to a potential illness threat (see Leventhal, Kelly, & Leventhal, in press a; Rothman & Kiviniemi,1998), but there is no need to assess perceived vulnerability to cancer when studying cancer patients; they know they have cancer.

New variables may need to be added and older ones redefined in each of our five domains as we attempt to model representations of potential illness threats. Causal factors may prove to be of greater importance for prevention than for illness behaviors, because causal hypotheses define pathways and procedures for intervention (Rothman & Kiviniemi,1998). For example, contact avoidance has long been recognized as a preventive factor for infectious diseases, although people's tendency to avoid physical contact with individuals suffering from noninfectious diseases (e.g., cancer patients and physically disabled persons; Rozin, Markwith, & McCauley, 1994) indicates that this common-sense outlook generalizes to situations for which it is totally irrelevant. Different time lines also will be salient for health and illness behaviors. Perceived time in life when a disease strikes and time needed for it to develop are likely to be more important for prevention, whereas health behaviors and time lines for illness duration and rehabilitation are more important for illness behavior.

The comparison between representations of illness behaviors and those for health behaviors brings the self-system to the fore. Given that illness creates problems in the here and now, it is possible to ignore the self and to stay within a problem solving approach when examining the processes involved in planning and executing procedures for illness management. It is more difficult to ignore the self, however, when examining prevention and health behaviors, because recognizing the possibility of illness is essentially a statement about vulnerability of the self. What is less clear, however, is what aspects of the self are important for motivating such future-oriented behavior. Although distinguishing between illness and health behaviors brings this issue into focus and is useful for organizing our text, we believe the distinction is artificial and less useful for the analysis of process, because the self also is involved in illness behavior. The nature of this involvement is for later discussion.

The Bilevel Nature of Attributes

The bilevel composition of attributes is the second area in which CSM variables differ from those of other models. Each attribute is represented in abstract and concrete or perceptual form. Thus, the *identity* of an illness is defined by its disease label and by its symptoms; its time line by clock time and felt time; its consequences by statements about physical change and by the experienced physical change, and so forth (see Figures 2 and 4). The importance of symptoms as a concrete referent for the presence or possible risk of illness is seen in the Lau et al. (1989) data, which show that over 90% of their subjects reported symptoms as the key feature of recent illnesses. Symptoms are also critical in the Meyer et al. (1985) study of hypertension: 90% of a group of patients who were in ongoing treatment believed they could tell when their blood pressure was elevated by their headaches, warm face, dizziness, and nervousness. In that same interview,

80% of these patients agreed with the statement that people can't tell when their blood pressure is elevated, and 64% of these respondents spontaneously said to the interviewer, "Don't tell my doctor what I said." That chronic blood pressure elevations have virtually no relationship to symptoms is of little consequence as far as patients' beliefs are concerned! Although the figures vary by study, anywhere from 50% to 90% of subjects believe their symptoms are reliable indicators of elevated blood pressure (Baumann & Leventhal, 1985; Blumhaugen, 1980; Lambert, 1996).

The data in support of the bilevel nature of identity led us to propose the symmetry hypothesis: People will seek and find labels to explain their symptoms and will seek and find symptoms to concretize (i.e., make sense of) their illness labels. This proposition generated experimental tests of the hypothesis that telling subjects they had elevated blood pressure would lead them to experience and report symptoms. In one such study, all participants had their blood pressures taken in preparation for an exercise task, and were randomly assigned to one of two types of feedback about their readings: a false, elevated reading in which the experimenter made a worried comment about the subject's blood pressure and asked the subject to complete some questionnaires while he or she consulted the professor before proceeding with the next task, and a normal reading for control subjects, who were asked to complete a set of questionnaires before going on with the next task (Baumann, Cameron, Zimmerman, & Leventhal, 1989). The questionnaire, which was completed as soon as the experimenter left the room, included a symptom check list that included items reported by patients with hypertension. Subjects who believed their blood pressure was elevated reported the very same symptoms as those reported by hypertensives; subjects in the control condition did not (see also studies by Croyle & Uretsky, 1987; Salovey & Birnbaum, 1989).

It appears, therefore, that the relationship of symptoms to labels is bidirectional; that is, that "there is a symmetrical relationship between symptoms and labels" (Leventhal, et al., 1980). We assume that the symmetry of illness identities is both a product of past experience with illness and a fundamental property of the representational process; that is, the mind anchors constructs in perceptual reality. Doing so is adaptive because it provides concrete indicators for self-regulation. Although our examples of the bilevel nature of CSM variables have focused on the identity attribute, variables in each of the five domains are bilevel. Time line provides an interesting example. We are all familiar with clock time, and it is likely that we also recognize "felt" time, the instances where time seems to drag on or speed by at a frightening pace; for example, the time that it seems to take before you are called from the waiting room and enter to see your doctor, or the time on the ticket line prior to boarding your plane. Felt time plays a role in Jamison's (1995; Jamison & Akiskal, 1983) discussion of patients' nonadherence to antidepressant medication:

Although they are told it will take weeks for medication to produce mood changes, patients feel that more than enough time has passed for the medications to do their work and regard the absence of mood changes as a sign of treatment failure. Their perception of failure is likely facilitated by the early onset of somatic but not mood changes induced by many antidepressants. These somatic indicators validate felt time; they make clear that enough time has elapsed to feel drug effects and conclude that the drugs are not working. In a later section, we argue that representations of the self have this same bilevel property as well as sharing the five content domains.

Representations Define Goals and Appraisal Criteria for Procedures

The close connection between representations and procedures was embodied in the second proposition of illness cognition, that representations define goals for procedures. Representations guide the choice of procedures, sustain procedures, and set the criteria for evaluating procedural efficacy. Thus, the identity of a disorder (e.g., its symptoms and location in the gut or head), its time line (e.g., how swiftly it developed and whether it is increasing or varying in intensity), its presumed consequences (e.g., interference with ongoing activities and elicitation of emotional distress), and expectations with respect to its cause (e.g., stress, virus, bacteria) and controllability (e.g., can be self-controlled, needs medical attention) play a central role in defining the plausibility of specific treatment procedures, influencing thereby the selection and maintenance of procedures and setting criteria for appraisal of efficacy.

One clear implication of this proposition is that the domains that define the attributes of illness representations will define the domains for the attributes of procedures. Thus, a procedure will have an identity (e.g., a label and concrete consequences or side effects), a time line (e.g., expected time to produce recovery), consequences (e.g., mastectomy will be seen to produce disfigurement), a causal route of application (e.g., self-applied, expert applied), efficacy, and controllability (e.g., ways to regulate its risks and benefits). Because the number of procedures is vast, it is essential to identify specific factors within these broader domains; for example, routes of causal action, types of consequence, and time frames (Horne, 1997).

V. COPING PROCEDURES: GENERALIZED FACTORS VERSUS IF–THEN RULES THAT INTEGRATE REPRESENTATIONS, PROCEDURES, AND APPRAISALS

The proposition that representations define goals and the selection and maintenance of specific procedures clearly implies that procedures may be numbered in the hundreds if not thousands: the billions of dollars spent on traditional medical care and the equal, if not greater, amount spent on alternative care, health foods, and so forth, testify to this diversity. Burning sensations in the gut call for different procedures than a bleeding thumb, and the experienced gut person may use different procedures to control burning sensations and cramps. By attending to the specific features of a vast array of procedures for disease management, the CSM departs from both the stress coping model of Lazarus and Folkman (1984) and the self-regulation model of Carver and Scheier (1981), because the factorial approaches used by these investigators led them to settle on one (Lazarus & Folkman, 1984) or two (Carver, Scheier, & Weintraub,1989) factors for problem-focused coping. We suspect these simple solutions arose because their items were phrased to fit multiple situations and ignored the particulars features of any single, specific problem representation. Ignoring situational particulars can be seen as an effort to generate scientifically sound generalizations, but doing so ignores differences among procedures that are conceptually important. For example, a severe headache can lead to coping procedures ranging from taking a warm bath, aspirins, rest and sleep, or calling a doctor, and different beliefs about the causes of headaches and procedures appropriate for their control may underlie each of these reactions. For example, warm baths or showers may be preferred by people who believe both that headaches are due to stress and that medication is dangerous (those who do not will use aspirin), while those who believe their headaches are surface reflections of an underlying illness and that their bodies need strengthening may attempt to strengthen their immune systems with a good night's sleep or go to their doctors for diagnosis and treatment if they believe the illness might be serious and are strong believers in the value of modern medicine. In sum, the product of the factorial approach for problem-based coping will seem deficient if one believes that scientific generalizations should encompass and explain situational particulars (Bandura, 1977a; Lewin, 1935).

It is interesting to note that the factorial approaches used by stress and coping researchers generated many more factors for managing affective reactions than for managing real world problems. Factors such as positive thinking, distraction or avoidant coping, monitoring, and self-medication emerged from factorial studies of coping (Lazarus & Folkman, 1984). The diversity of factors very likely reflects the similarity across situations of subjective experiences and somatic expressions of affective reactions such as fear; hence the items to tap fear control procedures can address the particular features of the affective response independent of context. The contrast between the paucity of factors for problem-based coping and the more robust number for affective-based coping suggested that an attempt to develop a psychometrically sound coping scale to measure problem-based coping was premature and not the best way to increase our understanding of process. This decision was made even though the CSM framework was the first to differentiate sharply between the same two classes of coping as did the stress coping model; that is, danger control and fear control (Leventhal, 1970) and problem-focused and emotion-focused coping (Lazarus & Launier, 1978).

Procedures: The Active Components in the Constructive Process

Having decided for the moment against the use of factorial methods, we searched for an alternative model for the analysis of procedures for threat management. The approach that seemed to best describe the position we had adopted on the connections between representations and procedures was Anderson's (1987, 1993) formulation of representations and procedures as if–then rules. In the CSM framework, the if component stands for the goals set by the representation of the health threat, and the then stands for the procedures to be performed to achieve a particular outcome or appraisal. Procedures are the covert thoughts and overt acts that test, elaborate, and construct representations. They are the active components in the if–then rules that integrate representations and outcome appraisals. For example, if I have a stress headache, then I will expect two aspirins to remove it in 20 to 30 minutes. The procedure tests the presumed cause, time line, and controllability of my identity of stress headache. I can retain this identity in the absence of an expected outcome if I assume that it is an especially bad headache and effect a cure by taking more aspirin. Alternatively, I can consider another procedure (e.g., a stronger analgesic) or an alternative identity (e.g., migraine, stroke, brain tumor, etc.).

How procedures are involved in constructing illness representations can be examined by entertaining how they might operate in the presence of a somatic disturbance of unknown origin and nature (e.g., ambiguous conditions such as joint pain). As a first step, one might fall back on general rules or accepted practices such as "do something until you can figure out what is going on!" This activity is justified by the expectation that it will lead to a hypothesis as to the identity, time line, and consequences of the sensations. Such conditions are not uncommon, for example, when the initiating event, in this case the somatic experience, does not conform to prior experience or when it has no known time frame because its cause and onset were not observed, and clues are lacking as to its likely consequences or potential for control. Not knowing whether something does or does not need to be done, general procedures or strategies will take over with mixed expectations; that is, the hope that it will all work out and/or that its cause and properties will eventually be made clear. If the joint distress continues or worsens, the individual may review his or her immediate history (e.g., did I overextend myself in yesterday's workout or do I have other symptoms (e.g., running nose), suggesting I'm coming down with a cold?) and try specific, previously effective treatments related to specific causal hypotheses, such as applying ointments to ease exercise-induced distress or drinking more fluid and resting to handle an incipient cold (see Conner & Norman, 1998, for a related discussion of expansion for the theory of planned behavior). If self-care fails and the disturbance remains undefined, advice seeking and medical care seeking may result (Leventhal & Crouch, 1997). The process is ongoing and circular, each step designed both to eliminate the disturbance and clarify its meaning.

Examples of If–Then Rules

The value of if–then rules is readily apparent when using them to clarify the meaning of a more general strategy such as social comparison. Social comparisons can be undertaken to meet a wide range of informational needs (Leventhal, Hudson, & Robitaille, 1997) and if–then rules provide a useful way to clarify their specific goals. For example, Ditto and Jemmott (1989) made use of the prevalence rule (Kahneman & Tversky, 1973) to test the hypothesis that an experimental subject who perceived himself or herself as alone in being at risk for a serious disease when others were not (if) would be more likely to believe the disease was serious (then) in comparison to someone who was one of many who were at risk (See Croyle & Jemmott, 1991). The participants in this study tested their saliva for a fictitious antigen that was claimed to indicate risk for pancreatic disease. Participants were randomly assigned to one of two conditions: They either were the only person in a group with a positive antigen test or were part of a group that tested positive. Participants who were alone in testing positive were expected to judge the disorder to be more serious than it was judged by participants who thought their peers also tested positive: The data confirmed these expectations. The impact of prevalence on subjects' ratings of the seriousness of this fictitious pancreatic disorder showed that an if–then heuristic such as the prevalence rule can help to refine the meaning of social comparison.

A second rule, the stress–illness rule, was uncovered in a study by Cameron, Leventhal, and Leventhal (1995). Their study examined older persons' use of primary care in response to ambiguous symptoms (e.g., tiredness) in comparison to symptoms that were distinct indicators of possible illness (e.g., green phlegm). They hypothesized that if people were experiencing a life stress that was of fairly recent onset (i.e., less than 3 weeks duration), then they would attribute their ambiguous symptoms to the stressor rather than to illness and would not seek medical care. If the duration of the life stress exceeded 3 to 4 weeks, they would then assume that the stressor was making them ill and they would seek care in response to ambiguous symptoms. The data showed that participants experiencing ambiguous symptoms and life stress of short duration attributed their symptoms to stress and were unlikely to seek care; care seeking was more frequent among participants experiencing ambiguous symptoms in the context of prolonged life stress. Life stress had no effect on rates of care seeking for participants whose symptoms were unambiguous signs of illness. In summary, symptoms led to an environmental search and the information gleaned from the search moderated care-seeking behavior in the context of an if–then rule (i.e., am I stressed or am I sick?).

Regulation or Self-Regulation in Existent If–Then Rules

Although both the prevalence and stress–illness rules are environmentally oriented and the self is the referent for evaluating these environmental checks, the self is treated much like any other environmental object, suggesting that the behavior is best defined as problem solving. Prevalence leads one to ask, "Do others have the X factor that I have?" Stress–illness leads one to ask, "Has my environment been more stressful than usual for the past few weeks?" The regulatory activities that emerge from these comparisons is the definition (i.e., seeking more information about pancreatic disorders; Croyle, 1992; Ditto & Jemmott, 1989) and control of a disease threat (i.e., seeking medical care; Cameron et al., 1995; Leventhal & Leventhal, 1995). Treating these informational searches as problem solving rather than self-regulation is consistent with the perception that the targets regulated are symptoms and the pathogens presumed to underlie them, and not the self. Indeed, medical prescriptions directed toward the self (e.g., a physician's recommendation to take fluids and rest rather than prescribing an antibiotic for a viral cold) are often resisted. In the CSM view of illness, fluid and rest fail to take direct aim at the pathogen.

VI. THE SELF SYSTEM

How does the self system enter the regulatory process? Can the self influence regulation without being a target in the self-regulatory stream? How might the self become a target for change? Parallel to the CSM distinction between representation and procedures, the self has been described as a multifaceted knowledge structure (e.g., representations of self or self-identities) linked to a multifaceted set of procedures (Cantor & Kihlstrom, 1987) ranging from tactics for solving specific problems to higher-order strategies used across problem domains (e.g., conserve resources and avoid risk; exercise to enhance physical strength to fight disease; see Ashmore & Jussim, 1997). As with illness representations, self-identities have time lines, causes, consequences (i.e., developmental histories and anticipated futures; Hooker, 1992; Markus & Nurius, 1986; e.g., the current self as athlete and the future self as old and ill), and are perceived as more or less susceptible to control. Thus, the CSM approach requires that we define content domains and content variables for the self system as well as for illnesses. Second, each of these domains is abstract (healthy self; the self sensitive to medications), and concrete and experiential (image of a well self when others are ill; image of aversive reactions to medications). The objective is to identify the match between disease-related and self-related variables from specific domains to determine how and when the self factors influence the disease factors and vice versa.

There are at least three ways to integrate the CSM with an expanded view of the self system. First, we can treat the self as a system that underlies and moderates goal setting and selection of procedural strategies for problem solving (the matching process described previously). Second, we can treat the self as a biopsychological mechanism that must be modulated and maintained to function effectively; that is, as a system of declarative and procedural knowledge that needs to be primed, focused, and occasionally rested if it is to solve problems. Third, we can regard the self, its identities, and procedures as targets for change; that is, as a set of entities undergoing renovation and reconstruction. Each of these three broadly defined approaches subsumes a variety of self-involvements with the regulatory system. The mode and complexity of this involvement will differ for prevention (i.e., in the absence of symptoms or signs of disease) and for disease management. The nature of self-involvement will also vary as a function of the specific disease threat and how it interacts with current and future life goals.

A. SELF AS A FACTOR THAT UNDERLIES AND MODERATES THE PROBLEM SPACE

Whereas the self system consists of multiple levels, where abstract executive processes are at the top and automatic procedures for the management of environmental events are at the bottom (Johnson & Multhaup, 1992), the self can directly influence and thereby moderate goals and problem solving strategies from the top down and from the bottom up (DeSteno & Salovey, 1997). The top-down influence involves the effects of representations of the self and models and/or procedures for problem solving on goal setting and the selection of strategies and tactics for solving illness-related problems. The bottom-up processes involve the self as an "automatic alert system," where disease threats directly activate emotional processes for self-protection. Examples of these processes can be generated for both illness (response to symptoms and signs) and health promotive behaviors (preventive behaviors in the absence of disease signs). We also propose that the self system serves as an integrative mechanism at the base of self-regulative action.

Top-Down Effects: Identities and Self-Regulative Procedures (Models) for Solving Illness Problems

It is not difficult to generate examples of how self-identities and procedural characteristics can direct goal setting and target selection in the domain of illness cognition if the focus is on disease-related identities. For example, an individual whose family history has created a self-identity as susceptible to cardiac disease and stroke rather than cancer may interpret stress-induced headaches and fatigue as possible indicators of a cerebral vascular accident, whereas someone with a different history and vulnerability identity may interpret the same ambiguous symptoms as signs of cancer (Brownlee, 1997; Easterling & Leventhal, 1989). Illness identities sensitize and bias the individual's interpretation of specific classes of symptoms, call forth specific procedures for symptom management, and set different goals and criteria for evaluating outcomes.

Broader aspects of the self, both disease related and not disease related, also can affect the attribute selected as a target for regulation and the level or criterion for a successful outcome. For example, for individuals differing in levels of self-described optimism (Scheier & Carver, 1985, 1992), both a self-declared optimist and a self-declared pessimist may take aspirin to control a headache that is interfering with preparation for an important and stressful examination. We would expect the optimist to anticipate and notice relief in a relatively short time frame, whereas the pessimist focuses on each pain and interprets it as a sign that the analgesia has failed, and that he will be unable to concentrate and, consequently, will fail his examination. The pessimist's response pattern will create a positive feedback loop that sustains stress and amplifies the headache. Positive feedback loops of this sort have been identified and labeled as ruminative coping in studies of adaptation to arthritis (Keefe, Brown, Wallston, & Caldwell, 1989; Park, 1994), test anxiety (Mandler, 1964; Mandler & Watson, 1966; Zeidner, 2000, this volume), and depression (Nolen-Hoeksema, 1997).

Disease-related aspects of the self broader than specific self-defined illness vulnerabilities hold considerable promise for understanding both health and illness behaviors, but they have been explored little, the possible exception being self-efficacy (e.g., Holman & Lorig, 1992; Lorig, 1998). Although it is a judgment of a self-attribute and is used in many studies of health and illness behavior, self-efficacy is not a general self-attribute: It is the perception of one's ability to perform a specific treatment or preventive response (e.g., taking medication daily or quitting smoking; Bandura, 1977b). Individuals have working models of their procedural capacities, that is, of their resources to perform complex strategies to manage illness threats and expectations of the efficacy of these strategies or self-regulative procedures. For example, many elderly persons perceive themselves as needing to conserve their limited resources and prefer, therefore, to place the burden of decision making and coping with illness on professionals rather than place the burden on themselves. This limited resource view of the working self encourages a strategy of rapid care seeking for any somatic symptom that exceeds a relatively low threshold of seriousness or severity (Leventhal & Crouch, 1997; Leventhal, Leventhal,

Schaefer, & Easterling, 1993). Although a conservation strategy of this type may facilitate swift detection and treatment of potential illness threats, it may discourage the expenditure of effort needed to replace activities that are given up in the face of more serious, chronic illness (Duke, 1998). Thus, the same procedural self-appraisal can benefit or harm adjustment and quality of life, depending on the context. Other, procedurally related self-identities, such as the belief that one's body reacts negatively to manufactured chemicals but tolerates natural substances, can result in resistance to medication and preference for alternative treatments for disease management (Horne, 1997). In sum, beliefs about the somatic system and models as to how it can best be regulated will affect symptom interpretation and the selection of procedures for symptom and disease management.

Bottom-Up Effects: Automatic Goal Setting

In contrast to the top-down effects of self-identities and procedural capacities, the self system possesses low-level automatic competencies that can set goals from the bottom up (Gibbons, Gerrard, Ouellette, & Burzette, 1998). Automatic, affective reactions, such as the pain and distress induced by severe injury, and the disgust and nausea generated by gastrointestinal pathogens, can activate coping procedures prior to complex, interpretive reactions (Scherer, 1988). A severe toothache of sudden onset will stimulate a variety of manipulations of the jaw (e.g., touching, bathing the mouth in warm water) and eventual care seeking, regardless of the meaning ascribed to the injury. The meaning, however (e.g., cancer of the jaw versus decay that reached a nerve), may add more than a touch of panic to the response. Although potent somatic stimuli and their associated affective and coping reactions emerge from the self and create a focus on the self, automatic reactions of this sort might be regarded best as problem-focused responses to symptoms rather than as self-regulation. How we categorize these reactions matters less, however, than our ability to develop models of their underlying mechanisms.

Identities, Goal Setting, and Procedural Models
for Promoting Health Behaviors

Although numerous studies have examined the adoption of protective health actions as a function of attitudes, perceived normativeness, and intentions to act (see Conner & Norman, 1998), few studies have explored how the self system affects these attitudes, perceptions, and intentions. This is somewhat surprising because self-identities and procedural skills are likely more salient in the representation and adoption of preventive action for prospective health threats than in the processes involved in managing illness behaviors. Consider, for example, efforts to persuade suburban high school students to engage in safe sex practices (e.g., use of condoms) to avoid AIDS. For the majority of these students, AIDS is a media problem: They are unlikely to know anyone with AIDS or to perceive AIDS-infected persons among their actual or potential sexual partners. To increase the vividness and human side of AIDS intervention programs, AIDS patients (e.g., gay males and/or intravenous drug users) are sometimes recruited as communicators. Investigators find that messages from these sources are likely to be seen as irrelevant because of the perceived discrepancy between the lifestyle of the average teenaged recipient and the image of the lifestyle of the source (Misovich, Fisher, & Fisher, 1997). Differences in self-identity associated with imagined differences in sexual practices perceived to cause the spread of AIDS create a gulf between source and recipient. Gump and Kulik (1995) have shown that increased acceptance of AIDS risk is associated with increased similarity between source and recipient.

The AIDS studies indicate that the acceptance of recommendations for health actions are affected by identities, consequences, implications for control, and time frames for the self system of the source and the recipient. We would add that the significance of these shared features depends on their overlap with the representation of the recommended health action. An early study from our group illustrates this point. It examined acceptance of two quite different recommendations by pregnant women approaching the date of childbirth: to adopt rooming-in while in the hospital (i.e., keeping the baby with them) and to adopt breast feeding to enhance the infant's resistance to disease (Mazen & Leventhal, 1972). Although we did not assess the representations of these two different actions, it is clear that they have very different time lines and different consequences that may be more or less controllable by the mother-to-be. Breast feeding is a long-term commitment that is carried out in the home environment and has implications for relationships to work and family. Rooming-in is a short-term in-hospital affair. Four female communicators delivered the two recommendations. Because half the expectant mothers were white and half were black, two of the communicators were white and two were black. All four communicators were also expectant mothers, and all four delivered their messages to half of the participants when they also were very pregnant and to the other half of the participants after they had delivered their own babies. The data, therefore, allowed us to examine the effects of similarity in race and similarity in pregnancy on acceptance of these two behaviors. The results were clear: Similarity in pregnancy enhanced acceptance of rooming-in; similarity in race and, possibly, a common, postpartum social environment affected acceptance of breast feeding. In short, acceptance was greatest when the source, the recipient, and the recommended action shared relevant attributes. Thus, the very same individual could be an effective source for one action and not for another at the same point in time.

The paucity of data examining the moderating effects of self-identities on health behavior should encourage the formulation of hypotheses as to how both stable and transient features of the self can moderate the selection and ongoing use of procedures for promoting health and avoiding illness. There is no need to give examples of how observations of someone similar in age and lifestyle struggling with the diagnosis of cancer or cardiovascular disease can activate feelings of vulnerability to the self and stimulate protective actions and screening behavior in the absence of known illness. Less is known about the variables that might maintain these behaviors. A variety of factors, including the nature and durability of the interpersonal relationship or perceived similarities of physical makeup and constitutional temperament, might determine whether behavioral changes stimulated by observations of another are temporary or become part of one's permanent repertory of reactions (see Aspinwall, 1997; Suls, Martin, & Leventhal, 1997). In a recent paper, we suggested that the representation of health threats (i.e., their perceived causes, consequences, control, etc.) can have a major impact on social comparison processes, the content of the representation establishing the relevance of specific dimensions for social comparison (Leventhal et al., 1997). The meaning of the information gleaned from a comparison is framed by the representation of the disease. To diagnose whether one's gut upset is due to food poisoning, a virus, or something worse, it makes sense to compare oneself to someone who has eaten the same food during the past 24 hours. The fear of a patient about to undergo bypass surgery (cause of pain, threat of death, unknown time frame for recovery, etc.) is more likely reduced by rooming with two or three postsurgical patients in robust condition than with a similarly frightened group of expectant others (Kulik & Mahler, 1987, 1997). The substance of the representation of treatment, self, and other give meaning to observed reality.

B. REDEFINING AND REORGANIZING THE SELF AND MODIFYING ITS PROCEDURES

Self-regulation moves to the construction and reorganization of the self when problem solving is focused on the modification, reorganization, and creation of identities and procedural skills. In each of the following cases, that is, the redefinition of old identities, the creation of new ones, the reprioritizing of identities, and the addition or remodeling of existent procedures for managing the self and illness threats, a component of the self is the focus of problem solving. In these cases, response feedback adds or modifies facets of self and adds, deletes, and/or modifies existent procedures. Conceptualizing these mechanisms poses a special challenge for theory.

Identity and Self-Organization

Numerous studies suggest that chronic illness leads to major changes in affect, specifically depression, and quality of life. Depression is a frequent accompaniment to Parkinson's disease (Cummings, 1992), is common in patients suffering from myocardial infarction (MI) and a predictor of post-MI mortality (Frasure-Smith, Lespérance, & Talajic, 1993, 1995), and is a sequela of illness-related physical dysfunction (Mirowsky & Ross, 1992; Zeiss, Lewinsohn, Rohde, & Seeley, 1996).

Although it seems plausible that increments in depressive affect are mediated by the impact of illness on the self system, relatively few empirical studies have documented that illness-induced changes in the self are responsible for these affective outcomes, and fewer still have examined the process by which these changes come about. One interesting study by Heidrich, Forsthoff, and Ward (1994) suggests that declines in positive affect and quality of life in cancer patients are mediated by the impact of the representation of cancer on the self system. Their data showed that those cancer patients who had a poorer quality of life represented their cancer as having a chronic rather than an acute time line. Their analyses showed that the impact of the cancer time line was mediated by the self system; that is, the negative effect of chronicity on quality of life was accounted for by the discrepancy between patients' current and former self-concepts. Their data, however, were cross sectional and do not identify the sequence in which the changes occurred. For example, cancer time line and self system time lines might be reciprocally related: Newly diagnosed cancer patients who perceive their cancer as chronic experience a threat to the duration (time line) of the self and a decline in positive affect. The decline in positive affect and perception of imminent loss of life activities associated with a newly defined, temporally restricted time line for the self could increase the perceived severity of cancer or increase the perception of cancer as uncontrollable, and these changes could feed back and alter self-identity (self as victim) and impact negatively on perceived self-regulatory procedures.

Substantial data on social comparison processes also suggests that the self plays a critical role in adaptation to chronic illness, although once again, it is unclear whether the self is involved as a relatively stable entity that moderates coping or as a set of identities and procedures that change from feedback generated from the management of chronic disease (see Suls et al., 1997; Wood & VanderZee, 1997). However, we cannot rely upon affect indicators as evidence of change in the self system, because increases in depressive affect may be direct reactions to illness and be unmediated by change in self-concept. This is clearly likely given that depression is a common reaction to mild (Aneshensel, Frerichs, & Huba, 1984) as well as to severe physical illnesses (Cummings, 1992), and there is little evidence of change in the self system in the former case and frankly not a great deal more in the latter. Indeed, a direct path from chronic illness to depressive affect and/or anhedonia may be an increasingly common route for the elicitation of depression among elderly persons (Leventhal, Patrick-Miller, Leventhal, & Burns, 1997).

Case Examples of the Dynamics of Self-Change in Response to Chronic Illness

Individual accounts of encounters with life-threatening cancer and coronary disease provide dramatic examples of redefinitions and reorganizations of the self, and compensate somewhat for the limited number of empirical findings in the quantitative literature (for overviews, see Charmaz, 1991; Leventhal et al., 1999). Price's (1982) account of his encounter with a cancerous tumor provides one such example. Price's first indication of the presence of a tumor was a disruption of his gait. This initial difficulty in walking was a concrete, functional indicator, what Jones, Farina, Hastorf, Markus, & Scott (1984) term as a "mark" of yet more physical and psychological changes to come. As the tumor enlarged and increased its pressure on the spinal cord, unrelenting pain and loss of the ability to walk were added to the symptom picture: Price's symptoms were joined by a label (spinal tumor), establishing the identity of his condition. As his condition worsened, his attention was focused on primary, everyday functions (e.g., walking, getting in and out of bed, and climbing steps) that were all previously automatic actions of the self that absorbed little or no space in working memory. These deficits disrupted more complex activities including driving, food shopping, and teaching. Thus, simple actions that were neither unique to Price nor self-defining were consequences of a disease with an unknown time line and limited control (surgery was impossible because the tumor was intertwined with the nerves of his spinal cord). The rapid pace of these disruptions required swift redefinition of self-competencies; for example, seeing the self as a patient, as physically compromised, dependent upon others, and needing new ways (procedures) to manage daily life.

Changes in physical function were not the only inputs shaping Price's reconstruction of his identities and skills; his social environment made important additions. His surgeon had confirmed that a cancerous tumor in the spinal cord was responsible for the functional deficits, and added that the tumor could be removed only partially and would remain a permanent if unwelcome visitor. The surgeon's prognosis and the functional and subjective changes Price was experiencing were mutually confirming, adding to Price's acceptance that major changes were happening, with more to come. The pressure for self-change likely would have been far less had laser surgery been available, because it would have permitted near complete removal of the tumor. It is interesting to speculate whether this would have reduced the pressure for reconstruction of the self. However, lasers were not available at that time and the increasing pain and functional disability that Price experienced along with his surgeon's prognosis required extensive reconstruction of the self.

A Hierarchy of Signals for Self-reorganization

In Price's (1982) case (also see reports by Frank, 1991, 1995), the initial encounter with chronic illness began as a bottom-up process (i.e., with changes in somatic sensations and movement). These marks were noticed, did not match existent schemata for self-structure or function, and were interpreted as threats to the self. In each case, we can see how the interaction of bottom-up and top-down processes in the form of fundamental if–then questions (e.g., if the disordered gait is not serious, why doesn't it go away?) led to seeking advice and assistance from family members, and finally to seeking expert diagnosis and treatment. Many features of this sequence mimic the way in which the immune system manages intruders. The primary defense cells of the immune system identify pathogens as alien, and break them down into components that are then held up as marks or flags that signal other immune cells to the attack. If the signals activate the immune system's memory (i.e., its acquired skills), it can destroy the intruders relatively quickly. The immune system analogy is valuable because it reveals the limited nature of our psychological knowledge. Immunologists have identified the cells that hold up the flags, the actual shape of the flags, and the type of cells and the shape of their receptor sites that recognize the flags. Answers are lacking to parallel psychological questions; for example, what are the schemata that identify somatic change as non-self, what is the physical and temporal "shape" of the marks, what cognitive or procedural schemata identify these marks and what attributes (receptor sites?) or procedures are involved in the identification, what elements lead to seeking expert help, and what changes in the self are needed to speed the detection and control of threat, and how do these changes in the self occur? These questions call for further differentiation of constructs and processes involved in the generation of representations both of disease and the self.

Insight into these self-regulatory and constructive processes also can be gained from observing events in reverse order; that is, when they are initiated from the top down. Feedback from diagnostic tests (e.g., an abnormal pap smear or a rise in prostate-specific antigen) can indicate the presence of a pathogen in the absence of symptoms, and these top-down sequences may be associated with signs of puzzlement and disbelief that rarely are found when self-regulation begins from the bottom up. Remarks such as, "I feel fine! How can I be sick? Maybe it's a mistake!," reflect the incredulity a person experiences when given a diagnostic label in the absence of symptoms. The anxiety, anger, and depression elicited by such information may create the concrete, somatic changes and symptoms (fatigue, distress) to confirm that one is sick. Common sense is uncomfortable when a diagnostic label fails to match perceptual experience. Construction of the self and the development of motivation for skill acquisition involve, therefore, a hierarchical control system with low-level concrete markers detecting discrepancies in form and function from the normal self, and higher-order, acquired knowledge elaborating upon the meaning (identity, time line, consequences, perceived cause, control) and implication of these changes for the self system. These processes initiate a complex problem solving process that includes procedures to defeat disease and procedures to generate new skills and acquiring new self-identities.

C. THE SOCIAL ENVIRONMENT

Both physical changes and diagnostic tests are but the beginning of an evolving, psychological process that can lead to the identification of disease and the alterations of self-identities and procedures for living (Figure 5). The evolution of these processes is clearly influenced by the social environment and the ability of an individual to make use of its informational and technical resources. Price's story illustrates the vital role of institutional and social factors in his self-reconstruction. His identity as a prominent author and professor of English at a major university provided access to powerful colleagues at a world-class medical school, insuring resources for treatment (medical insurance) and multiple opportunities for alternative modes of functioning. Family and former student colleagues managed the daily tasks of food shopping, housekeeping, and transportation, and served as intermediaries, when needed, with the medical care system. These environmental and social factors, what Greeno (1998) labeled affordances, provided a supportive framework for enactment of the procedures that allowed Price to construct new and reshape existent self-identities. Price's intelligence, persistence, and religious faith provided personal resources for these enactments, and his professorial role provided the self-regulative strategies to form working relationships with former students that mirrored the mutual supportiveness that is part of effective faculty–graduate student relationships. He was able to acquire alternative skills for maneuvering about his environment, skills that helped him shape a new sense of self with respect to dependence while confirming and expanding his views of the people whose complementary roles afforded the opportunity for self-change. The actions involved in acquiring the skills needed for successful functioning in the face of severe, physical compromise were the active elements responsible for the formation of Price's new identities, and the confirmation and reshaping of existent identities; for example, the confirmation of his spiritual self and the acceptance of new areas of

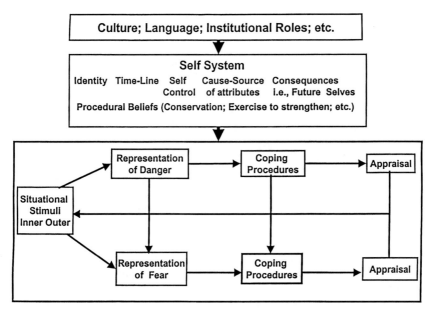

FIGURE 5 The full representation of the Common Sense Model embeds the mental model for solving health and illness problems, the CMS, in a multilevel context defined by personal (self), social, and cultural factors. The five domains of illness representation provide a provisional set of substantive domains for the representation of the self system. Thus, the meaning of each self-identity or role is elaborated by factors from each of the five domains; for example, self as a spouse or patient has features describing the role identity (label and concrete features), role time frame, role cause, role consequences, and control. The text presents some speculations as to how procedural activity constructs and revises self-identities and skills by creating, identifying, and removing matches and mismatches between the features of representations of illness and self-representations.

functional dependency. Whereas Price's performances had identities, perceived causes (self vs. other), control, consequences, and time lines, their concrete physical and social feedback conveyed information in each of the five domains of both illness and self-representation. These performances, both covert (mental) and overt, were the active elements that generated change in both the self and the illness system.

The interchange between the chronically ill and the social environment is not always smooth. Differences in perspectives or goals can generate a sense of alienation; that is, that one's suffering is not fully appreciated (Wortman & Lehman, 1985) and that one is a burden to others. Data suggest that differences in perspective may be based on differences in the representation of a disease. For example, Heijmans, deRidder, and Bensing (in press) found impaired adjustment in chronically ill Addison's disease patients whose spouses minimized the impact of the symptoms and consequences of this illnesses. Spouses are likely to overestimate how well an Addison's patient is doing because medication controls many of the overt features of this life-threatening illness. This effect was absent for chronic fatigue patients because there are no effective treatments for it and its impact is visible to both spouse and patient. Thus, poor adjustments to chronic illness are correlated with differences in the illness representations of patient and spouse, and the consequences of these discrepancies for patient adjustment differ by disease. Representations are more similar for patient and spouse for identity (symptoms) and consequences when the effects of the illness are clearly visible.

Incongruity between patient and physician representations of a disease can have serious effects. In the Meyer et al. (1985) study, patients who were beginning hypertension treatment for the first time were much more likely to drop out in the following months if they told their physicians that they used their symptoms to monitor blood pressure changes. By expressing an opinion at variance with their physician's belief that hypertension is asymptomatic, they put discrepant models on the table and created the possibility of conflict and an eventual loss of confidence in their doctor. Differences between patient and physician illness representations can impact the self and in some cases lead to new, unpleasant identities. When the surgeon described Price's (1982) spinal cord and tumor in technical terms and omitted discussion of their concrete, experiential aspects, Price experienced both the tumor and himself as objects: the tumor as a disease and himself as an organic system in distress rather than as a complex human being.

The extent to which differences in viewpoints and goals can generate alienation appears to reflect two sets of factors: the ability of the outside observer to communicate a sense of understanding of the patient's subjective world (i.e., the patient's representation of disease and self at an experiential level) and the ability of the patient to link his longer-term needs to the goals and perspective of the external observer. Mutual understanding means, therefore, sharing subjective views of the illness' identity (both concrete experience as well as its label), time frame and consequences (the experience of time and effort to perform everyday tasks over longer time frames), and the notions of its susceptibility to control and concerns about the means of control (hospitalization, anesthesia, and high risk surgery). Understanding involves intuition as to the cognitive and affective meanings of disease and treatment in relationship to the patient's self. Not surprisingly, this level of understanding is often best communicated by long-standing family and friends; they possess the empathic skills and patience to sustain trust and are typically the first people to be sought out in times of physical ambiguity and duress (Cohen & Syme, 1985; Zola, 1972). Price's story illustrates the importance of being able to mesh immediate and long-term goals (fears of treatment, reduction of pain, and return of function) respecting disease and treatment with those held by others, in this case, his surgeon's view of the need for and possibility of relief by surgical treatment. His ability to deal with differences in disease and self-representations, particularly at the concrete, experiential level, was bolstered by the trust he developed in his surgeon and strengthened by the support of knowledgeable and trusted family members and the institutional framework (the university) within which he lived.

Price's example suggests that the activity of the chronically ill patient involves a blend of solving a series of problems, some set by the disease and by other persons (problem solving) and some set by one's self (regulation of attention and energy expenditure), in conjunction with performances leading to the reshaping of existent identities and procedures and the acquisition of new ones (reconstruction of the self). Problem solving, self-regulation, and self-construction are heavily influenced by the individual's common-sense model of disease and by the social context in which problem solving, self-regulation, and self-construction take place. These processes can be initiated from the bottom up (i.e., by indicators, or signs and symptoms) or from the top down (i.e., by social feedback); the two paths typically act simultaneously. An individual's representation of the mechanisms underlying somatic changes creates expectations regarding the possibility for control and suggests specific procedures for achieving desired outcomes and criteria for their appraisal. Appraisal may go no further than examining the subjective feedback from a coping procedure (e.g., did taking this medication reduce my pain) or it may require a social procedure such as the selection of a relevant other for social comparison. For example, if we find it difficult to recall the details of a lecture and wonder if advancing age is causing comprehension and/or memory loss, we may compare our recall to that of the very sharp, younger colleague who was also in attendance. If we do as well as our colleague, we can attribute our difficulties to the abstruseness of the topic or the poverty of the presentation. In short, the hypothesis, or model-driven comparison, allows us to disconfirm the pathogenic implication of the memory indicator.

All of our examples treat the individual as an active problem solver in a supportive, social environment. The relationship of the chronically ill to their environment is often far less positive because the individual may lack economic resources and may be coping with a disease that is stigmatized. Stigmatization, or the negative evaluation and avoidance of a disease and its victims, is often accompanied by fear, disgust, and repulsion (Jones et al., 1984), and at times by violence and murder. Many of the negative reactions defining stigmatization appear to depend on the visible, aesthetic properties of a disease. Aesthetic properties associated with noticeable birth defects, severe injuries, and extensive wounds induce fear in primates, including humans (Hebb, 1946). Socially held representations of specific diseases are also sources of stigmatization and avoidance. For example, beliefs about the cause of AIDS (e.g., as retribution for sin) and beliefs about contagion or fear of "catching" AIDS and cancer encourage avoidance and separation from those who are ill rather than involvement and support (Rozin, Markwith, & McCauley, 1994).

Stigmatization, a problem we have barely touched upon, is a serious problem for the chronically ill. The CSM framework is strengthened, however, by the overlap between the five domains of illness representations and the six dimensions of stigmatization elaborated upon by Jones et al. (1984, p. 25):

1. Timeline, identified in Jones et al. as the course or pattern of change over time,
2. Consequences, identified with two dimensions: disruptiveness (hampering interaction and communication) and peril (perceived danger posed by the illness).
3. Cause, identified as the origin of the condition with particular reference to self-responsibility.
4. Identity, similar to the Jones et al. dimension of the aesthetic qualities, the extent to which the symptoms and/or signs are "ugly" and generate repulsion.
5. Control, similar to their sixth dimension of concealability, or managing the social representation of a stigmatized disorder.

More germane to our current discussion of the self is the way in which stigmatization affects the representation of the self system in the social environment. Specifically, does stigma remain an external, social problem, something the marked person views as "a problem for others" that calls for procedures such as concealment, or does the stigma become an internal problem or facet of a now degraded self?

Stigmatization is but one of many ways in which the ill self can be regarded by others and by one's self. Patients living with and defying the morbidities of life-threatening diseases can be seen as possessing "guts," their hopes and commitment to fully involved living tempered by their realistic views of their life expectancies, presenting a combination that can define courage. Effective problem solving and self-management are undoubtedly facilitated by positive self-identities, and it is likely that effective disease and self-management in the face of pain and anticipated death strengthen and encourage their development. The individual's social network will play an important role in determining the emergence of a denigrating or enhancing self-image during health crises, the contribution of the network depending in part on its representation of the individual, the illness, and the treatments for disease control. The substance of the representations held by patients and critical others, whether these representations are shared or discrepant with regard to time line, expected consequences, affective valence, and so forth, and whether the sharing involves experiential content, is a fascinating domain for theoretical and empirical work.

VII. SUMMARY AND CONCLUDING COMMENTS

Our approach to understanding behavior for managing current and avoiding future disease has emphasized the distinction between problem solving or environmental regulation, self-regulation, and construction of the self. Creating new identities and altering old ones, and adding and modifying procedures for problem solving are not the typical reactions to confrontations with illness. Most illnesses are time limited and managed with an available repertoire of treatments. Reconstruction of the self begins when illness poses novel problems, and extensive redefinition of the self is more likely for illnesses that are represented and experienced both as highly disruptive and long lasting. The goal-directed processes involved in adaptation to illness, whether goals are set by the self or by experts and involve or do not involve reconstruction of the self, are heavily influenced by the biological properties of the disease (e.g., level of pain, functional disability, visibility of damage) and by individual and societal models of the disease process.

Broad, abstract terms such as those that defined the CSM model in its early stages (e.g., danger coping versus fear coping; Leventhal, 1970) provided a highly limited understanding of self-regulation and adaptation to disease threats. Fortunately, the model has moved toward increasing specificity. Although the development has not been rapid, the steps are clear. Having recognized the existence of parallel cognitive and affective processing, and differentiated the representational and action-plan or procedural components of each arm, as did others, we next differentiated abstract, conceptual processes and concrete, perceptual processes in both cognitive and affective processing (Epstein, 1993a; Leventhal, 1984). This latter distinction led to research in medical and laboratory settings that showed that different behaviors could be promoted by each level, automatic coping and affective responses being heavily influenced by concrete experience (e.g., Johnson, 1975).

The next phase involved multiple steps. The first, the identification of the five attributes of illness representations, identity, time line, consequences, cause, and control, might be better described as the identification of five domains for differentiation, because multiple factors may reside in each category (Bishop, 1991). Next was recognition that variables within each of the five attributes or categories needed to be represented at both abstract and perceptual levels. Our first mental heuristic, the symmetry rule, emerged at this time: people seek illness labels for symptoms and find symptoms for illness labels. Recognition of the existence of a vast number of procedures for goal attainment (i.e., for regulating the goals or set points established by illness representations) led to our next rule, that is, that representations shape the selection and guide the performance and evaluation of procedures. A variety of specific procedures or rules were identified to describe the differentiation being made by an active, mental system (e.g., the stress–illness rule and the aging–illness rule).

Our increased awareness of the dynamic and evolving nature of illness representations led us to segment illness episodes into appraisal stages, illness stages, and utilization stages. These differentiations, although not intrinsically theoretical, proved useful for the analysis of the change process for care seeking (Safer et al, 1979; Leventhal et al., 1993). Horne and Weinmann's work (Horne, 1997) developed the theme that procedures have attributes that overlap with those of illness representations. Thus, procedures have identities (names and side effects), time lines, and consequences (cure, addiction to medication), and are more or less susceptible to control. Finally, we defined a domain of individual differences involving higher-order procedural strategies or belief systems respecting self-management (as you get older, you conserve energy and avoid risks to health) as distinct from tactics or specific responses to reach particular goals (e.g., take aspirin to reduce headache; Leventhal & Crouch, 1977).

The emphasis on the dynamic aspect of illness cognition, the temporal evolution and the interaction of affective and cognitive processes, led us to reemphasize what may well be our most basic proposition: Specifically, people's judgments as to whether they are sick or well are based on appraisals of concrete perceptual experiences of somatic change and physical, affective, and cognitive function, and the appraisals reflect the action of decision heuristics or rules tied to schemata of illness, life events, and the self (e.g., the symmetry rule: If I'm ill, I will have symptoms; Am I sick or stressed by life events?; Am I sick or old?). The focus on the evolution of illness representations and the role of heuristics has opened the final phase of our work, which involves the complexities surrounding the interaction of representations of illness with representations of the self. How we regulate our environments and manage illness threats is the first of a series of questions concerning goal setting; that is, are we self-regulating (choosing our own goals) or being regulated (following doctors orders), or are we reconstructing the self system, that is, are we altering our identities (adopting new roles and modifying old ones) and acquiring new and modifying existent procedural skills?

The current, and possibly temporary, minimization of threat from infectious disease has extended our life-spans and we now live long enough to experience diseases caused by the dysregulation of basic biological systems (e.g., diabetes, endocrine disorders, cardiovascular diseases, and cancer; Dingle, 1973). Currently, there are neither magic bullets nor guaranteed cures for many of these ills. Experts can only guide us in the lifelong process of problem solving to control disease and the construction of self-identities and procedures useful for living in ways that reduce both the likelihood of chronic illness and its morbidity when it strikes. Thus, many of these diseases are problems to be managed and lived with rather than cured, and new models of the self with illness are needed. The movement for patient empowerment is a reflection of this change. Everyday management of disease involves a wide range of decisions, most of which should reflect the individual's personal goal structure and not just goals set by health professionals or the impositions of the biology of a particular disease. Investigations that delineate the details of the processes underlying regulation, self-regulation, and construction of the self will add to our knowledge and our ability to empower people to act to improve function, minimize morbidity, and enhance quality of life.

ACKNOWLEDGMENT

Preparation of this chapter was supported by grants AG 03501 and AG 12072.

REFERENCES

Ajzen, I. (1991). The theory of planned behavior. *Organizational Behavior and Human Decision Processes, 50*, 179–211.

Ajzen, I., & Fishbein, M. (1972). Attitudes and normative beliefs as factors influencing behavioral intentions. *Journal of Personality and Social Psychology, 21*, 1–9.

Ajzen, I., & Fishbein, M. (1977). Attitude–behavior relations: A theoretical analysis and review of empirical research. *Psychological Bulletin, 84*, 888–918.

Ajzen, I., & Fishbein, M. (1980). *Understanding attitudes and predicting social behavior.* Englewood Cliffs, NJ: Prentice-Hall.

Anderson, J. R. (1987). *The architecture of cognition.* Cambridge, MA: Harvard University Press.

Anderson, J. R. (1993). *The adaptive character of thought.* Hillsdale, NJ: Erlbaum.

Aneshensel, C. S., Frerichs, R. R., & Huba, G. J. (1984). Depression and physical illness: A multiwave, nonrecursive causal model. *Journal of Health and Social Behavior, 25*, 350–371.

Ashmore, R. D., & Jussim, L. (1997). Toward a second century of the scientific analysis of self and identity. In R. D. Ashmore & L. Jussim (Eds.), *Self and identity: Fundamental issues* (Vol. 1, pp. 3–19). New York: Oxford University Press.

Aspinwall, L. G. (1997). Future-oriented aspects of social comparisons: A framework for studying health-related comparison activity. In B. P. Buunk & F. X. Gibbons (Eds.), *Health, coping, and well-being: Perspectives from social comparison theory.* (pp. 125–165). Hillsdale, NJ: Erlbaum.

Baer, J. S., Kamarck, T., Lichtenstein, E., & Ransom, C. C. (1989). Analyses of temptations and transgressions after initial cessation. *Journal of Consulting and Clinical Psychology, 57*, 623–627.

Bandura, A. A. (1969). *Principles of behavior modification.* New York: Holt, Rinehart & Winston.

Bandura, A. A. (1977a). *Social learning theory*. Englewood Cliffs, NJ: Prentice-Hall.

Bandura, A. A. (1977b). Self-efficacy: Toward a unifying theory of behavioral change. *Psychological Review, 84,* 191–215.

Baumann, L. J., Cameron, L. D., Zimmerman, R. S., & Leventhal, H. (1989). Illness representations and matching labels with symptoms. *Health Psychology, 8,* 449–469.

Baumann, L. J., & Leventhal, H. (1985). I can tell when my blood pressure is up, can't I?, *Health Psychology, 4,* 203–218.

Becker, M. H. (1974). The health belief model and personal health behaviors. *Health Education Monographs, 2,* 376–423.

Becker, M., & Maiman, L. A. (1975). Sociomedical determinants of compliance with health and medical care recommendations. *Medical Care, 13,* 10–24.

Bishop, G. D. (1991). Understanding the understanding of illness: Lay disease representations. In J. A. Skelton & R. T. Croyle (Eds.), *Mental representation in health and illness*. (pp. 32–59). New York: Springer-Verlag.

Bishop, G. D (1994). *Health psychology: Integrating mind and body*. Boston, MA: Allyn & Bacon.

Bishop, G. D., & Converse, S. A. (1986). Illness representations: A prototype approach. *Health Psychology, 5,* 95–114.

Blumhagen, D. (1980). Hyper-tension: A folk illness with a medical name. *Culture, Medicine, and Psychiatry, 4,* 197–227.

Brownlee, S. (1997). *Perceived vulnerability to illness*. Unpublished doctoral dissertation, Rutgers, the State University of New Jersey, New Brunswick, NJ.

Buunk, B., & Gibbons, F. X. (1997). *Social comparisons, health, and coping*. Hillsdale, NJ: Erlbaum.

Cameron, L. C., Leventhal, E. A., & Leventhal, H. (1995). Seeking medical care in response to symptoms and life stress. *Psychosomatic Medicine, 57,* 37–47.

Cantor, N., & Kihlstrom, J. F. (1987). *Personality and social intelligence*. Englewood Cliffs, NJ: Prentice-Hall.

Carver, C. S., & Scheier, M. F. (1981). *Attention and self-regulation: A control-theory approach to human behavior*. New York: Springer-Verlag.

Carver, C. S., & Scheier, M. F. (1982). Control theory: A useful conceptual framework for personality-social, clinical, and health psychology. *Psychological Bulletin, 92,* 111–135.

Carver, C. S., & Scheier, M. F. (in press). *On the self regulation of behavior*. New York: Cambridge University Press.

Carver, C. S., Scheier, M. F., & Weintraub, J. K. (1989). Assessing coping strategies: A theoretically based approach. *Journal of Personality and Social Psychology, 56,* 267–283.

Chapman, G. B. (1998) Sooner or later: The psychology of intertemporal choice. In *The psychology of learning and motivation*. (Vol. 38) New York: Academic Press.

Charmaz, K. (1991). *Good days, bad days: The self in chronic illness*. New Brunswick, NJ: Rutgers University Press.

Cohen, S., & Syme, S. L. (1985). *Social support and health*. Orlando, FL: Academic Press.

Conner, M., & Norman, P. (1988). Social cognition models in health psychology [Special issue]. *Psychology & Health, 13,* 179–385.

Croyle, R. T. (1992). Appraisal of health threats: Cognition, motivation, and social comparison. *Cognitive Therapy and Research, 16,* 165–182.

Croyle, R. T., & Barger, S. D. (1993). Illness cognition. In S. Maes, H. Leventhal, & M. Johnston (Eds.), *International Review of Health Psychology*, (Vol. 2, pp. 29–49). Chichester, UK: Wiley.

Croyle, R. T., & Jemmott, J. B., III. (1991). Psychological reactions to risk factor testing. In J. A. Skelton & R. T. Croyle (Eds.), *Mental representation in health and illness* (pp. 85–107). New York: Springer-Verlag.

Croyle, R. T., & Uretsky, M. B. (1987). Effects of mood on self-appraisal of health status. *Health Psychology, 6*, 239–253.

Cummings, J. L. (1992). Depression and Parkinson's disease: A review. *American Journal of Psychiatry, 149*, 443–454.

Cunningham, L. L. C., Lauren, L. C., Andrykowski, M. A., Wilson, J. F., McGarth, P. C., Sloan, D. A., & Kennedy, D. E. (1998). Physical symptoms, distress, and breast cancer risk perceptions in women with benign breast problems. *Health Psychology, 17*, 371–375.

D'Andrade, R. G., Quinn, N. R., Nerlove, S. B., & Romney, A. K. (1972). Categories of disease in American-English and Mexican-Spanish. In A. K. Romney, R. N. Shepard, & S. B. Nerlove (Eds.), *Multidimensional scaling: Theory and applications in the behavioral sciences.* (Vol. II, pp. 9–54). New York: Seminar Press.

DeSteno, D., & Salovey, P. (1997). Structural dynamism in the concept of self: A flexible model for a malleable concept. *Review of General Psychology, 1*, 389–409.

Dingle, J. H. (1973). The ills of man. *Scientific American, 229*, 77–84.

Ditto, P. H., & Jemmott, J. B., III. (1989). From rarity to evaluative extremity: Effects of prevalence information on evaluations of positive and negative characteristics. *Journal of Personality and Social Psychology, 57*, 16–26.

Dollard, J., & Miller, N. E. (1950). *Personality and psychotherapy.* New York: McGraw-Hill.

Duke, J. (1998). *Replacing losses due to illness.* Unpublished master's thesis, Rutgers, the State University of New Jersey, New Brunswick, NJ.

Easterling, D. E., & Leventhal, H. (1989). The contribution of concrete cognition to emotion: Neutral symptoms as elicitors of worry about cancer. *Journal of Applied Psychology, 74*, 787–796.

Epstein, S. (1973). The self concept revisited: Or a theory of a theory. *American Psychologist, 28*, 404–416.

Epstein, S. (1993a). Emotion and self-theory. In M. Lewis & J. M. Haviland, (Eds.), *Handbook of emotions* (pp. 313–326). New York: Guilford.

Epstein, S. (1993b). Implications of cognitive–experiential self-theory for personality and developmental psychology. In D. C. Funder, & R. Parks, (Eds.), *Studying lives through time: Personality and development* (pp. 339–438). Washington, DC: American Psychological Association.

Fishbein, M., & Ajzen, I. (1974). Attitudes towards objects as predictors of single and multiple behavioral criteria. *Psychological Review, 81*, 59–74.

Frank, A. W. (1991). *At the will of the body.* Boston: Houghton Mifflin.

Frank, A. W. (1995). *The wounded storyteller: Body, illness and ethics.* Chicago: University of Chicago Press.

Frasure-Smith, N., Lespérance, F., & Talajic, M. (1993). Depression following myocardial infarction: Impact on 6-month survival. *Journal of the American Medical Association, 270*, 1819–1825.

Frasure-Smith, N., Lespérance, F., & Talajic, M. (1995). The impact of negative emotions on prognosis following myocardial infarction: Is it more than depression? *Health Psychology, 14*, 388–398.

Gibbons, F. X., Gerrard, M., Ouellette, J. A., & Burzette, R. (1998). Cognitive antecedents to adolescent health risk: Discriminating between behavioral intention and behavioral willingness. *Psychology & Health, 13*, 319–339.

Gonder-Frederick, L. A., & Cox, D. J. (1991). Symptom perception, symptom beliefs, and blood glucose discrimination in the self-treatment of insulin-dependent diabetes. In J. A. Skelton & R. T. Croyle, (Eds.), *Mental representation in health and illness* (pp. 220–246). New York: Springer-Verlag.

Greeno, J. G. (1998). The situativity of knowing, learning, and research. *American Psychologist, 53*, 5–26.

Greenwald, A. G. (1981). Self and memory. In G. H. Bower (Ed.), *The psychology of learning and motivation*. (Vol. 15, pp. 201–236). New York: Academic Press.

Gump, B. B., & Kulik, J. A. (1995). The effect of a model's HIV status of self-perceptions: A self-protective similarity bias. *Personality and Social Psychology Bulletin, 21*, 827–833.

Hampson, S. E., Glasgow, R. E., & Zeiss, A. (1994). Personal modes of osteoarthritis and their relation to self-management and quality of life. *Journal of Behavioral Medicine, 17*, 143–158.

Hebb, D. O. (1946). On the nature of fear. *Psychological Review, 53*, 259–276.

Hecker, B. L., & Ajzen, I. (1983). Improving the prediction of health behavior: An approach based on the theory of reasoned action. *Academic Psychology Bulletin, 5*, 11–19.

Heidrich, S. M., Forsthoff, C. A., & Ward, S. E. (1994). Psychological adjustment in adults with cancer: The self as mediator. *Health Psychology, 13*, 346–353.

Heijmans, M., & deRidder, D. (1998a). Assessing illness representations of chronic disease: Explorations of their disease-specific nature. *Journal of Behavioral Medicine. 21*, 485–503.

Heijmans, M., & deRidder, D. (1998b). Structure and determinants of illness representations in chronic disease: A comparison of Addison's disease and chronic fatigue syndrome. *Journal of Health Psychology, 3*, 523–537.

Heijmans, M., deRidder, D., & Bensing, J. (in press). Dissimilarity in patients' and spouses' representations of chronic disease: Explorations of relations to patient adaptation. *Psychology and Health*.

Hochbaum, G. M. (1958). *Public participation in medical screening programs: A sociopsychological study*. Washington, DC: U.S. Government Printing Office.

Holman, H. R., & Lorig, K. (1992). Perceived self-efficacy in self-management of chronic diseases. In R. Schwartzer (Ed.), *Self-efficacy: Thought control of action* (pp. 305–323). Washington, DC: Hemisphere.

Hooker, K. (1992). Possible selves and perceived health in older adults and college students. *Journals of Gerontology, 47*(2), 85–95.

Horne, R. (1997). Representations of medication and treatment: Advances in theory and measurement. In K. J. Petrie & J. A. Weinman (Eds.), *Perceptions of health and illness: Current research and applications* (pp. 155–188). London: Harwood Academic Press.

Jamison, K. R. (1995). *An unquiet mind*. New York: Knopf.

Jamison, K. R., & Akiskal, H. S. (1983). Medications compliance in patients with bipolar disorder. *Psychiatric Clinics of North America, 6*, 175–192.

Janis, I. L. (1969). Effects of fear arousal on attitude change: Recent developments in theory and experimental research. In L. Berkowitz (Ed.), *Advances in experimental social psychology*, (Vol. 3, pp. 166–224). New York: Academic Press.

Janis, I. L., & Feshbach, S. (1953). Effects of fear-arousing communications. *Journal of Abnormal & Social Psychology, 48*, 78–92.

Janis, I. L., & Feshbach, S. (1954). Personality differences associated with responsiveness to fear-arousing communications. *Journal of Personality, 23*, 154–166.

Johnson, J. E. (1975). Stress reduction through sensation information. In I. C. Sarason & C. O. Speilberger (Eds.), *Stress and anxiety* (Vol. 2). Washington: Hemisphere.

Johnson, J. E., & Leventhal, H. (1974). The effects of accurate expectations and behavioral instructions on reactions during a noxious medical examination. *Journal of Personality and Social Psychology, 29*, 710–718.

Johnson, M. K., & Multhaup, K. S. (1992). Emotion and MEM. In S. A. Christianson (Ed.), *The handbook of emotion and memory: Current research and theory* (pp. 33–66). Hillsdale, NJ: Erlbaum.

Jones, E. E., Farina, A., Hastorf, A. H., Miller, D. T., & Scott, R. A. (1984). *Social stigma: The psychology of marked relationships*. New York: Freeman.

Kahneman, D., & Tversky, A. (1973). On the psychology of prediction. *Psychological Review, 80*, 237–251.

Kasl, S. V., & Cobb, J. (1966). Health behavior, illness behavior and sick-role behavior. *Archives of Environmental Health*, *12*, 531–541.

Keefe, F. J., Brown, G. K., Wallston, K. A., & Caldwell, D. S. (1989). Coping with rheumatoid arthritis pain: Catastrophizing as a maladaptive strategy. *Pain*, *37*, 51–56.

Kornzweig, N. D. (1967). *Behavior change as a function of fear arousal and personality.* Unpublished doctoral dissertation, Yale University, New Haven, CT.

Kulik, J. A., & Mahler, H. I. M. (1987). The effects of preoperative roommate assignment on preoperative anxiety and postoperative recovery from bypass surgery. *Health Psychology*, *6*, 525–543.

Kulik, J. A., & Mahler, H. I. M. (1997). Social comparison, affiliation, and coping with acute medical threats. In In B. P. Buunk & F. X. Gibbons (Eds.), *Health, coping, and well-being: Perspectives from social comparison theory* (pp. 227–262). Hillsdale, NJ: Erlbaum.

Lacroix, J. M. (1991). Assessing illness schemata in patient populations. In J. A. Skelton & R. T. Croyle (Eds.), *Mental representation in health and illness* (pp. 193–219). New York: Springer-Verlag.

Lacroix, J. M., Martin, B., Avendano, M., & Goldstein, R. (1991). Symptom schemata in chronic respiratory patients. *Health Psychology*, *10*, 268–273.

Lambert, J. F., (1996). *Illness representations among African-American hypertensives: Relationship to adherence and blood pressure control.* Unpublished master's thesis, Rutgers, the State University of New Jersey, New Brunswick, NJ.

Lau, R. R., Bernard, T. M., & Hartman, K. R. (1989). Further explorations of common sense representations of common illnesses. *Health Psychology*, *8*, 195–219.

Lau, R. R. & Hartman, K. R. (1983). Common sense representations of common illnesses. *Health Psychology*, *2*, 167–185.

Lazarus, R. S. (1966). *Psychological stress and the coping process.* New York: McGraw-Hill.

Lazarus, R. S., & Folkman, S. (1984). *Stress, appraisal, and coping.* New York: Springer.

Lazarus, R. S., & Launier, R. (1978). Stress-related transactions between person and environment. In L. A. Pervin & M. Lewis (Eds.), *Perspective in interactional psychology* (pp. 287–327). New York: Plenum.

Lazarus, R. S., Spiesman, J. C., Mordkoff, A. M., & Davison, L. A. (1962). A laboratory study of psychological stress produced by a motion picture film. *Psychological Monographs*, *76*, (34, whole No. 553).

Leventhal, E. A., & Crouch, M. (1997). Are there differences in perceptions of illness across the lifespan? In K.J. Petrie & J. A.Weinman (Eds.), *Perceptions of health and illness: Current research and applications* (pp. 77–102). London: Harwood Academic Press.

Leventhal, E. A., Leventhal, H., Schaefer, P., & Easterling, D. (1993). Conservation of energy, uncertainty reduction and swift utilization of medical care among the elderly. *Journal of Gerontology: Psychological Sciences*, *48*, P78–P86.

Leventhal, E. A., Leventhal, H., Shacham, S., & Easterling, D. V. (1989). Active coping reduces reports of pain from childbirth. *Journal of Consulting and Clinical Psychology*, *57*, 365–371.

Leventhal, H. (1970). Findings and theory in the study of fear communications. *Advances in Experimental Social Psychology*, *5*, 119–186.

Leventhal, H. (1984). A perceptual–motor theory of emotion. *Advances in Experimental Social Psychology*, *17*, 117–182.

Leventhal, H., & Diefenbach, M. (1991). The active side of illness cognition. In J. A. Skelton & R. T. Croyle (Eds.), *Mental representation in health and illness* (pp. 247–272). New York: Springer-Verlag.

Leventhal, H., Diefenbach, M., & Leventhal, E. A. (1992). Illness cognition: Using common sense to understand treatment adherence and affect cognition interactions. *Cognitive Therapy and Research*, *16*, 143–163.

Leventhal, H., Easterling, D. V., Coons, H., Luchterhand, C., & Love, R. R. (1986). Adaptation to chemotherapy treatments. In B. Andersen (Ed.), *Women with cancer*, (pp. 172–203). New York: Springer-Verlag.

Leventhal, H., Hudson, S., & Robitaille, C. (1997). Social comparison and health: A process model. In B. Buunk and F. X. Gibbons (Eds.), *Health, coping and well being: Perspectives from social comparison theory* (pp. 411–432). Hillsdale, NJ: Erlbaum.

Leventhal, H., Idler, E., & Leventhal, E. A. (1999). The impact of chronic illness on the self system. In R. Ashmore, L. Jussim, & R. Contrada (Eds.), *Self, social identity, and physical health: Interdisciplinary explorations. Second Rutgers Symposium on self and social identity.* (pp. 185–208). New York: Oxford.

Leventhal, H., Kelly, K., & Leventhal, E. (in press a). Perceived risk, motivation, and cancer preventive behavior. *Journal of the National Institutes of Health.*

Leventhal, H., Leventhal, E. A., & Cameron, L. (in press b). Representations, procedures and affect in illness self regulation: A perceptual-cognitive model. In A. Baum, T. Revenson, & J. Weinman (Eds.), *Handbook of health psychology.* Hillsdale, NJ: Erlbaum.

Leventhal, H., Leventhal, E. A., & Contrada, R. J. (1998b). Self regulation, health, and behavior: A perceptual–cognitive approach. *Psychology & Health. 13,* 717–733.

Leventhal, H., Leventhal, E. A., & Robitaille, C. (1998c). The role of theory for understanding the process of self care: A self regulation approach. In M. Ory & G. DeFriese (Eds.), *Self care in later life: Research, programs and policy perspectives* (pp. 118–141). New York: Springer Publishing.

Leventhal, H., Meyer, D., & Nerenz, D. (1980). The common sense representation of illness danger. In S. Rachman (Ed.), *Contributions to medical psychology* (Vol. II, pp. 7–30). New York: Pergamon.

Leventhal, H., & Nerenz, D. R. (1983). A model for stress research with some implications for the control of stress disorders. In D. Meichenbaum & M. Jaremko (Eds.), *Stress reduction and prevention* (pp. 5–38). New York: Plenum.

Leventhal, H., Patrick-Miller, L., Leventhal, E. A., & Burns, E. A. (1997). Does stress-emotion cause illness in elderly people? In K. W. Schaie & M. P. Lawton (Eds.). *Annual Review of Gerontology and Geriatrics: Focus on emotion and adult development.* (Volume 17, pp. 138–184). New York: Springer.

Leventhal, H., Rosenstock, I. M., Hochbaum, G. M., & Carriger, B. K. (1960). Epidemic impact on the general population in two cities. In *The impact of Asian influenza on community life: A study in five cities* (Publication No. 766). Washington, DC: U.S. Department of Health, Education, and Welfare, the Public Health Service.

Leventhal, H., Singer, R., & Jones, S. (1965). Effects of fear and specificity of recommendations upon attitudes and behavior. *Journal of Personality and Social Psychology, 2,* 20–29.

Leventhal, H., Watts, J. C., & Pagano, F. (1967). Effects of fear and instructions on how to cope with danger. *Journal of Personality and Social Psychology, 6,* 313–321.

Leventhal, H., Zimmerman, R., & Gutmann, M. (1984). Compliance: A self-regulation perspective. In W. D. Gentry (Ed.), *Handbook of behavioral medicine* (pp. 369–436). New York: Guilford.

Lewin, K. (1935). *A dynamic theory of personality.* New York: McGraw-Hill.

Linz, D., Penrod, S., Leventhal, H., & Siverhus, S. (1981). *The cognitive organization of disease and illness among lay persons.* Unpublished manuscript, University of Wisconsin at Madison.

Lorig, K. (1998). Arthritis self-efficacy scales measure self-efficacy. *Arthritis Care & Research, 11*(3), 155–157.

Mandler, G. (1964). The interruption of behavior. In D. Levine (Ed.), *Nebraska Symposium on Motivation.* (Volume 12). Lincoln: University of Nebraska Press.

Mandler, G., & Watson, D. L. (1966). Anxiety and interruption of behavior. In C. D. Speilberger (Ed.), *Anxiety and behavior.* New York: Academic Press.

Mandler, J. M. (1992). How to build a baby: II. Conceptual primitives. *Psychological Review*, *99*, 587–604.

Markus, H., & Nurius, P. (1986). Possible selves. *American Psychologist*, *41*, 954–969.

Mazen, R., & Leventhal, H. (1972). The influence of communicator–recipient similarity upon the beliefs and behavior of pregnant women. *Journal of Experimental Social Psychology*, *8*, 289–302.

Meyer, D., Leventhal, H., & Gutmann, M. (1985). Common-sense models of illness: The example of hypertension. *Health Psychology*, *4*, 115–135.

Millar, M. G., & Millar, K. (1995). Negative affective consequences of thinking about disease detection behaviors. *Health Psychology*, *14*, 141–146.

Millar, M. G., & Millar, K. (1996). The effects of anxiety on response times to disease detection and health promotion behaviors. *Journal of Behavioral Medicine*, *19*, 401–413.

Miller, G. A., Galanter, E., & Pribram, C. (1960). *Plans and the structure of behavior*. New York: Holt, Rinehart & Winston.

Miller, N. E. (1951). Learnable drives and rewards. In S. S. Stevens (Ed.), *Handbook of experimental psychology*. (pp. 435–472). New York: Wiley.

Mirowsky, J., & Ross, C. E., (1992). Age and depression. *Journal of Health & Social Behavior*, *33*, 187–205.

Misovich, S. J., Fisher, W. D., & Fisher, J. D. (1997). Social comparison as a factor in AIDS risk and AIDS preventive behavior (pp. 95–123). In B. Buunk & R. Gibbons (Eds.), *Health, coping and social comparison*. Hillsdale, NJ: Erlbaum

Moss-Morris, R., Petrie, K. J., & Weinman, J. (1996). Functioning in chronic fatigue syndrome: Do illness perceptions play a regulatory role? *British Journal of Health Psychology*, *1*, 15–25.

Nerenz, D. R., & Leventhal, H. (1983). Self-regulation theory in chronic illness. In T. G. Burish & L. A. Bradley (Eds.), *Coping with chronic disease: Research and applications* (pp. 13–37). New York: Academic Press.

Nolen-Hoeksma, S. (1997). Chewing the cud and other ruminations. In R. S. Wyer, (Ed.), *Ruminative thoughts. Advances in social cognition* vol. 9, (pp. 135–144). Hillsdale, NJ: Erlbaum.

Ory, M., & DeFriese, G. (1998). *Self care in later life*. New York: Springer Publishing.

Park, D. C. (1994). Self-regulation and control of rheumatic disorders. In S. Maes, H. Leventhal, & M. Johnston, (Eds.), *International review of health psychology* (Vol. 3, pp. 189–217). New York: Wiley

Peak, H. (1958). Psychological structure and psychological activity. *Psychological Review*, *65*, 325–347.

Pescosolido, B. A. (1992). Beyond rational choice: The social dynamics of how people seek help. *American Journal of Sociology*, *97*, 1096–1138.

Petrie, K. J., & Weinman, J. A. (1997). *Perceptions of health and illness: Current research and applications*. Amsterdam: Harwood Academic Publishers.

Powers, W. T. (1973). *Behavior: The control of perception*. Chicago: Aldine.

Price, R., (1982). *A whole new life: An illness and a healing*. New York: Penguin.

Rogers, R. W. (1983). Cognitive and physiological processes in fear appeals and attitude change: A revised theory of protection motivation. In J. T. Cacioppo & R. E. Petty (Eds.), *Social psychophysiology: A source book* (pp. 153–176). New York: Guilford.

Rosenberg, M. J., Hovland, C. I., McGuire W. J., Abelson, R. P., & Brehm, J. W. (1960). *Attitude organization and change*. New Haven, CT: Yale University Press.

Rosenstock, I. M. (1974). The health belief model and preventive health behavior. *Health Education Monographs*, *2*, 354–386.

Rosenstock, I. M., Hochbaum, G. M., & Leventhal, H. (1960). *The impact of Asian influenza on community life: A study in five cities* (Publication No. 766). Washington, DC: U.S. Department of Health, Education, and Welfare, the Public Health Service.

Rothman, A. J., & Kiviniemi, M. T. (1998). *Treating people with health information: An analysis and review of approaches to communicating health risk information.* Unpublished manuscript, University of Minnesota, Minneapolis.

Rozin, P., Markwith, M., & McCauley, C. (1994). Sensitivity to indirect contacts with other persons: AIDS aversion as a composite of aversion to strangers, infection, moral taint, and misfortune. *Journal of Abnormal Psychology, 103,* 495–505.

Safer, M., Tharps, Q., Jackson, T., & Leventhal, H. (1979). Determinants of three stages of delay in seeking care at a medical clinic. *Medical Care, 17,* 11–29.

Salovey, P., & Birnbaum, D. (1989). Influence of mood on health-relevant cognitions. *Journal of Personality and Social Psychology, 57,* 539–551.

Sarason, I. G. (1960). Empirical findings and theoretical problems in the use of anxiety scales. *Psychological Bulletin, 57,* 403–415.

Scharloo, M., & Kaptein, A. (1997). Measurement of illness perceptions in patients with chronic somatic illness: A review. In K. J. Petrie & J. A. Weinman (Eds.), *Perceptions of health and illness: Current research and applications* (pp. 103–1154). London: Harwood Academic Press.

Scheier, M. F., & Carver, C. S. (1985). Optimism, coping and health: Assessment and implications of generalized outcome expectancies. *Health Psychology, 4,* 219–247.

Scheier, M. F., & Carver, C. S. (1992). Effects of optimism on psychological and physical well-being: Theoretical overview and empirical update. *Cognitive Therapy and Research, 16*(2), 201–228.

Scherer, K. R. (1988). Criteria for emotion–antecedent appraisal: A review. *Cognitive perspectives on emotion and motivation.* Dordrecht, The Netherlands: Kluwer.

Schiaffino, K. M., & Cea, C. D. (1995). Assessing chronic illness representations: The implicit models of illness questionnaire. *Journal of Behavioral Medicine, 20,* 531–549.

Schiaffino, K. M., & Revenson, T. A. (1992). The role of perceived self-efficacy, perceived control and causal attributes in adaptation to rheumatoid arthritis: Distinguishing mediator vs moderator effects. *Personality & Social Psychology Bulletin, 18,* 709–718.

Silverman, C. (1999). *Psychological adjustment top uncertain outcomes: The threat of cancer recurrence.* Unpublished dissertation, University of Illinois, Champaign-Urbana.

Skelton, J. A., & Croyle, R. T. (1991). *Mental representation in health and illness,* New York: Springer-Verlag.

Stoller, E. P. (1998). Medical self care: Lay management of symptoms by elderly people. In M. G. Ory, & G. DeFriese, *Self care in later life* (pp. 24–61). New York: Springer Publishing.

Suls, J., Martin, R., & Leventhal, H. (1997). Social comparison, lay referral, and the decision to seek medical care. In B. Buunk and F. X. Gibbons (Eds.), *Social comparisons, health, and coping* (pp. 195–226). Hillsdale, NJ: Erlbaum.

Tolman, E. C. (1938). The determiners of behavior at a choice point. *Psychological Review, 45,* 1–41.

Wood, J. V., & VanderZee, K. (1997). Social comparisons among cancer patients: Under what conditions are comparisons upward and downward? In B. Buunk and F. X. Gibbons, (Eds.), *Social comparisons, health, and coping* (pp. 299–328). Hillsdale, NJ: Erlbaum.

Wortman, C. B., & Lehman, D. R. (1985). Reactions to victims of life crises: Support attempts that fail. In I. Sarason and B. Sarason, *Social support: Theory, research and applications.* Dordrecht, The Netherlands: Nijhoff.

Zeidner, M., Boekaerts, M., & Pintrich, P. R. (2000). Self-regulation: Directions and challenges for future research. In M. Boekaerts, P. R. Pintrich, & M. Zeidner, *Handbook of self-regulation* (Chap. 23). San Diego, CA: Academic Press. (This volume)

Zeiss, A. M., Lewinsohn, P. M., Rohde, P., & Seeley, J. R. (1996). Relationship of physical disease and functional impairment to depression in older people. *Psychology & Aging, 11,* 572–581.

Zola, I. K. (1972). Studying the decision to see a doctor. In Z. V. Lipowski (Ed.), *Psychosocial aspects of physical illness* (pp. 216–236). Basel, Switzerland: Karger.

13

SELF-REGULATED LEARNING

FINDING A BALANCE BETWEEN LEARNING GOALS AND EGO-PROTECTIVE GOALS

MONIQUE BOEKAERTS[1] AND
MARKKU NIEMIVIRTA[2]

[1]Leiden University, Leiden, The Netherlands
[2]Helsinki University, Helsinki, Finland

I. INTRODUCTION

In the traditional school setting, students tend to depend on their teachers for the acquisition of information. They expect their teachers to provide learning material, to motivate them, and to take responsibility for the learning process. It is accepted, even expected, that teachers should be largely in control of what is being learned, how it is learned, when it is learned, and to what extent. The generally accepted role pattern wherein teachers convey declarative and procedural knowledge and students must find a way to comprehend, store, and activate that knowledge leads to a situation in which students lack sufficient opportunity to organize and regulate their own learning. A question that should be raised is, "Are teachers well equipped to create conditions that will foster the development of effective self-regulatory skills?" To answer this question we need a clear definition of self-regulation and an understanding of how students and teachers interpret their complementary roles.

Copyright © 2000 by Academic Press.
All rights of reproduction in any form reserved.

Zimmerman and Schunk (1989) defined self-regulated learning (SRL) as students' self-generated thoughts, feelings, and actions, which are systematically oriented toward attainment of their goals. This definition implies that for effective self-regulation to develop, students should be allowed to work in a context in which they can create their own learning episodes according to their own goals. Three constructs are central to this definition of self-regulated learning, namely, learning episodes, self-set learning goals, and goal processes. In the first section of this chapter, we define learning episodes and explain how natural learning episodes differ from teacher-set learning episodes. Self-set goals are compared and contrasted with teacher-set goals. In the second section, we demonstrate that self-regulation processes originate in the identification, interpretation, and appraisal of an opportunity to learn. The Model of Adaptable Learning is presented briefly and later extended to include two new constructs: chronic goals and intentionally induced goals. In the third and fourth sections, goal setting and goal striving are addressed as sequential stages in SRL. Finally, we argue that SRL is not a unitary construct, but refers to a system concept that integrates activity in different control systems.

II. WHAT TURNS A POTENTIAL LEARNING OPPORTUNITY INTO A SITUATION THAT THE STUDENT IDENTIFIES AS SUCH?

Drawing on Ford (1995), who assumes that virtually all human activity is organized in behavior episode form, Boekaerts (1996a) introduced the term "learning episode" and defined it as a situation in which a person is invited, coached, or coaxed to display context-specific, goal-directed learning behavior. If the learner accepts this invitation, his or her learning behavior unfolds over time until one of the following conditions is met: (1) the learning goal that organized the learning episode is attained, (2) the learning goal is attained only partially, but this state of affairs is accepted by the learner, (3) the learning goal is reappraised as unattainable, unattractive, or irrelevant, or (4) another goal takes precedence. In the context of the present discussion it is important to make a clear distinction between learning episodes that occur in a natural context and those that occur in the classroom. The former type of learning episodes differ from the latter on a number of grounds. First, natural learning episodes are often self-initiated or occur spontaneously. Second, they are cumulative, thus creating ongoing and unfolding learning experiences. Third, this type of learning is always socially situated. Fourth, it is driven by personal goals and therefore consequential in nature and affectively charged.

As many educational psychologists have pointed out, most learning initiated in traditional classrooms is neither cumulative nor goal directed in the true sense of these words. In a traditional scholastic context, learning episodes tend to be fragmented, indirect experiences, steered by teacher-set goals. These deliberately and systematically planned learning experiences may or may not capture the students' interest, meaning that information provided during these episodes may or may not be used by students to activate prior knowledge and to steer the learning process.

There are a number of reasons why self-regulation may be harder to realize in a classroom context than in a natural context. First, most students consider it to be the teacher's role to provide relevant resources and to motivate them to engage in the learning activity. They also expect teachers to monitor their performance carefully and to provide relevant feedback. Such role beliefs are hard to change and inhibit the self-regulation process, mainly because most students do not have a clear conception of their own needs and aspirations concerning the acquisition of new knowledge and skills. They mostly do not feel an urgent need to acquire new knowledge and skills. What usually happens is that teachers must convince students that the opportunity they offer is a unique chance to acquire a valuable skill. Such teacher communications convey a triple message: first, that one should make an effort to acquire a new skill; second, that all other goals should be set aside in favor of this urgent teacher-set goal; and third, that such commitment will be rewarded with teacher regulation and support.

A. WHEN OPPORTUNITY AND FELT NECESSITY COINCIDE

When working with students, one can easily observe that most teacher-provided learning opportunities do not automatically create "felt necessity." Some students may not attach value to the new skill, whereas others may view the skill as valuable, yet do not feel like practicing it on command. Our line of argument is that although most teachers may think that they provide plenty of opportunities for self-regulated learning to develop, in reality the opportunities they create do not guarantee that effective self-regulation will develop. Optimal conditions for the development of self-regulated learning exist when students are given the chance to establish and pursue personal, nontrivial goals. The point being made is that providing opportunity is different from seeking opportunity. For example, accepting the teacher's statement that learning to write in cursive script is a necessary skill is not the same as feeling the need to acquire that skill. Consider the following example as an illustration of natural learning episodes.

When Elaine was two years old, her baby sister, Mia, was born. Elaine went to the hospital with her grandmother and immediately sensed that there was a new rival. As she grew older, Elaine took great pride outsmarting her baby sister. She deliberately used her reading and writing skills to communicate messages to parents, grandparents, and visitors, realizing all too well that Mia could not share the experience. When Mia was 5 years old, she also started reading words and phrases. Elaine did not like this new development. One day she asked her grandmother whether she could have her birthday present a few months in advance. She explained that she wanted a book that would teach her to write in cursive script. The reason why she wanted such a book was that she assumed that it would take Mia quite a while to learn to read and write printed letters, and in the meantime she could still outsmart her by using a code that Mia would not be able to understand. Elaine designed her own way to acquire the skill of writing in cursive script. She asked older children or relatives to rewrite texts or letters she had printed herself, using the cursive letters as models for her practice sessions. She also found a way to monitor her progress. Whenever she finished copying a text, she asked somebody to read out loud what she had written and used her printed version of the text to check whether she had correctly copied the cursive letters.

These observations illustrate that very young children may set personal goals and design their own learning episodes in accordance with these goals. This example also shows that children are able to represent an immediate or urgent need mentally and link it to their higher-order goals and to specific scripts that they have available in their repertoire (see also Carver & Scheier, 2000, this volume). Elaine used her knowledge of developmental differences in various domains to make a mental representation of her higher-order goal ("I want to outsmart my baby sister") and to transform this abstract goal into various action plans. Using her knowledge about the reading and writing acquisition process, she established a specific short-term goal: "I want to communicate a written message without Mia being able to read it." Elaine realized that such a learning goal called for action. She therefore asked her grandmother to buy her a book. She also designed learning episodes herself. These episodes included copying texts, as well as asking parents, grandparents, and older children to provide feedback on her progress. It is evident that Elaine's behavior was driven by a personal goal. Her learning episodes were self-initiated and she designed them in accordance with her own wishes, expectations, and needs. Moreover, the learning episodes she planned built successively upon one another, making her learning cumulative and making the knowledge and skills she acquired available for use. This example also draws attention to the essential difference between motivational and cognitive accounts of goal-directed behavior. Indeed, Elaine was able to set her own learning targets in accordance with her needs and wishes, developing clear expectancies about the positive and negative consequences of her actions and about the effort required. She also realized that she needed some standard to guide and evaluate her own and other people's performance: "Grandma, Mia can do it if she really tries hard, but then you have to hold the paper upright and not put it on the table."

This example illustrates that powerful environments for the development of SRL arise when opportunity and felt necessity coincide. When individuals feel a need to extend or adapt their existing scripts, while at the same time perceiving an opportunity to acquire those scripts, they will feel inspired to seek or create learning opportunities based on their own wishes, needs, and expectations. We assume that knowledge and skills acquired in this manner will become an integral part of the network of goals that steer and direct an individual's behavior. An interesting question to raise in the present context is, "Where do personal goals come from?"

B. GOALS VIEWED AS KNOWLEDGE STRUCTURES THAT GUIDE BEHAVIOR

Currently, most theoretical accounts cast goals as concrete anchor points for directing our actions in fulfillment of our needs. Goals are viewed as guiding principles that people consciously and intentionally set to effectively steer their behavior (Austin & Vancouver, 1996). Many authors view the self as a key component in understanding an individual's goal setting and goal striving. Some researchers use the terms "ideal self" or "possible self" when talking about a person's aspirations and strivings. For example, Higgins (1987) contrasted the actual self to the "ideal self" (a presentation of the attributes that a person would like to possess) and the "ought self" (the attributes that a person thinks he or she should possess). Markus and Nurius (1986) contrasted the self that is currently on-line in information processing to "possible selves." Possible selves, ought selves, and ideal selves are viewed by these authors as self-directive standards, goals, or acquired self-guides.

Powers (1973) used the goal construct in a slightly different sense. He described the self as a coherent structure of principles or higher-order goals and proposed a goal hierarchy in which goals are described at several levels of abstraction. Powers's "principle control" is akin to Markus and Nurius' "possible selves," Higgins's "ideal self," and Carver & Scheier's (2000) "be goals." The principles specified in Powers's higher-order goals provide the lower-level goals with a reference value, because they specify the quality of the acts that a person wishes to perform. These higher-order goals are connected to action programs that specify *how* the acts should be performed. When the course of action is adapted to a local context, the term "script" is used. Examples of goal hierarchies are given later in this chapter.

Most theorists assume that goals are not equivalent in their relevance to a person. The higher a goal is situated in the hierarchy, the more it contributes to the person's sense of self, yet the more abstract it is (see Carver & Scheier, 2000). Also, goals that are connected to multiple higher-order goals tend to be more highly valued. Several authors (Austin & Vancouver, 1996; Vallacher & Wegner, 1987) have argued that movement in the hierarchy can be top-down or bottom-up. *Top-down movement* means that subgoals have been derived from higher-order goals, implying that action programs and scripts have been consciously and intentionally chosen. *Bottom-up movement* refers to goal processes that reflect the individual's motivation to do something because the environmental conditions are just right or to refrain from doing things because environmental conditions pose an impediment.

Kruglanski (1996) proposed that goals should be viewed as knowledge structures that apply to desirable and undesirable future end states. His conceptualization of goals enables us to borrow the general principles that have been well documented in other areas of psychology, particularly cognitive psychology and text processing (e.g., Wilson & Anderson, 1986), and apply them to the study of goal processes (examples of such processes are preattentional processes, knowledge acquisition processes, knowledge accessibility). Although the exact nature of goal processes is still open to debate, recent research suggests many similarities between goal processing and text processing. For example, Locke and Latham (1990) pointed out that some goals are conscious, whereas others are unconscious; some are internal, whereas others are external to the individual. However, each goal represents a specific content that differentiates it from other goals. Goals must be activated to have an impact on actions. Bargh's (1990) position is that goal activation can be automatic or deliberate and Bargh and Barndollar (1996) demonstrated that some goals may be activated or triggered directly by environmental cues, outside the awareness of the individual. They used the term"auto-motives" to refer to these preattentional goal processes and suggested that a goal may become preconsciously activated, provided it has been encoded in a highly accessible knowledge structure.

Following this line of reasoning, it could be argued that goals are interconnected knowledge structures that differ with respect to their accessibility. Some of these knowledge structures have been "automatized" through being set often and regularly as part of a frequently and consistently repeated action pattern. As a consequence, these knowledge structures become chronic goals, in the sense that they can be discharged readily when a student attends to a specific perceptual category. Bargh and his colleagues proposed that such chronically triggered goals should be distinguished from goals that are intentionally constructed. We will come back to this issue after we have discussed identification, interpretation, and appraisal processes.

III. SELF-REGULATED LEARNING ORIGINATES IN THE IDENTIFICATION, INTERPRETATION, AND APPRAISAL OF AN OPPORTUNITY TO LEARN

An issue that has received little attention in the educational literature is that students may pursue many goals simultaneously and that these goals may be either in harmony or in disharmony (see Wenzel, 1994, for an exception). We already have pointed out that not all teacher-set goals are equivalent in their relevance to the students. A related yet distinct point is that learning goals communicated by the teacher may not tap affectively charged themes. Even worse, these goals may activate negative scenarios that direct the students' attention away from the learning goal (avoidance goals).

Our argument is not that students are unwilling to adopt teacher-set goals and practice strategies that the teacher deems important. Fortunately, many students do adopt teacher-set goals and carry out the required action plans. Rather, our argument is that most goals that students pursue in the context of the classroom are not intentionally constructed on the basis of personal strivings or aspirations to comprehend the dynamics of unfolding learning episodes in the context of the classroom and to understand individual differences in the perception, interpretation, and appraisal of those episodes, consider the following example:

Lia, Bob, and Tim are seventh graders in the same mathematics class. Both Lia and Bob do fairly well in math, whereas Tim's performance usually falls slightly below average. Pat, the mathematics teacher, views both Lia and Bob as active and enthusiastic students. However, she perceives some qualitative differences in the way they approach school tasks. Lia seems to be more concerned with understanding what she is doing, whereas Bob is more interested in getting the job done—and the sooner the better. He likes to show off in front of the class and often makes public announcements about how fast he can do the assignments. Yet, he is very sensitive to social comparisons and fears making mistakes in public. When he does make a mistake, he quickly finds an excuse or makes a funny remark to draw the others' attention away from his mistake. By contrast, Lia is often so focused on a specific problem that she forgets to participate in routine classroom activities. Also, she does her work so meticulously that she often cannot finish it in time and has to take it home. Tim differs from both these students: he cares less about mathematics and is very quiet in the classroom, mostly minding his own business. The teacher has noted that he is very insecure and always in doubt about whether he will or will not be able to complete a task. She knows that whenever Tim feels emotionally threatened, he either withdraws mentally or reacts with suppressed aggression. Despite Tim's low interest in mathematics and his mindless attitude toward school tasks in general, the math teacher thinks that he has the capacity to do well in mathematics: he lacks only the self-confidence and social support to realize his full potential.

Pat is a very friendly and supportive person who wants to create optimal learning opportunities for her students. Last week, she attended an in-service training program and learned that surprise quizzes are a good tool to keep students alert and make them do their homework. Yesterday, she announced her first surprise quiz: she asked her students to finish their exercises, put their gear in their bags and get ready for the quiz. An increase in the noise level informed her that her students were upset. Some students told her that it is not fair to evaluate students' performance without prior warning. Pat quickly declared that it was not her intention to grade their performance on the quiz, but that she simply wanted to gain more insight into their progress. However, this modifying statement did not decrease the noise level in the classroom.

Let us take a closer look at the way Tim, Bob, and Lia define desirable and undesirable end states that may serve as concrete anchor points for directing their attention and actions. Tim did not pay any attention to the teacher's qualifying statement. The announcement of the quiz, the fact that they had to clear their tables, and the loud complaints from his fellow learners convinced him that this was a test situation. He felt out of control because he had not prepared for the exam. He also felt depressed. When the teacher noticed his passivity, she asked what was the matter. He started complaining that he had a headache and that he could not concentrate on the task. In contrast, both Lia and Bob clearly heard that the teacher had qualified the nature of the assessment episode. This information made Bob focus on the positive consequences of the quiz: He felt confident that he could solve the problems that would be given. The fact that there would be no grading encouraged him to take more risks to show the teacher and his classmates that he is very fast and competent in mathematics. Lia simply welcomed the quiz, viewing it as an opportunity to get feedback on her progress in solving algebraic equations.

We trust that it has become clear that every learning opportunity is unique. A task or an invitation to solve a problem or learn a new skill is always situated in a specific content circle, but also in a wider social context. Perceptions of the content of a task, as well as of contextual factors, will affect a student's reaction to a learning situation. However, the manner in which the same learning situation is interpreted varies across different students, leading to different action patterns.

A. IDENTIFICATION OF A LEARNING SITUATION

It is important to realize that the objective meaning of a (surprise) quiz differs from the subjective meaning that Bob, Tim, and Lia assigned to it. Students' situational construals are not restricted to the perception of the situation as such (i.e., data-driven or bottom-up processing). As many authors have pointed out (e.g., Bargh & Gollwitzer, 1994; Higgins, 1990), the assignment of subjective meaning involves integration of current informational input with relevant prior knowledge. Much of the significance of events, situations, and other social objects derives from how individuals categorize them. Identification refers to the recognition of an input as an instance of a class of situations, such as an instance of the class of achievement situations, stressful situations, or socially unacceptable situations.

We view the identification process as akin to pattern or template recognition (Neuman, 1984) in the sense that it proceeds smoothly and without much conscious attention. In various areas of psychology evidence is accumulating that implicates precoded information in such categorization processes (Bargh & Gollwitzer, 1994). Drawing on Fodor (1985) and Zajonc (1980), Boekaerts (1987) argued that emotions elicited in a learning context could be conceptualized as the outcome of a primitive data-driven computational unit. This unit detects stimulus features in the input that have been labeled threatening or aversive in the past. Once such a computational unit has been established, it acts as a sentry, watching out for danger signals. If such signals are detected in the input (i.e., a threshold is exceeded), an alarm bell rings (increased level of arousal) and prepares the individual for action.

For example, when the quiz was announced, all students recognized the stimulus configuration immediately as an instance of a previously established class of events, namely, as a test situation. The salient features of such a situation are that it is highly structured, requires students to demonstrate their knowledge and skills, to abide by the rules, and to suffer negative consequences if their performance is below standard. It is assumed that detection of the perceptual knowledge category "test situation" triggers particular behavioral patterns or scripts in all students: They are supposed to work fast, quietly, and independently, and are not supposed to look at each other's work. However, the identification of a learning situation always occurs in a wider context, and aspects of that context will contribute to accurate assessement of the situation. Recall that the teacher provided extra information at the beginning of the classroom episode, and that this additional information should have turned the test situation into a natural assessment situation without personal consequences. Yet, not all students paid close attention to the teacher's remarks, leading to an incorrect identification of the learning situation. What underlies such biased perception? Individual differences in knowledge about the essential features or inherent properties of a situation, as well as the students' past learning history may give rise to biased situation construals. In turn, these construals affect students' attention to salient contextual properties and restrict the number of action paths that are available, accessible, and perceived as applicable.

Several researchers have pointed to salient properties or dimensions of an individual's situation construal (e.g., Forgas, 1982; Frijda, 1986; Zajonc, 1980). Forgas (1982) showed that social episodes are perceived and cognitively represented in terms of a limited number of connotative attribute dimensions. He found (Forgas, 1985) that individuals interpret social situations in terms of three basic dimensions: intensity of the situation (serious vs. fun situations), interest in the situation (pleasantness), and the social anxiety elicited by the situation (self-confidence). The relative weight that individuals gave to these three relatively independent dimensions was related to the level of their social skills. Forgas reported that social anxiety dominated the episode representation of those who had low social skills. These individuals paid little attention to the potential interestingness of the social episode. Individuals with high social skills paid far more attention to the intensity and interest dimensions and far less to the social anxiety dimension.

In our judgment, learning episodes also can be perceived and cognitively represented in terms of a limited number of connotative attribute dimensions. All of the students in Pat's class view exams as strictly structured situations whose form and implementation lie largely or entirely outside their personal control. However, there are clear individual differences in how students might identify a particular quiz (Trope, 1986), that are rooted in differences in self-regulatory focus and, hence, have implications for the course of subsequent action. We could speculate, then, that Tim failed to take account of the contextual information because his data-driven computational units triggered a generalized response pattern: He felt emotionally threatened and anxious, which made him want to withdraw from the situation. It is highly likely that Tim's identification process activated negative scenarios (Bandura, 1993) that made him anticipate a negative course of action with concomitant negative cognitions and feelings. Higgins and his colleagues proposed that the secondary phase of situation construal should be partioned conceptually into two tightly interwoven processes, namely, the interpretation process and the appraisal process.

B. INTERPRETATION AND APPRAISAL

Higgins, Strauman, and Klein (1986) argued that interpretation and appraisal of an event are distinct from mere identification in that these processes are often, if not always, related to some kind of internal standard, point of reference, ideal self, or ought self. Higgins (1990) stated that during the interpretation process, personal meaning is assigned to an event. The individual draws inferences about the implications of an event in terms of desirable or undesirable outcomes. Higgins viewed the appraisal process as inherently evaluative: Individuals estimate the personal significance of a situation, thus bringing their hopes, needs, expectations, obligations, and fears to bear on the situation. Other authors have referred to the postidentification process with terms such as "interpretations" (Schachter & Singer, 1962), "meaning analysis" (Mandler, 1984), and "appraisals" (Frijda, 1986). Frijda (1988) argued that events appraised in terms of their meanings are "the emotional piano player's finger strokes; available modes of action readiness are the keys that are tapped; changes in action readiness are the tones brought forth" (p. 351). He also suggested that such situational meaning structures are unique and emotion-specific.

In a similar vein, Lazarus and Smith (1988) referred to processes of evaluating particular relational harms or benefits with the term "appraisals," viewing them as mediators between a situation and subsequent actions. They emphasized that appraisals should be distinguished from the knowledge structures on which they are based. Lazarus and Folkman (1984) described appraisals at two levels: primary and secondary. Primary appraisal concerns the questions, "What is this situation about? Is it benign, neutral, or threatening for my well being?" Secondary appraisal deals with the question, "What is required to deal with the situation and can I handle it under the present conditions?" Following Lazarus and Folkman's theorizing, Boekaerts (1992) assumed that students continuously judge whether a learning situation is benign, neutral, or threatening for their well-being. She defined appraisals as nonstop evaluation processes that result in emotions/action readiness of upcoming and ongoing learning activities. A central role was assigned to these appraisals in her Model of Adaptable Learning. This model was developed in the last decade in an attempt to integrate and extend the fragmented research and theory in the domains of learning, motivation, anxiety, coping with stress, and action control (Boekaerts, 1992, 1996a). In the next section we provide an overview of this model, and thereafter we further discuss and extend it in light of our present discussion, thus representing identification, interpretation, and control processes explicitly in the model.

C. THE MODEL OF ADAPTABLE LEARNING: FINDING A BALANCE BETWEEN PARALLEL GOALS

The Model of Adaptable Learning is a holistic framework that allows us to explore the interaction between intertwined aspects of SRL. Over the years, a number of interrelated processes have been differentiated, including metacognitive control, motivation control, emotion control, and action control. This analytical decomposition of self-regulated learning into different forms of control made it possible to focus on a particular aspect of self-regulation, while keeping the "one reality perspective" manageable.

An important assumption of the model is that individuals inherently self-regulate their behavior in terms of two basic priorities. On the one hand, they want to extend their knowledge and skills so that they can expand their personal resources. On the other hand, they wish to maintain their available resources and to prevent loss, damage and distortions of well-being. It is further assumed that the information processing modes that underlie these two basic priorities coexist, but may fight for dominance in the individual's goal hierarchy. In the original model, a central role was given to the appraisal construct. It was theorized that each learning situation triggers a network of highly specific connotations, because it impinges on a learner's personal strivings and vulnerabilities. This is represented by links between the appraisal process and the contents of a dynamic internal working model (WM), which is constantly fed information from three main sources (cf. Figure 1). The first source of information is the perception of the learning situation, including the task, the instructions given by the teacher, and the physical and social context (component 1). The second source of information concerns activated domain-specific knowledge and skills, including declarative and procedural knowledge, cognitive strategies that have been successful in that domain, and metacognitive knowledge relevant to the learning situation (component 2). The third source refers to aspects of the students' self-system, including their goal hierarchy (ideal and ought selves), values, and motivational beliefs pertaining to the domain that is activated by the situation (component 3).

Although several other models also emphasize that students' expectancies and their goal setting is influenced jointly by situation variables and person variables (e.g., Rheinberg, Vollmeyer, & Rollett, 2000, this volume), the Model of Adaptable Learning differs from this and similar models on many grounds. An important difference that concerns us here is that the Model of Adaptable Learning explicitly differentiates between two types of person variables, namely, those that reflect the individual's metacognition and interact with the content of the task (component 2) and those that reflect the individual's self and motivational beliefs (component 3) (see Boekaerts, 1996a, for a more detailed account). As we explain shortly, this distinction allows us to separate two types of interpretation processes and distinguish between different types of higher-order control processes, including metacognitive control and motivational control.

A student's appraisal of a particular learning situation is considered to be unique because the information stemming from the three sources differs for every learning opportunity, thus eliciting specific experiential states (positive and negative affects) and specific behavioral intentions. In the original model it was assumed that the students' unique appraisals steer and direct their behavior in the classroom, including their goal setting (learning or coping intentions) and their goal striving (activity in

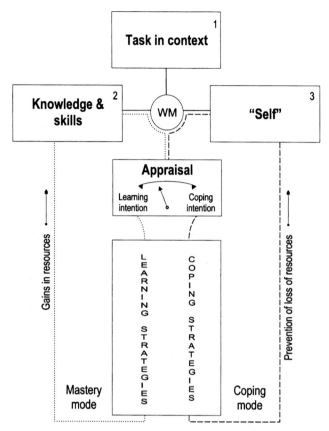

FIGURE 1 The original model of adaptable learning. From "Coping with stress in childhood and adolescence." In M. Zeidner & N. S. Endler (Eds.), *Handbook of Coping. Theories, Research, Application* (pp. 452–484). New York: Wiley. Copyright 1996 by John Wiley & Sons, Inc. Reprinted with permission.

the mastery mode or the well-being mode). Boekaerts and her colleagues hypothesized that positive appraisals are evoked when the information in the dynamic working model is primarily positive, either because relevant scripts are available (domain-specific input from component 2) or because the activity that has to be performed is inherently linked to personally relevant goals and personal gains (input from component 3). By contrast, it was hypothesized that negative appraisals arise when no relevant scripts can be located (input from component 2) or when the learner is not inclined to invest energy in the task (input from component 3).

Empirical work based on the model, featuring children in different age groups doing tasks in different subject-matter areas, has revealed that the joint effect of positive and negative task judgments influences the students' intention to learn (formation of a learning goal) and their experiential state (cf. Boekaerts, 1999; Boekaerts, Seegers, & Vermeer, 1995). More specifically, task attraction is a crucial aspect of a student's situation construal. It is directly influenced by activated positive and negative scenarios (measured at the middle level; goal orientation, achievement motivation, fear of failure), by value-related perceptions of the situation at hand (e.g., its relevance and importance), and by perceived subjective competence (which includes perception of difficulty, success expectation, and self-efficacy). A negative emotional state (feeling anxious, tense, and not happy) during the formation of a learning intention was influenced directly by unfavorable appraisals (low task attraction, low perceived relevance, and low subjective competence).

The Model of Adaptable Learning further assumes that predominantly positive appraisals steer and direct students' attention and energy to adaptive payoffs (increase in competence and other resources; left pathway in Figure 1), whereas largely negative appraisals urge students to protect their ego or restore their well-being (prevention of loss of resources; right pathway in Figure 1). These two parallel processing modes are referred to as (1) the mastery or learning mode and (2) the coping or well-being mode. Pioneering work in relation to these two processing modes was carried out by Diener and Dweck (1978). In a series of studies, they examined children's reactions to failure in academic settings that followed a successful performance. Based on their prior work on learned helplessness, Dweck and her colleagues classified these subjects into two groups: a group that was likely to adopt a pattern of engagement that reflects helplessness and another group that tended to exhibit mastery behavior. Interestingly, these children, who shared the same ability level, did not show any differences in strategy use or reported interest when they experienced success. However, after the children had been through a failure experience, two clearly different behavioral patterns emerged. The helpless group began to express negative emotions and engaged in task-irrelevant verbalizations. They also began to attribute their failure to lack of competence and insufficient skills, and tried to compensate the noted failure by speaking about their abilities in other domains. In contrast, the mastery group demonstrated more enthusiasm when facing obstacles and new challenges set by difficult tasks: They became more involved with the procedure and increased their effort expenditure. In addition to more careful planning and monitoring, students who belonged to the mastery group engaged in intense motivation control and maintained their positive attitude toward the performance situation despite the failure context.

These striking differences only occurred after failure and this finding neatly illustrate the situationally sensitive nature of children's reactions. In the present context, we go one step further and argue that children may generalize either one of these engagement patterns to all situations they have come to define as functionally equivalent. In addition to our own studies (Boekaerts, Seegers, & Vermeer, 1995; Niemivirta, 1998, 1999), a substantial body of experimental and correlational evidence supports this assumption (see Jagacinski, 1992; Pintrich, Marx, & Boyle, 1993; Kuhl & Beckmann, 1994).

It is important to note that in the original model of adaptable learning, the distinction between the two fundamentally different types of processing modes was largely categorical. It was argued that the action patterns that students display when in one of the two processing modes may differ. However, it was not made clear why students' action patterns take on different forms. Current conceptualizations of identification and interpretation processes allow us to connect students' perceptions of situational constraints and the availability and accessibility of personal resources to their self-regulatory focus. In light of these conceptualizations, the model has been extended to include the strength of the associations between an action plan (learning or coping strategies) and (1) knowledge associated with a given perceptual category (identification process), (2) knowledge structures in component 2 (interpretation process based on activated domain-specific knowledge and skills), and (3) knowledge structures in component 3 (interpretation process based on motivational beliefs). In the next two sections we focus on the hypothetical relationships between, on the one hand, the origins of the goal processes (identification, interpretation, and appraisal processes) and, on the other, goal setting and goal striving.

IV. GOAL SETTING: AN ESSENTIAL ASPECT OF SELF-REGULATED LEARNING

It is clear, that the same learning situation may be interpreted differently by different students and that this may lead to diverse action patterns. As several authors have argued, there are various ways (means) leading to the attainment of a goal. However, not all students perceive a choice among alternative action paths. We have hinted that those who do may have an advantage over those who do not by initiating a self-directed learning episode. It is evident from the work of motivation researchers such as Deci and Ryan (1985) and Ford (1995) that goal setting, choice of goals, and goal striving are essential aspects of goal-directed behavior, because these constructs link goals to action plans. As early as the 1940s, Lewin, Dembo, Festinger, and Sears (1944) made a distinction between goal setting and goal striving. Later, Kuhl (1984) described the process of making decisions about which goals to adopt as "motivation" and used the term "volition" to refer to the phase where the choice has been made and the individual initiates and executes the actions that lead to goal attainment. A model that deals explicitly with choice and personal preferences is the Action Phase Model (Heckhausen & Gollwitzer, 1987; Gollwitzer,

1990). It goes beyond the conceptual distinction of goal setting and goal striving, providing a coherent framework for bridging the gap between motivation and volition. Four phases are distinguished, namely, the predecisional, preactional, actional, and postactional phases. These phases are separated by particular transition points, namely, making a decision, initiating the action, and perceiving the action outcomes.

During the predecisional or motivational phase, individuals translate their needs, expectations, and wishes into intentions. They weigh the feasibility and desirability (Heckhausen & Gollwitzer, 1987), in other words, the outcome expectancy and outcome-consequence expectancy of alternative goals, using their own criteria (see also Winne, 1997; Winne & Perry, 2000, this volume). They make a choice among alternative goals, which leads to a goal intention. This choice represents a leap from a state of uncertainty about the goal to a commitment to a desired end state (cf. Gollwitzer, 1990).

Although several researchers (e.g., Smith & Lazarus, 1993) have described the predecisional phase as one where individuals deliberately scan alternatives, Kruglanski (1996) has argued convincingly that out-of-consciousness factors also may affect goal formation. He pointed out that need for closure may affect the extent of information processing in forming a goal, although it may not figure officially as a reason for a person's choice among alternatives. Our point is that the predecisional stage necessitates some degree of open mindedness and heightened receptivity to incoming information (data-driven processing), lest subjectively relevant information be activated from memory that biases accurate perception, information processing, and goal setting. As we have argued previously, not all students attend automatically to relevant clues. Gollwitzer and his colleagues (e.g., Bargh & Gollwitzer, 1994; Gollwitzer, 1996; Gollwitzer, Heckhausen, & Ratajczak, 1990) demonstrated in a series of studies that goal congruent information becomes readily accessible and is processed effectively when individuals are striving for desirable goals. A lot less is known about situations where goals remain implicit or where externally set goals are in conflict with personal strivings and vulnerabilities.

In our opinion, the Model of Action Phases seems to be most applicable to situations that allow several alternative routes to goal attainment, thus dealing with choice and personal preferences. We are not so sure that the model works equally well in situations where habitual engagement and/or externally set goals are prominent. For example, in the test situation that Lia, Bob, and Tim encountered, limited goal choice is offered. The task is assigned by the teacher, thus providing both an externally set goal and a framework for action. In other words, the students' alternatives are limited. They have to concentrate on the set task, deciding whether they are going to engage seriously (mindfully) in the quiz or not.

Let us return to the Model of Adaptable Learning. As already explained, this model gives a central position to appraisals. Appraisal processes are considered to be based on activated domain-specific knowledge and skills, including knowledge about how things work in general, and in the present context in particular (component 2), and beliefs about the self, including a student's goal hierarchies and the consequences of specific actions in the present context (component 3). Boekaerts (1992, 1996a, 1996b) took the position that students' appraisals of a learning situation affect their goal setting (learning or coping intention) and goal striving (learning and coping strategies) in important ways. As can be seen in Figures 2 and 3, our present approach is slightly different. Two generalized action patterns (a, b and a', b') originate in component 1 and map automatically onto specific emotions (component 4) and modes of action readiness (component 7). Please note that these generalized action patterns bypass secondary appraisal (component 5) and goal setting (component 6). These fast processing, or "curtailed," goal paths will be discussed next. In Figure 3, several control processes are depicted. These slower processing paths draw heavily on interpretation processes and secondary appraisal, and pass through the goal setting and goal striving components.

A. CURTAILED GOAL PATHS

We have explained already that goals may become preconsciously activated, provided they have been encoded in a highly accessible knowledge structure. We speculate further that interactive episodic confrontations with specific learning situations in the past, for example with testlike situations, may result in data-driven computational units, capable of triggering a generalized response pattern. Bargh and Gollwitzer (1994) state, "It is assumed that the habitual serving of a goal within a given situation not only connects the goal with the situation but also those goal-directed behaviors that have been effective in satisfying the goal in the past" (p. 78). Such direct links are depicted in Figure 2 as connections between components 1 and 4 (identification process; paths a and b), leading to component 7 and feeding back to components 2 and 3 (generalized action pattern; paths a' and b'). Tim's identification of the quiz as a member of the class of threatening situations produced arousal that was labeled negatively, thus activating a network of knowledge structures that represents his preconceptions and vulnerabilities (situational meaning structure represented by component 4). Tim curtails the goal setting phase because he relies predominantly on a fast estimate of the personal significance of the learning episode in terms of well-being without considering mindfully what is required to deal with the situation and whether or not he can handle it under the present conditions. His primary appraisal maps onto goal striving, which is oriented to restore well-being. More specifically, Tim uses

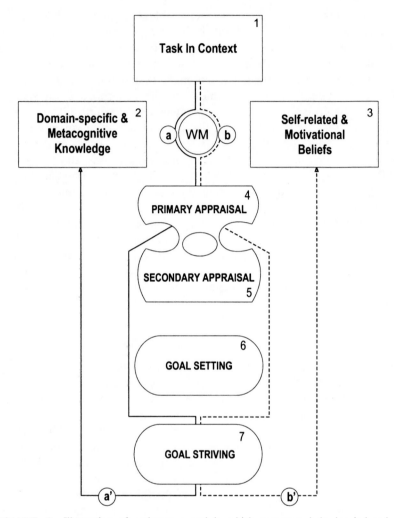

FIGURE 2   Illustration of pathways a and b, which represent behavior induced by situational identification (chronic goals). Please note that the origins of these goal processes are in box 1, leading to primary appraisal.

mental withdrawal or suppressed aggression (b') to control his own actions and bring them in line with his self-related and motivational beliefs (component 3). It is important to note that the other fast processing path, labeled a', feeds back to component 2. Activity in this fast path may be initiated, for example, when a teacher-set task triggers knowledge structures that are congruent with the students' learning goal and other available resources.

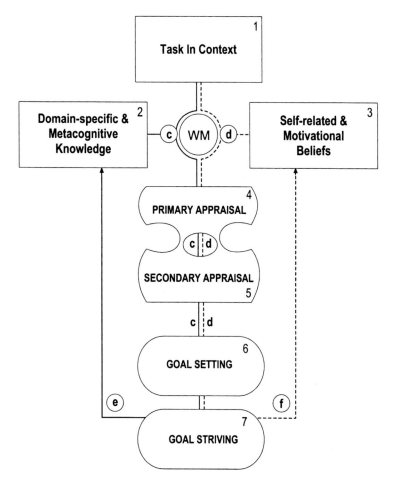

FIGURE 3 Illustration of pathways c, d, e, and f, which represent behavior induced by interpretation processes (intentionally induced goals). Please note that the origins of these goal processes are in boxes 1, 2, and 3, leading to secondary appraisal, goal setting, and goal striving. Goal setting is based on c, task-focused interpretation, and d, self-focused interpretation. Goal striving can move in two directions: e, problem-focused actions to continue or discontinue ongoing behavior to achieve gains (positive goals); f, emotion-focused actions to continue or discontinue ongoing behavior to prevent losses (negative goals).

As already described, some classroom behaviors may be initiated "mind-lessly" by the environmental cues or situational features. Even though such habitual or automatic processes play an important role in students' goal-directed activities, most learning situations require conscious control and deliberation. For a student to engage in action effectively, he or she must not have only an idea of what is needed to attain a goal, but also believe that he or she has access to the means needed and that the goal can be attained under the current conditions (see Skinner, 1995; Chapman, Skinner, and Baltes, 1990). The impact of such representations on further action is discussed next. At this point, we want to emphasize the crucial role of task-focused and self-focused interpretation processes in SRL.

B. GOAL SETTING BASED ON TASK-FOCUSED AND SELF-FOCUSED INTERPRETATION

Interpretation processes feed and influence upcoming and ongoing appraisal processes, thus affecting goal setting as well as goal striving. We differentiate between task-focused and self-focused interpretation. The former refers to the process of assigning meaning to a task (activity, situation, event) based on one's mental representation of the inherent properties of the task and one's metacognitive knowledge about it (component 2). Self-focused interpretation refers to the activation of one's current goals, ideal selves, and ought selves, and using this information to make a mental representation of the perceived valence, relevance, congruence, and control of a task and its context (component 3). We focus, first, on the effect of interpretation processes on goal setting, turning to goal striving in the next section.

Unlike Tim, who is inclined to identify test situations as "problematic" and approach them in a generic way, Bob and Lia's behavior is more situationally and momentarily dynamic. Their goal setting is represented in Figure 3 by several pathways, connecting components 1, 2, and 3 to primary appraisal (component 4), and then further to secondary appraisal (component 5). It is noteworthy that even though both Lia's and Bob's major goal is to do well, they use different interpretative frameworks to assign meaning to the quiz situation: Their goal structures are similar in some respects and different in others. For example, they share the higher-order goal "I want to do well at school." Lia wants to acquire understanding (action program) by using scripts, such as using elaborate strategies and asking the teacher for feedback. In contrast, Bob wants to perform well in tests (action program) by using scripts, such as avoiding help and be the first to hand in the test.

Tim's goal hierarchy, which is totally different, shows that goals can be treated as organizing structures of students' behavior. Knowledge of a student's goals can indeed help us understand how they perceive and approach a quiz (see Figure 4). However, goals are but one component in a student's situation construal. At this point, we want to add a layer of complexity and illustrate that the outcome of a student's interpretation process influences goal setting to a considerable extent. Recall that Lia is often so focused on a specific problem that she forgets to participate in routine classroom activities. She likes mathematics and does her work

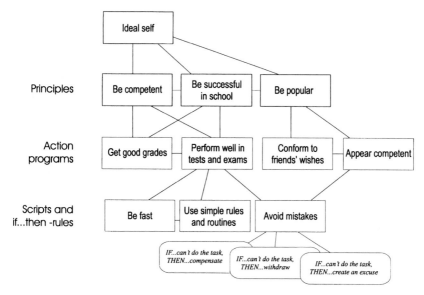

FIGURE 4 Bob's goal structure.

meticulously, often losing track of time. When faced with a mathematics problem, she usually is aware of the availability and accessibility of domain-specific knowledge and relevant scripts, and she also has a clear idea of the strategies that will and will not be effective (means–ends beliefs; metacognitive knowledge in component 2). She feels confident that she will know what to do and will not lose confidence in her problem-solving capacity (agency beliefs in component 3), even when faced with a difficult problem or with an interruption of her plan. Her usual approach is to orient herself to the problem mindfully, breaking it into parts and searching for available scripts. We have represented these content-based control processes in Figure 3 by a path that connects component 2 (domain-specific knowledge and metacognition) to secondary appraisal (component 5). Our position is that Lia's self-regulation process in the goal setting stage is primarily governed by task-focused interpretation (path c), which we consider to be an aspect of metacognitive control.

Let us now focus on Bob's interpretative framework in the goal setting stage. Two interesting aspects of his interpretation process need to be mentioned: First, teacher-set goals are not always congruent for him. Second, he explicitly judges his personal resources to do a task before he commits himself. Bob's self-regulation seems to originate in self-focused interpretation processes (path d). In relation to this particular learning episode, he perceives the goal as desirable, even though his feasibility judgment is biased by the possibility of failure. We postulate that Bob's self-regulation process in the goal setting stage is governed by self-focused interpretation as an important aspect of motivation control. In other words, his motivational beliefs (including his self-efficacy judgment, attributions, goal orientation, and attitudes) shape his goal setting.

In short, there are similarities and differences in these students' situation construals. For both Lia and Bob the situation is motivationally relevant (although for different reasons) and congruent (they both want to succeed). Also, the situation has positive valence for both of them: an opportunity to get feedback for Lia and an opportunity to demonstrate ability for Bob. The fundamental difference between Lia's and Bob's goal setting processes is captured in their expectancy pattern: Lia uses activated metacognitive knowledge to estimate the probability of success. She uses her own reference norms, which means that activity-related incentives guide her performance. In contrast, Bob uses social reference norms, thus focusing primarily on the consequences of his action. Our main message here is that even though Lia's and Bob's situation construals are based on a positive categorization of the learning situation (i.e., they are perceived as controllable), their secondary appraisal is different because it is fed by different interpretation processes. Lia's interpretation process is primarily based on the inputs from component 2, whereas Bob's interpretation process is essentially fueled by the contents of component 3.

There is abundant evidence that supports this view. The literature on goal orientation (Dweck, 1986, and Niemivirta, 1998, 1999) shows that learning-focused goals are associated with specific means–end beliefs and that performance goals are connected to ability-related beliefs. Also, there is accumulating evidence that instructional practices that force students to demonstrate ability (Nicholls, 1990), encourage the use of social reference norms (Rheinberg, 1989), or emphasize evaluation procedures (Boggiano et al., 1989) automatically increase self-focus, thus biasing the interpretation process. Rheinberg and his colleagues reported that students who are encouraged to estimate the probability of success on the basis of their own reference norms, rather than on the basis of social reference norms, are more likely to use activity-related incentives when they are confronted with a learning situation. Interestingly, they found that activity-related incentives decreased as a function of the value students attach to the consequences of an action. In light of this evidence, it is not surprising that most students do not find quizzes and exams motivating, mainly because these classroom episodes force them to focus on the consequences of their actions.

In conclusion, we adopt the view that SRL does not proceed in a linear way through the different phases of the model. Students may or may not become aware of certain dimensions of the unfolding learning episode and this awareness may prompt them to backtrack to a previous phase or to bypass components. Accordingly, we proposed that Tim used a shortcut, thus jumping several phases. Both Lia and Bob accessed the information in components 2 and 3 to make a mental representation of the learning goal and to orient themselves on the quiz. Lia's mental representation is the result of mindful activation of information in component 2 and reflection on it (metacognitive control), whereas Bob's mental representation is predominantly based on the contents of component 3: His main focus is on the actions that are necessary and sufficient to demonstrate ability (motivation control). Both these mental representations will be used in the postdecision stage to steer and direct their actions. These are discussed in the next section.

V. SELF-REGULATED LEARNING IMPLIES GOAL STRIVING

Let us now turn to goal striving. In the Action Phase Model, the postdecisional phase begins when the goal has been set. The student then shifts from the motivational to the volitional stage. Kuhl and Goschke (1994) illustrated that good intentions (component 6) do not necessarily lead to goal striving and goal attainment, even though they may have been strong in the predecisional stage. Some further planning is required. Also, the individual needs to reflect on his or her actions while performing them, and to maintain motivation and goal striving.

A. IMPLEMENTATION INTENTIONS

In the preaction phase, decisions concerning when, where, and how to get started are made. Gollwitzer (1993) referred to these decisions as implementation intentions: These decisions support goal intentions and set the stage for the transformation of a learning intention into a series of "self-set tasks," which require different metacognitive and motivation control processes. According to Gollwitzer (1996), implementation intentions not only help people to get started with their goal-directed actions, they also increase their commitment to goal intentions. It is important to note that involvement in creating an action plan and preparing for the execution of the successive steps induces a state of cognitive tuning that is different from the deliberate mindset of the predecisional phase. Gollwitzer's studies (1996) warrant this conclusion. He found that an "implementation mindset" facilitates a person's perceptual and behavioral readiness to take in goal-relevant information while simultaneously lowering the likelihood of attending to expectancy-value cues that are typical of the predecisional phase.

In other words, effective planning of an action involves the activity itself as well as the monitoring processes that are necessary to direct one's striving. It is beyond the scope of this chapter to discuss the problem-solving processes that are part and parcel of the planning process. Suffice it to say here that problem-solving theories primarily describe search processes, how individuals construct alternative problem-solving paths, and how they specify various subgoals. In the educational literature these processes are described under the general heading of metacognitive skills, which include identifying the problem, examining and comparing solutions, executing the action plan, and monitoring (cf. Pintrich, 2000, this volume).

Apart from searching for and generating relevant problem-solving plans, students should also be aware of the conditions that facilitate and restrict their learning in a specific domain. Indeed, SRL implies that students are mindful to situational cues that provide information on the conditions that surround the implementation path. Gollwitzer, Heckhausen, and Ratajczak (1990) asked students to name unresolved personal problems that needed to be handled (for example, continuing or changing one's major). They found that students who committed themselves to a specific implementation path progressed better in these personal projects than subjects who only considered alternative routes or imagined the positive consequences of fulfilling their wishes. Other researchers (Carver & Scheier, 1989; Gollwitzer 1996; Taylor & Gollwitzer, 1995) have shown that an implementation mindset supports goal commitment by bolstering self-confidence, control perceptions, and optimistic expectations concerning goal achievement.

B. DEALING WITH STRATEGY FAILURE

Up to now, we have kept the discussion relatively simple by pretending that our three students monitor the environment and their own performance in relation to a single goal (e.g., doing well on the test). We shift our attention now to multiple goals, focusing more explicitly on conflict between goals. Students may pursue different goals simultaneously, even though they are not always aware of it. Their ever-changing goal structure may be consciously perceived when they experience incoherence in their goal system. Boekaerts (1998a, 1998b) argued that students may experience a feeling of disconnection, incoherence, or a conflict between goals when they are asked to accomplish a goal that they find unappealing, uninteresting, too difficult or too easy, threatening, or boring. Likewise, incongruence or disconnection may be experienced when students' self-defined goals are thwarted or when they experience strategy failure. Incoherence in the goal striving phase, particularly in relation to strategy failure, calls for different forms of control.

Kuhl and Goschke (1994) described a number of control mechanisms that underlie goal striving, including attention and intention control, motivation and emotion control, action control, and volitional control.

Attention and intention control refer to the maintenance of an intention in terms of selectively activating supporting representations in the form of either selectively activating action-related knowledge or selectively processing intention-relevant external information. *Emotion and motivation control* refer to both the processes of inhibiting emotional states that may undermine the efficiency of current engagement and the processes of generating action-related emotions that increase the evaluative strength of an intention and the degree of initiative. *Action control* refers to the inhibition of counterintentional impulses. *Volitional control* refers to a set of functions that mediate both the maintenance of goals in the face of distractions or competing action tendencies and the disengagement from an intention.

Winne (1997; Winne & Perry, 2000) pointed out that adaptive self-regulatory processes are necessary to strike a balance between maintaining and shifting goals on the basis of a constant monitoring of the current situation with respect to prior reference values. He articulated how children detect and search for regularities in their intentions, behaviors, and corresponding outcomes. In the course of development, they acquire implicit rules, such as working carefully and diligently on a math task produces more correct answers. However, in novel situations where the strategy does not apply directly (e.g., when speed is rewarded more than accuracy), disengaging from the current strategy and implementing another strategy requires the enactment of effective forms of control.

Boekaerts (1998a) argued that students who have formed a learning intention need several forms of control to continue their striving, particularly when they encounter strategy failure. Strategy failure calls for a change of strategy, for a coping response, a reconsideration of the goal, and for a decision concerning whether more or less effort is in order. This conceptualization of goal striving implies that there are multiple pathways along which self-regulation in this stage of the learning episode materializes. Boekaerts differentiated between five basic ways to react to strategy failure, namely, (1) mindful effort, (2) disengagement, (3) danger control, (4) self-handicapping, and (5) avoidant behavior. Students who engage in mindful effort differ in important ways from those who use other forms of control. First, they are likely to label an increase in the level of arousal in terms of goal-congruent emotions (e.g., surprise that the strategy does not work, curiosity, challenge and anticipated pleasure, or pride). In other words, perception of increased arousal is viewed as a signal that close monitoring is in order, rather than as a danger signal. This positive interpretation (task-focused reinterpretation) results in an increased rate of task-relevant (meta) cognitions, including reflections on the source of difficulty and the amount of effort needed to solve the problem (path e). The outcome of this reflection process is the decision to continue with the current scripts and pay more attention, or to decide that alternative scripts should be selected from the action hierarchy because the ones that had been selected before cannot do the job. When these students consider it meaningful to invest resources, they will continue striving, investing effort to adapt the action plan so that it will fit the local conditions better (see Figure 3, path e).

Imagine that Lia encounters strategy failure and cannot retrieve an adequate solution strategy, despite her feeling of knowing. She may then feel an urge to move on to the next problem so as not to lose too much time. However, her feeling of knowing may force her to concentrate better on the task. She may heuristically try different alternatives to help her retrieve knowledge more effectively. It is important to note, however, that this sort of redirected and intensified engagement is likely to occur only through supportive secondary appraisals, meaning that the outcome of the secondary appraisal process should be that the task is difficult but still solvable. Boekaerts, Seegers, and Vermeer (1995) found that primary school students who feel confident that they know how to solve a problem in the goal setting stage deal swiftly with an interruption of a concrete action plan in the action stage. These students treat the noted imbalance and the concomitant increase in the level of arousal as a signal that close monitoring is in order or that a change of plan should be contemplated. Girls experienced more imbalance in the goal setting stage than boys did, even when controlled for their competence level. No differences were noted in the goal striving phase. Efklides, Samara, and Petropoulou (1997) provided evidence that the feeling of difficulty that students may report before, during, and after doing a mathematics problem refers to a complex experience that becomes progressively differentiated during the problem-solving process.

It is interesting to note that students also may opt to disengage temporarily from the behavior that caused the disturbance. Researchers and teachers should differentiate between students who disengage from a task on rational grounds and those who avoid the task on emotional grounds. Students who have access to metacognitive knowledge that helps them to represent strategy failure mentally may realize what it takes to overcome the perceived difficulties (cf. Winne, 1997), yet they may consider the current conditions suboptimal and judge it better to postpone effort investment until later. In other words, disengagement is a form of volitional control (path e) that should be separated from various forms of emotion control (path f) that may look similar to the untrained observer.

C. CURTAILED GOAL STRIVING SHOULD NOT BE EQUATED WITH FAILURE OF SELF-REGULATION

It is important to note that students who lack the metacognitive knowledge and skills to interpret strategy failure may find it difficult to determine which forms of control are needed to protect the self from esteem-threatening situations. When faced with a difficult problem or with an obstacle during the implementation process, the possibility of losing face may surface and cause a switch in a student's goal structure. The student may then concern himself or herself with the question, "Can I do something to prevent loss of face?" Rather than spend time to find out what the source of the difficulty is (metacognitive control or problem-focused actions), students may opt to attempt to protect their egos (emotion control or emotion-focused actions), because they have lost confidence in their problem-solving capacity (agency beliefs in component 3). Many studies stemming from the literature on goal orientation (Dweck, 1986; Nicholls, 1990; Niemivirta, 1998, 1999), coping with stress (Boekaerts, 1998a; Compas, Malcarne, & Fondacaro, 1988), and learned helplessness (Seligman, 1975) support this view.

Jones and Berglas (1978) and Covington (1992) described a form of emotion control that is characterized by deliberate attempts to withhold effort and even put obstacles in one's own performance path. This self-handicapping strategy is considered to be maladaptive by most teachers. It refers to individuals' attempts to strategically control their attributions to save face by externalizing the source of possible failure. Deliberately withdrawing effort during a test or attending a party the night before an exam are illustrations of self-handicapping. Tim's behavior is an attempt to provide an acceptable explanation for potential failure at the onset of the quiz. From his vantage point, the criteria for a successful course of action are not based on the actual task outcomes, but on his success in dealing with the disturbance itself. Once he believes that the teacher will attribute his low performance to his headache rather than to low capacity, he feels safe and can discharge tension (see Figure 4).

Interestingly, most teachers and parents praise increased effort in reaction to strategy failure or any other interruption of plan. As a result, many students display increased quantitative effort after strategy failure, reflected in working faster, producing more material, increasing the number of responses, repeating answers randomly, and blind substitution of scripts. There is abundant evidence in the literature on mathematical problem solving that describes such mindless or undirected effort (Lester, Garofalo, & Krole, 1989). Leventhal (1980) labeled this coping strategy "danger control," explaining that individuals who are inclined to focus on the changed demand–capacity ratio tend to restore the noted imbalance by increasing rather than decreasing effort. Their focus is on reallocating resources to control the danger (protecting their ego) rather than on the activity itself. Importantly, this form of control (emotion control; path f) produces rumination, which interferes with the learning process itself and may lead to an increase rather than a decrease in the level of anxiety. It is easy to imagine that Bob may use different types of coping strategies when he is confronted with an interruption of plan. He may adopt a danger control strategy when he feels the need to prevent negative outcomes from occurring. Also, when Bob realizes that he cannot find a solution fast, the task may no longer be congruent with his major goal to be the first to hand in the quiz sheet. Because Bob believes that quick performance is a sign of competence, he may monitor his progress and his rate of progress simultaneously (cf. Carver & Scheier, 1990). The mere observation that some of his classmates have finished the quiz would trigger negative affect and emotion control.

Leventhal contrasted danger control with anxiety control, which has the potential to reduce anxiety, simply because the source of stress is ignored, avoided, or attenuated. Avoidant behavior occurs when students no longer perceive a link between their action and the outcome of their actions. They may then give up on the activity or task and turn their attention to other activities, thus communicating to teacher and peers that they do not even care about the negative outcomes. None of the students in our quiz example demonstrated this behavior. However, all students may be inclined to avoid some activities.

Similar to what has been described in relation to goal setting, we propose that goal striving does not proceed in a linear fashion: Awareness of different dimensions of the unfolding learning episode may initiate different forms of monitoring and control. It is important to realize, though, that some forms of control are considered maladaptive forms of engagement by the teacher. However, from the perspective of the student, each form of control may be highly adaptive because it serves different functions, such as selective perception of external and internal information, inhibiting emotional states, increasing or decreasing the evaluative strength of an intention, and protecting one's self-esteem and well-being.

In conclusion, we adopt the view that SRL does not proceed in a linear way through the different phases of the model. Students may or may not become aware that their goal striving is not in accordance with their goal setting. Those who closely monitor the unfolding learning episode may backtrack several times to a previous phase, meaning that the mental representations they formed in the preactional phase are used in the postdecisional phase to steer and direct their actions. For example, students who formulate the intention to invest effort in a task, yet decide to disengage from the task later because it is too easy (or not personally relevant) or because they do not have access to the necessary recources (path e, in Figure 3) are mastery oriented. Their mental representation in the preaction stage is congruent with their actions in the postdecisional phase. In contrast, students who started mindfully and diligently on a task, but later deliberately withhold effort to feel safe (self-handicapping) or use danger control (path f in Figure 3) are switching from the mastery to the ego-protective mode. These students experience difficulty in finding a balance between learning and ego-protective goals. Much more research is needed to document this nonlinear process.

VI. CONCLUSIONS AND FUTURE DIRECTIONS

In this chapter, we defended the view that for effective self-regulation to develop, students should be allowed to work in a learning context in which they can create their own learning episodes according to their own goals. We argued that identification, interpretation, and appraisal processes are the gateways to self-regulation. In light of present conceptualizations of goal processes, the model of adaptable learning was extended to include an identification process, two interpretation processes (task-focused interpretation and self-focused interpretation), and primary and secondary appraisal processes. We focused on the hypothetical relationships between these five key processes of a student's interpretative framework and theorized how these processes may affect goal setting and goal striving. We also pointed to different levels of awareness and differentiated between different forms of control that interact while the learning process is unfolding over time.

A central message throughout this chapter is that SRL is not a unitary construct. Rather, it has been presented as a generic term used for a number of phenomena, each of which is captured by a different control system. In our judgment, self-regulation is a system concept that refers to the overall management of one's behavior through interactive processes between these different control systems (attention, metacognition, motivation, emotion, action, and volition control). We adopted the view that no single control system is appropriate to explain all the phenomena of control that are at work in SRL. In the past decade, researchers involved in educational research have concentrated mainly on activity in one control system—the metacognitive control system—thus ignoring the interplay between the metacognitive control system and other control systems. However, it is evident that the different control systems share information and processing capacity with the metacognitive control system and that resources may flow freely from one control systems to another.

In our opinion, three issues should be addressed in future research on SRL. First, we need to know in what ways students who are capable of regulating their learning efficiently differ from those who are less efficient. More specifically, we need to know how they integrate information stemming from the interconnected control systems. Researchers should go beyond the mere description of activity in control systems, specifying the properties that emerge from the interaction of these control systems. Only through the investigation of these mutual influences will new properties of the system, as a whole, be revealed.

Second, it follows from the adoption of SRL as a system construct that single feedback loop systems are insufficient to explain SRL. Multiple feedback systems provide information about the learning activity that is going on. We need to know how these interacting feedback loops operate and how students learn to integrate this information and act upon it. Carver and Scheier described positive and negative feedback loops that are part of the self-regulation process. Positive feedback loops lead to change, growth, and development, whereas negative feedback loops provide information about discrepancies between desirable states (a standard of performance) and the present state. This information allows the individual to keep activity in a control system within reasonable bounds. It is important that researchers pay attention to the feedback loops that operate within each control system. They should seek further insight into the way students plan an activity, monitor that activity, and use feedback to modify the activity. However, they also should examine how feedback processes operate between control systems. This will help them to understand how different forms of control are achieved and how the interacting processes are coordinated (overall self-regulation). A good starting point for the study of these multiple feedback loops is Powers's (1973) goal hierarchy. He views the goals for a given unit in his model as the output of higher-order units, thus positioning feedback loops within the configuration of hierarchically arranged loops (see Vancouver, 2000, this volume, and also Figure 4).

Third, future research should address the dynamics of the interacting control systems that affect each student's learning process as well as his or her relationship with significant others. If students are not aware that their attempts at self-regulation are situated within a social context with changing personal and social goals, they may never learn to regulate their learning in an optimal way. Very little is known about the nature of conflicting goal processes in a classroom context. Boekaerts (1998a) addressed this issue and raised a number of questions. She argued that students are also part of larger groups, such as families, peer groups, communities of learners, school, and youth cultures. When students interact in the context of these larger groups, they influence each other, leading to changes in the functioning and interaction of the different control systems. As such, the study of self-regulated learning should also involve the effect of social forces (social control) on the individual's learning.

REFERENCES

Austin, J. T., & Vancouver, J. B. (1996). Goal constructs in psychology: Structure, process, and content. *Psychological Bulletin, 120*, 338–375.

Bandura, A. (1993). Perceived self-efficacy in cognitive development and functioning. *Educational Psychologist, 28*, 117–148.

Bargh, J. A. (1990). Auto-motives. Preconcious determinants of social interaction. In E. T. Higgins & R. M. Sorrentino (Eds.), *Handbook of motivation and cognition. Foundations of social behavior* (pp. 93–103). New York: Guilford.

Bargh, J. A., & Barndollar, K. (1996). Automaticity in action: The unconscious as repository of chronic goals and motives. In P. M. Gollwitzer & J. A. Bargh (Eds.), *The psychology of action: Linking cognition and motivation to behavior* (pp. 457–481). New York: Guilford.

Bargh, J. A., & Gollwitzer, P. M. (1994). Environmental control of goal-directed action: Automatic and strategic contingencies between situations and behavior. In W. Spaulding (Ed.), *Nebraska Symposium on Motivation. Integrative views of motivation, cognition, and emotion, 41* (pp. 71–124). Lincoln: University of Nebraska Press.

Boekaerts, M. (1987). Die Effekte von state- und trait-motivationaler Orientierung auf das Lernergebnis [Effects of state and trait motivational orientation on learning outcome]. *Zeitschrift für Pädagogische Psychologie, 1*, 29–43.

Boekaerts, M. (1992). The adaptable learning process: Initiating and maintaining behavioural change. *Journal of Applied Psychology: An International Review, 41*, 377–397.

Boekaerts, M. (1996a). Personality and the psychology of learning. *European Journal of Personality, 10*, 377–404.

Boekaerts, M. (1996b). Coping with stress in childhood and adolescence. In M. Zeidner & N. S. Endler (Eds.), *Handbook of coping. Theories, research, applications* (pp. 452–484). New York: Wiley.

Boekaerts, M. (1998a). Coping in context: Goal frustration and goal ambivalence in relation to academic and interpersonal goals. In E. Frydenberg (Ed.), *Learning to cope: Developing as a person in complex societies* (pp. 175–197). Oxford, UK: Oxford University Press.

Boekaerts, M. (1998b). Boosting students' capacity to promote their own learning: A goal theory perspective. *Research Dialogue, 1*(1), 13–22.

Boekaerts, M. (1999). Motivated learning: The study of student * situation transactional units. *European Journal of Psychology of Education, 14*(4), 41–55.

Boekaerts, M., Seegers, G., & Vermeer, H. (1995). Solving math problems: Where and why does the solution process go astray? *Educational Studies in Mathematics, 4*, 1–23.

Boggiano, A. K., Main, D. S., Flink, C., Barrett, M., Silvern, L., & Katz, P. A. (1989). A model of achievement in children: The role of controlling strategies in helplessness and affect. In R. Schwarzer, H. M. van der Ploeg, & C. D. Spielberger (Eds.), *Advances in test anxiety research* (pp. 13–26). Amsterdam: Swets & Zeitlinger.

Carver, C. S., & Scheier, M. F. (1989). Expectancies and coping: From test anxiety to pessimism. In R. Schwarzer, H. M. van der Ploeg, & C. D. Spielberger (Eds.), *Advances in test anxiety research* (pp. 3–11). Amsterdam: Swets & Zeitlinger.

Carver, C. S., & Scheier, M. F. (1990). Origins and functions of positive and negative affect: A control-process view. *Psychological Review, 90*, 19–35.

Carver, C. S., & Scheier, M. (2000). On the structure of behavioral self-regulation. In M. Boekaerts, P. R. Pintrich, & M. Zeidner (Eds.), *Handbook of self-regulation* (Chap. 3) San Diego, CA: Academic Press. (This volume)

Chapman, M., Skinner, E. A., & Baltes, P. B. (1990). Interpreting correlations between children's perceived control and cognitive performances: Control, agency, or means-ends beliefs? *Developmental Psychology, 26*, 246–253.

Compas, B. E., Malcarne, V. L., & Fondacaro, K. (1988). Coping with stressful events in older children and young adolescents. *Journal of Consulting and Clinical Psychology, 56*, 405–411.

Covington, M. V. (1992). *Making the grade. A self-worth perspective on motivation and school reform.* Cambridge, UK: Cambridge University Press.

Deci, E. L., & Ryan, R. M. (1985). *Intrinsic motivation and self-determination in human behavior.* New York: Plenum.

Diener, C. I., & Dweck, C. S. (1978). An analysis of learned helplessness: Continuous changes in performance, strategy and achievement cognitions following failure. *Journal of Personality and Social Psychology, 36*, 451–462.

Dweck, C. S. (1986). Motivational processes affecting learning. *American Psychologist, 41*, 1040–1048.

Efklides, A., Samara, A., & Petropoulou, M. (1997). *Feeling of difficulty: At the junction of monitoring and control.* Paper presented at the 7th European Conference for Research on Learning and Instruction, Athens, Greece.

Fodor, J. A. (1985). Précis of "the modularity of mind." *The Behavioral and Brain Sciences, 8,* 1–15.

Ford, M. E. (1995). Intelligence and personality in social behavior. In D. H. Saklofske & M. Zeidner (Eds.), *International handbook of personality and intelligence* (pp. 125–142). New York: Plenum.

Forgas, J. P. (1982). Episode cognition: Internal representation of interaction routines. In L. Berkowitz (Ed.), *Advances in experimental social psychology* (pp. 59–101). New York: Academic Press.

Forgas, J. P. (1985). Cognitive representations of interaction episodes and social skill. In G. D'Ydewalle (Ed.), *Cognition, information processing, and motivation* (pp. 321–344). Amsterdam: North-Holland.

Frijda, N. H. (1986). *The emotions.* Cambridge, UK: Cambridge University Press.

Frijda, N. H. (1988). The laws of emotion. *American Psychologist, 43,* 349–358.

Gollwitzer, P. M. (1990). Action phases and mind-sets. In E. T. Higgins & R. M. Sorrentino (Eds.), *Handbook of motivation and cognition: Foundations of social behavior* (pp. 52–92). New York: Guilford.

Gollwitzer, P. M. (1993). Goal achievement: The role of intentions. In W. Stroebe & M. Hewstone (Eds.), *European review of social psychology* (pp. 141–185). Chichester, UK: Wiley.

Gollwitzer, P. M. (1996). The volitional benefits of planning. In P. M. Gollwitzer & J. A. Bargh (Eds.), *The psychology of action: Linking cognition and motivation to behavior* (pp. 287–312). New York: Guilford.

Gollwitzer, P. M., Heckhausen, H., & Ratajczak, H. (1990). From weighing to willing: Approaching a change decision through pre- or postdecisional mentation. *Organizational Behavior and Human Decision Processes, 45,* 41–65.

Heckhausen, H., & Gollwitzer, P. M. (1987). Thoughts contents and cognitive functioning in motivational versus volitional stages of mind. *Motivation and Emotion, 11,* 101–120.

Higgins, E. T. (1987). Self-discrepancy: A theory relating self and affect. *Psychological Review, 94,* 319–340.

Higgins, E. T. (1990). Personality, social psychology, and person-situation relations: Standards, and knowledge activation as a common language. In L. A. Pervin (Ed.), *Handbook of personality: Theory and research.* New York: Guilford.

Higgins, E. T., Strauman, T., & Klein, R. (1986). Standards and the process of self-evaluation: Multiple affects from multiple stages. In E. T. Higgins & R. M. Sorrentino (Eds.), *Handbook of motivation and cognition: Foundations of social behavior* (pp. 229–264). New York: Guilford.

Jagacinski, C. M. (1992). The effects of task involvement and ego involvement on achievement-related cognitions and behaviors. In D. H. Schunk & J. L. Meece (Eds.), *Student's perceptions in the classroom: Causes and consequences.* Hillsdale, NJ: Erlbaum.

Jones, E. E., & Berglas, S. (1978). Control of attributions about the self through self-handicapping strategies: The appeal of alcohol and the role of underachievement. *Personality and Social Psychology Bulletin, 4,* 200–206.

Kruglanski, A. W. (1996). Goals as knowledge structures. In P. M. Gollwitzer & J. A. Bargh (Eds.), *The psychology of action: Linking cognition and motivation to behavior.* New York: Guilford.

Kuhl, J. (1984). Volitional aspects of achievement motivation and learned helplessness: Toward a comprehensive theory of action control. In B. A. Maher & W. B. Maher (Eds.), *Progress in experimental personality research* (pp. 99–171). New York: Academic Press.

Kuhl, J., & Beckmann, J. (1994). *Volition and personality: Action versus state orientation.* Göttingen, Germany: Hogrefe & Huber.

Kuhl, J., & Goschke, T. (1994). A theory of action control: Mental subsystems, models of control, and volitional conflict-resolution strategies. In J. Kuhl & J. Beckmann (Eds.), *Volition and personality: Action versus state orientation.* Göttingen, Germany: Hogrefe & Huber.

Lazarus, R. S., & Folkman, S. (1984). *Stress, appraisal and coping.* New York: Springer-Verlag.

Lazarus, R. S., & Smith, C. A. (1988). Knowledge and appraisal in the cognition–emotion relationship. *Cognition and Emotion, 2,* 281–300.

Lester, F. K., Garofalo, J., & Krole, D. L. (1989). Self-confidence, interest, beliefs, and metacognition: Key influences on problem-solving behavior. In D. B. McLeod & V. M. Adams (Eds.), *Affect and mathematical problem-solving* (pp. 75–88). New York: Springer-Verlag.

Leventhal, H. (1980). Toward a comprehensive theory of emotion. In L. Berkowitz (Ed.), *Advances in experimental social psychology* (pp. 140–208). New York: Academic Press.

Lewin, K., Dembo, T., Festinger, L. A., & Sears, P. S. (1944). Level of aspiration. In M. J. Hunt (Ed.), *Personality and the behavior disorders* (pp. 333–379). New York: Ronald Press.

Locke, E. A., & Latham, G. P. (1990). *A theory of goal setting and task performance.* Englewood Cliffs, NJ: Prentice-Hall.

Mandler, G. (1984). *Mind and body: Psychology of emotion and stress.* New York: Norton.

Markus, H., & Nurius, P. (1986). Possible selves. *American Psychologist, 41,* 954–969.

Neuman, O. (1984). Automatic processing: A review of recent findings and a plan for an old theory. In W. Printz & A. Sanders (Eds.), *Cognition and motor processes.* Berlin: Springer-Verlag.

Nicholls, J. G. (1990). What ability and why are we mindful of it? A developmental perspective. In R. J. Sternberg & J. Kolligan, Jr. (Eds.), *Competence considered* (pp. 11–40). New Haven, CT: Yale University Press.

Niemivirta, M. (1998). Individual differences in motivational and cognitive factors affecting self-regulated learning—A pattern-oriented approach. In P. Nenniger, R. S. Jäger, A. Frey, & M. Wosnitza (Eds.), *Advances in motivation* (pp. 23–42). Landau, Germany: Verlag Empirische Pädagogik.

Niemivirta, M. (1999). Motivational and cognitive predictors of goal setting and task performance. *International Journal of Educational Research, 31.*

Pintrich, P. R. (2000). The role of goal orientation in self-regulated learning. In M. Boekaerts, P. R. Pintrich, & M. Zeidner (Eds.), *Handbook of self-regulation* (Chap. 14). San Diego, CA: Academic Press. (This volume)

Pintrich, P. R., Marx, R. W., & Boyle, R. A. (1993). Beyond cold conceptual change: The role of motivational beliefs and classroom contextual factors in the process of conceptual change. *Review of Educational Research, 63,* 167–199.

Powers, W. T. (1973). *Behavior: The control of perception.* Chicago: Aldine.

Rheinberg, F. (1989). *Zweck und Tätigkeit* [Purpose and action]. Göttingen, Germany: Hogrefe.

Rheinberg, F., Vollmeyer, R., & Rollett, W. (1999). Motivation and action in self-regulated learning. In M. Boekaerts, P. R. Pintrich, & M. Zeidner (Eds.), *Handbook of self-regulation* (Chap. 15). San Diego, CA: Academic Press. (This volume)

Schachter, S., & Singer, J. E. (1962). Cognitive, social and psychological determinants of emotional state. *Psychological Review, 69,* 379–399.

Seligman, M. E. P. (1975). *Helplessness: On depression development and death.* San Francisco: Freeman.

Skinner, E. A. (1995). *Perceived control, motivation, and coping.* Thousand Oaks, CA: Sage.

Smith, C. A., & Lazarus, R. S. (1993). Appraisal components, core relational themes, and the emotions. *Cognition and Emotion, 7,* 233–269.

Taylor, S. E., & Gollwitzer, P. M. (1995). The effects of mind-sets on positive illusions. *Journal of Personality and Social Psychology, 69,* 213–226.

Trope, Y. (1986). Identification and inferential processes in dispositional attribution. *Psychological Review, 93,* 239–257.

Vallacher, R. R., & Wegner, D. M. (1987). What do people think they're doing? Action identification and human behavior. *Psychological Review, 94,* 3–15.

Vancouver, J. B. (2000). Self-regulation in organizational settings: A tale of two paradigms. In M. Boekaerts, P. R. Pintrich, & M. Zeidner (Eds.), *Handbook of self-regulation* (Chap. 10). San Diego, CA: Academic Press. (This volume)

Wenzel, K. R. (1994). Relations of social group pursuit to social acceptance, classroom, behavior, and perceived social support. *Journal of Educational Psychology, 86,* 173–182.

Wilson, P. T., & Anderson, R. C. (1986). What they don't know will hurt them: The role of prior knowledge in comprehension. In J. Orasanu (Ed.), *Reading comprehension: From research to practice.* Hillsdale, NJ: Erlbaum.

Winne, P. H. (1997). Experimenting to bootstrap self-regulated learning. *Journal of Educational Psychology, 89,* 1–14.

Winne, P. H., & Perry, N. E. (2000). Measuring self-regulated learning. In M. Boekaerts, P. R. Pintrich, & M. Zeidner (Eds.), *Handbook of self-regulation* (Chap. 16). San Diego, CA: Academic Press. (This volume)

Zajonc, R. B. (1980). Feeling and thinking: Preference need no inference. *American Psychologist, 35,* 151–175.

Zimmerman, B. J., & Schunk, D. H. (1989). *Self-regulated learning and academic achievement: Theory, research, and practice.* New York: Springer-Verlag.

14

THE ROLE OF GOAL
ORIENTATION IN
SELF-REGULATED
LEARNING

PAUL R. PINTRICH

The University of Michigan, Ann Arbor, Michigan

Self-regulated learning concerns the application of general models of regulation and self-regulation to issues of learning, in particular, academic learning that takes places in school or classroom contexts. There are a number of different models of self-regulated learning that propose different constructs and different conceptualizations (e.g., Boekaerts & Niemivirta, 2000, this volume; Butler & Winne, 1995; Corno, 1993; Pintrich & De Groot, 1990; Pintrich, Wolters, & Baxter, in press; Pressley, 1986; Schunk, 1994; Schunk & Zimmerman 1994; Winne, 1995; Zimmerman, 1986; 1989; 1990; 1998a, 1998b, 2000, this volume), but all of these models share some general assumptions and features. One purpose of this chapter is to discuss some of the common features of these models to provide a synthetic overview and general framework for theory and research in self-regulated learning.

At the same time, a number of different motivational constructs have been linked to the processes of self-regulation (Pintrich, Marx, & Boyle, 1993; Pintrich & Schrauben, 1992) and there is a need for models of self-regulated learning that include both motivational and cognitive processes. Accordingly, a second purpose of this chapter involves a discussion of how motivational constructs, specifically goal orientation, may be related to processes of self-regulated learning. To accomplish these two

Copyright © 2000 by Academic Press.
All rights of reproduction in any form reserved.

general goals, a general framework for self-regulated learning is discussed first, followed by a summary of different goal orientations and how they may be linked to the different components of self-regulated learning. As part of this discussion of goal orientations, a taxonomy of goal orientations is presented to help organize the research. Given the nature of this handbook and space constraints for all the chapters, these two sections are not intended to be comprehensive reviews of all the extant research on self-regulated learning and goal orientation, but rather an integrative review with citations to illustrative research. This chapter concludes with some suggestions for future theory and research.

I. A GENERAL FRAMEWORK FOR SELF-REGULATED LEARNING

There are many different models of self-regulated learning that propose different constructs and mechanisms, but they do share some basic assumptions about learning and regulation. One common assumption might be called the *active, constructive assumption*, which follows from a general cognitive perspective. That is, all the models view learners as active, constructive participants in the learning process. Learners are assumed to actively construct their own meanings, goals, and strategies from the information available in the external environment as well as information in their own minds (the internal environment). Learners are not just passive recipients of information from teachers, parents, or other adults, but rather active, constructive meaning makers as they go about learning.

A second, but related, assumption is the *potential for control assumption*. All the models assume that learners can potentially monitor, control, and regulate certain aspects of their own cognition, motivation, and behavior as well as some features of their environments. This assumption does not mean that individuals will or can monitor and control their cognition, motivation, or behavior at all times or in all contexts; rather, just that some monitoring, control, and regulation is possible. All of the models recognize that there are biological, developmental, contextual, and individual difference constraints that can impede or interfere with individual efforts at regulation.

A third general assumption that is made in these models of self-regulated learning, as in all general models of regulation stretching back to Miller, Galanter, & Pribram (1960), is the *goal, criterion, or standard assumption*. All models of regulation assume that there is some type of criterion or standard (also called goals or reference value) against which comparisons are made in order to assess whether the process should continue as is or if some type of change is necessary. The commonsense example is the thermostat operation for the heating and cooling of a house. Once a desired temperature is set (the goal, criterion, standard), the thermostat monitors the temperature of the house (monitoring process) and then turns the heating or air conditioning units (control and regulation processes) on or off to reach and maintain the standard. In a parallel manner, the general example for learning assumes that individuals can set standards or goals to strive for in their learning, monitor their progress toward these goals, and then adapt and regulate their cognition, motivation, and behavior to reach their goals.

A fourth general assumption of most of the models of self-regulated learning is that self-regulatory activities are *mediators* between personal and contextual characteristics and actual achievement or performance. That is, it is not just individuals' cultural, demographic, or personality characteristics that influence achievement and learning directly, or just the contextual characteristics of the classroom environment that shape achievement, but the individuals' self-regulation of their cognition, motivation, and behavior that mediate the relationships between the person, context, and eventual achievement. Most models of self-regulation assume that self-regulatory activities are directly linked to outcomes such as achievement and performance, although much of the research examines self-regulatory activities as outcomes in their own right.

Given these assumptions, a general working definition of self-regulated learning is that it is an active, constructive process whereby learners set goals for their learning and then attempt to monitor, regulate, and control their cognition, motivation, and behavior, guided and constrained by their goals and the contextual features in the environment. These self-regulatory activities can mediate the relationships between individuals and the context, and their overall achievement. This definition is similar to other models of self-regulated learning (e.g., Butler & Winne, 1995; Zimmerman, 1989, 1998a, 1998b, 2000). Although this definition is relatively simple, the remainder of this section outlines in more detail the various processes and areas of regulation, and their application to learning and achievement in the academic domain that reveals the complexity and diversity of the processes of self-regulated learning.

Table 1 displays a framework for classifying the different phases and areas for regulation. The four phases that make up the rows of the table are processes that many models of regulation and self-regulation share (e.g., Zimmerman, 1998a, 1998b; 2000) and they reflect goal-setting, monitoring, and control and regulation processes. Of course, not all academic learning follows these phases, because there are many occasions for students to learn academic material in more tacit or implicit or unintentional ways without self-regulating their learning in such an explicit manner as suggested in the model. These phases are suggested as a heuristic to

TABLE 1 Phases and Areas for Self-Regulated Learning

Phases	Areas for regulation			
	Cognition	Motivation/affect	Behavior	Context
1. Forethought, planning, and activation	Target goal setting	Goal orientation adoption	[Time and effort planning]	[Perceptions of task]
	Prior content knowledge activation	Efficacy judgments	[Planning for self-observations of behavior]	[Perceptions of context]
	Metacognitive knowledge activation	Ease of learning judgements (EOLs); perceptions of task difficulty		
		Task value activation		
		Interest activation		
2. Monitoring	Metacognitive awareness and monitoring of cognition (FOKs, JOLs)	Awareness and monitoring of motivation and affect	Awareness and monitoring of effort, time use, need for help	Monitoring changing task and context conditions
			Self-observation of behavior	
3. Control	Selection and adaptation of cognitive strategies for learning, thinking	Selection and adaptation of strategies for managing motivation and affect	Increase/decrease effort	Change or renegotiate task
			Persist, give up	Change or leave context
			Help-seeking behavior	
4. Reaction and reflection	Cognitive judgments	Affective reactions	Choice behavior	Evaluation of task
	Attributions	Attributions		Evaluation of context

organize our thinking and research on self-regulated learning. Phase 1 involves planning and goal setting as well as activation of perceptions and knowledge of the task and context and the self in relationship to the task. Phase 2 concerns various monitoring processes that represent metacognitive awareness of different aspects of the self or task and context. Phase 3 involves efforts to control and regulate different aspects of the self or task and context. Finally, Phase 4 represents various kinds of reactions and reflections on the self and the task or context.

The four phases do represent a general time-ordered sequence that individuals would go through as they perform a task, but there is no strong assumption that the phases are hierarchically or linearly structured such that earlier phases always must occur before later phases. In most models of self-regulated learning, monitoring, control, and reaction can be ongoing simultaneously and dynamically as the individual progresses through the task, with the goals and plans being changed or updated based on the feedback from the monitoring, control, and reaction processes. In fact, Pintrich et al. (in press) suggest that much of the empirical work on monitoring (phase 2) and control/regulation (phase 3) does not find much separation of these processes in terms of people's experiences as revealed by data from self-report questionnaires or think-aloud protocols.

The four columns in Table 1 represent different areas for regulation that an individual learner (the personal self) can attempt to monitor, control, and regulate. The first three columns of cognition, motivation/affect, and behavior reflect the traditional tripartite division of different areas of psychological functioning (Snow, Corno, & Jackson, 1996). As Snow et al. (1996) noted, the boundaries between these areas may be fuzzy, but there is utility in discussing them separately, particularly because much of traditional psychological research has focused on the different areas in isolation from the others. These first three areas in the columns in Table 1 represent aspects of the individual's own cognition, motivation/affect, and behavior that he or she can attempt to control and regulate. These attempts to control or regulate are "self-regulated" in that the individual (the personal self) is focused on trying to control or regulate his or her own cognition, motivation, and behavior. Of course, other individuals in the environment such as teachers, peers, or parents can try to "other" regulate an individual's cognition, motivation, or behavior as well, by directing or scaffolding the individual in terms of what, how, and when to do a task. More generally, other task and contextual features (e.g., task characteristics, feedback systems, evaluation structures) can facilitate or constrain an individual's attempts to self-regulate his or her learning.

The cognitive column in Table 1 concerns the different cognitive strategies individuals may use to learn and perform a task as well as the metacognitive strategies individuals may use to control and regulate their cognition. In addition, both content knowledge and strategic knowledge are included in the cognitive column. The motivation and affect column concerns the various motivational beliefs that individuals may have about themselves in relation to the task such as self-efficacy beliefs and values for the task. In addition, interest or liking of the task would be included in this column as well as positive and negative affective reactions to the self or task. Finally, any strategies that individuals may use to control and regulate their motivation and affect would be included in this column. The behavior column reflects the general effort the individual may exert on the task as well as persistence, help seeking, and choice behaviors.

The fourth column in Table 1, context, represents various aspects of the task environment or general classroom or cultural context where the learning is taking place. Given that this column concerns the external environment, attempts to control or regulate it would not be considered self-regulating in some models because the context is not assumed to be part of the individual. In these models, self-regulation usually refers only to aspects of the self that are being controlled or regulated. On the other hand, individuals do try to monitor and control their environment to some extent and, in fact, in some models of intelligence (e.g., Sternberg, 1985) attempts to selectively control and change the context are seen as very adaptable. In the same manner, in this model, it is assumed that individual attempts to monitor and control the environment are an important aspect of self-regulated learning, because the self or person tries to actively monitor and regulate the context. It is the self or person who is acting on the context and attempting to change it as well as adapt to it that makes attempts to regulate the context a part of self-regulated learning. In this case, it is not the area that is being regulated that determines the label "self-regulating," but the fact that the personal self is involved and the strategies the individual person is using to monitor, control, and regulate the context that makes it an important aspect of self-regulated learning.

This general description of the rows and columns of Table 1 provides an overview of how the different phases of regulation relate to different areas for regulation. The next section describes in more detail the cells in the table, organized by column.

A. REGULATION OF COGNITION

Table 1 displays the four general phases of self-regulation that can occur, and within the column for cognition, there are four cells that represent how these different phases may be applied to various aspects of cognition. Each cell is discussed separately for rhetorical and logical reasons, including ease of presentation, although as noted previously, the phases may overlap or occur simultaneously with multiple interactions among the different processes and components. There is no strong assumption of a simple linear, static process with separable noninteracting components.

Cognitive Planning and Activation

As shown in Table 1, there are three general types of planning or activation: (1) target goal setting, (2) activation of relevant prior content knowledge, and (3) activation of metacognitive knowledge. Target goal setting involves the setting of task-specific goals that can be used to guide cognition in general and monitoring in particular (Harackiewicz, Barron, & Elliot, 1998; Pintrich et al., in press; Pressley & Afflerbach, 1995; Schunk, 1994; Zimmerman, 1989; Zimmerman & Martinez-Pons, 1986, 1988). As noted before, the goal acts as a criterion against which to assess, monitor, and guide cognition, just as the temperature setting of a thermostat guides the operation of the thermostat and the heating–cooling system. Of course, goal setting is most often assumed to occur before starting a task, but goal setting actually can occur at any point during performance. Learners may begin a task by setting specific goals for learning, goals for time use, and goals for eventual performance, but all of these can be adjusted and changed at any time during task performance as a function of monitoring, control, and reflection processes.

The second aspect of forethought and planning involves the activation of relevant prior knowledge. At some level, this process of activation of prior knowledge can and does happen automatically and without conscious thought. That is, as students approach a task in a particular domain, for example, mathematics, some aspects of their knowledge about mathematics will be activated automatically and quickly without conscious control. This type of process would not be considered self-regulatory and involves general cognitive processing, because it is not under the explicit control of the learner. At the same time, students who are more self-regulating or metacognitive, actively can search their memory for relevant prior knowledge before they actually begin performing the task. This prior knowledge can include content knowledge as well as metacognitive knowledge about the task and strategies (Alexander, Schallert, & Hare, 1991; Flavell, 1979; Pintrich et al., in press).

The activation of prior knowledge of the content area can happen automatically, but it also can be done in a more planful and regulatory manner through various prompts and self-questioning activities, such as asking oneself, "What do I know about this domain, subject area, topic, problem type, etcetra?," as well as the construction of better problem representations. It appears that both domain experts and self-regulating learners do engage in these type of planning activities (cf. Chi, Feltovich, & Glaser, 1981; Larkin, McDermott, Simon, & Simon, 1980; Zimmerman & Martinez-Pons, 1986).

The third entry in the cell in Table 1, the activation of metacognitive knowledge, includes the activation of knowledge about cognitive tasks and cognitive strategies, and seems to be useful for learning (Pintrich et al., in press; Schneider & Pressley, 1997). Again, as with prior content knowledge, this activation can be rather automatic, stimulated by individual, task, or contextual features, or it can be more controlled and conscious. Metacognitive task knowledge includes knowledge about how task variations can influence cognition. For example, if there is more information provided in a question or a test, then it generally will be more easily solved than when there is little information provided. Most students come to understand this general idea and it becomes part of their metacognitive knowledge about task features. Other examples include knowing that some tasks, or the goals for the task, are more or less difficult, like trying to remember the gist of a story versus remembering the story verbatim (Flavell, 1979).

Knowledge of strategy variables includes all the knowledge individuals can acquire about various procedures and strategies for cognition, including memorizing, thinking, reasoning, problem solving, planning, studying, reading, writing, and so forth. This is the area that has seen the most research and is probably the most familiar category of metacognitive knowledge. Knowledge that rehearsal strategies can help in recalling a telephone number or that organizational and elaboration strategies can help in the memory and comprehension of text information are examples of strategy knowledge.

Metacognitive knowledge has been further broken down into declarative, procedural, and conditional metacognitive knowledge (Alexander et al., 1991; Paris, Lipson, & Wixson, 1983; Schraw & Moshman, 1995). Declarative knowledge of cognition is the knowledge of the *what* of cognition and includes knowledge of the different cognitive strategies, such as rehearsal or elaboration, that can be used for learning. Procedural knowledge includes knowing *how* to perform and use the various cognitive strategies. It may not be enough to know that there are elaboration strategies like summarizing and paraphrasing; it is important to know how to use these strategies effectively. Finally, conditional knowledge includes knowing *when* and *why* to use the various cognitive strategies. For example, elaboration strategies may be appropriate in some contexts for some types of tasks (learning from text); other strategies such as rehearsal may be more appropriate for different tasks or different goals (trying to remember a telephone number). This type of conditional knowledge is important for the flexible and adaptive use of various cognitive strategies.

Cognitive Monitoring

Cognitive monitoring involves the awareness and monitoring of various aspects of cognition and is an important component of what is classically labeled metacognition (Baker 1979; Baker 1989; Brown, Bransford, Ferrara, & Campione, 1983; Flavell, 1979; Koriat & Goldsmith, 1996; Nelson, 1996; Pintrich et al., in press; Schraw & Dennison 1994; Schraw, Dunkle, Bendixen & Roedal, 1995; Schneider & Pressley, 1997). In contrast to metacognitive knowledge, which is more static and "statable" (individuals can tell if they know it or not), metacognitive judgments and monitoring are more dynamic and process oriented, and reflect metacognitive awareness and ongoing metacognitive activities individuals may engage in as they perform a task.

One type of metacognitive judgment or monitoring activity involves *judgments of learning* (JOLs) and comprehension monitoring (Nelson & Narens, 1990; Pintrich et al., in press). These judgments may manifest themselves in a number of activities, such as individuals becoming aware that they do not understand something they just read or heard, or becoming aware that they are reading too quickly or slowly given the text and their goals. Judgments of learning also would be made as students actively monitor their reading comprehension by asking themselves questions. Judgments of learning also could be made when students try to decide if they are ready to take a test on the material they just read and studied or in a memory experiment as they try to judge whether they have learned the target words (Nelson & Narens, 1990). Pressley & Afflerbach (1995) provided a detailed listing of monitoring activities that individuals can engage in while reading. In the classroom context, besides reading comprehension or memory judgments, JOLs could involve students making judgments of their comprehension of a lecture as the instructor is delivering it or whether they could recall the lecture information for a test at a later point in time.

Another type of metacognitive awareness process is termed the *feeling of knowing* (FOK; Nelson & Narens, 1990; Koriat, 1993). A typical instance of FOK occurs when a person cannot recall something when called upon to do so, but knows he or she knows it, or at least has a strong feeling that he or she knows it. In colloquial terms, this experience is often called the tip of the tongue phenomenon and it occurs as a person attempts to recall something. In the Nelson and Narens (1990) framework, FOKs are made after failure to recall an item and involve a determination of whether the currently unrecallable item will be recognized or recalled by the individual at a later point in time. Koriat (1993) points out that there is evidence that FOK judgments are better than chance predictors of future recall performance, albeit not a perfect correlate. In a reading comprehension task, FOKs would involve the awareness of reading something in the past and having some understanding of it, but not being able to recall it on demand. FOKs in the classroom context could involve having some recall of the teacher lecturing on the material or the class discussing it, but not being able to recall it on the exam.

Cognitive Control and Regulation

Cognitive control and regulation includes the types of cognitive and metacognitive activities that individuals engage in to adapt and change their cognition. In most models of metacognition and self-regulated learning, control and regulation activities are assumed to be dependent on, or at least strongly related to, metacognitive monitoring activities, although metacognitive control and monitoring are conceived as separate processes (Butler & Winne, 1995; Nelson & Narens, 1990; Pintrich et al., in press; Zimmerman, 1989, 1994). As in any model of regulation, it is assumed that attempts to control, regulate, and change cognition should be related to cognitive monitoring activities that provide information about the relative discrepancy between a goal and current progress toward that goal. For example, if a student is reading a textbook with the goal of understanding (not just finishing the reading assignment), then as the student monitors his or her comprehension, this monitoring process can provide the student with information about the need to change reading strategies.

One of the central aspects of the control and regulation of cognition is the actual selection and use of various cognitive strategies for memory, learning, reasoning, problem solving, and thinking. Numerous studies have shown that the selection of appropriate cognitive strategies can have a positive influence on learning and performance. These cognitive strategies range from the simple memory strategies very young children through adults use to help them remember (Schneider & Pressley, 1997) to sophisticated strategies that individuals have for reading (Pressley & Afflerbach, 1995), mathematics (Schoenfeld, 1992), writing (Bereiter & Scardamalia, 1987), problem solving, and reasoning (see Baron, 1994; Nisbett, 1993). Although the use of various strategies is probably deemed more cognitive than metacognitive, the decision to use them is an aspect of metacognitive control and regulation as is the decision to stop using them or to switch from one strategy type to another.

In research on self-regulated learning, the various cognitive and learning strategies that individuals use to help them understand and learn the material would be placed in this cell. For example, many researchers have investigated the various rehearsal, elaboration, and organizational strategies that learners can use to control their cognition and learning (cf. Pintrich & De Groot, 1990; Pintrich, Smith, Garcia, & McKeachie, 1993; Pressley & Afflerbach, 1995; Schneider & Pressley, 1997; Weinstein & Mayer, 1986; Zimmerman & Martinez-Pons, 1986). These strategies include the use of imagery to help encode information on a memory task as well as imagery to help one visualize correct implementation of a strategy (e.g., visualization in sports activities as well as academic ones; cf. Zimmerman, 1998a). The use of mnemonics also would be included in this cell as well as various strategies like paraphrasing, summarizing, outlining, networking, constructing tree diagrams, and notetaking (see Weinstein & Mayer, 1986).

Cognitive Reaction and Reflection

The processes of reaction and reflection involve learners' judgments and evaluations of their performance on the task as well as their attributions for performance. As Zimmerman (1998b) pointed out, good self-regulators do evaluate their performance in comparison to learners who avoid self-evaluations or are not aware of the importance of self-evaluation in terms of the goals set for the task. In addition, it appears that good self-regulators are more likely to make adaptive attributions for their performance (Zimmerman, 1998b). Adaptive attributions are generally seen as making attributions to low effort or poor strategy use, not lack of general ability (e.g., I did poorly because I'm stupid or dumb.) in the face of failure (Weiner, 1986; Zimmerman & Kitsantas, 1997). These adaptive attributions have been linked to deeper cognitive processing and better learning and achievement (Pintrich & Schrauben, 1992) as well as a host of adaptive motivational beliefs and behaviors such as positive affect, positive efficacy and expectancy judgments, persistence, and effort (Weiner, 1986).

B. REGULATION OF MOTIVATION AND AFFECT

In the same manner that learners can regulate their cognition, they can regulate their motivation and affect. However, there is not as much research on how students can regulate their motivation and affect as there has been on regulation of cognition, given all the research on metacognition and academic learning by cognitive and educational psychologists. The area of motivational regulation has been discussed more by personality, motivational, and social psychologists (e.g., Kuhl, 1984, 1985), not educational psychologists (for exceptions, see Boekaerts, 1993; Cantor & Kihlstrom 1987; Corno, 1989, 1993; Garcia, McCann, Turner, & Roska, 1998), but this trend is changing as researchers on learning and self-regulation recognize the importance of motivation in general and attempts to regulate motivation in the classroom (Wolters, 1998).

Regulation of motivation and affect includes attempts to regulate various motivational beliefs that have been discussed in the achievement motivation literature (see Pintrich & Schunk, 1996; Wolters, 1998) such as goal orientation (purposes for doing task) and self-efficacy (judgments of competence to perform a task), as well as task value beliefs (beliefs about the importance, utility, and relevance of the task) and personal interest in the task (liking the content area, domain). Kuhl (1984, 1985) as well as Corno (1989, 1993) discussed, under the label of volitional control, various strategies that individuals might use to control their motivation. They also included in their more global construct of volitional control, strategies for emotion control, as did Boekaerts (1993), which includes coping strategies for adapting to negative affect and emotions such as anxiety and fear.

Accordingly, some of the volitional control strategies discussed by these researchers are included in the motivation/affect column in Table 1. However, rather than introduce another term, "volition" or "volitional control," it seems more parsimonious to just discuss regulation of motivation and affect, paralleling the discussion of the regulation of cognition. In the same manner, there is a literature on metacognition that is fairly well established on the awareness of and control of cognition, but there is little on "metamotivation" (but see Boekaerts, 1995), which would include student awareness of and attempts to control motivation. Again, in the interests of parsimony, the term "metamotivation" will not be used, but the model does include motivational self-awareness and control. Finally, although goal orientation is listed in Table 1 in the cell for activation of motivation, it will not be discussed in the current section, because it is the central focus of the second half of this chapter.

Motivational Planning and Activation

In terms of the phases in Table 1, planning and activation of motivation involve judgments of efficacy as well as the activation of various motivational beliefs about value and interest. In terms of self-efficacy judgments, Bandura (1997) and Schunk (1989, 1991, 1994) have shown that individuals' judgments of their capabilities to perform a task have consequences for affect, effort, persistence, performance, and learning. Of course, once a learner begins a task, self-efficacy judgments can be adjusted based on actual performance and feedback, as well as individual attempts to actively regulate or change one's efficacy judgments (Bandura, 1997).

In the cognitive research on memory, individuals can make determinations of the difficulty level of the task such as how hard it will be to remember or learn the material, which, in the Nelson and Narens (1990) framework is called ease of learning judgments (EOL). These EOL judgments draw on both metacognitive knowledge of the task and metacognitive knowledge of the self in terms of past performance on the task. In the classroom context, students could make these EOL judgments as the teacher introduces a lesson or assigns a worksheet, project, or paper. These EOL judgments are similar to self-efficacy judgments, although the emphasis is on the task rather than the self. In this sense, EOL judgments and self-efficacy judgments reflect the task difficulty perceptions and self-competence perceptions from expectancy-value models (e.g., Eccles, 1983).

Along with judgments of competence, learners also have perceptions of the value and interest the task or content area has for them. In expectancy-value models (Eccles, 1983; Wigfield, 1994; Wigfield & Eccles, 1992), task value beliefs include perceptions of the relevance, utility, and importance of the task. If students believe that the task is relevant or important for their future goals or generally useful for them (e.g., chemistry is important because I want to be a doctor; math is useful because I need it to be a good consumer), then they are more likely to be engaged in the task as well as choose to engage in the task in the future (Wigfield, 1994; Wigfield & Eccles, 1992). In terms of a model of self-regulated learning, it seems likely that these beliefs can be activated early on, either consciously or automatically and unconsciously, as the student approaches or is introduced to the task by teachers or others. In addition, in the current model of self-regulated learning, it is assumed that students can attempt to regulate or control these value beliefs (e.g, Wolters, 1998).

Beside value beliefs, learners also have perceptions of their personal interest in the task or in the content domain of the task (e.g., liking and positive affect toward math, history, and science). The research on personal interest suggests that it is a stable enduring characteristic of an individual, but that the level of interest can be activated and can vary according to situational and contextual features; this construct is labeled the psychological state of interest (Krapp, Hidi, & Renninger, 1992; Schiefele, 1991). In addition, this research has shown that interest is related to increased learning, persistence, and effort. Although the research on interest has been pursued from both an expectancy-value framework (Wigfield, 1994; Wigfield & Eccles, 1992) and from intrinsic motivation or needs-based models (see Deci & Ryan, 1985; Renninger, Hidi, & Krapp, 1992), it seems clear that interest can be activated by task and contextual features and that learners also can try to control and regulate it (Sansone, Weir, Harpster, & Morgan, 1992; Wolters, 1998).

Finally, just as interest can be a positive anticipatory affect, learners also can anticipate other more negative affects such as anxiety or fear. In the academic learning domain, test anxiety would be the most common form of anxiety and the most researched in terms of its links with learning, performance, and achievement (Hembree 1988; Hill & Wigfield, 1984; Wigfield & Eccles, 1989; Zeidner, 1998). Students who anticipate being anxious on tests and worry about doing poorly even before they begin the test can set in motion a downward spiral of maladaptive cognitions, emotions, and behaviors that lead them to do poorly on the exam (Bandura, 1997; Zeidner, 1998). In this way, the anticipatory affects such as anxiety or fear can influence the subsequent learning process and certainly set up conditions that require active and adaptive self-regulation of cognition, motivation, and behavior.

Motivational Monitoring

In terms of monitoring motivation and affect, there is not as much research on how individuals become aware of their motivation and affect as there is on metacognitive awareness and monitoring, but it is implied in the research on individuals attempts to control and regulate their motivation and affect. That is, as in the cognitive research, it can be assumed that for individuals to try to control their efficacy, value, interest, or anxiety, they would have to be aware of these beliefs and affects, and monitor them at some level. In fact, paralleling the cognitive strategy intervention research (Pressley & Woloshyn, 1995), research on interventions to improve motivation often focus on helping students become aware of their own motivation and adapting it to the task and contextual demands. For example, in the research on self-efficacy, the focus is on having individuals become aware of their own efficacy levels and self-doubts, and then changing their efficacy judgments to make them more realistic and adaptive (Bandura, 1997). Research on attributional retraining attempts to help individuals become aware of their maladaptive attributional patterns and then change them (Foersterling, 1985; Peterson, Maier, & Seligman, 1993). In the test anxiety research, in addition to attempts to change the environmental conditions that increase anxiety, there are a host of suggested coping strategies that individuals can adopt that include monitoring both the emotionality (negative affect) and cognitive (negative self-thoughts and doubts) components of anxiety (Hill & Wigfield, 1984; Tryon, 1980; Zeidner, 1998). In all these cases, the monitoring of motivation and affect is an important prelude to attempts to control and regulate motivation and affect.

Motivational Control and Regulation

There are many different strategies that individuals can use to control motivation and affect; not as many perhaps as have been discussed by cognitive researchers investigating strategies to control cognition, but still there are a fair number of different motivation and emotion control strategies. Kuhl (1984, 1985), Corno (1989, 1993), and Boekaerts (1993; Boekaerts & Niemivirta, 2000) all have discussed various strategies for motivation and emotion control.

These strategies include attempts to control self-efficacy through the use of positive self-talk (e.g., I know I can do this task; see Bandura, 1997). Students also can attempt to increase their extrinsic motivation for the task by promising themselves extrinsic rewards or making certain positive activities (taking a nap, watching TV, talking with friends, etc.) contingent on completing an academic task (Wolters, 1998; called self-consequenting in Zimmerman and Martinez-Pons, 1986, and incentive escalation in Kuhl, 1984). Wolters (1998) also found that college students intentionally would try to evoke extrinsic goals such as getting good grades to help them maintain their motivation. Students also can try to increase their intrinsic motivation for a task by trying to make it more interesting (e.g., make it into a game; Sansone et al., 1992; Wolters, 1998) or to maintain a more mastery-oriented focus on learning (Wolters, 1998). Finally, Wolters (1998) also found that students would try to increase the task value of an academic task by attempting to make it more relevant or useful to them or their careers, experiences, or lives. In all these cases, students are attempting to change or control their motivation in order to complete a task that might be boring or difficult.

In other cases, students may use a self-affirmation strategy whereby they decrease the value of a task to protect their self-worth, especially if they have done poorly on the task (Garcia & Pintrich, 1994). For example, students who fail on an academic task might try to affirm their self-worth by saying it does not matter to them and that school is not that important compared to other aspects of their lives that they value more. Steele (1988, 1997) suggested that self-affirmation and disidentification with school (devaluing school in comparison to other domains) might help explain the discrepancy between African–American students' achievement and their self-esteem.

In addition, there are strategies that students can use to try to control their emotions that might differ from those that they use to control their efficacy or value (Boekaerts, 1993; Boekaerts & Niemivirta, 2000; Corno, 1989, 1993; Kuhl, 1984, 1985; Wolters, 1998). Self-talk strategies to control negative affect and anxiety (e.g., don't worry about grades now, don't think about that last question, move on to the next question) have been noted by anxiety researchers (Hill and Wigfield, 1984; Zeidner, 1998). Students also may invoke negative affects such as shame or guilt to motivate them to persist at a task (Corno, 1989; Wolters, 1998). Defensive pessimism is another motivational strategy that students can use to actually harness negative affect and anxiety about doing poorly to motivate them to increase their effort and perform better (Garcia & Pintrich, 1994; Norem & Cantor, 1986). Self-handicapping, in contrast to defensive pessimism, involves the decrease of effort (little or no studying) or procrastination (only cramming for an exam, writing a paper at the very end of the deadline) to protect self-worth by attributing the likely poor outcome to low effort, not low ability (Baumeister & Scher, 1988; Berglas, 1985; Garcia & Pintrich, 1994; Midgley, Arunkumar, & Urdan, 1996).

Motivational Reaction and Reflection

After the students have completed a task, they may have emotional reactions to the outcome (e.g., happiness at success, sadness at failure) as well as reflect on the reasons for the outcome; that is, make attributions for the outcome (Weiner, 1986). Following attribution theory, the types of attributions that students make for their success and failure can lead to the experience of more complicated emotions like pride, anger, shame, and guilt (Weiner, 1986, 1995). As students reflect on the reasons for their performance, both the quality of the attributions and the quality of the emotions experienced are important outcomes of the self-regulation process. Individuals actively can control the types of attributions they make to protect their self-worth and motivation for future tasks. Many of the common attributional biases identified by social psychologists (Fiske & Taylor, 1991) may be used rather automatically (e.g., the fundamental attribution error, or the actor–observer bias), but they could also be more intentional strategies used to protect self-worth (e.g., the self-serving or hedonic bias or the self-centered bias; see Fiske & Taylor, 1991; Pintrich & Schunk, 1996).

In fact, much of the attributional retraining literature is focused on helping individuals change their attributions or attributional style to have more adaptive cognitive, motivational, affective, and behavioral reactions to life events (Peterson et al., 1993; Foersterling, 1985). Finally, these reflections and reactions can lead to changes in the future levels of self-efficacy and expectancy for future success, as well as value and interest (Pintrich & Schunk, 1996; Weiner, 1986, 1995). In this manner, these potential changes in efficacy, value, and interest from phase 4 flow back into phase 1 and become the entry level motivational beliefs that students bring with them to new tasks.

C. REGULATION OF BEHAVIOR

Regulation of behavior is an aspect of self-regulation that involves individuals' attempts to control their own overt behavior. Some models of regulation would not include this as an aspect of self-regulation, because it does not explicitly involve attempts to control and regulate the personal self and would just label it behavioral control. In contrast, the framework in Table 1 follows the triadic model of social cognition (Bandura, 1986; Zimmerman, 1989), where behavior is an aspect of the person, albeit not the internal self that is represented by cognition, motivation, and affect. Nevertheless, individuals can observe their own behavior, monitor it, and attempt to control and regulate it, and, as such, these activities can be considered self-regulatory for the individual.

At the same time, as signaled by the brackets for the cell that represents the intersection of the row for phase 1—forethought, planning, and activation—and the column for behavior, this cell for time and effort planning really represents cognitions. In this sense, it could be placed in the cell that reflects the intersection of forethought and cognition. That is, there may not really be any behavioral planning that is not also cognitive. However, there are models of intentions and intentional planning (e.g., Gollwitzer, 1996) that do conceptualize behavioral intentions as an aspect of volitional and regulatory control. Accordingly, in terms of the structure of the taxonomy in Table 1, it seems reasonable to place students' attempts to intentionally plan their behavior in this cell and to discuss them as part of the column for behavioral regulation.

Behavioral Forethought, Planning, and Activation

Models of intentions, intentional planning, and planned behavior (e.g., Ajzen, 1988, 1991; Gollwitzer, 1996) have shown that the formation of intentions is linked to subsequent behavior in a number of different domains. In the academic learning domain, time and effort planning or management would be the kinds of activities that could be placed in this cell in Table 1. Time management involves making schedules for studying and allocating time for different activities, which are classic aspects of most learning and study skills courses (see Hofer, Yu, & Pintrich, 1998; McKeachie, Pintrich, & Lin, 1985; Pintrich, McKeachie, & Lin, 1987; Simpson, Hynd, Nist, & Burrell, 1997). Zimmerman and Martinez-Pons (1986) have shown that self-regulating learners and high achievers do engage in time management activities. In addition, Zimmerman (1998a) discussed how expert writers, musicians, and athletes also engage in time management activities, not just students. As part of time management, students also may make decisions and form intentions about how they will allocate their effort and the intensity of their work. For example, students might plan to study regularly 1 or 2 hours a night during the semester, but during midterms or finals intend to increase their effort and time spent studying.

Zimmerman (1998a, 2000,) also has discussed how individuals can observe their own behavior through various methods and then use this information to control and regulate their behavior. For example, writers can record how many pages of text they produce in a day and record this information over weeks, months, and years (Zimmerman, 1998b). To enact these self-observational methods, some planning must be involved to organize the behavioral record keeping. Many learning strategy programs also suggest some form of behavioral observation and record keeping in terms of studying so as to provide useful information for future attempts to change learning and study habits. Again, the implementation of these self-observational methods requires some planning and the intention to actually implement them during learning activities.

Behavioral Monitoring and Awareness

In phase 2, students can monitor their time management and effort levels, and attempt to adjust their effort to fit the task. For example, in phase 1, students may plan to spend only 2 hours reading two textbook chapters for the course, but once they begin reading, they realize that it is more difficult than they foresaw and that it will take either more time or more concentrated effort to understand the chapter. They also could realize that although they set aside 2 hours for reading the chapters in the library, they spent 1 hour of that time talking with friends who were studying with them. Of course, this type of monitoring should lead to an attempt to control or regulate their effort (e.g., set aside more time, do not study with friends; the next cell in Table 1). This type of monitoring behavior is often helped by formal procedures for self-observation (e.g., keeping logs of study time, diaries of activities, and record keeping) or self-experimentation (Zimmerman, 1998a, 2000). All of these activities will help students become aware of and monitor their own behavior, which provides information that can be used to actually control or regulate behavior.

Behavioral Control and Regulation

Strategies for actual behavioral control and regulation are many as attested to by the chapters in this volume that address issues of behavioral control of physical health, mental health, work behaviors, and social relationships with others, as well as behavioral control of activities for academic learning. As noted in the previous section, students may regulate the time and effort they expend studying two textbook chapters based on their monitoring of their behavior and the difficulty of the task. If the task is harder than they originally thought, they may increase their effort, depending on their goals, or they may decrease effort if the task is perceived as too difficult. Another aspect of behavioral control includes general persistence, which is also a classic measure used in achievement motivation studies as an indicator of motivation. Students may exhort themselves to persist through self-talk (keep trying, you'll get it) or they may give up if the task is too difficult, again depending on their goals and monitoring activities.

The motivational strategies mentioned earlier such as defensive pessimism and self-handicapping included attempts to control anxiety and self-worth, but also had direct implications for an increase in effort (defensive pessimism) or decrease in effort (self-handicapping). As such, these strategies are also relevant to behavioral control efforts. One aspect of self-handicapping is procrastination, which is certainly behavioral in nature in terms of putting off studying for an exam or writing a paper until the last minute. Of course, because effort and persistence are two of the most common indicators of motivation, most of the motivational strategies mentioned in the earlier section will have direct implications for the behaviors of effort and persistence.

Another behavioral strategy that can be very helpful for learning is help seeking. It appears that good students and good self-regulators know when, why, and from whom to seek help (Karabenick & Sharma, 1994; Nelson-Le Gall, 1981, 1985; Newman, 1991, 1994, 1998a, 1998b; Ryan & Pintrich, 1997). Help seeking is listed here as a behavioral strategy because it involves the person's own behavior, but it also involves contextual control because it necessarily involves the procurement of help from others in the environment and as such is also a social interaction (Ryan & Pintrich, 1997). Help seeking can be a dependent strategy for students who are seeking the correct answer without much work or who wish to complete the task quickly without much understanding or learning. In terms of this goal of learning and understanding, dependent help seeking would be a generally maladaptive strategy, in contrast to adaptive help seeking where the individual is focused on learning and is only seeking help to overcome a particularly difficult aspect of the task.

Behavioral Reaction and Reflection

Reflection is a more cognitive process and so there may be no behavioral reflection per se, but just as with forethought, the cognitions an individual has about behavior can be classified in this cell. For example, reflections on actual behavior in terms of effort expended or time spent on task can be important aspects of self-regulated learning. Just as students can make judgments or reflect on their cognitive processing or motivation, they can make judgments about their behaviors. They may decide that procrastinating studying for an exam may not be the most adaptive behavior for academic achievement. In the future, they may decide to make a different choice in terms of their effort and time management. Certainly, in terms of reaction, the main behavior is choice. Students cannot decide only to change their future time and effort management; they also may make choices about what classes to take in the future (at least for high school and college students) or, more generally, what general course of study they will follow. This kind of choice behavior results in the selection of different contexts and leads us into the last column in Table 1.

D. REGULATION OF CONTEXT

As previously noted, Table 1 includes the individual's attempts to monitor, control, and regulate the context as an important aspect of self-regulated learning, because the focus is on the personal self or individual who is engaged in these activities. Given that it is the active, personal self who is attempting to monitor, control, and regulate the context, it seems important to include these activities in a model of self-regulated learning.

Contextual Forethought, Planning, and Activation

This cell in Table 1 includes individuals' perceptions of the task and context. As in the behavioral column, this cell is in brackets because these perceptions are really cognitions, not aspects of the context, but the focus of the perceptions is outward, away from the individual's own cognition or motivation, and toward the tasks and contexts. In a classroom context, these perceptions can be about the nature of the tasks in terms of the classroom norms for completing the task (e.g., the format to be used or the procedures to be used to do the task, such as working with others is permitted or is considered cheating), as well as general knowledge about the types of tasks and classroom practices for grading in the classroom (Blumenfeld, Mergendoller, & Swarthout, 1987; Doyle, 1983).

In addition, perceptions of the classroom norms and classroom climate are important aspects of the students' knowledge activation of contextual information. For example, when students enter a classroom, they may activate knowledge about general norms or perceive certain norms (talking is not allowed, working with others is cheating, the teacher always has the correct answer, students are not allowed much autonomy or control, etc.) that can influence their approach to the classroom and their general learning. Other aspects of the classroom climate, such as teacher warmth and enthusiasm as well as equity and fairness for all students (e.g., no bias on the basis of gender or ethnicity), can be important perceptions or beliefs that are activated when students come into a classroom (Pintrich & Schunk, 1996). Of course, these perceptions can be veridical and actually represent the classroom dynamics, but there is also the possibility that the students can misperceive the classroom context because they are activating stereotypes without reflecting on the actual nature of the classroom. For example, there may be occasions when females accurately perceive a male math teacher's bias against females in math, but there also can be cases where this is a more stereotypical perception that is not reflected in the teacher's behavior. In any case, these perceptions, veridical or not, offer opportunities for monitoring and regulation of the context.

Contextual Monitoring

Just as students can and should monitor their cognition, motivation, and behavior, they also can and should monitor the task and contextual features of the classroom. In classrooms, just as in work and social situations, individuals are not free to do as they please; they are involved in a social system that provides various opportunities and constraints that shape and influence their behavior. If students are unaware of the opportunities and constraints that are operating, then they will be less likely to be able to function well in the classroom. Awareness and monitoring of the classroom rules, grading practices, task requirements, reward structures, and general teacher behavior are all important for students to do well in the classroom. For example, students need to be aware of the different grading practices and how different tasks will be evaluated and scored for grades. If they are not aware that format can count (e.g., good penmanship in early grades) or that original thinking is important in a report, not just summarizing material from books or encyclopedias, then they will be less likely to adjust their behavior to be in line with these requirements. In college classrooms, entering freshmen often have difficulty in their first courses because they are not monitoring or adjusting their perceptions of the course requirements to the levels expected by the faculty. Many college learning strategy or study skills courses attempt to help students become aware of these differences and adjust their strategy use and behavior accordingly (Hofer et al., 1998; Simpson et al., 1997).

Contextual Control and Regulation

Of course, as with cognition, motivation, and behavior, contextual monitoring processes are intimately linked to efforts to control and regulate the tasks and context. In comparison to control and regulation of cognition, motivation, and behavior, control of the tasks or context may be more difficult because they are not always under direct control of the individual learner. However, even models of general intelligence (e.g., the contextual subtheory; see Sternberg, 1985) often include attempts to shape, adapt, or control the environment as one aspect of intelligent behavior. Models of volitional control usually include a term labeled environmental control, which refers to attempts to control or structure the environment in ways that will facilitate goals and task completion (Corno, 1989, 1993; Kuhl, 1984, 1985). In terms of self-regulated learning, most models include strategies to shape, control, or structure the learning environment as important strategies for self-regulation (Zimmerman, 1998a).

In the traditional classroom context, the teacher controls most of the aspects of the tasks and context and therefore, there may be little opportunity for students to engage in contextual control and regulation. However, students often may attempt to negotiate the task requirements downward (can we write 5 pages instead of 10?; can we use our books and notes on the exam?; etc.) to make them simpler and easier for them to perform (Doyle, 1983). This kind of task negotiation probably has been experienced by all teachers from elementary through graduate school faculty and does represent one attempt by students to control and regulate the task and contextual environment even in classrooms with high levels of teacher control.

In more student-centered classrooms, such as communities of learners classrooms and project-based instruction (e.g., Blumenfeld, et al., 1991; Brown, 1997), students are asked to do much more actual control and regulation of the academic tasks and classroom climate and structure. They often are asked to design their own projects and experiments, design how their groups will collect data or perform the task, develop classroom norms for discourse and thinking, and even work together with the teacher to determine how they will be evaluated on the tasks. These types of classrooms obviously offer a great deal more autonomy and responsibility to the students and they provide multiple opportunities for contextual control and regulation. Of course, this does not mean that developmentally all students, especially those in the early elementary years, are able to regulate the academic tasks, classroom context, and themselves, but these types of classrooms do highlight the potential types of contextual regulation that is possible in the classroom context.

In postsecondary settings, students have much more freedom to structure their environment in terms of their learning. Much of the learning that goes on takes place outside the college lecture hall or classroom, and students have to be able to control and regulate their study environment. Monitoring of their study environment for distractions (music, TV, talkative friends or peers) and then attempts to control or regulate their study environment to make it more conducive for studying (removing distractions, having an organized and specific place for studying) can facilitate learning and seems to be an important part of self-regulated learning (Hofer et al., 1998; Zimmerman, 1998a). Zimmerman (1998a) also discusses how writers, athletes, and musicians attempt to exert contextual control over their environment by structuring it in ways that facilitate their learning and performance.

Contextual Reaction and Reflection

Finally, in terms of contextual reaction and reflection, students can make general evaluations of the task or classroom environment. These evaluations can be made on the basis of general enjoyment and comfort, as well as more cognitive criteria regarding learning and achievement. In some of the more student-centered classrooms, there is time set aside for occasional reflection on what is working in the classroom and what is not working in terms of both student and teacher reactions (Brown, 1997). As with cognition and motivation, these evaluations can feed back into phase 1 components when the student approaches a new task.

In summary, the four phase by four area taxonomy for regulation in Table 1 represents a general framework for conceptualizing self-regulated learning in the academic domain. It provides a taxonomy of the different processes and components that can be involved in self-regulated learning. The format of the taxonomy also allows for the integration of much of the research on self-regulated learning that has spawned a diversity of terms and constructs, but organizes it in such a manner that the similarities and differences can be seen easily. As researchers traverse the different areas of self-regulated learning, the taxonomy allows them to locate their own efforts within this topography as well as to spy underexplored territories in need of further investigation and examination. The next section of this chapter turns to how the adoption of different goal orientations can influence self-regulated learning.

II. GOAL ORIENTATION AND SELF-REGULATED LEARNING

As noted before, a key assumption of all models of regulation is that some goal, standard, criterion, or reference value exists that can serve as a gauge against which to assess the operation of the system and then guide regulatory processes. In self-regulated learning research, two general classes of goals have been discussed under various names such as target and purpose goals (e.g., Harackiewicz et al., 1998; Harackiewicz & Sansone, 1991) or task-specific goals and goal orientations (e.g., Garcia & Pintrich, 1994; Pintrich & Schunk, 1996; Wolters, Yu, & Pintrich, 1996;

Zimmerman & Kitsantas, 1997). The general distinction between these two classes of goals is that target and task-specific goals represent the specific outcome the individual is attempting to accomplish. In academic learning contexts, it would be represented by goals such as wanting to get 8 out of 10 correct on a quiz or trying to get an A on a midterm exam. These goals are specific to a task and are most similar to the goals discussed by Locke and Latham (1990) for workers in an organizational context such as wanting to make 10 more widgets an hour or to sell 5 more cars in the next week. They also are probably most similar to the goals discussed in many of the chapters in this volume on self-regulation (e.g., trying to stay physically healthy, trying to lose weight, and trying to stay mentally healthy).

In contrast, purpose goals or goal orientations reflect the more general reasons an individual does a task and are related more to the research on achievement motivation (Elliot, 1997; Urdan, 1997): it is an individual's general orientation (or schema or theory) for approaching the task, doing the task, and evaluating their performance on the task (Ames, 1992; Dweck & Leggett, 1988; Pintrich, in press). In this case, purpose goals or goal orientations refer to *why* individuals want to get 8 out of 10 correct, *why* they want to get an A, or *why* they want to make more widgets or sell more cars as well as the standards or criteria (8 out of 10 correct, an A) they will use to evaluate their progress toward the goal. The inclusion of the reasons why an individual is pursuing a task allows for an integration of the achievement motivation literature into our models of self-regulated learning, because the achievement motivation literature is concerned with what, why, and how individuals are motivated to achieve in different settings (Pintrich & Schunk, 1996). The what, why, and how of motivation forms a general theory or orientation to the task that can influence many of the different processes of self-regulation (Meece, 1994). For example, if individuals are motivated to master and learn the material, then they should orient their monitoring processes to cues that show progress in learning and invoke certain types of cognitive strategies for learning (e.g., deeper processing strategies) so as to make progress toward their goal of learning and mastery. In contrast, if they are oriented to demonstrating their superiority over others in terms of grades or scores on academic tasks, then their monitoring and control processes may be qualitatively different because they monitor others' work and grades, and attempt to regulate their motivation and cognition to demonstrate their superiority.

Moreover, a focus on broader purpose goals or goal orientations may offer more potential for generalizability, as well as specific implications for practice, in contrast to a focus on more specific target goals. Given that there are an infinite number of specific target goals that individuals can adopt, it is not clear how a focus on the specific goal contents will offer much direction for educational practice, beyond the usual suggestion that setting specific proximal goals is generally positive for learning and performance (Pintrich & Schunk, 1996). In contrast, a focus on general goal orientations might offer some parsimonious, but powerful and useful, ways to characterize individuals' motivation and how their motivation is linked to their self-regulated learning. In turn, these generalizations should lead to some specific suggestions for the improvement of educational practice (e.g., Maehr & Midgley, 1996). Finally, there has been a fair amount of research on how goal orientations are linked to various self-regulatory processes in the academic learning and achievement motivation literatures. The remainder of this section discusses two general goal orientations that have been proposed in different models and how different approach and avoidance forms of these goals may be linked to the different self-regulatory processes that were outlined in Table 1.

A. MODELS OF GOAL ORIENTATION

There are a number of different models of goal orientation that have been advanced by different achievement motivation researchers (cf. Ames, 1992; Dweck & Leggett, 1988; Harackiewicz et al., 1998; Maehr & Midgley, 1991; Nicholls, 1984; Pintrich, 1989; Wolters et al., 1996). These models vary somewhat in their definition of goal orientation and the use of different labels for similar constructs. They also differ on the proposed number of goal orientations and the role of approach and avoidance forms of the different goals. Finally, they also differ in the degree to which an individual's goal orientations are more personal, based on somewhat stable individual differences, or the degree to which an individual's goal orientations are more situated or sensitive to the context and a function of the contextual features of the environment. Most of the models assume that goal orientations are a function of both individual differences and contextual factors, but the relative emphasis along this continuum does vary between the different models. Much of this research also assumes that classrooms and other contexts (e.g., business or work settings and laboratory conditions in an experiment) can be characterized in terms of their goal orientations (see Ford, Smith, Weissbein, Gully, & Salas, 1998, for an application of goal orientation theory to a work setting), but for the purposes of this chapter the focus will be on individuals' personal goal orientation. All of these differences have made integration of the findings somewhat difficult across different research programs.

Most models propose two general goal orientations that concern the reasons or purposes individuals are pursuing when approaching and engaging in a task. In Dweck's model, the two goal orientations are labeled *learning* and *performance* goals (Dweck & Leggett, 1988), where learning goals reflect a focus on increasing competence and performance goals involve either the avoidance of negative judgments of competence or the attainment of positive judgments of competence. Ames (1992) labels these orientations *mastery* and *performance* goals, where mastery goals orient learners to "developing new skills, trying to understand their work, improving their level of competence, or achieving a sense of mastery based on self-referenced standards" (p. 262). In contrast, performance goals orient learners to focus on their ability and self-worth, to determine their ability with reference to besting other students, surpassing others, and receiving public recognition for their superior performance (Ames, 1992).

Maehr and Midgley and their colleagues (e.g., Anderman & Midgley, 1997; Kaplan & Midgley, 1997; Maehr & Midgley, 1991, 1996; Middleton & Midgley, 1997; Midgley, et al., 1996; Midgley et al., 1998;) mainly have used the terms *task* goals and *performance* goals in their research program, and these terms parallel the two main goals from Dweck and Ames. Task-focused goals involve an orientation to mastery of the task, increasing one's competence, and progress in learning, all of which are similar to the learning and mastery goals of Dweck and Ames. Performance goals involve a concern with doing better than others and demonstrating ability to the teacher and peers, similar to the performance goals discussed by Dweck and Ames.

In a similar, but somewhat different vein, Nicholls and his colleagues (Nicholls, 1984, 1989; Thorkildsen & Nicholls, 1998) have proposed *task-involved* and *ego-involved* goals or *task orientation* and *ego orientation*. In this research, the focus and operationalization of the goals has been on when individuals feel most successful, which is a somewhat different perspective than the more general reasons or purposes learners might adopt when approaching or performing a task. Nevertheless, they are somewhat similar to the goals proposed by others in that task-involved goals are defined as experiencing success when individuals learn something new, gain new skills or knowledge, or do their best. Ego-involved goals involve individuals feeling successful when outperforming or surpassing their peers or avoiding looking incompetent.

Finally, Harackiewicz and Elliot and their colleagues (e.g., Elliot, 1997; Elliot & Church, 1997; Elliot & Harackiewicz, 1996; Harackiewicz et al., 1997, 1998) have investigated two general goal orientations, a *mastery orientation* and a *performance orientation*. In their work, a mastery goal orientation reflects a focus on the development of knowledge, skill, and competence relative to one's own previous performance and thus is self-referential. Performance goals concern striving to demonstrate competence by trying to outperform peers on academic tasks. These two general orientations are in line with the other definitions of goals discussed in this chapter. More importantly, however, Elliot and his colleagues (e.g., Elliot, 1997; Elliot & Church, 1997) also made a distinction between two different types of performance goals: a *performance-approach* goal and a *performance-avoidance* goal. They suggest that individuals can be positively

motivated to try to outperform others and to demonstrate their competence and superiority, which reflects an approach orientation to the
general performance goal. In contrast, individuals also can be negatively
motivated to try to avoid failure and to avoid looking dumb, stupid, or
incompetent, which they label an avoidance orientation to the performance goal.

In the same vein, Midgley and her colleagues (Middleton & Midgley,
1997; Midgley et al., 1998) have separated out both approach and avoid
ability goals, which parallels the work by Elliot and his colleagues on
approach- and avoidance-performance goals. Other researchers (e.g.,
Wolters et al., 1996; Urdan, 1997) have examined what they have called
relative ability goals, but this construct seems to reflect the same construct
as the approach-performance goal of Elliot and his colleagues. Finally,
Skaalvik and his colleagues (Skaalvik, 1997; Skaalvik, Valas, & Sletta,
1994) also have proposed two dimensions of performance or ego goals, a
self-enhancing ego orientation, where the emphasis is on besting others and
demonstrating superior ability, as in the approach-performance goal, and
self-defeating ego orientation, where the goal is to avoid looking dumb or to
avoid negative judgments, as in the avoidance-performance orientation.
The approach-performance orientation focused on besting others and
superior performance relative to peers is similar to the performance and
ego orientation in the models of Dweck, Ames, and Nicholls. In addition,
although not formally separated as two distinct performance or ego goals
in the models of Dweck and Nicholls, both of those models did include
concerns of avoiding judgments of incompetence or feeling dumb or stupid
in their conceptualizations of performance and ego orientations, similar to
the avoidance-performance orientation of Elliot and Midgley or the self-
defeating ego orientation of Skaalvik.

Research on goal orientation also has revealed a number of other goals
that students might adopt in classroom settings. For example, Pintrich and
his colleagues (Pintrich 1989; Pintrich & De Groot, 1990; Pintrich &
Garcia, 1991; Pintrich, Roeser, & De Groot, 1994; Pintrich et al., 1993;
Wolters et al., 1996), as well as others (e.g, Urdan, 1997), have discussed an
extrinsic orientation to the classroom where the focus is on getting good
grades or seeking approval or avoiding punishment from teachers or other
adults. This extrinsic orientation is most similar to extrinsic motivation as
discussed in self-determination theory (Deci & Ryan, 1985). Nicholls and
his colleagues have found two other goals, beyond ego- and task-involved
goals, which they labeled work avoidance and academic alienation (Nicholls,
1989; Nicholls, Cheung, Lauer, & Patashnick, 1989). Work avoidant goals
concern feeling successful when work or tasks are easy, whereas academic
alienation goals are defined in terms of feeling successful when the
students feel they can fool around and not do their school work and get
away with it. Meece, Blumenfeld, & Hoyle (1988) also discussed work

avoidant goals in terms of a desire to complete school work without putting forth much effort, a goal of reducing effort. Urdan (1997; Urdan & Maehr, 1995) and Wentzel (1991a, 1991b) have discussed the role of social goals, where the focus is on seeking friendships or being socially responsible, and how these goals are linked to self-regulation and achievement.

Given all these different goals and orientations, which share some similar and some different features, future research needs to clarify the relations among these goals and their links to self-regulated learning. At the same time, given space considerations in this chapter, the remaining discussion will focus on the role of mastery and performance goals, and their approach and avoidance forms, which seems appropriate given that most of the research has addressed these two general goals. There is clearly a role for extrinsic, work avoidant, and social goals in self-regulated learning given some of the extant research, but that discussion will not be the focus here.

To organize the literature on mastery and performance goals, it seems helpful to propose a general framework that allows for the classification of the two goals and their approach and avoidance versions. Table 2 represents one attempt at such a taxonomy. The columns in Table 2 reflect the general approach–avoidance distinction that has been a hallmark of achievement motivation research (Atkinson, 1957; McClelland, Atkinson, Clark, & Lowell, 1953; Elliot, 1997) since its inception, as well as more

TABLE 2 Two Goal Orientations and Their Approach and Avoidance Forms

	Approach focus	Avoidance focus
Mastery orientation	Focus on mastering task, learning, understanding	Focus on avoiding misunderstanding, avoiding not learning or not mastering task
	Use of standards of self-improvement, progress, deep understanding of task (Learning goal, task goal, task-involved goal)	Use of standards of not being wrong, not doing it incorrectly relative to task
Performance orientation	Focus on being superior, besting others, being the smartest, best at task in comparison to others	Focus on avoiding inferiority, not looking stupid or dumb in comparison to others
	Use of normative standards such as getting best or highest grades, being top or best performer in class	Use of normative standards of not getting the worst grades, being lowest performer in class
	(Performance goal, ego-involved goal, self-enhancing ego orientation, relative ability goal)	(Performance goal, ego-involved goal, self-defeating ego orientation)

recent social cognitive perspectives on approaching and avoiding a task (e.g., Covington & Roberts, 1994; Harackiewicz et al., 1998; Higgins, 1997). In particular, recent social cognitive models of self-regulation such as Higgins (1997) explicitly use this distinction of approach–avoidance (or promotion–prevention focus in his terms) to discuss different self-regulatory processes. An approach or promotion focus leads individuals to move toward positive or desired end states and to try to promote their occurrence, whereas an avoidance or prevention focus leads individuals to move away from negative or undesired end states and to prevent them from occurring (Higgins, 1997). As such, there should be some important distinctions between approaching and avoiding certain goals with concomitant influences on self-regulated learning. For example, a promotion or approach orientation might be expected to have some generally positive relations with cognition, motivation, and behavior, whereas a prevention or avoidance orientation should be negatively related to these aspects of self-regulated learning.

The rows in Table 2 reflect two general goals that students might be striving for and represent the general goals of mastery and performance that have been proposed by every one of the different models discussed here. The cells included in parentheses in Table 2 give some of the different labels that have been proposed for the two main goal orientations in different models. All the models agree that mastery goals (learning, task, task involved) are represented by attempts to improve or promote competence, knowledge, skills, and learning, and that standards are self-set or self-referential with a focus on progress and understanding. In all the models discussed, mastery goals have been discussed and researched only in terms of an approach orientation, that is, that students were trying to approach or attain this goal, not avoid it. As such, most models have proposed only the first cell in the first row in Table 2; it is not clear if there is an avoidance-mastery goal theoretically, and there has been no explicit empirical research on an avoidance-mastery goal.

On the other hand, there may be occasions when students are focused on avoiding misunderstanding or avoiding not mastering the task. Some students who are more "perfectionistic" may use standards of not getting it wrong or doing it incorrectly relative to the task. These students would not be concerned about doing it wrong because of comparisons with others (an avoidance-performance goal), but rather in terms of their own high standards for themselves. Future empirical research will have to be done to determine if avoidance-mastery goals exist or if adopting avoidance-mastery goals leads to differential predictive relations with other motivational, cognitive, and affective outcomes (such as those outlined in Table 1) in comparison to avoidance-performance goals.

The second row in Table 2 reflects the general performance goal orientation that all the models propose, but the approach and avoidance columns allow for the separation of the goal of trying to outperform or best others using normative standards from the goal of avoiding looking stupid, dumb, or incompetent relative to others. This distinction was formally made in the work of Elliot, Midgley, Skaalvik, and their colleagues, and all the studies have shown that there are differential relations between other motivational and cognitive outcomes and an approach-performance goal and an avoidance-performance goal (Harackiewicz et al., 1998; Middleton & Midgley, 1997; Midgley et al., 1998: Skaalvik, 1997). In Dweck's model, the performance orientation included both trying to gain positive judgments of the self as well as trying to avoid negative judgments (Dweck & Leggett, 1988). In Nicholls's model, ego-involved or ego orientation also included both feeling successful when doing better than others or avoiding looking incompetent (Nicholls, 1984; Thorkildsen & Nicholls, 1998). Accordingly, most of the models did recognize the possibility that students could be seeking to gain positive judgments of the self by besting or outperforming others as well as trying to avoid looking stupid, dumb, or incompetent, although Dweck and Nicholls did not separate the constructs conceptually as did Elliot, Midgley, and Skaalvik. In this case, within this performance row in Table 2 and in contrast to the mastery row in Table 2, there is no doubt that both approach and avoidance goal orientations are possible, that students can adopt them, and that they can have differential relations to other motivational or cognitive outcomes.

The remainder of this section applies the four cells of Table 2 to the various areas for regulation from Table 1. The purpose is to discuss how the different types of goal orientations may be differentially related to aspects of self-regulation. If the proposed four cells of the taxonomy in Table 2 are to be theoretically productive and useful, they should result in differential predictions for how they are linked to motivation, cognition, and behavior. In addition, the review will point out gaps in the literature where there is little or no research on how the different goals are linked to self-regulation.

B. MASTERY GOALS AND SELF-REGULATED LEARNING

Given that all the different models of goal orientation have included approach-mastery goals in their empirical research, there is a good deal of converging evidence on the positive influence mastery goals have on the different components of self-regulated learning. Whereas all models of self-regulated learning include some goal construct, a general goal or focus on mastery, improvement, and learning should be propaedeutic for learning. That is, if individuals set their general criterion or standard for academic tasks to be learning and improving, then as they monitor their performance and attempt to control and regulate it, this standard should guide them toward the use of more self-regulatory processes. In fact, the vast majority of the empirical evidence from both experimental laboratory studies and correlational classroom studies suggests just such a stable generalization. Students who adopt or endorse an approach-mastery goal orientation do engage in more self-regulated learning than those who do not adopt or endorse to a lesser extent a mastery goal (Ames, 1992; Pintrich & Schrauben, 1992; Pintrich & Schunk, 1996).

Mastery Goals and Cognitive Self-Regulation

In terms of the four phases of the model presented in Table 1, most of the research in the cognitive column has focused on phases 2 through 4. There has been less research on the linkages between mastery goals and activation of content knowledge or metacognitive knowledge. This is certainly an area for future research, because there has been little investigation of how goal orientations, once adopted, result in the activation of different kinds of knowledge. This is an area where there is a need for more experimental research on knowledge representation and how it can be influenced by different goals and, reciprocally, how knowledge representations and activation may influence the adoption of different goals.

In terms of phases 2 through 4 in the cognitive column in Table 1, the research suggests that students who adopt a mastery goal are more likely to report monitoring and attempting to control their cognition through the use of various learning and cognitive strategies. Much of this research is based on self-report data from correlational classroom studies, although Dweck and Leggett (1988) summarized data from experimental studies. The classroom studies typically assess students' goal orientations and then measure students' reported use of different strategies for learning either at the same time or longitudinally. Although there are some problems with the use of self-report instruments for measuring self-regulatory strategies (see Pintrich et al., in press), these instruments do display reasonable psychometric qualities. Moreover, the research results are overwhelmingly consistent in terms of mastery goals accounting for between 10% to 30% of the variance in the cognitive outcomes. Studies have been done with almost all age groups from elementary to college students and have assessed students' goals for school in general as well as in the content areas of English, math, science, and social studies.

The studies have found that students who endorse a mastery goal are more likely to report attempts to self-monitor their cognition and to seek ways to become aware of their understanding and learning (phase 2) such as checking for understanding and comprehension monitoring (e.g., Ames & Archer, 1988; Dweck & Leggett, 1988; Meece, et al., 1988; Meece & Holt, 1993; Middleton & Midgley, 1997; Nolen, 1988; Pintrich & De Groot, 1990; Pintrich & Garcia, 1991; Pintrich et al., 1994; Pintrich & Schrauben, 1992; Wolters et al., 1996). In addition, this research consistently has shown that students' use of various cognitive strategies (phase 3) is positively related to mastery goals. In particular, this research has shown that students reported use of deeper processing strategies, such as the use of elaboration strategies (i.e., paraphrasing, summarizing) and organizational strategies (networking, outlining), is positively correlated with the endorsement of mastery goals (Ames & Archer, 1988; Bouffard, Boisvert, Vezeau, & Larouche, 1995; Graham & Golen, 1991; Kaplan & Midgley, 1997; Meece et al., 1988; Pintrich & De Groot, 1990; Pintrich & Garcia, 1991; Pintrich et al., 1993, 1994; Wolters et al., 1996).

Finally, in some of this research, mastery goals have been negatively correlated with the use of less effective or surface processing strategies (i.e., rehearsal), especially in older students (Anderman & Young, 1994; Kaplan & Midgley, 1997; Pintrich & Garcia, 1991; Pintrich et al., 1993). In contrast to this research on the use of various self-regulatory and learning strategies, there has not been much research on how mastery goals are linked to the use of other problem solving or thinking strategies. This is clearly an area that will be investigated in the future.

Although there has been no research on avoidance mastery goals formally, it would be predicted that they would be less helpful in self-regulated learning than approach mastery goals. It could be that avoidance-mastery goals would lead to less adaptive monitoring processes because the student would focus on not making mistakes, rather than on learning and progress. This might lead to the use of less deep processing strategies and perhaps more memorization of the material because the student tries to not be incorrect and relies on the text or content material to define what is correct. Avoidance-mastery goals also would seem to lead to less risk taking or less willingness to explore the material using different types of cognitive or thinking strategies. These are predictions that need to be tested in empirical research, but they do suggest that approach- and avoidance-mastery goals could set up different ways to approach and engage in an academic task in terms of cognition.

Mastery Goals and Motivational Regulation

There has been a great deal of research on how mastery goals are linked to other motivational beliefs such as efficacy, value, interest, attributions, and affect. Much of this research is not necessarily in a paradigm of research on self-regulated learning and has not explicitly conceptualized motivational beliefs as components that can be controlled and regulated. Rather, the research has been generated from a general achievement motivation paradigm and it investigated how goal orientations can give rise to different patterns of motivation, attributions, interest, and affect. Nevertheless, within the framework of this chapter, this research is relevant for building theoretical linkages between goals and motivational regulation.

Again, as in the cognitive domain, summarizing the research on approach-mastery goals and how they are related to other motivational constructs is fairly straightforward. Generally, the research shows that adopting a mastery goal has positive implications for self-efficacy, task value, interest, attributions, and affect. In one of the original formulations of mastery goals, Dweck and Leggett (1988) summarized mainly laboratory research that showed that students who were oriented to mastery and learning were able to maintain positive and adaptive efficacy beliefs and perceptions of competence in the face of difficult tasks. Other more correlational classroom research also has shown the same general pattern (e.g., Ames, 1992; Kaplan & Midgley, 1997; Middleton & Midgley, 1997; Pintrich & De Groot, 1990; Pintrich & Garcia, 1991; Pintrich et al., 1993; Thorkildsen & Nicholls, 1998; Wolters et al., 1996). Students who are focused on improving and learning would be more likely to interpret performance feedback in terms of the progress they have made, thereby supporting their efficacy beliefs.

Dweck and Leggett (1988) also showed that students who adopted a mastery goal were much more likely to make adaptive attributions for their performance. In fact, it was the search for factors that predicted why some individuals seemed to make adaptive attributions for failure and did not show a pattern of learned helplessness that generated some of the original goal theory research. In some of the early research, making certain kinds of attributions was seen as part of a general mastery goal orientation. Although it seems theoretically useful to separate goal orientations, which can be adopted at the start of a task, from attributions, which are reactive cognitions after task performance, the linkages between goals and attributions are strong. Most of the research repeatedly shows that students who adopt a mastery goal orientation are more likely to believe that effort will lead to success (positive effort–outcome covariation), that effort does not necessarily mean low ability (positive effort–ability covariation rather than inverse covariation), and that failure can be attributed to low effort or poor strategy selection (Ames, 1992; Dweck & Leggett, 1988; Nicholls, 1984; Pintrich & Schunk, 1996). This is an adaptive pattern of attributions for students who will often confront difficult tasks or tasks that they will fail, but with attributions to effort or strategy use, their future expectancies will not necessarily drop and their affect will remain positive, following the general findings in the attributional literature (Weiner, 1986).

In terms of the links between interest, task value, and mastery goals, the empirical research shows strong positive relations. In some cases, mastery goals have been measured in ways that are similar to personal interest or the mastery scales include items that reflect interest, but it is important for future research to separate these constructs conceptually. In general, the research shows that students who adopt an approach-mastery goal report more personal interest or intrinsic interest or enjoyment in the task (e.g., Butler, 1987; Harackiewicz, et al., 1998; Meece et al., 1988) as well as higher levels of task value in terms of ratings of the utility and importance of school work (e.g., Wolters et al., 1996). Future research needs to examine the causal ordering of these constructs because it may be that high levels of personal interest or task value for a domain or task may be part of the personal characteristics that give rise to mastery goals as would be suggested by interest and intrinsic motivation theories (Deci & Ryan, 1985; Renninger et al., 1992), rather than vice versa, as goal theory assumes.

The research on mastery goals and the use of motivational strategies is not as voluminous as that on mastery goals and cognitive strategy use. Studies of self-handicapping (e.g., Midgley et al., 1996) show little relation of mastery goals to self-handicapping, although it is positively related to performance goals. Wolters (1998) found that college students' adoption of a mastery goal was positively related to their attempts to regulate their efficacy, interest, and value, what he labeled regulation of intrinsic motivation. He also found that mastery goals were negatively related to the use of extrinsic regulation strategies such as the use of rewards for regulating effort and motivation.

The general positive influence of mastery goals also appears in studies that have examined affective reactions. Given that mastery goals seem to be tied closely to an adaptive attributional pattern as noted previously, it is not surprising, following the general principles and findings of attribution theory (Weiner, 1986), that mastery goals are linked to more positive affective reactions. Studies have found that mastery goals are associated with less anxiety and more pride and satisfaction (Ames, 1992; Dweck & Leggett, 1988; Jagacinski & Nicholls, 1984, 1987).

All of this research on mastery goals and motivation has examined only approach-mastery goals, not avoidance-mastery goals. Accordingly, research on the role of avoidance-mastery goals is needed. However, given the general predictions of goal theory and avoidance forms of motivation (Higgins, 1997), it is hypothesized that avoidance-mastery goals would give rise to some negative motivational beliefs and affect. First, given the focus on not being wrong, it is predicted that anxiety would be higher under an avoidance-mastery goal than under an approach-mastery goal. In addition, interest might be lower and self-efficacy also might be lower. Again, these predictions need to be tested in future empirical research, but they seem to follow the general model and may be more likely than the hypotheses offered for cognitive self-regulation in the previous section. It may be that avoidance-mastery goals may not interfere greatly with cognition, but have their costs in terms of student motivation and affect. The important issue is that the separation of these goals into approach and avoidance forms allows for the clarification of these potential differential relations.

Mastery Goals and Behavioral and Contextual Regulation

There has not been as much research on goals and how individuals regulate their own behavior or attempt to shape or control their environment. There is a clear need for more research on how both approach- and avoidance-mastery goals are related to behavioral and contextual regulation. Studies have shown that approach-mastery goals are more positively related to college students' attempts to manage their time and effort (Pintrich, 1989; Pintrich & Garcia, 1991; Pintrich et al., 1993), an important aspect of behavioral self-regulation. Research on help seeking has shown consistently that adopting a personal mastery goal is positively associated with adaptive help seeking (Newman, 1994, 1998a, 1998b; Ryan & Pintrich, 1997, 1998). Students who approach a task with a mastery orientation focused on learning would not see help seeking as a negative reflection on their ability (e.g., showing others that they are unable). They would be more likely to see help seeking as a strategy to help them learn (Newman, 1994, 1998a). Classroom research also shows that contexts that foster a mastery orientation in the classroom climate and structure lead to more adaptive help seeking (Newman, 1998b; Ryan, Gheen, & Midgley, 1998). In contrast, avoidance-mastery goals may lead to less adaptive help seeking and more dependent help seeking, because the student is only concerned with not being incorrect, not with actual mastery.

In summary, approach-mastery goals are generally related to positive outcomes, including the use of more self-regulatory strategies for cognition, positive motivational beliefs and strategies, and behavior. There is a need for research on how mastery goals are linked to the activation of knowledge about cognition as well as self-knowledge and the clarification of the causal relations between goals and other motivational constructs (i.e., interest). It seems likely that these relations are reciprocal, with mastery goals leading to interest and interest leading to mastery goals, but further specification of the dynamics of these reciprocal processes would be helpful for both theory and practice. For example, in terms of practice, goal theorists would concentrate on making classrooms more mastery and learning focused by changing the structural characteristics of the classrooms (feedback, opportunities for social comparison, reward structures, etc.), whereas interest theorists would focus on making the tasks more personally interesting to students. Of course, these intervention strategies are not mutually exclusive, but the example does highlight how practice might vary, depending on the causal relations expected by the different theories. Finally, there is a need for more research on the meaning and operation of an avoidance-mastery goal and if there are differential and more negative relations with self-regulation outcomes in comparison to an approach-mastery goal.

C. PERFORMANCE GOALS AND SELF-REGULATED LEARNING

The research on performance goals and self-regulated learning is not as easily summarized as the results for mastery goals. The original goal theory research generally found negative relations between performance goals and various cognitive, motivational, and behavioral outcomes (Ames, 1992; Dweck & Leggett, 1988; Pintrich & Schunk, 1996), although it did not discriminate empirically between approach- and avoidance-performance goals. The more recent research that has made the distinction between approach- and avoidance-performance goals does show some differential relations between approaching a task focused on besting others and approaching a task focused on trying not to look stupid or incompetent. In particular, the general distinction between an approach and an avoidance orientation suggests that there could be some positive aspects of an approach-performance orientation. If students approach a task by trying to promote certain goals and strategies, this might lead them to be more involved in the task than students who are trying to avoid certain goals, which could lead to more withdrawal and less engagement in the task (Harackiewicz et al., 1998; Higgins, 1997).

Performance Goals and Cognitive Regulation

Most of the research on performance goals that did not distinguish between approach and avoidance versions finds that performance goals are negatively related to students' use of deeper cognitive strategies (e.g., Meece et al., 1988; Nolen, 1988; cf., however, Bouffard et al., 1995). This would be expected given that performance goals that include items about besting others as well as avoiding looking incompetent would guide students away from the use of deeper strategies. Students focused on besting others may be less likely to exert the time and effort needed to use deeper processing strategies, because the effort needed to use these strategies could show to others that they lack the ability, given that the inverse relation between effort and ability is usually operative under performance goals, and trying hard in terms of strategy use may signify low ability. For students who want to avoid looking incompetent, the same self-worth protection mechanism (Covington, 1992) may be operating, whereby students do not exert effort in terms of strategy use so that they have an excuse for doing poorly, which can be attributed to lack of effort or poor strategy use.

However, more recent research with measures that reflect only an approach- or avoidance-performance goal suggests that there may be differential relations between these two versions of performance goals. For example, Wolters et al. (1996), in a correlational study of junior high students, found that, independent of the positive main effect of mastery goals, an approach-performance goal focused on besting others was positively related to the use of deeper cognitive strategies and more regulatory strategy use. However, Kaplan and Midgley (1997), in a correlational study of junior high students, found no relation between an approach-performance goal and adaptive learning strategies, but approach-performance goals were positively related to more surface processing or maladaptive learning strategies. These two studies did not include separate measures of avoidance-performance goals. In contrast, Middleton and Midgley (1997), in a correlational study of junior high students, found no relation between either approach- or avoidance-performance goals and cognitive self-regulation. Some of the differences in the results of these studies stem from the use of different measures, classroom contexts, and participants, making it difficult to synthesize the results. Clearly, there is a need for more theoretical development in this area and empirical work that goes beyond correlational self-report survey studies to clarify these relations.

Nevertheless, it may be that approach-performance goals could lead to deeper strategy use and cognitive self-regulation, as suggested by Wolters et al. (1996), when students are confronted with overlearned classroom tasks that do not challenge them, interest them, or offer opportunities for much self-improvement. In this case, the focus on an external criterion of besting others or being the best in the class could lead the students to be more involved in these boring tasks and to try to use more self-regulatory cognitive strategies to accomplish this goal. On the other hand, it may be that approach-performance goals are not that strongly related to cognitive self-regulation in either a positive or negative way as suggested by the results of Kaplan and Midgley (1997) and Middleton and Midgley (1997). Taken together, the conflicting results suggest that approach-performance goals do not have to be negatively related to cognitive self-regulatory activities in comparison to avoidance-performance goals. This conclusion suggests that there may be multiple pathways between approach- and avoidance-performance goals, cognitive strategy use and self-regulation, and eventual achievement. Future research should attempt to map out these multiple pathways and determine how approach- and avoidance-performance goals may differentially relate to cognitive self-regulation activities.

Performance Goals and Motivational Regulation

One factor that adds to the complexity of the results in discussing approach- and avoidance-performance goals is that in Dweck's original model (Dweck & Leggett, 1988), the links between performance goals and other cognitive, motivational, and achievement outcomes were assumed to be moderated by efficacy beliefs. That is, if students had high perceptions of their competence to do the task, then performance goals should not be detrimental for cognition, motivation, and achievement, and these students should show the same basic pattern as mastery-oriented students. Performance goals were assumed to have negative effects only when efficacy was low. Students who believed they were unable and who were concerned with besting others or wanted to avoid looking incompetent did seem to show the maladaptive pattern of cognition, motivation, and behavior (Dweck & Leggett, 1988).

Other more correlational research that followed this work did not always explicitly test for the predicted interaction between performance goals and efficacy, or did not replicate the predicted moderator effect. For example, neither Kaplan and Midgley (1997) nor Miller, Behrens, Greene, & Newman (1993) found an interaction between approach-performance goals and efficacy on cognitive outcomes such as strategy use. Harackiewicz et al. (1998), using both experimental and correlational designs, did not find moderator or mediator effects of efficacy in relation to the effects of approach mastery or approach-performance goals on other outcomes such as actual performance or intrinsic motivation.

Correlational studies also have revealed a mixture of findings with regard to the linear relations between performance goals and efficacy. For example, Anderman and Midgley (1997) showed that approach-performance goals were positively related to perceptions of competence for sixth graders, but unrelated to perceptions of competence for fifth grades. Wolters et al. (1996) found that approach-performance goals were positively related to self-efficacy for junior high students, but Middleton and Midgley (1997) found, in another sample of junior high students, that approach-performance goals were unrelated to efficacy, but avoidance-performance goals were negatively related to efficacy. In two studies of junior high students, Skaalvik (1997) showed that approach-performance goals were positively related to efficacy and avoidance-performance goals were negatively related to efficacy.

It seems possible that students who are focused on approach-performance goals would have higher perceptions of efficacy as long as they are relatively successful in besting others and demonstrating their high ability. Some of the conflicting findings might be due to differences in the samples and who is represented in the approach-performance groups (e.g., actual high vs. low achievers). In contrast, students oriented to avoiding looking incompetent or stupid would seem likely to have lower perceptions of self-efficacy. In fact, these students seem to have some consistent self-doubts or concerns about their own competence, reflecting a schema that should generate low efficacy judgments. In addition, it may be that this relation may be moderated by the classroom context. In many of the studies the positive relations are found in junior high classrooms, but not in elementary classrooms. The literature suggests that junior high classrooms are more performance oriented than elementary classrooms, which are generally more mastery oriented (see review by Midgley, 1993). In this case then, in junior high classrooms there may be good reasons for efficacy to be positively related to approach-performance goals, but not in elementary classrooms, which are generally more mastery oriented (Anderman & Midgley, 1997).

In terms of other motivational outcomes, like interest or value, the results for performance goals are also mixed. Harackiewicz et al. (1998)

have shown in both experimental and correlational studies that approach performance goals do not necessarily lead to less interest, intrinsic motivation, or task involvement in comparison to mastery goals. In their experimental studies of college students playing pinball games or solving puzzles, an approach-performance orientation did increase intrinsic motivation and task involvement, especially for students high in achievement motivation (a traditional personality measure of nAch) or in more competitive contexts (a situational variable). They suggest that both mastery and approach-performance goals can draw students into an activity, depending on the students' personal characteristics and the context in which they are doing the task. At the same time, it is noted that avoidance-performance goals generally have negative effects on intrinsic motivation and performance (e.g., Elliot, 1997).

Some of the correlational studies generally support this view of the positive relations between approach-performance goals and interest, intrinsic motivation, and task value, and the negative relationships between avoidance-performance goals and these outcomes (e.g., Skaalvik, 1997; Wolters et al., 1996). In addition, work that has examined affective reactions shows that students who are oriented to avoiding negative judgments of their competence are clearly more anxious about tests and their performance (Middleton & Midgley, 1997; Skaalvik, 1997), in line with the original research on a general performance orientation (Ames, 1992; Dweck & Leggett, 1988). In contrast, approach-performance goals are either uncorrelated with anxiety (Wolters et al., 1996) or show relatively low negative relations with anxiety (Middleton & Midgley, 1997; Skaalvik, 1997).

Performance Goals and Behavioral and Contextual Regulation

There has not been as much research on aspects of behavioral and contextual regulation activities as on cognition and motivation. However, the studies on self-handicapping show that students who are concerned with approach-performance goals are more likely to report using self-handicapping strategies such as procrastination and low levels of effort (Midgley et al., 1996). Studies of help seeking also suggest that students who are concerned with besting others or with not looking incompetent are less likely to seek help (Newman, 1991, 1994, 1998b; Ryan & Pintrich, 1997). These are more public displays of behavior in the classroom in contrast to the use of cognitive strategies (which are generally covert), so it is not surprising that students who are concerned about either approach- or avoidance-performance issues are less likely to engage in behavior that can reflect poorly on their ability.

In summary, the results for approach- and avoidance-performance goals cannot be summarized easily in a simple generalization as was done for approach-mastery goals. It does seem clear that an avoidance-performance orientation is not an adaptive approach to academic tasks in the classroom, as would be predicted by both goal theory as well as the general framework proposed here. Students who are concerned about looking dumb or incompetent generally show a maladaptive pattern of cognition, motivation, affect, and behavior. However, it appears that an approach-performance goal can have some positive relations with cognition and motivation, contrary to normative goal theory predictions, but in line with the general approach–avoidance framework presented here and by others (e.g., Elliot, 1997; Harackiewicz et al., 1998; Higgins, 1997). Students who are somewhat more competitive and trying to best others can engage tasks in a manner that involves some adaptive aspects of cognition (more use of strategies) and motivation (increased interest and value). At the same time, this focus on besting others can have some costs in terms of increases in anxiety and negative affect, as well as decreases in the use of some adaptive strategies such as help seeking. These results for approach-performance goals may be moderated by both personal characteristics (need for achievement, efficacy level, actual achievement level, or success) and situational features (the competition level of the classroom or context). There is a need for more research on the various factors that might moderate and mediate the relations between approach-performance goals and achievement.

III. CONCLUSIONS AND FUTURE DIRECTIONS FOR THEORY AND RESEARCH

The framework presented in this chapter and represented most explicitly in Tables 1 and 2 attempts to show how different self-regulatory processes and goal orientations can be categorized and then linked together to provide a comprehensive picture of the role of goal orientation in self-regulated learning. The review of the research suggests that self-regulated learning is a complex and multifaceted phenomenon and that the links to goal orientation are not simple. The taxonomy of goal orientations in Table 2 attempts to develop a framework for conceptualizing goals that allows for a more refined perspective on their role in self-regulated learning. The general proposal is that approach versions of goals can have some positive features, whereas avoidance versions are generally negative. Within this general principle, the exact type of goal orientation, mastery or performance, may have differential relations to adaptive or maladaptive cognition, motivation, or behavior. This framework suggests that different goal orientations are not simply good or bad, or that they always have the same costs and benefits. Instead, the proposal is that by tracing the linkages between the different types of goals and different cognitive, motivational, and behavioral mediators and outcomes, we will be able to develop a more complex, sophisticated, but realistic, view of goals and self-regulated learning.

For example, the research clearly suggests that approach-mastery goals are related to very adaptive patterns of cognition, motivation, and behavior. There is very little disagreement with this generalization in the literature. Whereas the cell involving avoidance-mastery goals is a new proposal, there is a clear need for research on the existence and operation of this form of a mastery goal and how it may be related to self-regulated learning. In contrast, the distinctions between approach- and avoidance-performance goals suggest that they can have both costs and benefits for students' self-regulated learning. It may be that adopting one kind of approach-performance goal may result in some benefit for cognition and motivation, but it also may come at the cost of increased anxiety or negative affect. We need more carefully designed research that builds upon the existing research and attempts to tease out when these different performance goals are adaptive and when they are maladaptive for self-regulated learning. The research needs to move beyond simplistic good–bad distinctions and investigate when these goals are adaptive, for what kinds of cognitive, motivational, or behavioral mediators and outcomes, for whom (different types of individuals, ages, genders, ethnic groups, cultures), and where and under what contextual conditions (types of tasks, classrooms, schools, other settings). This will help us clarify our theories and models, but it also will help us develop better applications and interventions to improve schooling.

Besides this general suggestion for research and the specific areas mentioned in the preceding sections, there are a number of general themes that can serve as directions for future research on the role of goal orientation and self-regulated learning. These include the following:

1. *Definition and measurement of goals and self-regulated learning processes.* As pointed out throughout this chapter, the research has used different definitions of goals and self-regulatory processes, different measures (self-reports, interviews, etc.), and different types of methodologies (experimental, correlational, observational, qualitative). For the field to advance, there needs to be more systematic attention to all of these theoretical and methodological issues. There is a clear need for goal theorists to agree on general definitions and a taxonomy of goal orientations so that future research can build on the existing research without inventing new terms and labels (Pintrich, in press). In the same manner, research on self-regulated learning could prosper from a careful consideration of definitions and terms. Whereas these definitional issues are not just theoretical, but also depend on empirical relations, more research of a multitrait, multimethod (MTMM) nature, such as Howard-Rose and Winne

(1993), would be helpful in clarifying the theoretical and methodological differences in this research area. The key issue for future research is to maintain distinctions between terms and constructs when they reflect important and real differences in the terms, theories, and supporting empirical data, but not to let terms proliferate when they signify distinctions without any real theoretical or empirical differences.

2. *The role of personal characteristics and potential moderator relations.* Most of the research discussed in this chapter has not explicitly examined the role of how different personal characteristics (e.g., personality, intelligence, etc.) or demographic factors (age, gender, ethnicity, socioeconomic status, etc.) may moderate the relations between self-regulation and goals (for an exception, see Harackiewicz et al., 1998). However, there may be important moderating differences in the relations and generalizations that depend on these personal characteristics. For example, Graham (1994) pointed out that African–American students often maintain high efficacy perceptions, even in the face of frequent academic failure. This lack of calibration between efficacy and performance may be detrimental from a self-regulatory perspective, because the students may not believe they need to change some of their self-regulatory and cognitive strategies for learning. However, the high efficacy beliefs can be adaptive in terms of helping the students maintain their general level of effort and persistence. This type of dynamic needs to be explored more so as to understand how these processes work for different types of students.

Beyond ethnicity, there may be other personal characteristics that might moderate the general findings on the relations between goals and self-regulated learning. Gender could play a role in moderating the relations, although many studies do not report gender differences in the overall levels of endorsement of mastery and performance goals (Pintrich & Schunk, 1996). Developmentally, the relations between goals and self-regulation may change with age or the development of expertise. It is clear that younger children are less likely to be metacognitive and self-regulating than older children and adults, but most of the models of self-regulation and goals are not explicitly developmental in nature. There may be important developmental variations in how goals are linked to self-regulatory processes. Moving beyond age and gender, there may be other more psychological characteristics of individuals that could moderate the relations between goals and self-regulated learning. The potential moderating role of self-efficacy already has been mentioned, and given the conflicting findings, more research is needed to clarify the relation. General levels of achievement or prior knowledge or expertise in a domain could also play a moderating role. Individuals who are high achievers or experts who have a depth of prior knowledge and skill in a domain may not be as adversely affected by performance goals as low achievers or novices in a domain.

Finally, personality characteristics such as general temperament or emotionality (see Snow et al., 1996) may create a context where the relations between goals and regulation are modulated or exacerbated. For example, an individual who is higher in emotionality in general and prone to higher levels of both positive and negative emotions may have to be more self-regulating in general and then different goals may make this emotional regulation task easier or harder.

3. *The role of multiple goals.* Related to this issue of the moderating effects of different personal characteristics is the role of multiple goals and how to conceptualize them and trace their operation. This chapter, for rhetorical reasons mainly, has discussed the role of the different goal orientations separately. However, it seems possible that students can adopt multiple goals for academic tasks. The experimental research usually induces goals and students are assigned to different goal groups, a design that does not allow for testing interactions between different goals. The correlational studies usually assess two or three different goal orientations at the same time. Much of this research has focused on the main effects of the different goals using regression analyses, and even when interactions were explicitly examined (e.g., Wolters et al., 1996), the results were not substantial or systematic. In other studies (e.g., Meece & Holt, 1993), cluster analyses have been used to create different groups of students that show different goal profiles and some different patterns of self-regulation and performance. There is a need for more empirical work that explicitly examines the potential interactions among goals, but there also is a need for more theoretical work that conceptualizes how students represent and react to the multiple goals they may have for academic tasks (Pintrich, in press). There may be a hierarchy of goal orientations or more dynamic cognitive processes (see Shah and Kruglanski, 2000, this volume) that allow students to switch between different goal orientations within a task with concomitant changes in self-regulation and processing. This is an important direction for future research.

4. *The role of control, regulation, intentionality, and automaticity.* All models of self-regulated learning assume that attempts to monitor and control one's own learning through various adaptive cognitive, motivational, or behavioral regulatory strategies are basically positive for learning and achievement. There is certainly a great deal of evidence to suggest that students who engage in these kinds of adaptive self-regulatory processes do better in school, learn more, and achieve at high levels. At the same time, there may be a limit to how far these regulatory models can take us in understanding academic learning. There are still a host of issues related to the role of automaticity in cognitive processing and learning, and how these automatic processes may support, constrain, or conflict with attempts to self-regulate learning. There just has not been that much

theoretical or empirical work that has tried to integrate the research on automatic, implicit, and even unconscious processes with the research on self-regulated learning.

In addition, there are problems with the role of intentionality in our models of self-regulated learning and how to characterize what is considered intentional and adaptive self-regulation. For example, most models assume that students construct personal goals for their learning in the classroom and then they try to monitor and regulate their learning to accomplish these goals. However, what if the goals are maladaptive for learning in the classroom (e.g., avoiding work or effort), but the student is quite good at regulating toward these maladaptive goals? Is this still adaptive self-regulation because it is in the service of the student's own goals? In contrast, if students adopt goals given to them by others, such as teachers and parents, and then regulate toward those goals, this may not be considered self-regulation in some models, because the goals are not the students' own goals. Although most models of self-regulation would not consider students to be self-regulating if they use regulatory strategies by luck, accident, or under the direct instruction or control of the teacher, there are still developmental issues regarding when a strategy that is taught by others becomes "internalized" or adapted by the student to be considered the students' own intentionally used strategy.

5. *The role of tasks, contexts, and environments.* Most of the research discussed in this chapter has not been focused on the role of the different tasks and contexts that students confront in classrooms. Self-regulated learning research is based on the social cognitive assumption that how students construct their own cognition, motivation, behavior and perceptions of the environment is central to understanding their academic performance and achievement. This can lead to a lack of attention to the contextual affordances and constraints in the environment. Of course, some research has investigated how different environments can teach or foster self-regulation formally through classroom or other types of interventions (see Schunk & Zimmerman, 1998), but there has not been as much research on how self-regulation develops in natural contexts, especially different types of classrooms. There is a clear need for more descriptive, ethnographic, and observational research on how different features of the context can shape, facilitate, and constrain self-regulated learning.

6. *Cross-cultural generalizability of models of self-regulated learning.* Much of the research on self-regulated learning has a distinct Western and even, North American, flavor to it. The emphasis on the individual and the self is certainly paramount in models of self-regulation. Nevertheless, there may be other cultures both within North America as well as externally with different values and perspectives, where our models may not generalize or at least operate in the same manner (see Betancourt & Lopez, 1993;

Boekaerts, 1998; Graham, 1992). There is a clear need for research on how well our models of goal orientation and self-regulated learning transfer when applied in different cultures. It would seem that some of the processes should be very similar, but there may be important differences in the relations between goals and self-regulation. An understanding of these potential cultural differences would help us refine our models and improve our own research and practice on these important issues.

In conclusion, current research on goal orientation and self-regulated learning has suggested a general framework for examining learning and motivation in academic contexts. Moreover, there are some important generalizations that are emerging from this research. It seems clear that an approach-mastery goal orientation is generally adaptive for cognition, motivation, learning, and performance. The roles of the other goal orientations need to be explored more carefully in empirical research, but the general framework of mastery and performance goals seems to provide a useful way to conceptualize the academic achievement goals that students may adopt in classroom settings and their role in facilitating or constraining self-regulated learning. There is much theoretical and empirical work to be done, but the current models and frameworks are productive and should lead to research on classroom learning that is both theoretically grounded as well as pedagogically useful.

ACKNOWLEDGMENTS

Special thanks to my colleagues at Michigan and around the world who took time out of their busy schedules to provide a number of very helpful and insightful comments on an earlier version of this chapter. The comments and guidance of Lynley Anderman, Monique Boekaerts, Elisabeth De Groot, Carol Dweck, Andrew Elliot, Judith Harackiewicz, Martin Maehr, Judith Meece, Carol Midgley, Christopher Wolters, and Moshe Zeidner improved the chapter immeasurably, but of course I take full responsibility for the ideas presented here.

REFERENCES

Ajzen, I. (1988). *Attitudes, personality, and behavior*. Chicago: Dorsey Press.
Ajzen, I. (1991). A theory of planned behavior. *Organizational Behavior and Human Decision Processes, 50*, 179–211.
Alexander, P., Schallert, D., & Hare, V. (1991). Coming to terms: How researchers in learning and literacy talk about knowledge. *Review of Educational Research, 61*, 315–343.
Ames, C. (1992). Classrooms: Goals, structures, and student motivation. *Journal of Educational Psychology, 84*, 261–271.
Ames, C., & Archer, J. (1988). Achievement goals in the classroom: Students' learning strategies and motivation processes. *Journal of Educational Psychology, 80*, 260–267.
Anderman, E., & Midgley, C. (1997). Changes in achievement goal orientations, perceived academic competence, and grades across the transition to middle-level schools. *Contemporary Educational Psychology, 22*, 269–298.

Anderman, E., & Young, A. (1994). Motivation and strategy use in science: Individual differences and classroom effects. *Journal of Research in Science Teaching, 31,* 811–831.

Atkinson, J. (1957). Motivational determinants of risk-taking behavior. *Psychological Review, 64,* 359–372.

Baker, L. (1979). Comprehension monitoring: Identifying and coping with text confusions. *Journal of Reading Behavior, 11,* 365–374.

Baker, L. (1989). Metacognition, comprehension monitoring, and the adult reader. *Educational Psychology Review, 1,* 3–38.

Bandura, A. (1986). *Social foundations of thought and action: A social cognitive theory.* Englewood Cliffs, NJ: Prentice-Hall.

Bandura, A. (1997). *Self-efficacy: The exercise of control.* New York: Freeman.

Baron, J. (1994). *Thinking and deciding.* New York: Cambridge University Press.

Baumeister, R. F., & Scher, S. J. (1988). Self-defeating behavior patterns among normal individuals: Review and analysis of common self-destructive tendencies. *Psychological Bulletin, 104,* 3–22.

Bereiter, C., & Scardamalia, M. (1987). *The psychology of written composition.* Hillsdale, NJ: Erlbaum.

Berglas, S. (1985). Self-handicapping and self-handicappers: A cognitive/attributional model of interpersonal self-protective behavior. In R. Hogan & W. H. Jones (Eds.), *Perspectives in personality: Theory, measurement, and interpersonal dynamics* (pp. 235–270). Greenwich, CT: JAI Press.

Betancourt, H., & Lopez, S. (1993). The study of culture, ethnicity, and race in American psychology. *American Psychologist, 48,* 629–637.

Blumenfeld, P., Mergendoller, J., & Swarthout, D. (1987). Task as a heuristic for understanding student learning and motivation. *Journal of Curriculum Studies, 19,* 135–148.

Blumenfeld, P., Soloway, E., Marx, R., Krajcik, J., Guzdial, M., & Palincsar, A. (1991). Motivating project-based learning: Sustaining the doing, supporting the learning. *Educational Psychologist, 26,* 369–398.

Boekaerts, M. (1993). Being concerned with well-being and with learning. *Educational Psychologist, 28,* 148–167.

Boekaerts, M. (1995). Self-regulated learning: Bridging the gap between metacognitive and metamotivation theories. *Educational Psychologist, 30,* 195–200.

Boekaerts, M. (1998). Do culturally rooted self-construals affect students' conceptualization of control over learning? *Educational Psychologist, 33,* 87–108.

Boekaerts, M., & Niemivirta, M. (2000). Self-regulated learning: Finding a balance between learning goals and ego-protective goals. In M. Boekaerts, P. R. Pintrich, & M. Zeidner (Eds.), *Handbook of self-regulation* (Chap. 13) San Diego, CA: Academic Press. (This volume).

Bouffard, T., Boisvert, J., Vezeau, C., & Larouche, C. (1995). The impact of goal orientation on self-regulation and performance among college students. *British Journal of Educational Psychology, 65,* 317–329.

Brown, A. L. (1997). Transforming schools into communities of thinking and learning about serious matters. *American Psychologist, 52,* 399–413.

Brown, A. L., Bransford, J. D., Ferrara, R. A., & Campione, J. C. (1983). Learning, remembering, and understanding. In J. H. Flavell and E. M. Markman (Eds.), *Handbook of child psychology: Cognitive development* (Vol. 3, pp. 77–166). New York: Wiley.

Butler, R. (1987). Task-involving and ego-involving properties of evaluation: Effects of different feedback conditions on motivational perceptions, interest, and performance. *Journal of Educational Psychology, 79,* 474–482.

Butler, D. L., & Winne, P. H. (1995). Feedback and self-regulated learning: A theoretical synthesis. *Review of Educational Research, 65,* 245–281.

Cantor, N., & Kihlstrom, J. F. (1987). *Personality and social intelligence*. Englewood Cliffs, NJ: Prentice-Hall.

Chi, M., Feltovich, P., & Glaser, R. (1981). Categorization and representation of physics problems by experts and novices. *Cognitive Science*, *5*, 121–152.

Corno, L. (1989). Self-regulated learning: A volitional analysis. In B. J. Zimmerman & D. H. Schunk, (Eds.), *Self-regulated learning and academic achievement: Theory, research and practice* (pp. 111–141). New York: Springer-Verlag.

Corno, L. (1993). The best-laid plans: Modern conceptions of volition and educational research. *Educational Researcher*, *22*, 14–22.

Covington, M. V. (1992). *Making the grade: A self-worth perspective on motivation and school reform*. Cambridge, UK: Cambridge University Press.

Covington, M. V., & Roberts, B. (1994). Self-worth and college achievement: Motivational and personality correlates. In P. R. Pintrich, D. R. Brown, & C. E. Weinstein (Eds.), *Student motivation, cognition and learning: Essays in honor of Wilbert J. McKeachie* (pp. 157–187). Hillsdale, NJ: Erlbaum.

Deci, E. L., & Ryan, R. M. (1985). *Intrinsic motivation and self-determination in human behavior*. New York: Plenum.

Doyle, W. (1983). Academic work. *Review of Educational Research*, *53*, 159–199.

Dweck, C. S., & Leggett, E. L. (1988). A social–cognitive approach to motivation and personality. *Psychological Review*, *95*, 256–273.

Eccles, J. S. (1983). Expectancies, values, and academic behaviors. In J. T. Spence (Ed.), *Achievement and achievement motives* (pp. 75–146). San Francisco: Freeman.

Elliot, A. J. (1997). Integrating the "classic" and "contemporary" approaches to achievement motivation: A hierarchical model of approach and avoidance achievement motivation. In M. L. Maehr & P. R. Pintrich (Eds.), *Advances in motivation and achievement*. (Vol. 10, pp. 143–179). Greenwich, CT: JAI Press.

Elliot, A. J., & Church, M. (1997). A hierarchical model of approach and avoidance achievement motivation. *Journal of Personality and Social Psychology*, *72*, 218–232.

Elliot, A. J., & Harackiewicz, J. M. (1996). Approach and avoidance achievement goals and intrinsic motivation: A mediational analysis. *Journal of Personality and Social Psychology*, *70*, 461–475.

Fiske, S., & Taylor, S. (1991). *Social cognition*. New York: McGraw-Hill.

Flavell, J. H. (1979). Metacognition and cognitive monitoring: A new area of cognitive-developmental inquiry. *American Psychologist*, *34*, 906–911.

Foersterling, F. (1985). Attributional retraining: A review. *Psychological Bulletin*, *98*, 495–512.

Ford, J. K., Smith, E., Weissbein, D., Gully, S., & Salas, E. (1998). Relationships of goal orientation, metocognitive activity and practice strategies with learning outcomes and transfer. *Journal of Applied Psychology*, *83*, 218–233.

Garcia, T., McCann, E., Turner, J., & Roska, L. (1998). Modeling the mediating role of volition in the learning process. *Contemporary Educational Psychology*, *23*, 392–418.

Garcia, T., & Pintrich, P. R. (1994). Regulating motivation and cognition in the classroom: The role of self-schemas and self-regulatory strategies. In D. H. Schunk & B. J. Zimmerman (Eds.), *Self-regulation of learning and performance: Issues and educational applications* (pp. 127–153). Hillsdale, NJ: Erlbaum.

Gollwitzer, P. (1996). The volitional benefits of planning. In P. Gollwitzer & J. Bargh (Eds.), *The psychology of action: Linking cognition and motivation to behavior* (pp. 287–312). New York: Guilford.

Graham, S. (1992). "Most of the subjects were White and middle class": Trends in published research on African Americans in selected APA journals, 1970–1989. *American Psychologist*, *47*, 629–639.

Graham, S. (1994). Motivation in African Americans. *Review of Educational Research, 64,* 55–117.

Graham, S., & Golan, S. (1991). Motivational influences on cognition: Task involvement, ego involvement, and depth of information processing. *Journal of Educational Psychology, 83,* 187–194.

Harackiewicz, J. M., Barron, K. E., Carter, S. M., Lehto, A. T., & Elliot, A. J. (1997). Predictors and consequences of achievement goals in the college classroom: Maintaining interest and making the grade. *Journal of Personality and Social Psychology, 73,* 1284–1295.

Harackiewicz, J. M., Barron, K. E., & Elliot, A. J. (1998). Rethinking achievement goals: When are they adaptive for college students and why? *Educational Psychologist, 33,* 1–21.

Harackiewicz, J. M., & Sansone, C. (1991). Goals and intrinsic motivation: You can get there from here. In M. L. Maehr & P. R. Pintrich (Eds.), *Advances in motivation and achievement: Goals and self-regulation* (Vol. 7, pp. 21–49). Greenwich, CT: JAI Press.

Hembree, R. (1988). Correlates, causes, effects and treatment of test anxiety. *Review of Educational Research, 58,* 47–77.

Higgins, E. T. (1997). Beyond pleasure and pain. *American Psychologist, 52,* 1280–1300.

Hill, K., & Wigfield, A. (1984). Test anxiety: A major educational problem and what can be done about it. *Elementary School Journal, 85,* 105–126.

Hofer, B., Yu, S., & Pintrich, P. R. (1998). Teaching college students to be self-regulated learners. In D. H. Schunk & B. J. Zimmerman (Eds.), *Self-regulated learning: From teaching to self-reflective practice* (pp. 57–85). New York: Guilford.

Howard-Rose, D., & Winne, P. (1993). Measuring component and sets of cognitive processes in self-regulated learning. *Journal of Educational Psychology, 85*(4), 591–604.

Jagacinski, C., & Nicholls, J. (1984). Conceptions of ability and related affects in task involvement and ego involvement. *Journal of Educational Psychology, 76,* 909–919.

Jagacinski, C., & Nicholls, J. (1987). Competence and affect in task involvement and ego involvement: The impact of social comparison information. *Journal of Educational Psychology, 79,* 107–114.

Kaplan, A., & Midgley, C. (1997). The effect of achievement goals: Does level of perceived academic competence make a difference? *Contemporary Educational Psychology, 22,* 415–435.

Karabenick, S., & Sharma, R. (1994). Seeking academic assistance as a strategic learning resource. In P. R. Pintrich, D. R. Brown, & C. E. Weinstein (Eds.), *Student motivation, cognition, and learning: Essays in honor of Wilbert J. McKeachie* (pp. 189–211). Hillsdale, NJ: Erlbaum.

Koriat, A. (1993). How do we know that we know? The accessibility model of the feeling of knowing. *Psychological Review, 100,* 609–639.

Koriat, A., & Goldsmith, M. (1996). Monitoring and control processes in the strategic regulation of memory accuracy. *Psychological Review, 103,* 490–517.

Krapp, A., Hidi, S., & Renninger, K. A. (1992). Interest, learning and development. In K. A. Renninger, S. Hidi, & A. Krapp (Eds.), *The role of interest in learning and development* (pp. 3–25). Hillsdale, NJ: Erlbaum.

Kuhl, J. (1984). Volitional aspects of achievement motivation and learned helplessness: Toward a comprehensive theory of action control. In B. Maher & W. Maher (Eds.), *Progress in experimental personality research* (Vol. 13, pp. 99–171). New York: Academic Press.

Kuhl, J. (1985). Volitional mediators of cognition–behavior consistency: Self-regulatory processes and action versus state orientation. In J. Kuhl & J. Beckman (Eds.), *Action control: From cognition to behavior* (pp. 101–128). Berlin: Springer-Verlag.

Larkin, J., McDermott, J., Simon, D., & Simon, H. (1980). Expert and novice performance in solving physics problems. *Science, 208,* 1335–1442.

Locke, E. A., & Latham, G. P. (1990). *A theory of goal setting and task performance.* Englewood Cliffs, NJ: Prentice-Hall.

Maehr, M. L., & Midgley, C. (1991). Enhancing student motivation: A school-wide approach. *Educational Psychologist, 26,* 399–427.

Maehr, M. L., & Midgley, C. (1996). *Transforming school cultures.* Boulder, CO: Westview Press.

McClelland, D., Atkinson, J. W., Clark, R. A., & Lowell, E. L. (1953). *The achievement motive.* New York: Appleton-Century-Crofts.

McKeachie, W. J., Pintrich, P. R., & Lin, Y. G. (1985). Teaching learning strategies. *Educational Psychologist, 20,* 153–160.

Meece, J. (1994). The role of motivation in self-regulating learning. In D. H. Schunk & B. J. Zimmerman (Eds.), *Self-regulation of learning and performance: Issues and educational applications* (pp. 25–44). Hillsdale, NJ: Erlbaum.

Meece, J., Blumenfeld, P., & Hoyle, R. (1988). Students' goal orientation and cognitive engagement in classroom activities. *Journal of Educational Psychology, 80,* 514–523.

Meece, J., & Holt, K. (1993). A pattern analysis of students' achievement goals. *Journal of Educational Psychology, 85,* 582–590.

Middleton, M., & Midgley, C. (1997). Avoiding the demonstration of lack of ability: An underexplored aspect of goal theory. *Journal of Educational Psychology, 89,* 710–718.

Midgley, C. (1993). Motivation and middle level schools. In M. L. Maehr & P. R. Pintrich (Eds.), *Advances in motivation and achievement: Motivation and adolescence* (Vol. 8, pp. 217–274). Greenwich, CT: JAI Press.

Midgley, C., Arunkumar, R., & Urdan, T. (1996). "If I don't do well tomorrow, there's a reason": Predictors of adolescents' use of academic self-handicapping strategies. *Journal of Educational Psychology, 88,* 423–434.

Midgley, C., Kaplan, A., Middleton, M., Maehr, M. L., Urdan, T., Anderman, L., Anderman, E., & Roeser, R. (1998). The development and validation of scales assessing students' achievement goal orientations. *Contemporary Educational Psychology, 23,* 113–131.

Miller, R., Behrens, J., Greene, B., & Newman, D. (1993). Goals and perceived ability: Impact on student valuing, self-regulation, and persistence. *Contemporary Educational Psychology, 18,* 2–14.

Miller, G., Galanter, E., & Pribram, K. (1960). *Plans and the structure of behavior.* New York: Holt.

Nelson, T. (1996). Consciousness and metacognition. *American Psychologist, 51,* 102–116.

Nelson, T., & Narens, L. (1990). Metamemory: A theoretical framework and new findings. In G. Bower (Ed.), *The psychology of learning and motivation* (Vol. 26, pp. 125–141). New York: Academic Press.

Nelson-Le Gall, S. (1981). Help-seeking: An understudied problem solving skill in children. *Developmental Review, 1,* 224–246.

Nelson-Le Gall, S. (1985). Help-seeking behavior in learning. *Review of research in education* (Vol. 12, pp. 55–90). Washington DC: American Educational Research Association.

Newman, R. (1991). Goals and self-regulated learning: What motivates children to seek academic help? In M. L. Maehr & P. R. Pintrich (Eds.), *Advances in motivation and achievement: Goals and self-regulatory processes* (Vol. 7, pp. 151–183). Greenwich, CT: JAI Press.

Newman, R. (1994). Adaptive help-seeking: A strategy of self-regulated learning. In D. H. Schunk & B. J. Zimmerman (Eds.), *Self-regulation of learning and performance: Issues and educational applications* (pp. 283–301). Hillsdale, NJ: Erlbaum.

Newman, R. (1998a). Adaptive help-seeking: A role of social interaction in self-regulated learning. In S. Karabenick (Ed.), *Strategic help-seeking: Implications for learning and teaching* (pp. 13–37). Hillsdale, NJ: Erlbaum.

Newman, R. (1998b). Students' help-seeking during problem solving: Influences of personal and contextual goals. *Journal of Educational Psychology, 90*, 644–658.

Nicholls, J. (1984). Achievement motivation: Conceptions of ability, subjective experience, task choice, and performance. *Psychological Review, 91*, 328–346.

Nicholls, J. (1989). *The competitive ethos and democratic education.* Cambridge, MA: Harvard University Press.

Nicholls, J., Cheung, P., Lauer, J., & Patashnick, M. (1989). Individual differences in academic motivation: Perceived ability, goals, beliefs, and values. *Learning and Individual Differences, 1*, 63–84.

Nisbett, R. (1993). *Rules for reasoning.* Hillsdale, NJ: Erlbaum.

Nolen, S. (1988). Reasons for studying: Motivational orientations and study strategies. *Cognition and Instruction, 5*, 269–287.

Norem, J. K., & Cantor, N. (1986). Defensive pessimism: Harnessing anxiety as motivation. *Journal of Personality and Social Psychology, 51*, 1208–1217.

Paris, S. G., Lipson, M. Y., & Wixson, K. K. (1983). Becoming a strategic reader. *Contemporary Educational Psychology, 8*, 293–316.

Peterson, C., Maier, S., & Seligman, M. (1993). *Learned helplessness: A theory for the age of personal control.* New York: Oxford University Press.

Pintrich, P. R. (1989). The dynamic interplay of student motivation and cognition in the college classroom. In C. Ames & M. L. Maehr (Eds.), *Advances in motivation and achievement: Motivation-enhancing environments* (Vol. 6, pp. 117–160). Greenwich, CT: JAI Press.

Pintrich, P. R. (in press). An achievement goal theory perspective on issues in motivation terminology, theory, and research. *Contemporary Educational Psychology.*

Pintrich, P. R., & De Groot, E. V. (1990). Motivational and self-regulated learning components of classroom academic performance. *Journal of Educational Psychology, 82*, 33–40.

Pintrich, P. R., & Garcia, T. (1991). Student goal orientation and self-regulation in the college classroom. In M. L. Maehr & P. R. Pintrich (Eds.), *Advances in motivation and achievement: Goals and self-regulatory processes* (Vol. 7, pp. 371–402). Greenwich, CT: JAI Press.

Pintrich, P. R., Marx, R., & Boyle, R. (1993). Beyond cold conceptual change: The role of motivational beliefs and classroom contextual factors in the process of conceptual change. *Review of Educational Research, 63*(2), 167–199.

Pintrich, P. R., McKeachie, W., & Lin, Y.-G. (1987). Teaching a course in learning to learn. *Teaching of Psychology, 14*, 81–86.

Pintrich, P. R., Roeser, R., & De Groot, E. (1994). Classroom and individual differences in early adolescents' motivation and self-regulated learning. *Journal of Early Adolescence, 14*, 139–161.

Pintrich, P. R., & Schrauben, B. (1992). Students' motivational beliefs and their cognitive engagement in classroom tasks. In D. Schunk & J. Meece (Eds.), *Student perceptions in the classroom: Causes and consequences* (pp. 149–183). Hillsdale, NJ: Erlbaum.

Pintrich, P. R., & Schunk, D. H. (1996). *Motivation in education: Theory, research and applications.* Englewood Cliffs, NJ: Prentice Hall Merrill.

Pintrich, P. R., Smith, D., Garcia, T., & McKeachie, W. (1993). Predictive validity and reliability of the Motivated Strategies for Learning Questionnaire (MSLQ). *Educational and Psychological Measurement, 53*, 801–813.

Pintrich, P. R., Wolters, C., & Baxter, G. (in press). Assessing metacognition and self-regulated learning. In G. Schraw (Ed.), *Metacognitive assessment.* Lincoln: University of Nebraska Press.

Pressley, M. (1986). The relevance of the good strategy user model to the teaching of mathematics. *Educational Psychologist, 21*, 139–161.

Pressley, M., & Afflerbach, P. (1995). *Verbal protocols of reading: The nature of constructively responsive reading.* Hillsdale, NJ: Erlbaum.

Pressley, M., & Woloshyn, V. (1995). *Cognitive strategy instruction that really improves children's academic performance*. Cambridge, MA: Brookline Books.

Renninger, K. A., Hidi, S., & Krapp, A. (1992). *The role of interest in learning and development*. Hillsdale, NJ: Erlbaum.

Ryan, A., Gheen, M., & Midgley, C. (1998). Why do some students avoid asking for help? An examination of the interplay among students' Academic efficacy, teachers' social-emotional role, and the classroom goal structure. *Journal of Educational Psychology, 90*, 528–535.

Ryan, A., & Pintrich, P. R. (1997). "Should I ask for help?" The role of motivation and attitudes in adolescents' help seeking in math class. *Journal of Educational Psychology, 89*, 329–341.

Ryan, A., & Pintrich, P. R. (1998). Achievement and social motivational influences on help-seeking in the class room. In S. Karabenick (Ed.), *Strategic help-seeking: Implications for learning and teaching* (pp. 117–139). Mahwah, NJ: Erlbaum.

Sansone, C., Weir, C., Harpster, L., & Morgan, C. (1992). Once a boring task, always a boring task? The role of interest as a self-regulatory mechanism. *Journal of Personality and Social Psychology, 63*, 379–390.

Schiefele, U. (1991). Interest, learning, and motivation. *Educational Psychologist, 26*, 299–323.

Schneider, W., & Pressley, M. (1997). *Memory development between 2 and 20*. Mahweh, NJ: Erlbaum.

Schoenfeld, A. (1992). Learning to think mathematically: Problem solving, metacognition, and sense making in mathematics. In D. Grouws (Ed.), *Handbook of research on mathematics teaching and learning* (pp. 334–370). New York: Macmillan.

Schraw, G., & Dennison, R. (1994). Assessing metacognitive awareness. *Contemporary Educational Psychology, 19*(4), 460–475.

Schraw, G., Dunkle, M., Bendixen, L., & Roedel, T. (1995). Does a general monitoring skill exist? *Journal of Educational Psychology, 87*, 433–443.

Schraw, G., & Moshman, D. (1995). Metacognitive theories. *Educational Psychology Review, 7*, 351–371.

Schunk, D. H. (1989). Social cognitive theory and self-regulated learning. In B. J. Zimmerman & D. H. Schunk (Eds.), *Self-regulated learning and academic achievement: Theory, research, and practice* (pp. 83–110). New York: Springer-Verlag.

Schunk, D. H. (1991). Self-efficacy and academic motivation. *Educational Psychologist, 26*, 207–231.

Schunk, D. H. (1994). Self-regulation of self-efficacy and attributions in academic settings. In D. H. Schunk & B. J. Zimmerman (Eds.), *Self-regulation of learning and performance: Issues and educational applications* (pp. 75–99). Hillsdale, NJ: Erlbaum.

Schunk, D. H., & Zimmerman, B. J. (1994). *Self-regulation of learning and performance: Issues and educational applications*. Hillsdale, NJ: Erlbaum.

Schunk, D. H., & Zimmerman, B. J. (1998). *Self-regulated learning: From teaching to self-reflective practice*. New York: Guilford.

Shah, J., & Kruglanski, A. (2000). Aspects of goal networks: Implications for self-regulation. In M. Boekaerts, P. R. Pintrich, & M. Zeidner (Eds.), *Handbook of self-regulation*: Theory, research, and applications. (Chap. 4). San Diego, CA: Academic Press.

Simpson, M., Hynd, C., Nist, S., & Burrell, K. (1997). College academic assistance programs and practices. *Educational Psychology Review, 9*, 39–87.

Skaalvik, E. (1997). Self-enhancing and self-defeating ego orientation: Relations with task avoidance orientation, achievement, self-perceptions, and anxiety. *Journal of Educational Psychology, 89*, 71–81.

Skaalvik, E., Valas, H., & Sletta, O. (1994). Task involvement and ego involvement: Relations with academic achievement, academic self-concept and self-esteem. *Scandinavian Journal of Educational Research, 38*, 231–243.

Snow, R., Corno, L., & Jackson, D. (1996). Individual differences in affective and cognative functions. In D. Berliner & R. Calfee (Eds.), *Handbook of educational psychology* (pp. 243–310). New York: Macmillan.

Steele, C. M. (1988). The psychology of self-affirmation: Sustaining the integrity of the self. *Advances in Experimental Social Psychology, 21,* 261–302.

Steele, C. M. (1997). A threat in the air: How stereotypes shape intellectual identity and performance. *American Psychologist, 52,* 613–629.

Sternberg, R. (1985). *Beyond IQ: A triarchic theory of intelligence.* New York: Cambridge University Press.

Thorkildsen, T., & Nicholls, J. (1998). Fifth graders' achievement orientations and beliefs: Individual and classroom differences. *Journal of Educational Psychology, 90,* 179–201.

Tryon, G. (1980). The measurement and treatment of test anxiety. *Review of Educational Research, 50,* 343–372.

Urdan, T. (1997). Achievement goal theory: Past results, future directions. In M. L. Maehr & P. R. Pintrich, (Eds.), *Advances in motivation and achievement* (Vol. 10, pp. 99–141). Greenwich, CT: JAI Press.

Urdan, T., & Maehr, M. L. (1995). Beyond a two-goal theory of motivation: A case for social goals. *Review of Educational Research, 65,* 213–244.

Weiner, B. (1986). *An attributional theory of motivation and emotion.* New York: Springer-Verlag.

Weiner, B. (1995). *Judgments of responsibility: A foundation for a theory of social conduct.* New York: Guilford.

Weinstein, C. E., & Mayer, R. (1986). The teaching of learning strategies. In M. Wittrock (Ed.), *Handbook of research on teaching and learning* (pp. 315–327). New York: Macmillan.

Wentzel, K. (1991a). Social and academic goals at school: Motivation and achievement in context. In M. L. Maehr & P. R. Pintrich (Eds.), *Advances in motivation and achievement: Goals and self-regulatory processes* (Vol. 7, pp. 185–212). Greenwich, CT: JAI Press.

Wentzel, K. (1991b). Social competence at school: Relation between social responsibility and academic achievement. *Review of Educational Research, 61,* 1–24.

Wigfield, A. (1994). Expectancy–value theory of achievement motivation: A developmental perspective. *Educational Psychology Review, 6,* 49–78.

Wigfield, A., & Eccles, J. (1989). Test anxiety in elementary and secondary school students. *Educational Psychologist, 24,* 159–183.

Wigfield, A., & Eccles, J. (1992). The development of achievement task values: A theoretical analysis. *Developmental Review, 12,* 265–310.

Winne, P. (1995). Inherent details in self-regulated learning. *Educational Psychologist, 30,* 173–187.

Wolters, C. (1998). Self-regulated learning and college students' regulation of motivation. *Journal of Educational Psychology, 90,* 224–235.

Wolters, C., Yu, S., & Pintrich, P. R. (1996). The relation between goal orientation and students' motivational beliefs and self-regulated learning. *Learning and Individual Differences, 8,* 211–238.

Zeidner, M. (1998). *Test anxiety: The state of the art.* New York: Plenum.

Zimmerman, B. J. (1986). Development of self-regulated learning: Which are the key subprocesses? *Contemporary Educational Psychology, 16,* 307–313.

Zimmerman, B. J. (1989). A social cognitive view of self-regulated learning and academic learning. *Journal of Educational Psychology, 81*(3), 329–339.

Zimmerman, B. J. (1990). Self-regulated learning and academic achievement: An overview. *Educational Psychologist, 25,* 3–17.

Zimmerman, B. J. (1994). Dimensions of academic self-regulation: A conceptual framework for education. In D. H. Schunk & B. J. Zimmerman (Eds.), *Self-regulation of learning and performance: Issues and educational applications* (pp. 3–21). Hillsdale, NJ: Erlbaum.

Zimmerman, B. J. (1998a). Academic studying and the development of personal skill: A self-regulatory perspective. *Educational Psychologist*, *33*, 73–86.

Zimmerman, B. J. (1998b). Developing self-fulfilling cycles of academic regulation: An analysis of exemplary instructional models. In D. H. Schunk & B. J. Zimmerman (Eds.), *Self-regulated learning: From teaching to self-reflective practice* (pp. 1–19). New York: Guilford.

Zimmerman, B. J. (2000). Attaining self-regulation: A social cognitive perspective. In M. Boekaerts, P. R. Pintrich, & M. Zeidner (Eds.), *Handbook of self-regulation* (Chap. 2) San Diego, CA: Academic Press. (This volume)

Zimmerman, B. J., & Kitsantas, A. (1997). Developmental phases in self-regulation: Shifting from process to outcome goals. *Journal of Educational Psychology*, *89*, 29–36.

Zimmerman, B. J., & Martinez-Pons, M. (1986). Development of a structured interview for assessing student use of self-regulated learning strategies. *American Educational Research Journal*, *23*, 614–628.

Zimmerman, B. J., & Martinez-Pons, M. (1988). Construct validation of a strategy model of student self-regulated learning. *Journal of Educational Psychology*, *80*(3), 284–290.

15

MOTIVATION AND ACTION IN SELF-REGULATED LEARNING

FALKO RHEINBERG, REGINA VOLLMEYER, AND
WOLFRAM ROLLETT

University of Potsdam, Potsdam, Germany

I. INTRODUCTION AND CONCEPTUAL FRAMEWORK

It is not particularly novel to state that people can learn without being forced and without direct tutoring. For example, Piaget (1936) described in detail how children gain a more realistic image of their environment by alternating between accommodation and assimilation—even if there is no instructing teacher. His student Aebli (1963) declared self-initiated learning to be a teaching principle: Students should be their own teachers.

The processes that direct this learning (accommodation, assimilation, curiosity driven attention, etc.) are quite basic in nature. Their initiation and regulation is partly automatic in that they do not require a deliberate decision by the learner to engage in learning. However, it is likely that goal-oriented and intentional learning increases in importance as the learner becomes older. Such self-directed conscious learning becomes necessary when acquiring competence with the more complex material of school or university. Consciousness is not restricted though to school learning: It is also required when training for a driver's license, acquiring athletic or artistic competence, learning how to work with a computer, and so on. We call such intentional learning activities that are not under a tutor's control, but under one's own direction, *self-regulated learning* (SRL). This rather general definition may be specified by additional components like self-regulated learning strategies, self-monitoring of effectiveness, and

Copyright © 2000 by Academic Press.
All rights of reproduction in any form reserved.

self-motivation (Schunk & Zimmerman, 1994; Zimmerman, 1995a). However, enriching the definition too much might create a problem in that we subsume many components under a normative concept instead of studying them empirically as effects of SRL. Thus we adhere to the more general definition just mentioned.

In SRL, a tutor's direct guidance and support is missing, so there are many learning options, but also many opportunities for distractions. Therefore, in SRL we are interested in at least two questions: First, why does a learner engage in learning activities at all instead of doing something else? The question of why people learn has been addressed under the topic of learning motivation and, under certain conditions, volition. Research concerning this first question conceives motivation–volition as dependent variables. The second question is how does motivation influence the learning process and the learning outcome? In this case, motivation–volition are understood as independent or mediating variables. Figure 1 presents a framework in which these and similar questions can be understood.

The diagram starts with the antecedents of current learning motivation and ends with the learning outcome achieved on a specific learning task in a specific learning episode. Following Lewin (1951), we assume that motivated behavior is always a function of the person and the situation. This fundamental assumption also holds for SRL. On the person side (box 1) we have to consider motivational traits, such as competence-related motives (e.g., Atkinson, 1957), personal interests (Krapp, 1992), superordinate goals (Heckhausen, 1977), self-efficacy beliefs (Bandura, 1977), motivational orientation (Dweck & Leggett, 1988; Nicholls, 1984), and similar variables that describe rather stable characteristics of the person. On the situation side (box 2) we have to consider task characteristics, such as the subject matter or the task's structure and difficulty. Furthermore, we have to take into account more general features of the learning situation, for example, the social setting (learning alone vs. learning within a group) and potential gains and losses the learner could face or anticipate in this situation. Possible gains may be new information about one's own ability, good marks, being in close contact with an appreciated subject matter, praise from relevant agents, prestige, prizes, or trophies for excellent results, the competence to use a powerful instrument such as a car or a computer, and so on. In some learning situations, certain aspects may be salient; in others, they may not.

It should not be supposed though that personal characteristics and situation are always independent in their impact on current motivation for SRL. Depending on the learners' motivational traits, some of these situational characteristics could rise in relevance and, therefore, have an impact on current motivation to SRL. More precisely, the interaction between personal and situational characteristics influences the goal setting, the

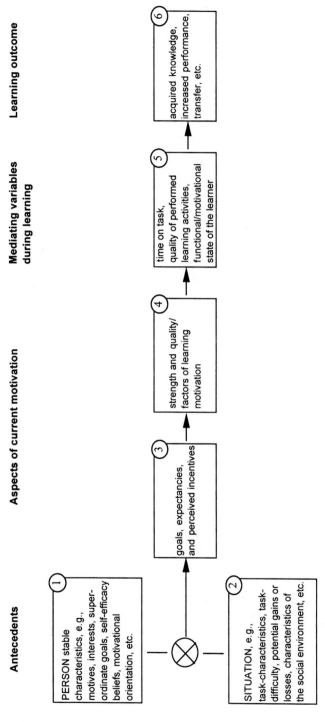

FIGURE 1 A framework for learning motivation and its effects on self-regulated learning.

expectancies, and the incentives the person perceives in this situation (see box 3). These variables determine both the strength of learning motivation and the quality of this motivation (box 4). The *quality of learning motivation* refers to the type of striving. For example, students may engage in text learning because they became very interested in the topic described in the text. On the other hand, they may enjoy the challenge of a very difficult task, anticipate applause from others, and so on. (In Section III of this chapter we report a way to measure such qualities as motivational factors.)

As previously mentioned, quality and strength of learning motivation depend on the person and the situation. If, for example, the learning task consists of a very simple routine (e.g., learning a couple of facts by heart), this situation creates no challenge. However, whether a potentially challenging task (like trying to handle a complex system) actually functions as an incentive for learning depends on a person's competence-related motives.

Until now we have restricted the discussion to motivational features. Certainly, motivation in the context of SRL is a very interesting and important topic to study. Nevertheless, we need to take the next step and ask how, in detail, do motivational variables influence learning and how can we understand the impact they can have on the learning outcome? These questions lead us to variables that mediate the influence motivation may (or may not!) have on learning (box 5). In the case of SRL, in which the learner has numerous degrees of freedom for how to learn, we assume that *time on task* and the quality of performed learning activities are relevant mediating variables. (The term "quality of learning activity" refers to things like reading relevant sections repeatedly, mapping schemata, writing down main ideas, learning by heart, speaking aloud difficult words, etc.; see Pintrich & De Groot, 1990.) A further mediating variable may be the student's *functional state* during learning. This variable can refer to activation or concentration during learning. Last, but not least, we think that the learner's motivational state during learning mediates the effects the initial motivation has on the learning outcome. The term *motivational state* refers to the momentary strength and quality of (learning) motivation that can be measured repeatedly during a learning phase (see Section III.B). Whereas the initial motivation (i.e., the motivation that led the student to start learning) may change considerably during a long learning period, it is not tautological to regard motivational state (during learning) as a mediating variable for the impact of initial motivation on learning outcome. Of course, there could be more mediators. For the moment, we restrict the list of mediators to those we studied in our research.

Learning outcome (box 6) marks the end of the functional chain presented in Figure 1. What kind of indicators for learning are used depends on the nature of the task and the questions the researcher is interested in. We should keep in mind that the effects motivation has on measured learning outcome may depend strongly on the performance measures we use. Under certain conditions, increasing motivation may, for instance, lead to increased quantity and, simultaneously, to decreased quality of performance (Schneider & Kreuz, 1979; see Heckhausen, Schmalt, & Schneider, 1985). Thus, two researchers may find opposite motivational effects in their experimental data if one of them used quantitative and the other more qualitative measures for learning outcome. Obviously such results may produce confusion and lead to ignorance of motivational variables in learning experiments by researchers who prefer to study simple models.

In the following part of this chapter, we first discuss questions of motivation and volition referred to in boxes 1 to 4 of Figure 1 (antecedence and aspects of current motivation to learn). Next, we step forward to boxes 5 and 6 in Figure 1 and discuss questions of how, in detail, initial motivation affects learning and learning performance (the effects motivation has on SRL).

II. AN ACTION MODEL FOR THE PREDICTION OF LEARNING MOTIVATION

A. RESEARCH STRATEGY

Even a quick glance at Figure 1 gives an impression of the spatial distance between a person's motivational traits (box 1) and the learning performance in a specific learning episode with a specific learning task (box 6). Thus it is not very surprising that the measured correlations between traitlike variables and learning are at best low: The common variance between personal interest, for example, and learning performance on the topic of interest, is about 9% on average (Krapp, 1992; Schiefele & Schreyer, 1994). Even if we take into account relevant situational factors (box 2), as was done in early achievement motivation research (e.g., Karabenick & Yousseff, 1968), we get at best results that may be useful for testing a theoretical model (e.g., the risk-taking model by Atkinson, 1957). However, these results are not sufficient to understand the motivational processes in such a way that we can successfully predict the learning motivation for a single person (Heckhausen et al., 1985; Schiefele & Rheinberg, 1997). To gain deeper insight and greater power in predicting individuals' motivation to learn, we must study the relationship between variables that lie closer together in our diagram presented in Figure 1. Thus, the gap to be bridged is smaller and there are fewer uncontrolled influences that obscure the relationship in question. In the following section we summarize a series of studies that explore the relationship between goals, expectancies, and incentives (box 3), and explore the strength of learning motivation (box 4). All were studies of intentional learning at home, a situation in which there was no guiding instructor and in which the students were free to do activities other than learning. In our opinion this is a typical condition for SRL.

B. A COGNITIVE MODEL OF MOTIVATION IN SELF-REGULATED LEARNING

Imagine a student who has just been told that an exam in a particular subject will be given next week. What are the conditions under which this student will study for this exam on his or her own? That is, when will SRL be engaged in? According to the general structure of expectancy-by-value models (Feather, 1982), two conditions must be fulfilled: First, the student has to believe that learning activities will improve the result he or she will receive in this exam (expectancy); second, receiving a good result in this exam has to be sufficiently important for her or him (value).

This simple structure of expectancy-by-value models becomes more differentiated if we start to ask, "On what does it depend, whether a good result is important to the student or not?" That is a question of what consequences the student expects from the result. Thus, we need to know each consequence perceived by the student and the subjective value (i.e., its incentive value) it has for her or him. Furthermore we have to know how certain the student is that this consequence actually will occur if the desired result is reached.

Obviously things become complex if we analyze learning motivation in real life settings. Therefore, a model would be helpful that specifies and links the different components (i.e., expectancies, consequences, incentive values) we have to consider in this context. Such a model was proposed by Heckhausen (1977, 1991, pp. 413–418) and specified for learning situations (Heckhausen & Rheinberg, 1980; Rheinberg, 1989).

We use this model to bridge the gap between boxes 3 and 4 in Figure 1. It helps us to organize the elements within box 3 in such a way that we can predict the strength of motivation in box 4. Figure 2 presents a modified version of this model.

The model subdivides a learning episode into a sequence of four stages: perceived situation, action, intended outcome–goal, and consequences. In the previously described exam example, the situation is created by the announcement of the exam and what this exam means to the student. *Action* is the activity or activities that the student believes will lead to a desired result in the exam (the goal). In the case of SRL, these activities are performed intentionally and under the student's own control. Intended *outcome–goal* refers to the desired result. The student's perception of the consequences follows from assumptions about the effects the intended outcome will probably have, once attained. Our studies with students

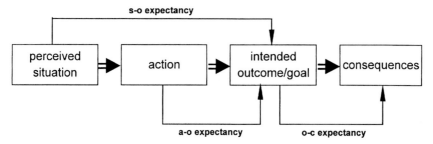

FIGURE 2   A modified version of the expanded cognitive model of motivation. *Note.* The incentives to act lie in the (evaluated) consequences. Abbreviations: s–o, situation → outcome; a–o, action → outcome; o–c, outcome → consequences. Adapted from Heckhausen and Rheinberg (1980), Lernmotivation im Unterricht, erneut betrachtet, *Unterrichts wissenschaft*, *8*, 7–47.

identified a number of such consequences, such as contentment–pride in the result (self-evaluation), praise and acceptance of teachers, parents, and classmates (other evaluation), good learning chances for the subsequent classes, increased chance of getting a good job or university place, profitable usage of the learned skills outside school (e.g., learning foreign languages), monetary rewards, certainty that a good result will decrease the need for further study of this subject, and so on (Rheinberg, 1989).

Whether these and other consequence are perceived depends on their salience in the situation (box 2 in Figure 1) as well as on the student's attentional focus. Such focus is directed by the student's motivational characteristics (box 1 in Figure 1). However, these motivational characteristics not only influence perception, but also the evaluation of the perceived consequences. A perceived consequence, for example, acceptance or admiration by classmates, may be quite irrelevant for student A, but an extremely important, desirable, and activating issue for student B. We refer to such evaluations with the term *incentive value*. This incentive value may be higher or lower and may be positive or, in the case of feared consequences, negative. Differing from Aktinson's well known way of indirect incentive assessment (1 minus the probability of success; Atkinson, 1957), we measured incentive values more directly when we analyzed students' motivation to learn: We asked them how many weeks without allowance each consequence was worth to them. As just mentioned, this incentive value is influenced by a student's motivational traits (see Figure 1, box 1). We found, for example, significant correlations between students' achievement motives (as measured by AMS; see Gjesme & Nygard, 1970) and the incentive value of self-evaluation and of superordinate goals (as measured by the week-without-allowance scale; Rheinberg, 1989).

The four stages of the model (situation, action, outcome, and consequence, see Figure 2) are bridged by three expectancies. The action →

outcome (a–o) expectancy is the subjective probability that one's own learning action will lead to the desired outcome. This kind of expectancy is quite similar to the probability of success in achievement motivation theory (Atkinson, 1957; Heckhausen, 1967) or Skinner's (1996) agency–outcome expectancy. It integrates Bandura's (1977) early concepts of self-efficacy and behavior–outcome expectancy: To have a high action → outcome expectancy, the person must be sure that action X can produce the intended outcome Y (Bandura's behavior–outcome expectancy). Simultaneously, the person must be sure that action X is under his or her control (Bandura's self-efficacy expectancy). Low action → outcome expectancy can arise from either low self-efficacy expectancy or low behavior-outcome expectancy, or can be due to both conditions.

The situation → outcome (s–o) expectancy is the (subjective) assumption that the just given situation will lead to the desired outcome on its own, without the need to take any action. This kind of expectancy usually is neglected by motivational psychologists, but, nevertheless, is important for learning motivation under everyday conditions. Bolles (1972) discussed this kind of expectancy as the $S - S^*$ component of the so-called *psychological syllogism*. (The other component is the $R - S^*$, which is quite similar to the action → outcome expectancy just mentioned.) The third expectancy is the outcome → consequence (o–c) expectancy (see Figure 2). It refers to the subjective probability that the outcome will actually have the specific consequences the learner desires. In the field of industrial psychology, this outcome → consequence expectancy is known as *instrumentality* (Vroom, 1964).

The three types of expectancies described in the preceding text do not really fit into the classification scheme Skinner (1996) proposed, because this scheme does not discriminate between outcome and consequences. Both are conceived as "ends" (Skinner, 1996, pp. 553, 554) and thus the substantial difference between action → outcome expectancy and outcome → consequence expectancy becomes blurred.

This expanded cognitive model fits situations in which a person has a certain action outcome as a goal (e.g., to get a good result in an exam, to understand the difficult instruction for a video recorder, to master a particular coordinated movement in sports). However, the goal's attractivity depends on the expectancy of all possible outcome consequences anticipated by the learner. Such goal-oriented situations often exist in everyday life, particularly in learning situations in which there is more to be gained than just the joy of increased competence or contact with a topic of interest.

The expanded cognitive model bridges the gap between boxes 3 and 4 (Figure 1) in predicting that learning motivation (i.e., the tendency to perform learning activities) is only strong enough to result in self-directed action if the following conditions are fulfilled: (1) The intended outcome–goal does not occur by itself (low s → o expectancy) and (2) can be influenced by one's own learning activity (high a → o expectancy); (3) the perceived outcome's consequences have a sufficiently high incentive value; (4) at the same time they are closely linked with the intended outcome (high o → c expectancy). These four conditions are presented as a flow diagram in Figure 3.

In a set of studies by Rheinberg (1989), this model was used to predict whether students voluntarily would prepare at home for an exam or, instead would use their free time to do something else. Whereas these learning activities were done intentionally and were self-directed, this was

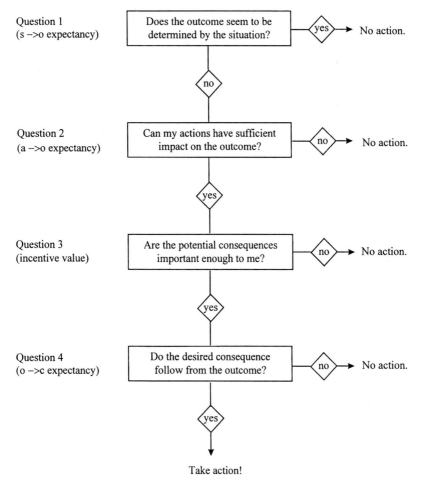

FIGURE 3 A flow diagram of questions and responses used by Heckhausen and Rheinberg (1980) and Rheinberg (1989) to evaluate the component of utility-centered motivation in SRL. For definition of the expectancies, see Figure 2.

a typical case of SRL as we defined it previously. To predict students' motivation, we measured the four parameters represented in the questions shown in Figure 3. The measurement was done one week before an announced exam was given. As a first step the students were asked what mark they were striving for in the announced exam. This was their intended outcome–goal. To assess the situation → outcome expectancy, students rated their probability to reach this mark without any further learning at home. This could be compared to their action → outcome expectancy; that is, the probability of reaching the desired mark if a maximum amount of self-regulated learning was engaged in at home (doing nothing else but preparing for this exam at home next week.). To predict sufficient motivation for SRL at home, the first expectancy had to stay below a critical value; the second one had to stay above.

To have adequate information concerning the consequences (Questions 3 and 4 in Figure 3) the students were asked what they thought would happen if they succeeded in reaching their desired mark. Each of these consequences was rated according to the outcome → consequence expectancy and its incentive value. For the latter, we used the previously mentioned week-without-allowance scale: The students rated how many weeks without allowance this consequence was worth.

On the basis of the question and answer sequence in Figure 3, it was predicted for each student whether she or he would be a case of no learning action or take learning action. To test these single case predictions, we assessed each student's preparation criteria immediately before the exam was given. Ten minutes before the exam took place, students reported how many hours of their free time they spent during the previous week preparing for the exam and whether or not they thought that this was enough to obtain the desired result. This last estimate was the main criterion against which the model was tested (preparation sufficient vs. unsure or insufficient; for further details, see Rheinberg, 1989). In five studies, 75% to 85% of the predictions came true (Rheinberg, 1989). At a first glance this seems to be extraordinarily high. However, we have to consider that the predictors have been developed specifically for this very episode and that they were valid exclusively for this single situation.

C. CONSEQUENCES FOR ENHANCING MOTIVATION IN CLASSROOMS

The flow diagram presented in Figure 3 indicates that there are at least four qualitatively different types of poor learning motivation (which result in no action). For each of these types we need quite different interventions to change the result no action to take action! Behavior modification programs in the tradition of Skinner (1968) try to influence Questions 3 and 4: They systematically induce desirable consequences (Question 3) that are contingent with a defined behavior outcome (Question 4).

In the 1970s, Rheinberg studied teaching strategies that increased action → outcome expectancies (Question 2) and simultaneously decreased situation → outcome expectancies (Question 1). Additionally, self-evaluation consequences (Question 3) were modified (Rheinberg, 1977; Rheinberg & Krug, 1993). The core concept for the interventions was the Reference Norm Orientation (Rheinberg, 1980). According to Heckhausen (1974) and Nicholls (1978) teachers (and students) can compare a student's learning outcome interindividually with the corresponding learning outcome of other students. This kind of comparison was called *social reference norm*. On the other hand, a student's learning outcome can be compared intraindividually with learning outcomes that the same student previously achieved on comparable tasks. This kind of comparison was called *individual reference norm* (Rheinberg, 1980).

It emerged that teachers who preferred individual reference norms created instructional conditions that were favorable for enhancing students' learning motivation. Students who received intraindividual feedback on their performance development had the experience that success (i.e., increase of performance) was very likely to occur if they practiced specific learning activities. Such experience leads to high action → outcome expectancy. Conversely, students experienced that without any learning activity, the probability to fail (i.e., stagnation or decline of performance) was quite high. Experiences such as these lead to low situation → outcome expectancy. Simultaneously these teachers trained their students to evaluate themselves on the basis of their own earlier performances and not on the basis of other people's results (Rheinberg, 1977; for further details see Rheinberg, 1983; Heckhausen et al., 1985). Up to now, 21 studies have found that teachers' use of individual reference norms has favorable consequences for their students' motivation to learn (Mischo & Rheinberg, 1995). Meanwhile, programs have been developed to train teachers to use individual reference norms in their classes (Rheinberg & Krug, 1993). Components of the individual vs. social reference norm orientation are also described in the more recent concepts of motivational orientation (Dweck & Leggett, 1988; Nicholls, 1984).

D. ACTIVITY-RELATED INCENTIVES

Looking back to the expanded motivational model presented in Figures 2 and 3, it is obvious that this model is utility centered. The incentives for action are anchored in the outcome consequences. Thus, learning motivation was conceived strictly instrumentally: Learning activity is performed to attain highly evaluated outcomes after successfully completing this activity. This is an important component of learning motivation, but not the only one.

A further component of learning motivation emerged in an interview study in which students explained episodes of exam preparation; in particular, why they sometimes prepared themselves well and sometimes they did nothing (Rheinberg, 1989, Study E). In the case of intensive preparation, nearly 85% of the given explanations referred to the expanded motivational model, whereas 55% of the explanations for omitted preparation were in line with this model. However, the students reported that the incentives for intensive or omitted preparations were not anchored only in consequences external to the learning activity. There are also incentives embedded in the activity itself—no matter what the outcome and the consequences that follow. Such incentives are generated by carrying out the activity and not by the results that follow after the activity is finished (within-action vs. postaction incentives).

Obviously we have to distinguish two types of incentives. The first concerns the consequences of the action outcome the person is striving for. These incentives refer to future events that are expected to happen when an action in question is finished successfully. They may become powerful and gain behavioral impact when the person anticipates or imagines these future events. The expanded model of motivation to learn described in Section II.B operates with this type of incentives. The second type of incentives refers to the activity itself. Someone may hate learning lots of isolated facts by heart, but may feel good when mapping systematic overviews or discussing a text's main idea with other students. Such activity-specific incentives can be anticipated, too. Moreover, they may even influence SRL immediately during learning, because the aversion or attractivity of a certain (learning) activity are felt when the activity is performed. These activity-specific incentives may strengthen or weaken the consequence-derived tendency to start and continue with learning. Thus the model was again expanded by allocating the two types of incentives just described (see Figure 4).

According to McReynolds (1971), the activity-specific incentives could be called intrinsic. However, the distinction between intrinsic and extrinsic motivation has been used in several quite different ways (Csikszentmihalyi, 1975; Deci & Ryan, 1985; Harlow, 1950; Heckhausen, 1991; Schneider, 1996; White, 1959). Thus we prefer the term activity-specific incentive, because it stimulates and/or maintains activity-related motivation (as opposed to consequence-related motivation). These incentives are not anchored primarily in objects or subject matters, but in the actual learning activity like reading, creating coherent structures, drawing schemata, systematizing information, learning by heart, watching videos, having group discussions, and taking part in educational role play.

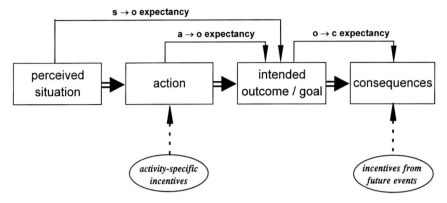

FIGURE 4   Two kinds of incentives in the expanded motivation model (Rheinberg, 1989).

Therefore, these incentives are not exactly the same that the educational *theory of interest* focuses on (Krapp, 1993; Renninger, Hidi, & Krapp, 1992), because this theory defines interest explicitly via the *specific object* or *subject matter* (interest in history, in cars, in insects, etc.). Someone may be very interested in history (i.e., the object of interest), but simultaneously hate to learn the data for the reigns of kings by heart (i.e., the learning activity). Thus, subject matters and learning activities can be independent sources of incentives to learn—both important, but sometimes different in nature. However, this distinction is analytic, and in everyday learning situations, both incentive sources may be correlated: Objects that are associated with many desirable activities are often interesting and activities done with desirable objects tend to be more pleasant. So, learning historical data by heart may be less aversive than, for example, learning chemical formulas by heart. In any case, incentives of activities and of objects–subject matters have one important quality in common: The incentive to learn is anchored within the learning process and not primarily in the consequences of learning outcome.

Further studies found that motivation during SRL is dependent both on the consequences and the activity-related incentives (Rheinberg, 1989). One important finding from these studies was that some learners were primarily consequence directed, whereas the focus of other learners was directed more by the immediate incentive of the activity itself. This interindividual difference can be measured with a questionnaire, namely, the Incentive Focus Scale (Rheinberg, 1989; Rheinberg, Iser, & Pfauser, 1997). These studies found that, depending on their dominant incentive focus, learners' performance was predicted better either by activity-related incentives or by the utility-centered structure of Heckhausen's (1977) expanded motivation model (i.e., the expected consequences of the outcome, see Rheinberg, 1989, Studies F and G).

However, the more (subjectively) important the consequences become, the less influential the activity-related incentives become (Rheinberg, 1988). To illustrate the underlying idea, think of monetary reward as a consequence of learning outcome. If reaching a specific performance level today (i.e., learning outcome) were rewarded with $10,000 (consequence), most students would perform even highly aversive activities as long as (only) these activities guaranteed success in achieving the crucial performance level: Very high consequence-related incentives may cause learners to overcome activity-specific aversions.

This hypothesis was confirmed by Rheinberg and Donkoff (1993), who found that incentives specific to the learning activity were the best predictors of learning activities for students who had a habitual tendency to focus on activity-related incentives, as long as the learning outcome was no more than moderately important. If the learning outcome was very important, however, then focus on activity-related incentives became less relevant, in that these students were more influenced by how efficient they expected the learning activity to be. Thus, they even used learning activities they regarded as aversive, just like students with a strong habitual tendency to focus on consequence-related incentives, as long as these activities seem to be highly efficient. (Momentarily, we ignore the issue that overcoming activity-specific aversions may reduce the actual efficiency of learning; see the next section.)

E. VOLITIONAL ASPECTS OF SELF-REGULATED LEARNING

Nevertheless, there are students who cannot force themselves to engage in aversive learning activities, even if the consequences of the learning outcome are very important. In this case, we do not have a problem of motivation, but of volition. Long ago, Ach (1910) studied volition in learning situations experimentally. However, his work was forgotten until Heckhausen and Kuhl (1985) and Kuhl (1985) revived Ach's idea that people may be more or less able to direct themselves to perform an activity that goes against their immediate motivational tendencies (i.e., to act against the activity-related incentives). Kuhl (1983, 1987) described some volitional control strategies, which are summarized in Table 1.

People use the strategies in Table 1 when they force themselves to control their actions in aversive activities (Kuhl, 1996). However, people differ in their ability to do so. Kuhl and Kraska (1993) developed a computer-based method for measuring interindividual differences in volitional action control. Corno (1992, 1995) and Zimmerman (1995b) proposed various methods that teachers might use to improve the volitional control strategies of their students. Some of these strategies are similar to those in Table 1.

TABLE 1   Six Self-Regulatory Strategies (Volitional Control Strategies; see Kuhl, 1985, 1987)

---

1. Attention control
   Active control of attentional focus so as to support the current intention and inhibit the processing of information supporting competing tendencies
2. Encoding control
   Selective encoding of those features of a stimulus that are related to the current intention and its purpose.
3. Emotion control
   Inhibiting emotional states that might undermine the efficiency of the protective function of volition
4. Motivation control
   Strengthening the feedback link from the self-regulatory processes to their own motivational basis
5. Environment control
   Manipulating the environment is a higher order strategy that supports emotion and motivation control strategies (e.g., making social commitments to create social pressure that may help maintain an intention)
6. Cognition control
   Parsimony of information processing and stopping rules to optimize the length of the decision making process, especially if further processing may reveal information that undermines the motivational power of the current intention

---

Given that time is limited and many leisure activities are usually more attractive than studying for an exam, students and adults often have to use volitional control processes. If they are lucky, new incentives arise while doing the activity (activity-related incentives, see Figure 4). For example, fast progress in learning can make the learning activity more attractive than initially expected (for details, see Rheinberg, 1996; see also Table 2). If no such positive incentives arise, then the learning activity has to be maintained continually with volitional control strategies: Learners have to remind themselves why learning is important (i.e., awareness of consequence-related incentives; Figure 4) and have to consciously use self-regulatory strategies. Such strategies can be like either those described in Table 1 or those described by Zimmerman and Martinez-Pons (1988), which are more specific to learning.

For aversive but unavoidable actions, such as quitting smoking or forcing oneself to do tedious physical training, a pure volitional control would be joyless, but possible. However, pure volitional control may be problematic for learning activities. Sokolowski (1993) found that students experienced volitional control as unpleasant and especially effortful. We suspect, that such tightly controlled learning is more inefficient, because the working memory is permanently loaded with self-regulatory strategies. Therefore, less working memory is available for the learning process per se. Evidence for this speculation might be found by directly comparing learning processes that are volitionally regulated with learning processes in which people experience flow (Csikszentmihalyi, 1975). When in flow, the learner becomes so absorbed by the learning activity that they no longer feel the passage of time and do not have any problems focusing on the task; thus, all of their working memory is devoted to the task. Thus, performing the same learning activities might have different effects on learning outcome depending on the learners' functional state during learning (see box 5 in Figure 1). However, this issue still needs a thorough empirical analysis. (For further details, see Rheinberg, 1996; Schiefele & Rheinberg, 1997.)

The more aversive the activity becomes, the more necessary are volitional control strategies. So it has become important to know what makes learning activities per se attractive or aversive. Currently, Rheinberg (1999) is studying the origins of positive and negative incentives in SRL. Table 2 gives the preliminary results of an interview study.

Table 2 presents only sources for those incentives that are effective during learning. Anticipated outcome consequences are not included. Of particular importance are increases in feelings of competence: While learning, the learner feels that doing the task is becoming smoother and easier, and that she or he is becoming better at it. Such feelings are often reported when participating in sports or playing music, but when learning cognitive material, these feelings seem to be less common: Our participants reported these feelings less frequently when they talked about learning on academic tasks. This could be due to the fact that the process of creating these feelings demands comparisons between the current and a previous state. From other studies, it is known already that comparisons

TABLE 2   Sources of Activity-Related Incentives in the Learning Process
(Examples from an Interview Study; Rheinberg, 1999)

Sources of positive incentives
- Learning situation fits the learner's motive structure (e.g., learning together with friends if the learner has a high affiliation motive)
- Learners evaluate the topic highly (fit between personal interest and learning topic)
- Learners feel an increase in competence while learning (requires a concise feedback system and free processing capacity)
- The mental interaction with the learning material makes a coherent structure out of many unlinked details; during learning things get simpler and clearer

Sources of negative incentives
- Learning material (e.g., a textbook) is incoherent
- Single issues do not make sense and have to be learned by heart
- The learning process is constantly interrupted because unknown things (e.g., words, formulas, etc.) have to be looked up and learned
- Intrusion of failing thoughts or emotions during the learning activity, such as when the learners notice that they cannot understand anything, or that even with a maximum effort, they do not succeed

during learning put a load on the working memory (Sweller, 1988). However, the working memory is fully involved in the learning activity itself. Thus, in the case of cognitive learning, it is difficult to perceive the increase in one's own competence during the learning activity and to enjoy such feelings. So, this learning may require additional support more frequently from positively evaluated consequences and volitional processes. Perhaps this is one (out of several) reason why, for many students, cognitive learning is less often a joyful activity in itself, unlike sports or playing an instrument, for example. If this assumption were verified, we would have to think about possibilities for how to improve the ease of evaluation during cognitive learning without interfering with the learning process as such.

III. MOTIVATION, LEARNING, AND PERFORMANCE

Until now we have dealt with questions regarding how motivation and volition arise in learning. Learning motivation even can be conceived as an educational goal that is important in itself (e.g., see Schiefele, Hausser, & Schneider, 1979). Additionally, we may ask how motivational factors influence the process and outcome of learning. We already know that there are only low to medium correlations between some indicators for motivation and some indicators for learning results (see Schiefele & Schreyer, 1994). Little is known, however, about the process by which motivation affects learning and its results. Of course, experts as well as laymen believe that motivation somehow positively influences learning—despite evidence that in some cases overmotivation can be detrimental (Atkinson, 1974; Yerkes & Dodson, 1908). Even if we disregard the latter fact, the question of how motivation in detail fosters learning remains. It could be that motivation and volition promote only contact between the self-regulated learner and the learning material, after which everything can be explained in terms of cognitive processes. Alternatively, could it be that motivational factors also determine how the material is learnt? Surprisingly little is known regarding these questions, perhaps because everybody was certain that motivation improves learning on a molar level, so there was thought to be little need to study the details of the process.

However, some researchers have begun to study how motivation affects the learning process—and not only the learning *result* (e.g., Pintrich & De Groot, 1990; Renkl, 1997; Schiefele, 1996; for a review, see Schiefele & Rheinberg, 1997). In our initial framework (see Figure 1), this research tries to link boxes 4, 5, and 6. The crucial question concerns box 5: What are the variables that mediate the effects motivation (box 4 in Figure 1) has on learning outcome (box 6) during the learning process?

A. MOTIVATIONAL INFLUENCES DURING THE LEARNING PROCESS: TOPIC INTEREST AND TEXT LEARNING

Schiefele (1996) studied this question for text learning. The motivational variable (box 4 in Figure 1) he measured was topic interest. The learning outcome variables (box 6) were based on van Dijk and Kintsch (1983) and were differentiated among verbatim vs. propositional vs. situational representations of the text. Several studies revealed that topic interest was related negatively to verbatim representations, but positively related to propositional representations (for details, see Schiefele, 1996; Schiefele & Rheinberg, 1997). Obviously, motivation (i.e., topic interest) does more than cause and maintain the contact between learner and text. In addition, motivation seems to influence, in some way or other, how the learner interacts with the text. However, what are the variables that mediate the relationship between motivation and performance? How can we understand the specific way topic interest influences text learning? Schiefele measured some affective variables (e.g., arousal, happiness, flow) during learning and some cognitive variables, such as learning strategies (elaboration, underlining, note-taking), attention, or concentration. According to our framework for learning motivation, these variables belong either to the category functional–motivational state of the learner or to the quality of performed learning activities (see Figure 1, box 5).

Schiefele (1996) showed that the affective variables during text learning indeed were related positively to topic interest. However, only one affective variable (i.e., arousal) out of five studies proved to have a significant mediating effect on learning outcome. With regard to cognitive variables, some of them were related to topic interest (e.g., elaborative strategies), whereas others were related to learning outcome (e.g., note-taking). However, for none of them could a significant mediating effect be found. Obviously, there can be no doubt that topic interest influences text learning, because there are reliable positive and negative relationships between these two variables. However, until now it was unclear via what specific variables this influence is mediated.

B. SELF-REGULATED LEARNING WITH A COMPLEX COMPUTER-SIMULATED SYSTEM

In our own research, we have studied motivational effects on learning when learners try to understand and control a complex computer-simulated system (the Biology Lab; Vollmeyer & Rheinberg, 1998; Vollmeyer, Rollett, & Rheinberg, 1997). During a learning phase, participants can detect the system's structure by manipulating input variables and analyzing the resulting effects on the output variables. Participants choose how they do this in detail and how long they work. However, participants know that they have to apply their knowledge after the learning phase. In this application phase, the participants receive goal states for the output variables that they have to reach by entering appropriate inputs. Although the learning situation is clearly structured, the learner is free to choose the activities used to learn how to reach the goal. According to our initial definition, this is a typical case of SRL.

Our experiments last between 1 and 4 hours, and allow repeated measurements of mediating variables during the learning phase. Whereas sophisticated analyses of motivational effects on learning outcome require a differentiation between specific qualities or factors of motivation (Schiefele & Rheinberg, 1997), we do not use a single indicator for learning motivation like strength of motivation or the just mentioned interest. Instead, we assess different motivational qualities with respective to factors of motivation with the Questionnaire for Current Motivation (QCM; Vollmeyer & Rheinberg, 1998). This questionnaire consists of 37 items that reflect motivational qualities participants can experience in this experimental setting (i.e., positive expectancies, fears, challenge, topic interest, etc.). In a series of studies (Vollmeyer & Rheinberg, 1998; Vollmeyer et al., 1997), four factors could be replicated: challenge ("This task is a real challenge for me" or "If I can do this task, I will feel proud of myself"); mastery confidence ("I think I am up to the difficulty of the task" or " I think everyone could do this task"); incompetence fear ("I'm a little bit worried" or "I'm afraid I will make a fool of myself"); interest ("After having read the instruction, the task seems to be very interesting" or "I would work on this task even in my free time"). These factors seem to be relevant for other experimental learning settings as well (e.g., Schoppek, 1997). They do not measure a person's generalized and stable characteristics (box 1 in Figure 1); instead, they assess situation-specific actualized motivation (box 4 in Figure 1).

If we relate these motivational factors to the expanded model of motivation (see Figures 2 and 4), we recognize that these empirically developed factors focus on specific parts of the model: The challenge factor reflects competence-related self-evaluation as a consequence of learning outcome; mastery confidence concerns high action → outcome expectancy; interest refers to object-specific incentives during learning (within-action vs. postaction incentives; see Section II.D); incompetence fear reflects low action → outcome expectancy combined with negative consequences of failure. In our experimental task, we expect positive effects on learning from the first three factors (challenge, mastery confidence, and interest), but negative effects from incompetence fear.

These four motivational factors measure *initial motivation*, that is, motivation when participants are instructed about the task, but have not started with the learning phase. Whereas the initial motivation can change dramatically after participants gain some experience with the task, we repeatedly measure the current motivational state with items such as, "The task is fun" or "I'm sure I will find the correct solution." Moreover, participants repeatedly rate their functional state during the learning phase (e.g., "I have no problems concentrating on the task"). A further repeatedly measured variable is the systematicity of the inputs' manipulations. It is known from earlier experiments (Vollmeyer, Burns, & Holyoak, 1996) that complex tasks like the Biology Lab demand a systematic approach to manipulating the inputs in order to analyze the outputs. However, to practice this systematic approach, learners have to invest some cognitive effort (i.e., for producing and controlling cognitions like hypotheses, complex comparisons, analytic plans, etc.). Unplanned trial-and-error operations require less cognitive effort. However, with this desultory surface strategy, there is no chance to detect the complex structure of the system that has to be controlled later on. In any case, systematicity of participants' approach to the task is repeatedly measured as a quality of performed learning activity. Thus, with the motivational and functional state and with the systematicity of the approach, we measured a set of variables that might mediate the effect initial motivation may have on learning outcome (see Figure 1, boxes 4, 5, and 6). The learning outcome variables are measured, on the one hand, as declarative knowledge about the system's structure and, on the other hand, as procedural competence in controlling the system.

For analyzing our data, mastery confidence and incompetence fear are usually combined into a latent variable that represents initial motivation, because they correlate negatively. Results from Structural Equation Modeling (EQS; Bentler, 1992) revealed that the effects of these latent variables on the acquired declarative knowledge were mediated via the motivational state during learning and the systematicity of the learners' approach. These two mediating variables were related: A positive motivational state during learning increased the probability that learners kept on using a systematic approach in spite of the cognitive effort this kind of learning demands (Vollmeyer et al., 1997). The functional state was more likely to mediate motivational effects on the performance when the acquired knowledge had to be applied (Vollmeyer & Rheinberg, 1998). Unexpectedly, time on task (see Figure 1, box 4) seemed to have no mediating effects in our experimental setting. Probably, this will not be true for SRL in everyday contexts (Helmke & Schrader, 1996).

Similar to other studies (Krapp, 1992, 1993), topic interest correlated with learning outcome (Vollmeyer et al., 1997). However, just as in Schiefele's (1996) studies on text learning, we failed to identify the mediating structure for this relationship, so it remains unknown via which mediators topic interest influences learning. The challenge factor of initial motivation usually had no direct effects on learning outcome. However, this variable seems to be a relevant moderator, at least for experimental settings: Correlations between initial motivation and learning outcome were stronger for learners who perceived the task as a high challenge compared to those perceiving a low challenge. For low-challenged learners, cognitive variables, (i.e., an ability measure and the systematicity) were better predictors for learning than the motivational variables (Rollett, Vollmeyer, & Rheinberg, 1997; similar results were reported by Schoppek, 1997, using a different learning task). Analyses based on dividing participants into different types revealed that there are subgroups of learners with different patterns of relationships between motivational and cognitive variables (Rheinberg & Vollmeyer, 1997).

The results of these and similar experiments have been obtained using specific types of learning tasks and situations. Therefore, they are valid only for comparable learning settings (Boekaerts, 1996). Changing the type of task (e.g., learning a foreign language instead of problem solving) or changing relevant situational features (e.g., salient consequences, distracting incentives of alternative activities, the possibility of postponing learning, etc.) may alter the way motivational factors influence learning and its outcome. Regardless, the reported results are valid at least for individual learners who must use self-regulation when trying to understand and control a complex system. This situation might not be too far from everyday life.

IV. TWO AIMS FOR FURTHER RESEARCH

A. SEARCH FOR MEDIATING VARIABLES IN DIFFERENT SITUATIONS AND LEARNING TASKS

The search for mediators in different situations and learning tasks is an important next step. There is a need to examine to what degree and in what way motivational effects on learning depend on the task and the situation. To state the mere existence of such a dependency is neither novel nor enlightening. In future research, it is necessary to vary systematically relevant characteristics of the task and the situation to study how these manipulations affect the predicted paths between motivation and learning outcome. Stability or change in the pattern of mediating variables may aid understanding of the more fundamental relationships between motivation and cognition.

By searching for mediators, it is possible to gain sophisticated knowledge about learning motivation that is not trivial and already known to everyone. The layman's statement, "Motivation fosters learning—some way or other," will be true for many situations. To go beyond laymen's intuitions, researchers must gain the ability to specify what exactly is meant by "some way or the other" with a specific task in a specific situation. Models that could guide the empirical studies have been presented by Kanfer and Ackerman (1989), Revelle (1989), Rheinberg (1988), Sanders (1983), and Schiefele (1996) (for an overview, see Schneider, Wegge, & Konradt, 1993).

B. HOW TO OVERCOME AVERSIVE LEARNING ACTIVITIES

The second aim for future research arises from the fact that (according to our definition) SRL concerns intentional and deliberate learning activities that are free from external guidance and supervision. Using Heckhausen's (1977) utility-centered model of motivation in SRL situations, we found students who failed to engage in learning activities in spite of highly valued consequences and in spite of favorable expectancies. The reason for such seemingly irrational behavior was found in the activity-specific incentives (see Section II.D). In contrast to instructional controlled learning in school or university, SRL usually has to be engaged in despite competition from perhaps more attractive leisure activities. Thus, the combination of important and reachable consequences of learning outcome with relatively unattractive or even aversive learning activities is likely to occur.

Such a combination causes problems, especially for learners who usually focus on incentives immediately related to learning activity (Rheinberg et al., 1997; see also Apter, 1989). These learners have difficulty forcing themselves to engage in unattractive activities. Research suggests two strategies that could help these learners: one that accepts the relative joylessness of learning activity as something to be worked around, and one that seeks to remove this joylessness. The first strategy flows from the work of Kuhl (1985, 1987), who identified volitional control strategies (see Table 1). Now that such control strategies have been identified, perhaps methods can be developed for training people in the use of such strategies (will training). Such training could provide learners with methods for making themselves do things that have to be done, but are no fun or even are aversive. As discussed already, SRL of this kind will not be only joyless, but also might function on a suboptimal level because the volitional control processes continuously put a load on the working memory and disturb those cognitive processes that lead to learning outcome (see Section II.E; functional state of the learner). Nevertheless, learning takes place. There may be situations in a student's career in which the latter is the only crucial issue.

Corno (1992) and Zimmerman (1995b) discussed methods by which teachers may help their students to increase their self-regulatory competence. These attempts could be enriched by transforming the results from volitional psychology (Heckhausen, 1987; Kuhl, 1996) to training programs for students (e.g., how to practice attention control or encoding control?). In our opinion flow experience (Csikszentmihalyi, 1975) is a powerful instrument to cover relative unattractive action periods, therefore, components of the flow concept should be considered in such training: Students should learn how to arrange the situation, the task, and the sequence of their inner and outer activities to create an opportunity for flow experience (Rheinberg, 1996). Developing and evaluating such standardizable training programs seems a solvable and important task for future research on SRL.

The issue of flow experience leads to the second strategy for overcoming unattractive learning activities. On this path, the aim is to change or enrich unattractive learning activities systematically with components that usually are experienced with highly attractive learning activities. This seems to be a more long-term goal for research, because our current knowledge about sources of positive incentives during learning is quite limited (see Table 2). Thus, the first step is to study and describe such positive incentives during SRL. Building on this knowledge, the second step would be to develop and to evaluate programs that teach students (and teachers) how to make unavoidable learning activities more attractive. For one single component, namely, the incentives of competence-related experience, this two-step strategy already has been carried out (Rheinberg & Krug, 1993; see also DeCharms, 1976).

ACKNOWLEDGMENTS

We thank Bruce Burns, Reinhold Kliegl, and the editors for their helpful comments on this paper. This research was supported by DFG Grant Vo 514/5 to Regina Vollmeyer and Falko Rheinberg and by DFG Grant Rh 14/3 to Falko Rheinberg.

REFERENCES

Ach, N. (1910). *Über den Willensakt und das Temperament* [On volition and temperament]. Leipzig, Germany: Quelle und Meyer.

Aebli, H. (1963). *Psychologische Didaktik* [Psychological didactic]. Stuttgart, Germany: Klett.

Apter, M. J. (1989). *Reversals theory. Motivation, emotion and personality.* London: Routledge.

Atkinson, J. W. (1957). Motivational determinants of risk-taking behavior. *Psychological Review, 64,* 359–372.

Atkinson, J. W. (1974). Strength of motivation and efficiency of performance. In J. W. Atkinson & J. O. Raynor (Eds.), *Motivation and achievement* (pp. 193–218). Washington, DC: Winston.

Bandura, A. (1977). Self-efficacy: Toward a unifying theory of behavior change. *Psychological Review, 84,* 191–215.

Bentler, P. M. (1992). *EQS: Structural equations program manual.* Los Angeles: BMDP Statistical Software.

Boekaerts, M. (1996). Personality and the psychology of learning. *European Journal of Personality, 10,* 377–404.

Bolles, R. C. (1972). Reinforcement, expectancy, and learning. *Psychological Review, 79,* 394–409.

Corno, L. (1992). Encouraging students to take responsibility for learning and performance. *Elementary School Journal, 93*, 69–83.

Corno, L. (1995). Comments on Winne: Analytic and systemic research are both needed. *Educational Psychologist, 30*, 201–206.

Csikszentmihalyi, M. (1975). *Beyond boredom and anxiety.* San Francisco: Jossey-Bass.

DeCharms, R. (1976). *Enhancing motivation: Change in the classroom.* New York: Irvington.

Deci, E. L., & Ryan, R. M. (1985). *Intrinsic motivation and self-determination in human behavior.* New York: Plenum.

Dweck, C. S., & Leggett, F. L. (1988). A social–cognitive approach to motivation and personality. *Psychological Review, 95*, 256–273.

Feather, N. T. (1982). *Expectations and actions: Expectancy-value models in psychology.* Hillsdale, NJ: Erlbaum.

Gjesme, T., & Nygard, R. (1970). *Achievement-related motives: Theoretical considerations and construction of a measuring instrument.* Unpublished manuscript, University of Oslo.

Harlow, H. F. (1950). Learning and satiation of response in intrinsically motivated complex puzzle performance by monkeys. *Journal of Comparative and Physiological Psychology, 43*, 289–294.

Heckhausen, H. (1967). *The anatomy of achievement motivation.* New York: Academic Press.

Heckhausen, H. (1974). *Leistung und Chancengleichheit* [Achievement and equality of chance]. Göttingen, Germany: Hogrefe.

Heckhausen, H. (1977). Achievement motivation and its constructs: A cognitive model. *Motivation and Emotion, 1*, 283–329.

Heckhausen, H. (1987). Perspektiven einer Psychologie des Wollens [Perspectives of psychology of volition]. In H. Heckhausen, P. M. Gollwitzer, & F. E. Weinert (Eds.), *Jenseits des Rubikon* [Beyond the Rubikon] (pp. 121–142). Berlin: Springer-Verlag.

Heckhausen, H. (1991). *Motivation and action.* Berlin: Springer-Verlag.

Heckhausen, H., & Kuhl, J. (1985). From wishes to action: The dead ends and short cuts on the long way to action. In M. Frese & J. Sabini (Eds.), *Goal-directed behavior: Psychological theory and research on action* (pp. 134–160). Hillsdale, NJ: Erlbaum.

Heckhausen, H., & Rheinberg, F. (1980). Lernmotivation im Unterricht, erneut betrachtet [Motivation to learn—reconsidered]. *Unterrichtswissenschaft, 8*, 7–47.

Heckhausen, H., Schmalt, H.-D., & Schneider, K. (1985). *Achievement motivation in perspective.* New York: Academic Press.

Helmke, A., & Schrader, F. W. (1996). Kognitive und motivationale Bedingungen des Studierverhaltens [Cognitive and motivational influences on learning behavior of students]. In J. Lompscher & H. Mandl (Eds.), *Lehr- und Lernprobleme im Studium* [Teaching and learning problems at university] (pp. 39–53). Bern: Switzerland: Huber.

Kanfer, R., & Ackerman, P. L. (1989). Motivation and cognitive abilities: An integrative aptitude–treatment interaction approach to skill acquisition. *Journal of Applied Psychology, 74*, 1125–1143.

Karabenick, S. A., & Yousseff, Z. I. (1968). Performance as a function of achievement level and perceived difficulty. *Journal of Personality and Social Psychology, 10*, 414–419.

Krapp, A. (1992). Das Interessenkonstrukt. Bestimmungsmerkmale der Interessenhandlung und des individuellen Interesses aus der Sicht einer Person-Gegenstands-Konzeption [The interest construct determinants of the interest-action and of individual interests from the perspective of a subject-object theory]. In A. Krapp & M. Prenzel (Eds.), *Interesse, Lernen, Leistung.* [Interest, learning, performance] (pp. 297–330). Münster, Germany: Aschendorff.

Krapp, A. (1993). Die Psychologie der Lernmotivation [Psychology of learning motivation]. *Zeitschrift für Pädagogik, 39*, 187–206.

Kuhl, J. (1983). *Motivation, Konflikt und Handlungskontrolle* [Motivation, conflict, and action control]. Berlin: Springer-Verlag.

Kuhl, J. (1985). Volitional mediators of cognition–behavior consistency: Self-regulatory processes and action versus state orientation. In J. Kuhl & J. Beckmann (Eds.), *Action control: From cognition to behavior* (pp. 101–128). Berlin: Springer-Verlag.

Kuhl, J. (1987). Action control: The maintenance of motivational states. In F. Halisch & J. Kuhl (Eds.), *Motivation, intention, and volition* (pp. 279–292). Berlin: Springer-Verlag.

Kuhl, J. (1996). Wille und Freiheitserleben. Formen der Selbststeuerung [Volition and autonomy. Kinds of self-regulation]. In J. Kuhl & H. Heckhausen (Eds.), *Motivation, Volition und Handlung. Enzyklopädie der Psychologie, C/IV/4* [Motivation, volition and action] (pp. 665–768). Göttingen, Germany: Hogrefe.

Kuhl, J., & Kraska, K. (1993). Self-regulation: Psychometric properties of a computer-aided instrument. *German Journal of Psychology, 17*, 11–24.

Lewin, K. (1951). *Field theory in social science*. New York: Harper & Row.

McReynolds, P. (Ed.). (1971). *Advances in psychological assessment*. Palo Alto, CA: Science and Behavior Books.

Mischo, C., & Rheinberg, F. (1995). Erziehungsziele von Lehrern und individuelle Bezugsnormen der Leistungsbewertung [Educational goals and teachers' preference of individual reference norms in evaluating academic achievement]. *Zeitschrift für Pädagogische Psychologie, 9*, 139–152.

Nicholls, J. G. (1978). The development of the concepts of effort and ability, perception of attainment, and the understanding that difficult tasks require more ability. *Child Development, 49*, 800–814.

Nicholls, J. G. (1984). Achievement motivation: Conceptions of ability, subjective experience, task choice, and performance. *Psychological Review, 91*, 328–346.

Piaget, J. (1936). *La construction de réel chez l'enfant* [The construction of reality in the child]. Neuchâtel, Switzerland: Delachaux & Niestlé.

Pintrich, P. R., & De Groot, E. V. (1990). Motivational and self-regulated learning components of classroom academic performance. *Journal of Educational Psychology, 82*, 33–40.

Renkl, A. (1997). *Intrinsic motivation, self-explanations, and transfer*. Paper presented at the annual meeting of the American Educationalist Research Association, Chicago.

Renninger, K. A., Hidi, S., & Krapp, A. (1992). *The role of interest in learning and development*. Hillsdale, NJ: Erlbaum.

Revelle, W. (1989). Personality, motivation, and cognitive performance. In R. Kanfer, P. L. Ackerman, & R. Cudeck (Eds.), *Abilities, motivation, and methodology: The Minnesota Symposium on Learning and Individual Differences* (pp. 279–341). Hillsdale NJ: Erlbaum.

Rheinberg, F. (1977). *Soziale und individuelle Bezugsnorm.* [Social and individual reference norms]. Unpublished dissertation, Department of Psychology, University of Bochum.

Rheinberg, F. (1980). *Leistungsbewertung und Lernmotivation* [Achievement evaluation and learning motivation]. Göttingen, Germany: Hogrefe.

Rheinberg, F. (1983). Achievement evaluation: A fundamental difference and its motivational consequences. *Studies in Educational Evaluation, 9*, 185–194.

Rheinberg, F. (1988). Motivation and learning activities: How research could proceed. *International Journal of Educational Research, 12*, 299–306.

Rheinberg, F. (1989). *Zweck und Tätigkeit* [Purpose and action]. Göttingen, Germany: Hogrefe.

Rheinberg, F. (1996). Von der Lernmotivation zur Lernleistung. Was liegt dazwischen? [From motivation to learn to learning outcome. What's between both?]. In J. Möller & O. Köller (Eds.), *Emotion, Kognition und Schulleistung* [Emotion, cognition, and academic achievement] (pp. 23–51). Weinheim, Germany: PVU.

Rheinberg, F. (1999). Eigenanreize des Lernens. Was Lernaktivitäten per se attraktiv vs. aversiv machen kann [Incentives of learning activity. What makes learning attractive or aversive?]. Manuscript in preparation.

Rheinberg, F., & Donkoff, D. (1993). Lernmotivation und Lernaktivität: Eine modellgeleitete Erkundungsstudie [Motivation and learning activity: A model guided pilot study]. *Zeitschrift für Pädagogische Psychologie, 7*, 117–124.

Rheinberg, F., Iser, I., & Pfauser, S. (1997). Freude am Tun und/oder zweckorientiertes Schaffen? Zur transsituativen Konsistenz und konvergenten Validität der AF-Skala [Doing something for fun and/or for gain? Transsituational consistency and convergent validity of the Incentive Focus Scale]. *Diagnostica, 2*, 174–191.

Rheinberg, F., & Krug, S. (1993). *Motivationsförderung im Schulalltag* [Motivational training at school]. Göttingen, Germany: Hogrefe.

Rheinberg, F., & Vollmeyer, R. (1997). *Motivation and learning in a computer-simulated system.* Paper presented at the 7th European Conference for Research on Learning and Instruction, Athens, Greece.

Rollett, W., Vollmeyer, R., & Rheinberg, F. (1997). *Situativ angeregte Herausforderung als Moderator für den Erklärungswert motivationaler Faktoren in Lernsituationen* [Challenge as moderator variable for the impact motivational factors have on learning]. Paper presented at the 16th Conference on Motivational Psychology, Potsdam, Germany.

Sanders, A. F. (1983). Towards a model of stress and human performance. *Acta Psychologica, 53*, 61–97.

Schiefele, H., Hausser, K., & Schneider, G. (1979). Interesse als Ziel und Weg der Erziehung [Interest as goal and way of education]. *Zeitschrift für Pädagogik, 25*, 1–20.

Schiefele, U. (1996). *Motivation und Lernen mit Texten* [Motivation and text learning]. Göttingen, Germany: Hogrefe.

Schiefele, U., & Rheinberg, F. (1997). Motivation and knowledge acquisition: Searching for mediating processes. In P. Pintrich & M. L. Maehr (Eds.), *Advances in motivation and achievement* (pp. 251–301). Greenwich, CT: JAI Press.

Schiefele, U., & Schreyer, I. (1994). Intrinsische Lernmotivation und Lernen [Intrinsic learning motivation and learning]. *Zeitschrift für Pädagogische Psychologie, 8*, 1–13.

Schneider, K. (1996). Intrinsisch (autotelisch) motiviertes Verhalten—dargestellt an den Beispielen des Neugierverhaltens sowie verwandter Verhaltenssysteme (Spielen und leistungsmotiviertes Handeln) [Intrinsic motivation: curiosity, play and achievement motivation]. In J. Kuhl & H. Heckhausen (Eds.), *Motivation, Volition und Handlung. Enzyklopädie der Psychologie C/IV/4.* [Motivation, volition and action] (pp. 119–153). Göttingen, Germany: Hogrefe.

Schneider, K., & Kreuz, A. (1979). Die Effekte unterschiedlicher Anstrengung auf die Mengen- und Güteleistung bei einer einfachen und schweren Zahlensymbolaufgabe [The effects of effort on quantitive and qualitative performance in a simple and difficult number symbol task]. *Psychologie und Praxis, 23*, 34–42.

Schneider, K., Wegge, J., & Konradt, U. (1993). Motivation und Leistung [Motivation and achievement]. In J. Beckmann, H. Strang, & E. Hahn (Eds.), *Aufmerksamkeit und Energetisierung. Facetten von Konzentration und Leistung* [Attention and energizing: Facets of concentration and performance] (pp. 101–131). Göttingen, Germany: Hogrefe.

Schoppek, W. (1997). Sollwertabweichung und Valenz bei der Handlungsregulation [Goal discrepancy, valence and the regulation of action]. In H.-P. Langfeldt (Ed.), *Tagung der Fachgruppe Pädagogische Psychologie* (Vol. 6, p. 139). Landau, Germany: Verlag Empirische Pädagogik.

Schunk, D. H., & Zimmerman, B. J. (1994). *Self-regulation of learning and performance.* Hillsdale, NJ: Erlbaum.

Skinner, B. F. (1968). *The technology of teaching.* New York: Appleton-Century-Crofts.

Skinner, E. A. (1996). A guide to constructs of control. *Journal of Personality and Social Psychology, 71*, 549–565.

Sokolowski, K. (1993). *Emotion und Volition* [Emotion and volition]. Göttingen: Germany: Hogrefe.

Sweller, J. (1988). Cognitive load during problem solving: Effects on learning. *Cognitive Science, 12,* 257–285.

van Dijk, T. A., & Kintsch, W. (1983). *Strategies of discourse comprehension.* Orlando, FL: Academic Press.

Vollmeyer, R., Burns, B. D., & Holyoak, K. J. (1996). The impact of goal specificity on strategy use and the acquisition of problem structure. *Cognitive Science, 20,* 75–100.

Vollmeyer, R., & Rheinberg, F. (1998). Motivationale Einflüsse auf Erwerb und Anwendung von Wissen in einem computersimulierten System [Motivational influences on the acquisition and application of knowledge in a simulated system]. *Zeitschrift für Pädagogische Psychologie 12,* 11–24.

Vollmeyer, R., Rollett, W., & Rheinberg, F. (1997). How motivation affects learning. In M. G. Shafto & P. Langley (Eds.), *Proceedings of the nineteenth annual conference of the Cognitive Science Society* (pp. 796–801). Mahwah, NJ: Erlbaum.

Vroom, V. H. (1964). *Work and motivation.* New York: Wiley.

White, R. W. (1959). Motivation reconsidered: The concept of competence. *Psychological Review, 66,* 297–333.

Yerkes, R. M., & Dodson, J. D. (1908). The relation of strength of stimulus to rapidity of habit-formation. *Journal of Comparative and Neurological Psychology, 18,* 459–482.

Zimmerman, B. J. (1995a). Self-regulated learning and academic achievement: An overview. *Educational Psychologist, 25,* 3–17.

Zimmerman, B. J. (1995b). Attaining reciprocality between learning and development through self-regulation. *Human Development, 38,* 367–372.

Zimmerman, B. J., & Martinez-Pons, M. (1988). Construct validation of a strategy model of student self-regulated learning. *Journal of Educational Psychology, 80,* 284–290.

16

MEASURING
SELF-REGULATED
LEARNING

PHILIP H. WINNE* AND NANCY E. PERRY[†]

*Simon Fraser University, Burnaby, Canada
[†]University of British Columbia, Vancouver, Canada

In the past quarter century, research has proliferated on self-regulation and, especially, on self-regulated learning (SRL). Cataloging and synthesizing this literature is now a substantial task, the scope of which is powerfully evidenced by the number and variety of chapters in this handbook. Both basic and applied research need to wrestle with questions about measuring constructs associated with SRL, including components such as metacognition, motivation, and strategic action. Measuring SRL and its components is the topic of this chapter.

Our chapter is divided into four sections. In the first section, we develop key points about measurement in general. In the second section, we describe a model of SRL and its components that researchers and practitioners seek to measure. Next, we survey protocols currently used to measure SRL, including questionnaires, structured interviews, teacher ratings, think aloud methods, error detection tasks, trace methodologies, and observations. In a final section, we constructively critique current protocols for measuring SRL and forecast what measurements of SRL might be like in the future.

Copyright © 2000 by Academic Press.
All rights of reproduction in any form reserved.

I. MEASURING INTERVENES IN
AN ENVIRONMENT

Measuring, except for genuinely unobtrusive measurements (Webb, Campbell, Schwartz, & Sechrest, 1966) and some traces (Winne, 1982), intervenes in a student's environment. We design measurement instruments with an intention to cause the student to recall or to generate a particular kind of response. In this view, instruments for measuring SRL and its components—a questionnaire item, a request to stop and talk about current thoughts, a chapter placed before a student with instructions to make any desired marks on pages of the chapter while studying it for a subsequent test—are, in principle, equivalent to an independent variable in an experiment. Interpreting measurement data, therefore, must attend to the same issues as those related to making valid interpretations of causal factors in general.

Cook and Campbell's (1979) typology of these issues has four main categories. First, issues of statistical conclusion validity concern factors that affect whether covariation between the intervention created by measuring and a student's response (a) can be detected, in the sense of having sufficient statistical power to avoid a false negative conclusion by wrongly declaring the absence of covariation between the measurement intervention and response because of a rare or inadequate sample, and (b) whether covariation has been falsely detected, in the sense of having sufficient statistical confidence to avoid claiming a relationship between the measurement intervention and response that is a false positive. Second, issues of internal validity concern the so-called third variable problem or confounding between the measurement intervention, other factors, and a response. When a response is given to a particular measuring instrument, is the response attributable to that intervention or to some other factor in the student's environment? Third, construct validity of putative causes and putative effects is a set of concerns about whether the instruments, as they are operationally defined, represent the components we intend to measure and not other components, and, whether the response reflects what we intend it to reflect. Finally, external validity or generalizability refers to factors that affect the degree to which the particular intervention and the specific observed response are representative of those in other circumstances or environments.

Messick's (1989) typology is another powerful set of lenses through which to view measurements as interventions. He focuses on issues of construct validity under two main headings. One is whether a construct is underrepresented in the sense that its components are not appropriately included in the measuring instrument and the environment in which that instrument is used to intervene. The other is whether the observed data reflect components that are irrelevant to the focal component.

At least two significant implications follow from characterizing measures of SRL as interventions in an environment. First, to adapt a maxim, no instrument is an island. Care should be exercised to map the environment in which measuring instruments intervene and the nature of the disturbance an instrument makes in that environment. We use this "intrusive" language deliberately because it reminds us that disturbances are, as Messick notes, issues to be investigated as experiments. When we measure, we change the environment.

This first inference leads directly to a second. It is that developers of measuring instruments must recognize they are operationally defining a theory of SRL in the instrument they develop. This is the topic of the next section on modeling SRL.

II. MEASUREMENTS OF SELF-REGULATED LEARNING REFLECT A MODEL OF SELF-REGULATED LEARNING

As the history of science shows, theory typically advances in reciprocal and recursive interaction with work to "engineer" measures related to theory. We believe this same interaction characterizes research and measurement of SRL. From the prior section, we also argue that theorizing should attend to factors of the environment into which measuring instruments are inserted because, if environmental factors are disturbed by measurement interventions, those effects may bear on internal validity and generalizability. Obviously, this complicates theorizing and, as well, work on developing measures of SRL.

A. COMPONENTS OF SELF-REGULATED LEARNING

The term "self-regulated" is associated with forms of learning that are metacognitively guided, at least partly intrinsically motivated, and strategic (Winne, 1995, 1997; Zimmerman, 1990). Metacognition is the awareness learners have about their general academic strengths and weaknesses, cognitive resources they can apply to meet the demands of particular tasks, and their knowledge about how to regulate engagement in tasks to optimize learning processes and outcomes. Intrinsic motivation refers to self-regulated learners' belief in incremental learning, a high value placed on personal progress and deep understanding as opposed to besting peers or impressing others, high efficacy for learning, and attributions that link outcomes to factors under their control (e.g., effective use of strategies). "Strategic" describes the way in which these learners approach challenging tasks and problems by choosing from a repertoire of tactics those they believe are best suited to the situation, and applying those tactics appropriately. From this description, it is plain that many facets of SRL are not readily observable. Therefore, one challenge in studying SRL is to find ways to document its components.

SRL has properties of an aptitude and an event (Winne, 1997; Winne & Stockley, 1998). An aptitude describes a relatively enduring attribute of a person that predicts future behavior. For example, a student answering a simple question about whether she or he adapts studying to the circumstances of assignments might say "Yes." On this basis, we might predict the student would study for tomorrow's quiz differently than when preparing an outline for a term project. Moreover, it should not matter whether the question is asked when the work is handed in or a week before, and it should not matter whether the quiz is about history and the project is on biology or vice versa.

An event is like a snapshot that freezes activity in motion, a transient state embedded in a larger, longer series of states unfolding over time. Although our everyday sense of time is one of an unbroken flow, measured time is not continuous. At fundamental physical levels and at levels that characterize SRL, time happens in discrete chunks. As a temporal entity, an event therefore has a beginning and an end; for example, an endpoint in an oscillating crystal or a decision to try a different tactic when studying does not seem to be progressing well enough that is made following deliberation. The event prior to the current one is like a brief-lived aptitude that may predict the next event. Two main features that differentiate aptitude measures of SRL from event-related measures of SRL are discussed throughout the next two sections: aggregation and the kind of information represented in the measurement.

B. SELF-REGULATED LEARNING AS APTITUDE

When SRL is measured as an aptitude, a single measurement aggregates over or abstracts some quality of SRL based on multiple SRL events. For instance, in the context of a student studying for a quiz, a researcher may be interested in metacognitive monitoring concerning a rehearsal tactic. The student's description of self-regulation might be recorded in several forms: a rating on a questionnaire item, an interviewer's classification of the student's response to a probe about what activities were used to study for the quiz, or the proportion of particular kinds of notes written in a textbook chapter. In each case, the student or the researcher abstracts over multiple events of monitoring to characterize the set of those events in a single datum generated in response to the measurement intervention. Measurements of SRL as aptitude often are used to predict whether a student will or will not, can or can not act on an SRL-related cognition such as a belief about performing a study tactic. In this sense, a measure-

TABLE 1   Components of Self-Regulated Learning as Aptitude

Metacognitive knowledge
- Knowledge of fine-grained cognitive operations that comprise cognitive tactics
- Knowledge about strategies that articulate cognitive tactics
- Procedural knowledge that enacts cognitive tactics
- Conditional knowledge about occasions to enact cognitive tactics
- Knowledge of tasks' parameters (e.g., resources, standards for success)
- Knowledge of self-parameters (e.g., interest, effort)

Metacognitive monitoring
- Difficulty in addressing the task (ease of learning, EOL)
- Match of achievement to standards (judgments of learning, JOL)
- Probability of retrieval from long-term memory (feeling of knowing, FOK)
- Confidence about the accuracy of monitoring

---

ment of SRL as aptitude is unary—it can stand alone, independent of other measurements.

The most common protocols for measuring SRL as an aptitude include questionnaires and structured interviews, although teacher ratings have been used also (Zimmerman & Martinez-Pons, 1988). When measured as an aptitude, SRL varies within individuals over relatively long time periods, within individuals across different tasks and settings, and across individuals (Pintrich, Wolters, & Baxter, in press; Winne, 1996). In Table 1 (modeled after Pintrich, Wolters, & Baxter, in press) we list facets of SRL as aptitude that have been examined in contemporary research.

C. SELF-REGULATED LEARNING AS EVENT

An event spans time, but is marked off along a timeline by a prior event and a subsequent event. We propose that SRL measured as an event has three successively more complex levels: occurrence, contingency, and patterned contingency.

An occurrence of SRL as event is observed when there is a transition from a first state, where an observable feature indicating SRL was not in existence, to a second state, where an indicator of SRL is present. For instance, suppose a student is solving a geometry problem and thinking aloud as the task unfolds. The student might muse aloud, "Wow, this is hard!" To have made that judgment, we presume the student monitored the current state of the task. Every monitoring event must use standards as points against which to monitor, and the standards used here might have been the number of steps taken so far, the time taken to reach this point in the task, or a revised estimate of the probability that the goal or endpoint of the task will be achieved (Winne, 1997). To count the student's report as SRL requires inferences that (a) one or more of those scales for judging task difficulty exceeded a threshold that had not been crossed previously, (b) the student thereby classified this task as "difficult," and (c) said so as a consequence of these cognitions. Note that the occurrence of metacognitive monitoring was not directly measured, but the student's report is interpreted as indirect evidence that it occurred.

SRL as a contingency has the form of a binary conditional relationship. It is often modeled in if–then form. Some data describe each of the ifs and other data describe the then. For example, if we observe the student who exclaimed, "Wow, this is hard!," to then take out note paper and make a note, there are two measurements—one of metacognitive monitoring of the difficulty of a task in progress and a second of metacognitive control exercised when the student made the note. This if–then contingency is an elemental cognitive tactic. Over repeated occurrences, the transition from the prior state—monitoring difficulty—to the subsequent state—exercising metacognitive control—can be quantified by a probability that the if transitions to a particular then. A probability of 1.0 indicates that the prior if is always followed by a specific then state. A transition probability less than 1.0 indicates the if state is followed by at least two then states. Whereas probabilities must sum to unity, the relative likelihood of each can be known. If a transition probability is less than 1.0 and only one then state is represented in the observer's measurement system, the system is incomplete, measurements of the if and then states are unreliable, or both.

SRL as a patterned contingency assembles several singular if–then contingencies into a structured ensemble (Corno, 1993; Winne, 1995, 1996, 1997). For example, several basic cognitive tactics might be arrayed as a cognitive strategy involving decision making (monitoring) that selects (controls) which particular tactics are applied in a task as a function of on-line feedback the student generates or receives from external sources (Butler & Winne, 1995; Winne, 1995). Graphic representations of SRL as a patterned contingency might resemble flow charts or path models (Winne, Gupta, & Nesbit, 1994), where the arrows or lines are labeled with probabilities of transitioning from a prior state to a subsequent one.

D. THE SELF-REGULATED LEARNING MODEL
OF WINNE AND HADWIN

A full view of SRL as an event spans three and sometimes four phases (Winne & Hadwin, 1997). Within a phase, cognitive operations, labeled as the Operation(s) box in Figure 1, construct a particular kind of product. Four kinds of products, enumerated in the box labeled Products, differentiate the four phases. In this model, information can play one of four roles: a condition, a product, an evaluation, or a standard. The arrows in Figure 1 represent paths along which information flows to update conditions, products, evaluations, and standards. Also depicted in Figure 1 are two events critical to SRL: metacognitive monitoring and metacognitive control.

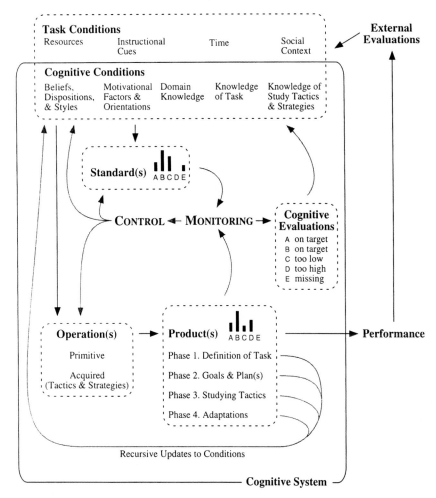

FIGURE 1   A four-stage model of self-regulated learning. From "Studying as self-regulated learning," by P. H. Winne and A. F. Hadwin, (1998), in D. J. Hacker, J. Dunlosky, & A. C. Graesser (Eds.), *Metacognition in Educational Theory and Practice*. Hillsdale, NJ: Erlbaum. Copyright 1998 by Lawrence Erlbaum Associates. Reprinted with permission.

Phase 1. Defining the Task

In Phase 1, the learner generates perceptions of the task at hand. These perceptions may be simple portraits, but they are more likely elaborate, multifaceted, personalized blends of information attended to in the environment plus memories about similar tasks experienced previously (Butler & Winne, 1995; Winne, 1997). There are two sources of information that contribute to these perceptions in Winne and Hadwin's model. Task conditions provide information about the task in the environment "as it is." Cognitive conditions are memorial representations of some features of similar past tasks. These features might include knowledge of the domain(s) of the task (e.g., spelling, searching the Internet), memories about self in relation to the task (e.g., attributions for qualities of prior achievements, interest), and memories about tactics and strategies applied in previous encounters with the same or similar tasks.

Cognitive operations such as searching memory work on conditions to create a definition of the task, thereby creating the first product listed in the Products box in Figure 1. We hypothesize that students generate at least two products in Phase 1. One is a default perception that characterizes the task if it is addressed using a standard or routine approach, whatever the student views that to be. The second perception is a hypothesis about what the task will be like if a nonstandard approach is taken. This hypothesis seems necessary on logical grounds: Even if there is just one tactic the student perceives as standard for the task, the student can exercise agency in Phase 3 to engage that tactic or to dismiss it (see Winne, 1997), the latter being the nonstandard approach. We conjecture that recognizing the existence of choices like this is one hallmark of SRL.

Phase 1 definitions of a task can be metacognitively monitored relative to standards. In Figure 1, five such standards are listed in the Standards box, abstractly labeled A, B, C, D, and E. Suppose the student is reading a chapter in an ecology text that has proved to be very demanding to understand and that standard B refers to amount of domain knowledge. This standard derives from a cognitive condition, a belief, the student holds. The height of the bar for standard B indicates the student believes that a lot of domain knowledge is required when studying this text.

The first sentence in the chapter, "Recall the model of the water cycle presented in the last chapter," is a task condition. By applying cognitive operations to this information, the student defines this task in terms of the domain knowledge it entails. This is represented by the tall bar associated with B in the Product box. If this product is monitored against its corresponding standard, the cognitive evaluation that results is a judgment about how equipped the student is to approach the task as he or she defined it, represented in the box of Cognitive Evaluations, where factor B is described as on target. If this were the only facet of the task considered, the student probably would exercise cognitive control to continue to Phase 2 because the perception generated about the task seems accurate enough to proceed.

Tasks are likely represented by more than a single facet of information, however. Other facets of this task—A, C, D, and E—constitute the student's full definition of the task. Monitoring the match of each of these products against their respective standards may lead to other forms of metacognitive control that recycle through Phase 1 to redefine the task. For example, suppose standard D refers to epistemological beliefs about the worth of spending effort to study ecology from the text. The student's initial standard for this was zero, but information available in the task's presentation, perhaps an indication of how significant the water cycle is to understanding conservation of rain forests, leads him or her to define the task as one involving a strong correlation between effort and worth. The student may be drawn to exercise metacognitive control in a form that reevaluates the task's conditions and to develop a new definition of the task. Similar flows of information occur within and between other phases of Winne and Hadwin's model.

Phase 2. Setting Goals and Planning How to Reach Them

Cognition in Phase 2 is decision making, supplemented by information retrieved from memory, to frame goals and assemble a plan for approaching them. In Figure 1, goals appear in the Standards box and are modeled as multivariate profiles of information (Butler & Winne, 1995; Winne & Hadwin, 1998). Each standard that makes up a goal profile is a value against which processes and products of engagement can be monitored. By cycling through this stage, the student may affirm precursors to goals that are initially developed in Phase 1 or the student may update a goal for the task that will have been generated during engagement with the task's central work, reserved for Phase 3. Once goals are active, memory may automatically retrieve tactics or strategies coupled to them (McKoon & Ratcliff, 1992). Plans constituted this way are a common sign of expertise.

As was the case with Phase 1, activities in Phase 2 may involve several cycles "around" the model when cognitive evaluations are not on target and lead the student to reframe cognitive conditions, or seek to change task conditions.

Phase 3. Enacting Tactics

Applying tactics and strategies identified in Phase 2 marks a transition into Phase 3, where tactics copy information into or construct information in working memory. Tactics are bundles of memories comprised of conditional knowledge (ifs that characterize a tactic's appropriateness) and cognitive operations (thens that change and construct information). Contemporary theory suggests that conditional knowledge consists of two classes of information. *Cold propositions* describe what a tactic is and does. *Hot propositions*—efficacy expectations, outcome expectations, incentives associated with completing (or failing to complete) a task, and attributions —are motivational beliefs that give rise or link to affect (Pintrich, Marx, & Boyle, 1993; Winne, 1995, 1997; Winne & Marx, 1989).

The cognitive and behavioral products that tactics create also are modeled as a multivariate profile. When the student monitors products, this generates internal feedback. If the products of Phase 3 are translated into overt behavior, external feedback also may be available from the environment when, say, a computer command fails to work or a peer remarks on qualities of a student's answer to a question.

Phase 4. Adapting Metacognition

Optionally, in Phase 4, the student makes major adaptations to those parts of the model under the student's control. This is accomplished (after Rumelhart & Norman, 1978) in three ways: by accreting (or deleting) conditions under which operations are carried out or by changing operations themselves, by tuning features that account for how tactics articulate as an event, or by significantly restructuring cognitive conditions, tactics, and strategies to create very different approaches to addressing tasks (Winne, 1997).

Although Figure 1 may imply that SRL unfolds as a linear sequence of phases, this is not likely the case. SRL is recursive in two ways. First, as illustrated for Phase 1, information generated in a particular phase may feed back into that same phase if metacognitive monitoring identifies a difference between the current state of cognition and a standard (goal). Second, the product of monitoring in a later phase may feed into a prior phase, as when a judgment about how well a "tried and true" tactic worked in Phase 3 invites the student to recalibrate initial perceptions about the task's difficulty or complexity available from Phase 1. In this sense, SRL is weakly sequenced. Once a first perception of a task is generated in Phase 1, information generated in that and any subsequent phase may jump phases or recurse to the same phase.

The Centrality of Monitoring and Feedback in Self-Regulated Learning

Metacognitive monitoring is the gateway to self-regulating one's learning (Butler & Winne, 1995; Winne, 1996, 1997) because without the cognitive evaluations it creates, there is no standard against which to enact regulation. Like other cognitive operations, monitoring produces information, a list of matches and mismatches between (a) the standards for a task and (b) a representation in working memory of the product(s) of (a phase of) a task. As illustrated earlier, when a student develops a definition of a task in Phase 1, that perception may be monitored relative to memories about similar prior tasks. In Phase 3, monitoring operations contrast the products that have been created so far in the task against standards (goals) framed in Phase 2. The products of monitoring, labeled cognitive evaluations in Figure 1, can update to any or all of (a) task conditions, for example, if the student is prompted to ask a question of the teacher that leads to a change in resources provided for the task, (b) cognitive conditions, for instance, when a student revises motivational elements that bear on the task, (c) standards (goals) the student assigns to the task, and (d) products generated in a first cycle of cognition or on the basis of recursive cognition, for instance, changing the tactics selected for approaching the goal. Within limits of cognitive resources—the student's cognitive conditions and working memory capacity—and given particular external task conditions—resources, instructional cues, time, and social factors—these updates afford potential for the student to exercise metacognitive control that adapts engagement in mid task.

E. SUMMARY AND PRELUDE TO MEASUREMENTS OF SELF-REGULATED LEARNING

Winne and Hadwin's (1998) model identifies four phases of a task's history that are differentiated by products created in each phase. Each product constitutes a different focus for metacognitive monitoring and metacognitive control that enact forms of self-regulation. Although monitoring is common across the phases as the trigger for cognitive control that enacts regulation, information monitored varies as a function of the product in a phase.

We believe this model affords views of SRL that suggest alternative approaches to measuring SRL as an aptitude and as an event. For example, think aloud protocols invite learners to describe unique task conditions and cognitive conditions within which they consider adapting a cognitive tactic based on cognitive evaluations of products created in Phase 3. Survey questions, in contrast, characterize a general or default set of conditions and, in reference to it, invite the student to construct or recollect a memory of some SRL event(s) that is (are) most probable (modal), significant (unique), or representative (median). In the former case, the data available allow measurements of elements in Phases 1 and 2. In the latter case, although elements of Phases 1 and 2 are not part of the observed measurement, they are nonetheless central to how the student responds. These kinds of differences open different windows onto views of SRL. In the next sections, we contrast these measurement approaches using features of Winne and Hadwin's model.

III. PROTOCOLS FOR MEASURING SELF-REGULATED LEARNING

This section describes seven protocols for measuring SRL. We group protocols according to whether they assess SRL as an aptitude or an event. Due to space limits, we have selected one or two well-known examples of each protocol and described them in detail. These protocols and measures focus on cognition and behavior related to learning in common educational settings such as schools, studying at home, or learning in computer environments.

A. MEASURING SELF-REGULATED LEARNING
AS AN APTITUDE

Self-Report Questionnaires

Self-report questionnaires are the most frequently used protocol for measuring SRL, perhaps because they are relatively easy to design, administer, and score. These measures inherently provide (a) information about learners' memories and interpretations of their actions and (b) their explanations of cognitive and metacognitive processes researchers cannot observe (Turner, 1995). Typically, self-report questionnaires measure SRL as an aptitude because items ask respondents to generalize their actions across situations rather than referencing singular and specific learning events while learners experience them.

A survey of conference programs and abstracting services will turn up scores of self-report questionnaires. We describe two of the most used of these, the Learning and Strategies Study Inventory (LASSI; Weinstein, Schulte, & Palmer, 1987) and the Motivated Strategies for Learning Questionnaire (MSLQ; Pintrich, Smith, Garcia, & McKeachie, 1991). Both are frequently used in research and, to our knowledge, are the only two self-report inventories that are accompanied by a manual. Other examples of inventories include the Index of Reading Awareness (Jacobs & Paris, 1987) and the Metacognitive Awareness Inventory (Schraw & Dennison, 1994).

Questionnaires are typically developed according to a three-slot script. First, after items are collected or written, an exploratory factor analysis of a sample's responses is done to examine correspondences between those responses and the model of SRL developers used to generate individual items. Second, reliability coefficients, almost always coefficients of internal consistency, are reported for the full scale and subscales, if there are any. Finally, the full scale and its subscales are correlated with external measures, almost always achievement. We use this script to describe the LASSI and the MSLQ.

Learning and Study Strategies Inventory (LASSI).   The LASSI (Weinstein et al., 1987) is a published, standardized, normed 77-item self-report inventory "designed to measure use of learning and study strategies" (Weinstein, 1987, p. 2) by undergraduate students. Items are simple declarations (e.g., I try to interrelate themes in what I am studying) and conditional relations (e.g., When work is difficult, I either give up or study only the easy parts). Students respond using a 5-point scale: not at all typical of me, not very typical of me, somewhat typical of me, fairly typical of me, and very much typical of me. Each of these options is elaborated by a sentence in instructions to students. For instance, "By fairly typical of me, we mean that the statement would be true of you about half the time."

The *LASSI User's Manual* (Weinstein, 1987) states that "no total score is computed since this is a diagnostic instrument" (p. 3). Uses for scores are suggested. For example, "If a student scores poorly on the Test Strategies Scale, she should be advised to concentrate at least part of her efforts on learning more about how to prepare for and take tests" (p. 3).

The LASSI can be self-administered and self-scored, and a scoring booklet is available for this purpose. It instructs a student how to compute subscale scores by adding items that form the subscale. On a separate page, the student places Xs in a column of numbers labeled by each subscale, then connects the Xs to draw a "learning and study strategies profile." The scores in each column are spaced to correspond to percentiles provided in the table's outside leftmost and rightmost columns. However, no instruction is given for interpreting a percentile other than to indicate it provides a comparison "in relation to other college students answering the same items."

Development of the LASSI included pilot testing of an initial pool of 645 items, interviewing students who took preliminary versions of the inventory, and eliminating items that correlated substantially ($\geq$ .50) with a scale of social desirability. Items on the 1987 version are grouped to form 10 nonoverlapping subscales. On a self-scoring guide, these are labeled (1) attitude and interest, (2) motivation, diligence, self-discipline, and willingness to work hard, (3) use of time management principles for academic tasks, (4) anxiety and worry about school performance, (5) concentration and attention to academic tasks, (6) information processing, acquiring knowledge, and reasoning, (7) selecting main ideas and recognizing important information, (8) use of support techniques and materials, (9) self testing, reviewing, and preparing for classes, and (10) test strategies and preparing for tests. The inventory has been normed on "a sample of 880 incoming freshman at a large southern university" (Weinstein, 1987, p. 5) and stability coefficients over a 3-week interval were calculated on a sample of 209 students in an introductory communications course. The *User's Manual* reports coefficients of internal consistency and test–retest coefficients for each subscale. Alphas range from .68 to .86 and stability coefficients range from .72 to .85.

Motivated Strategies for Learning Questionnaire (MSLQ). Pintrich and his colleagues developed the MSLQ (Pintrich et al., 1991) "to assess college students' motivational orientations and their use of different learning strategies for a college course" (p. 3). Items are simple declarations (e.g., I make good use of my study time for this course) and conditional relations (e.g., when reading for this course, I make up questions to help focus my reading). Students record answers to items using a 7-point scale anchored by not at all true of me (1) and very true of me (7). Instructions are to "answer the questions about how you study in this class as accurately as possible."

The inventory's 81 items manifest a hierarchical design, where subscales are nested within sections nested within one of two broad categories, motivation or learning strategies. The motivation category has a value section with three subscales—intrinsic goal orientation, extrinsic goal orientation, and task value—and an expectancy section that consists of three subscales—control of learning beliefs, self-efficacy for learning and performance, and test anxiety. The learning strategies category is divided into two sections. A cognitive and metacognitive strategies section includes subscales labeled rehearsal, elaboration, organization, critical thinking, and metacognitive self-regulation. A resource management strategies section has subscales of time and study environment, effort regulation, peer learning, and help seeking. Subscale scores are means of responses to subscale items after flipping some items that are worded contrary to the subscale's construct.

The authors provide examples of feedback sheets that can be returned to students. Each sheet provides a short paragraph describing the construct a subscale is intended to reflect; a list of items comprising the subscale; blanks to be filled in for the student's score, the class mean and scores at quartile boundaries (25th, 50th, and 75th percentiles); and a paragraph of suggestions about how to improve standing on that facet of motivation or learning strategy.

Development of the inventory spanned approximately 3 years, during which time items were tried and revised based on the results of factor analyses, reliability analyses, and correlations with measures of achievement. Because the MSLQ is designed to be used in individual courses, norms have not been developed. The inventory's manual reports subscale and item-level means, standard deviations, and correlations with final grade for a sample of university ($N = 356$) and community college ($N = 24$) students spanning 37 classrooms and 14 subject domains. Alpha internal consistency coefficients for subscales range from .52 to .92.

Separate confirmatory factor analyses have been computed for the motivation section and the learning strategies section using data from the aforementioned sample. The manual (Pintrich et al., 1991) reports that "while goodness of fit indices are not stellar, they are, nevertheless, quite reasonable values, given the fact that we are spanning a broad range of courses and subject domains" (pp. 79–80). We observe that coefficients from this analysis that are parallel to item–factor correlations often are less than a cutoff that the manual describes as appropriate for well-defined constructs. Among the six motivation subscales, phi values (interpreted like correlation coefficients) range from −.17 to .83. Phi coefficients among subscales in the learning strategies section range from .07 to .85. The authors conclude that "overall, the models show sound structures, and one can reasonably claim factor validity" (Pintrich et al., 1991, p. 80).

Structured Interviews

Interviews span a variety of protocols ranging from a simple query such as, "Tell me about how you ...," to highly structured scripts that list specific questions that are asked verbatim along with rules that control which particular following or follow-up question is posed conditional on information a student has just related. We differentiate interview protocols from a closely related protocol, think aloud (see the beginning of Section III.B), by a simple criterion: If the student is prompted to describe SRL while engaging with an authentic task, the method is a think aloud and SRL is measured as an event. In contrast, if the student is prompted to describe SRL based on memories about what is "typical" of behavior under a certain set of circumstances or to offer judgments about what probably would be typical behavior in a plausible future situation, the protocol is an interview and SRL is measured as an aptitude. Stimulated recall is an interview in which respondents describe their behaviors after completing a specific task and sometimes while reviewing records of engagement with that task, such as a videotape or worksheets. In this case, SRL may be construed either as an event or an aptitude, depending on particulars of the measurement intervention.

Interviews generate verbal descriptions. There are two fundamental alternative approaches to analyzing these descriptions: emergent and theory driven. Analyses that adopt an emergent method seek to identify classes or categories of SRL in the student's descriptions without enforcing a particular or a priori framework. This protocol is "bottom-up" in the sense that features in the material are the origins of classes or categories. We point out that it is not possible to be rid of all one's prior perceptions in applying an emergent method. To do so logically would prevent using any language or learned symbol system to examine, classify, and interpret emergent data. Rather, emergent methods strive to avoid prejudging what should be examined and how information should be classified. The alternative to emergent analyses are theory-guided analyses. These begin with a set of types or classes of data relative to which the students' description of SRL will be classified or quantified. It is a "top-down" approach. These two approaches are readily and often profitably combined in work that tests or extends a theory.

It is a misconception that emergent protocols are devoid of quantitative features. When unique instances of SRL are identified, these instances are assigned a count of 1. When interpretations characterize a class of SRL events as common (or rare), this entails comparing counts, that is, frequencies. If conditional relationships are described, a probability of the transition from condition to a particular following state is inherent in the description, even if it is not estimated with precision.

Self-Regulated Learning Interview Schedule (SRLIS).   The SRLIS was developed by Zimmerman and Martinez-Pons (1986, 1988) to explore SRL among high school students. It is a theory-guided, structured interview protocol. Table 2 lists 15 classes of SRL identified by the SRLIS in terms of Winne and Hadwin's (1998) model of SRL (Figure 1). Data about SRL-related behaviors are elicited by having students consider a contextualized but fictitious task. For example, two of six tasks included in the SRLIS are as follows: "Assume a teacher is discussing a topic with your class such as the history of the civil rights movement. He or she says that the class will be tested on the topic. Do you have a method to help you learn and remember what was discussed in class?" and "Most students find it necessary to complete some assignments or prepare themselves for class at home. Do you have any particular methods for improving your study at home?" (Zimmerman & Martinez-Pons, 1988, p. 285). If a student does not answer or indicates the protocol is not understood, a follow-up prompt is given: "What if you are having difficulty? Is there any particular method you use?" (Zimmerman & Martinez-Pons, 1988, p. 285).

TABLE 2   Classes of Self-Regulated Learning in the Self-Regulated Learning Interview Schedule

Class	Description relative to Winne & Hadwin's Model[a]
Self-evaluation	Monitoring products relative to standards
Organizing and transforming	Overt or covert rearrangement of resources
Goal setting and planning	Adopting or generating standards and planning the sequence, timing, and completion of activities
Seeking information	Searching for updates to conditions in nonsocial resources
Keeping records and monitoring	Logging information in an external form about conditions, operations, and products
Environmental structuring	Selecting or arranging task conditions
Self-consequences	Updating cognitive conditions (rewards and punishments) following monitoring of a product's standards
Rehearsing and memorizing	Overt or covert rehearsing
Seeking help from peers	Updating task conditions by asking peers for information
Seeking help from teachers	Updating task conditions by asking the teacher for information
Seeking help from adults	Updating task conditions by asking an adult (e.g., a parent) for information
Reviewing tests, notes and textbooks	Updating cognitive conditions, such as domain knowledge, and potentially cognitively operating on them again
Other	Unsolicited task-related information originating with an external source (e.g., peer, teacher, computer)

[a]All are student-initiated except behaviors falling in the Other class.

Three procedures have been used to score interviews (Zimmerman & Martinez-Pons, 1986, 1988). First, a dichotomous score describes whether a student uses a class of SRL. This is based on whether information referring to that class appears at least once in the transcript where the student describes how a task is addressed. Second, a frequency score is created by counting the number of instances of each class of SRL. In their 1986 study, Zimmerman and Pons observed that none of the classes of SRL was mentioned more than once in any of the six tasks, so this score reflected the number of tasks in which a particular class of SRL was used. A third method, yielding what Zimmerman and Martinez-Pons label a consistency score, is to ask students, after they have described how they address a task, to rate how consistently they use the classes of SRL they described. Ratings are made on a 4-point scale: seldom, occasionally, frequently, and most of the time. Although this consistency rating superficially resembles a questionnaire protocol (see the beginning of Section III.A), it differs in the SRLIS in that the student has just generated a description of how a context is addressed. In contrast, in almost all questionnaires, context and tasks within them are quite general such as "when you study" or "in this course."

A significant issue in scoring data generated by interviews is the degree to which scorers agree. After training raters on interview data gathered during pilot work, Zimmerman and Martinez-Pons (1986) reported that two scorers agreed at an 86% level when the number of categories scored identically was divided by the total number of unique categories identified by both scorers.

In the study by Zimmerman and Martinez-Pons (1986), participants attended schools that streamed students into an advanced achievement track or several other lower achievement tracks. The researchers used a dichotomous indication of ability, advanced track or other, as a criterion variable in a discriminant function analysis where predictors were scores on strategy use, strategy frequency scores, and strategy consistency ratings. The analysis was able to identify 91% of students correctly by track with a discriminant function that had standardized coefficients of $-.66$ for strategy use, .41 for strategy frequency, and 1.12 for strategy consistency rating (all coefficients $p < .001$).

Teacher Judgments

In their daily interactions with students, teachers are uniquely positioned to judge qualities of students' SRL. Typically, they base their judgments on event-related measures using trace methods and think aloud protocols that we describe later. In research, however, teacher judgments have been used infrequently as measures of students' SRL, perhaps because some researchers question the trustworthiness of these data (see Hoge & Butcher, 1984). A particular concern has been teachers' ability to distinguish between related constructs such as achievement and ability, or achievement and motivation. Reviews, however, indicate that teachers' judgments can avoid these shortcomings and serve as worthy assessments of students' achievement-related behaviors (Hoge & Coladarci, 1989; Perry & Meisels, 1996). According to Perry and Meisels, three conditions are required to achieve this status. First, judgment measures should be direct; that is, ask about distinctive observable student behaviors that reflect a small number of clear and distinct categories or constructs. Second, measures should be criterion-referenced or ask teachers to compare students to a familiar and stable norm group, such as comparing a target student to other students in their current class or to all students they have taught in the past. Third, teachers should be given specific and understandable metrics in terms of which to report judgments. Perry and Meisels also recommend triangulating teacher judgments with data gathered by other protocols.

Rating Student Self-Regulated Learning Outcomes: A Teacher Scale. Zimmerman and Martinez-Pons (1988) posited that teachers are uniquely positioned to observe students' SRL during daily classroom activities, and they developed an instrument that meets Perry and Meisels' (1996) criteria. Zimmerman and Martinez-Pons investigated relationships between students' reported use of SRL strategies, teachers' observations of students' SRL in classroom activities, and students' performance on a standardized achievement test, the Metropolitan Achievement Test (MAT). Zimmerman and Martinez-Pons predicted that teachers' ratings of students' SRL would correlate substantially with students' reported use of SRL strategies and moderately with students' performance on the MAT, because standardized measures assess aspects of students' abilities/learning that are distinct from SRL.

In their study, 80 grade 10 students (44 boys, 36 girls) that represented a range of achievement levels first described their SRL in an interview using the SRLIS protocol described previously. When students described one or more strategies for a given task, they were asked to rate the consistency with which they used each one on a 4-point scale.

Three teachers (two males) were asked to rate their own students' SRL as they had observed it in their classrooms using the Rating Student Self-Regulated Learning Outcomes: A Teacher Scale. The 12 items on this protocol were based on the same 14 categories of SRL in the SRLIS (Zimmerman & Martinez- Pons, 1986). Some strategies in the SRLIS are not reflected in the teacher judgment measure because they reflect self-regulating behaviors that typically occur outside the presence of teachers, such as structuring the environment to complete a homework assignment.

Items on the teacher judgment scale were worded as questions about observable behaviors; for example, "Does this student solicit additional information about the exact nature of forthcoming tests?" Teachers were instructed to rate individual students on each item according to a 5-point scale: 1 = never; 5 = always. Some items referred to students' direct use of a strategy, such as seeking teacher assistance, seeking information, and self-evaluating. Other strategies, such as organizing and transforming information or goal setting and planning, required teachers to judge observable outcomes of strategy use, such as whether the student completed assignments on or before a specified deadline and whether the student set goals and made plans. The three teachers represented three disciplines—English, social studies, and mathematics—and no two teachers shared students.

The reliability of the teachers' ratings, according to the Kuder–Richardson formula 20, was .95. An obvious issue in teachers' judgments of their students' SRL is whether students' observable behavior reveals enough of the students' cognitions. To examine this concern, Zimmerman and Martinez-Pons correlated the teachers' ratings of students' SRL with students' self-reports about using SRL strategies. The correlation was $r = .70$. Although this correlation cannot reveal whether teachers' judgments matched the frequency of students' SRL, it does show strong proportionality. Consistent with the researchers' hypotheses, teachers' ratings correlated moderately with students' MAT scores, $r = .43$.

B. MEASURING SELF-REGULATED LEARNING AS AN EVENT

Think Aloud Measures

The think aloud is a protocol in which a student reports about thoughts and cognitive processes while performing a task. Teachers long have used this method when they request of students, "Explain your work." The think aloud protocol can be as unstructured as that or it can follow a formal, conditional script that dynamically adjusts which questions or comments an observer makes depending on how the student behaves or whether the student mentions particular information.

A detailed scientific consideration of think aloud protocols and the data they generate was provided by Ericsson and Simon (1984/1993), but the protocol has been used for several thousand years according to Boring (1953). The area in which think aloud approaches to measuring SRL have been most popular is reading. Pressley and Afflerbach (1995) compiled and examined findings from 38 primary think aloud studies dealing with metacognition and SRL in reading. A notable feature of the set of studies they reviewed is diversity: Samples ranged from fourth-grade students to university professors; topics spanned almanacs, poetry, excerpts from short stories and novels, scholarly research publications, and computer programs. Methodologies also varied. Readers were set a variety of goals at the outset, the two most common being preparing for a test and reading as one normally would to be able to use the information afterward.

In some studies that Pressley and Afflerbach reviewed, the reader's thinking aloud was generated concurrently while reading. There were several variations about when readers were to provide descriptions: whenever the reader wanted (which signals at least that monitoring occurred); retrospectively at points within a task chosen by the observer, as when readers were interrupted every 2 minutes or upon completing each sentence or a section of text; or upon completing an entire reading assignment. Pressley and Afflerbach also noted that the studies they reviewed provided varying instructions about what readers were to report. This feature varied from the observer modeling the procedure of thinking aloud in general, to providing no guidance about what the reader was to report, to naming specific types of events or information (e.g., elaborations, predictions) that were targets of an investigation.

Verbal accounts generated by think alouds are analyzed subsequently using a protocol like that described by Zimmerman and Martinez-Pons (1986). The primary purpose for using think aloud protocols is to map out models of SRL. Except for seeking to determine whether raters agree on assigning readers' descriptions to categories, there is little other standard information about measurement properties of the think aloud protocol.

Error Detection Tasks

As noted earlier, metacognitive monitoring that identifies discrepancies between a goal and a current state of a task is the trigger for SRL. Cognitive evaluations produced by metacognitive monitoring then serve as a basis for deciding how to proceed with the task, thus exercising metacognitive control. To measure the monitoring that is a precursor to control, researchers have sometimes introduced errors into materials that students study or use in a task and then observed whether (a) the errors are detected and (b) what students do when they detect them. This protocol is known as the error detection method (Baker & Cerro, in press; Garner, 1987). Several variations of error detection have been developed with respect to (a) the context within which students report errors and (b) measurements that reflect detection (monitoring) of errors and subsequent exercise of metacognitive control.

Regarding contexts for reporting errors, students can be informed about the presence of errors in material after they study it or before. When students are not told about the presence of errors in the material, the context is plausibly more typical of everyday studying, because students justifiably should be able to assume that materials they use in learning have not purposefully been corrupted. In both contexts, it has been shown that a critical feature of measurement is information given to the student about the nature of errors. For instance, students can be given a very general description of error as "something that might confuse people or something that people might have trouble understanding" (Baker & Zimlin, 1989, p. 342). Alternatively, they can be thoroughly instructed, including being given criterion-referenced tests to validate the effects of that intervention, about types of errors that might appear in material, such as external consistency (created by replacing a word in a sentence with one that makes the meaning implausible or untrue), structural cohesiveness (adding information that fits the general theme of materials, but is irrelevant to the task at hand), and incompleteness (deleting information) (Baker & Zimlin, 1989).

Indicators that students monitor materials for errors have taken several forms including asking students to underline or otherwise mark spots where there is an error. Provided the student limits underlining to these instances, this identifies the extent to which a student discriminates errorful from error-free information. Another kind of data used to indicate monitoring has been eye fixations. This protocol requires an assumption that the duration of a fixation indicates monitoring versus other cognitive operations such as decoding. However, indications of monitoring alone are not sufficient to imply SRL. There also must be an indication of control.

In studies of reading comprehension, students' tendencies to engage in SRL have proven to be a drawback in measuring students' ability to detect errors. For instance, in her inaugural study of monitoring while reading a text that was corrupted with errors, Baker (1979) observed that adults who were not informed about the presence of errors appeared quite incompetent in locating them. After the study period, her readers could identify an average of only 38% errors overall and, more importantly, they reported noticing only 25% of the errors while they were studying the material in the first place. On examining recall measures, Baker observed that readers did not misrepresent or omit information, as might have been expected due to errors added to the study material. She interpreted that readers exercised control after recognizing errors by applying automatic fix-up tactics to repair them. In other words, it was because they engaged in SRL while studying that the readers were relatively unable to recall, recreate, or classify errors in the material they studied. In this sense, accurate recall of information in study material that contained an error indicates that SRL was applied provided that reconstructive memory was not the source of correct information appearing in the recall. Moreover, when the student cannot remember that an error was repaired, this plausibly indicates that monitoring and control were automatic, beneath levels of conscious inspection (see Winne, 1995).

Trace Methodologies

Traces (Winne, 1982) are observable indicators about cognition that students create as they engage with a task. When a student underlines or highlights material in a text, for example, this creates a trace signaling that the student discriminated marked content from other information. If the student writes material in the margin that labels or comments about particular marked text, the information provided by that annotation may allow an inference about standards the student used for selecting the marked text. Such annotations also may provide information about metacognitive control exercised. For instance, if the note contained a recognizable mnemonic that was not provided in the text, this reveals the student sought to control the likelihood of subsequent retrieval of information.

To make interpretations about standards used in metacognitive monitoring and cognitive operations applied in exercising metacognitive control, traces must be coupled with a model of cognition. For instance, suppose the student writes "See p. 23" in the margin next to some underlined text on page 30. Under Winne and Hadwin's (1998) model of SRL (Figure 1), this indicates that one of student's current goals is to off-load into that permanent comment an otherwise challenging demand on memory to remember that a comparison tactic should be applied to the highlighted information at a later time, say, during review of the material for a test. It might be plausible to infer further qualities about cognitive conditions, such as that the student holds (a) a belief that such demands on memory are likely to exceed capabilities and (b) has an epistemological view that effort applied to link material across pages 23 and 30 has value.

Under current models of memory search (e.g., McKoon & Ratcliff, 1992), the trace just described also implies that the student searched memory for a particular kind of information, namely, comparative information. When one or several candidates were retrieved, monitoring was applied to judge whether its attributes could be compared to information marked by the underline. Because we (presumably) know how the subject matter is organized, it also may be possible to infer standards the student used to monitor the success of the memory search.

Howard-Rose and Winne (1993) described trace methods in a study of SRL. Some traces they observed were unobtrusive. When students underlined, put a check near a block of information (e.g., a cell in a table), or inserted an asterisk into material, they inferred the student had discriminated that marked information from surrounding material. When students copied information into notes from a text or other resources, this was taken to indicate they had rehearsed that information. If the student wrote in their notes a phrase such as, "Think I'll ask the others in the group what they did for this part," it was inferred that students held a belief that a social or a material resource could help in addressing the task at hand. Students also were observed to write phrases in notebooks that signaled they were assembling information into larger units, such as when they developed a summary of material or drew a personal analogy to material they studied. They also tallied instances when students wrote comments about tactical planning, such as "How much of this activity will I need to do?," and monitoring, such as "This task is confusing." (All these examples of student statements were reported in Howard-Rose & Winne, 1993, p. 594.)

One trace in Howard-Rose and Winne's (1993) study was intrusive in the sense that students were instructed to monitor task engagement in ways that were not natural and to record perceptions about that engagement. It concerned attending to thoughts or events not relevant to the task at hand (e.g., I wonder what Joey's doing now?). Students wrote an "A" in the margin of the materials they used when they noticed off-task thoughts or behavior.

Except for concern about observer agreement in coding traces, an issue that is well known and understood, there is little information about measurement issues and uses of trace methods.

Observations of Performance

Recently, research on SRL has expanded to investigate relationships between contexts for learning and student behaviors. This reflects contemporary, sociocognitive views of learning that prompt researchers to consider how features that constitute contexts for learning, such as task structures, authority structures, and evaluation practices, influence students' beliefs about themselves as learners, their goals and expectations, and their decisions about how to regulate their behavior in learning activities (Perry, 1998; Pintrich, Marx, & Boyle, 1993).

Observations have three strengths as measurements in research on SRL (Turner, 1995). First, like trace protocols, they reflect what learners do versus what they recall or believe they do. Second, observations allow links between learners' behaviors to task conditions, especially those where feedback is available within the boundaries of a task. Finally, observations can ameliorate difficulties associated with assessing young children's SRL such as positive response bias and the children's limited language for describing cognitive processes.

Turner (1995) observed SRL events to investigate how classroom reading tasks influence young students' use of reading and learning strategies, persistence, and volitional control among average achieving students in first-grade classrooms. The observation system was divided into three sections. The first recorded identifying data: the name of the child being observed, their classroom, and the date and time span of observation. In the second section, observers used narrative protocols to describe students' behaviors and the instructional context as field notes. The third section provided checklists regarding five broad categories of reading strategies that Turner developed inductively by observing students engaged in reading tasks over a 3-month pilot study, and deductively by matching those records to research on motivation and strategic action. The categories of strategies were decoding (e.g., using graphophonemic or context cues), comprehension (e.g., predicting, summarizing), general learning (e.g., rehearsing, elaborating, organizing), volitional control (e.g., preventing or ignoring distractions), and persistence (e.g., through a difficult task, to correct errors). Observation data were supplemented by student interviews and detailed field notes collected over 5 consecutive days in each participating classroom to characterize teachers' approaches to reading instruction (whole language or basal) and reading tasks/activities in each classroom.

A time sampling procedure was used to collect observation data about SRL. Over the course of a reading or literacy activity, occurrences of any predefined SRL events were marked as present or absent at the end of each successive 3-minute segment. The frequencies of marks over the course of the activity were then dichotomized to reflect the presence or absence of each SRL event within the activity; that is, the measurement protocol was a sign system. Observers sat near target students and recorded in the narrative section frequencies of particular student behaviors as well as verbalizations, facial expressions, gestures such as finger pointing, eye movements, and writing. Immediately following each observed activity, observers interviewed students about the task they had just completed. The interview protocol included four open-ended questions designed to assess students' awareness of two key facets of SRL: the purposes of particular tasks and thinking during task engagement. Two tests of reliability were applied to student observation data: coder speed agreement, which reflected whether observers recorded the same number of behaviors for the same child, and coder category agreement, which addressed the extent to which observers agreed on the category assignment for individual behaviors. Coder speed agreement was 99% and coder category agreement was 89%.

Perry (1998) used Turner's (1995) measurement design as a model for her observational procedures to investigate young children's SRL in select writing contexts. Perry's observation instrument also had three sections. The first section recorded identifying data. The second section was a specimen system (Evertson & Green, 1986), where observers kept a running record of what was going on, including verbatim transcripts of teachers' and students' speech. SRL events were subsequently coded as present or absent.

In Phase 1 of Perry's three-phase study, the third section was a checklist of features of classroom contexts theorized to promote SRL, including items describing students' choices, control over challenge, opportunities for self-evaluation, and teacher and peer support. In Phase 3 of the study, the third section was a checklist of items describing behaviors associated with SRL such as writing strategies, portfolio strategies, executive strategies (e.g., modifying tasks or the environment to control challenge), and evidence of persistence. After each observation period, events and actions recorded in the running record were matched to items on the checklist. In Phase 1, a rating of 0, 1, or 2 was assigned to items on the checklist to code presence and quality in the observed activity. For example, if students had no choice concerning what to write, the "choice about what" item was rated 0. If student choices were relatively unconstrained, a rating of 2 was recorded. In Phase 3, behaviors associated with SRL were coded present or absent. A second rater was used to test interobserver agreement. Agreement between raters was 88% for Phase 1 observations and 97% for Phase 3 observations.

Turner's (1995) and Perry's (1996) observation systems take first steps toward providing data amenable to examining relationships among instructional contexts, the task conditions in Winne and Hadwin's (1998) model, and forms of SRL observable in students' engagements with tasks. In particular, they illustrate measurement protocols for assessing young children's motivation and competence as self-regulated learners in naturalistic contexts. By combining qualitative and quantitative methods, they also couple descriptions of an individual student's processes with general trends for larger groups (Many, Fyfe, Lewis, & Mitchell, 1996). Finally, they illustrate good practice by triangulating observations with measurements from questionnaires, interviews, and samples of students' work.

IV. ISSUES IN MEASURING SELF-REGULATED LEARNING

Although protocols for measuring SRL are new, principles regarding the validity of measurements are not. By and large, the measures of SRL we reviewed here have been well examined in terms of these principles (see also Pintrich et al., in press). Moreover, in general, each instance of the seven methodologies we reviewed provided models and useful starting points for furthering understandings about SRL as aptitude and as event. Beyond these accomplishments, there remain significant issues to address in striving to advance the quality of measures of SRL and thereby enhance understandings about SRL itself. We consider these issues in five main categories.

A. TARGETS FOR MEASUREMENT

Measurements grow out of a view about what to measure and about a metric for measurements. Along with Pintrich et al. (in press) and Schraw (in press) and Schraw, Wise, and Roos (in press), we note that much basic research remains to develop better models of SRL as guides for developing measures of SRL. However, as we noted earlier, this is a recursive bootstrapping process. Models of empirical phenomena depend on empirical feedback about their validity. Empirical feedback is gathered by measuring phenomena using protocols that are structured by models as well as measurement issues.

We adopted Winne and Hadwin's (1998) model of SRL as a basis for considering measures of SRL because it synthesizes from the current research literature a wide range of targets that can be measured to achieve a full view of SRL (Figure 1). Some targets—elements of task conditions, performance, and external feedback—are observable in the environment of a self-regulating student. Other targets—elements of cognitive conditions, standards used in monitoring, cognitive representations of stages that describe a task, primitive and acquired operations carried out that constitute engagement with the task, and cognitive evaluations—are constructs that must be inferred on the basis of externally observable behaviors.

We know of no measure of SRL that simultaneously and fully represents all these targets for measurement. Instead, what is practiced and practical is to focus on one or a small set of targets while controlling for others in an immediate periphery and while ignoring yet others outside that periphery that a model labels as extraneous relative to interpretations to be drawn from measurements. For example, a questionnaire protocol typically presumes that students have knowledge of the various study tactics and strategies mentioned in items that ask students to rate a tactic's or strategy's frequency of use or importance. In making their judgments about a tactic or strategy, students are directed to use a peripheral context such as "in this course" (Pintrich et al., 1991) that sets some task conditions to a constant value, but excludes others. Extraneous factors are presumed to "zero out" in group data due to randomization, but they remain as complications to interpreting data about an individual.

Boundaries that separate focal targets from peripheral targets from extraneous components are created by one's model of SRL. Issues of how effectively a measurement intervention operationalizes those boundaries, such that the measurement protocol causes data to be generated that can reflect focal targets validly, are those Cook and Campbell (1979) and Messick (1989) describe in their typologies of factors that affect drawing valid causal inferences. In both systems, the root of these factors is the model of SRL. We take it as obvious that the field must continue to bootstrap models of SRL concomitantly with developing better measures of SRL.

B. METRICS

Skirting the mathematical basis of measurement theory (e.g., see Cliff, 1982; Michell, 1990), a metric involves two basic qualities: a unit in terms of which a phenomenon is measured and rules by which measurements can be manipulated. For instance, Turner's (1995) and Perry's (1998) classroom observation systems for recording students' SRL defined a unit as acts differentiated by breaks in a stream of behavior. Subsequently, acts were categorized.

The operation of categorizing assumes a quality of equivalence among members of the category, specifically, that one instance can be substituted for another with neither loss of information nor introduction of irrelevant variance. This assumption allows a counting rule to be applied to acts within a category that aggregates them unit by unit to form a sum of counts or frequencies. In practice, it is almost always assumed further that a unit in one category is comparable to a unit in another category. This allows frequencies of acts to be compared across categories. It is rare for those who develop protocols for measuring SRL in any of the seven methodologies we reviewed to be this specific in defining measurements. Although such examinations should not consume research efforts, more attention could be given to issues of metrics.

Regarding the unit of a metric, Howard-Rose and Winne (1993) raise questions about the grain size of units. Grain size issues concern the dimensions of a datum that constitutes a unit. For instance, a trace in which a student circles a clause and draws an arrow connecting that circle to a term in a preceding paragraph is a small grain unit relative to a questionnaire item such as "I link up different bits of information." The labels of tactic and strategy also reflect differences in grain size, the latter being larger grained in two senses: it requires multiple tactics and it involves decision making to select those alternative tactics (Winne, 1995). Another variant of the grain size issue is the time span of a unit. An occurrence event occupies a briefer span of time than a contingency or a patterned contingency. An aptitude is theorized to be enduring, at least over the course of a research investigation that may span a few weeks.

We observe that models of SRL commonly characterize events as small grain units, whereas aptitudes and contextual factors, such as prior knowledge and classroom climate, respectively, are quite large grained. Care needs to be taken when metrics for measurements vary. Now that many macroelements of SRL—planning, monitoring, evaluating—are well documented, researchers are turning attention to more in-depth and fine-grained investigations of individuals' processes as they navigate specific learning activities (Many, et al., 1996; Winne, Hadwin, McNamara, J. K & Chu, 1998a). Assuming normal arithmetic operations are valid within a metric, as is almost always done in research on SRL, researchers need to examine whether usual transformations that standardize units are appropriate for units that originate within metrics of quite different grain size. This issue requires blending basic principles of metrics with other assumptions that underlie statistical treatments of data, and it merits further study given current models of SRL.

Finally, our notion of SRL as event (Winne, 1997; Winne & Stockley, 1998) introduces new issues in measuring SRL. Patterned contingencies that represent dynamic SRL events can be described using statistics adapted from graph theory (Winne et al., 1994), but units can become quite complicated when multiple, fine-grained if–then pieces are aggregated to characterize larger grained SRL strategies. The measurement properties of such large grain patterns are not known. Whereas every model of SRL of which we know includes targets like this, this area needs much work. A first step is to gather extensive descriptions about SRL as events in forms that allow studies of patterned contingencies. Computer-supported learning environments (e.g., see Winne, 1989; Winne & Field, 1998; Winne et al., 1998a) that constitute authentic contexts for studying as they gather trace data about SRL events are promising tools for these efforts.

C. SAMPLING

Every measurement is a sample of behavior. Two fundamental questions should be addressed based on this fact. First, what are characteristics that define the population from which the sample is drawn? Second, what qualities of the population are reflected in the obtained sample, to what degree, and how accurately?

Issues about characterizing the population from which a sample is drawn are evident in measurement protocols where the student's responses are selections of information from memory. Self-report questionnaires, structured interviews, and teacher judgments are three such protocols. To our knowledge, there are no well founded understandings about attributes of the personal "historical" database of events that a student searches as the basis for generating responses to questions.

The same issue applies to measurement protocols such as think aloud, traces, and classroom observations. For example, if a student does not carry out a SRL event, does this reflect (a) absence of critical components for that act of self-regulation, (b) a production deficiency, wherein those components are available to the student but not retrieved and brought into working memory to be topics of metacognitive monitoring and control, or (c) an act of self-regulation, wherein the student exercised metacognitive monitoring and control to omit a potential self-regulating act? Each of these options implies a different population from which measurements are sampled and, thus, has implications that bound valid interpretations about SRL.

A parallel issue concerns contextuality or its opposite, generalizability. To the extent that tasks differ and thereby shape perceptual and other cognitive processing that constitutes SRL, measurements will reflect contextuality. While the model portrayed in Figure 1 represents a range of factors that might constitute context, there is little work to date on how such differences affect measurements of SRL beyond documenting that students rate components of SRL differently as a function of task (e.g., Hadwin, Winne, Stockley, Nesbit, & Woszczyna, 1997). We recommend that measurements of SRL include more information than most now do about the products of Phase 1 in self-regulating learning, the definition of the task.

A further issue about individual differences in SRL concerns interactions between domain knowledge, the substance worked on in a task, and SRL per se. Expertise sidesteps some elements of self-regulation because knowledge in the domain of expertise encodes what a novice would need to "directly" self-regulate (Winne, 1995, 1997). We suggest that measurements of SRL should pay more attention to qualities of a student's domain knowledge to tease apart, as much as possible, SRL events from expertise.

In measuring achievement and some other variables, a distinction can be made between measures of maximum ability and typical ability. A questionnaire item might ask students to rate "how true is it of you" that "I try to play around with ideas of my own related to what I am learning in this course" (item 66, MSLQ, Pintrich et al., 1991). A trace protocol might count "blocks" of handwritten text in the margin of a textbook chapter where the student is judged to do the same. Are these measurements of typical ability or would data differ if students were asked or instructed to do this as often or as well as they could? Measures of SRL should distinguish whether they describe typical or maximum ability, a point Baker and Cerro (in press) also noted about error detection methods in general.

Features of the sample itself vis-à-vis the population also need attention. For instance, when asked to judge categorical features of SRL, such as the presence or absence of various self-regulating acts, how fully is the population of memories searched that are relevant to this question? A particularly interesting issue from our point of view is how the student assigns a value to an instance or description of self-regulation, such as its importance or frequency. What algorithm does the student use: averaging, ordinal dominance reflecting the most frequent or salient category, recency of occurrence, or some other rule? These questions concern calibration, the accuracy with which perceptions correspond to actual SRL events. They all concern decision making because whenever there are options about responses, the student must make a decision about how to match response options to a memory. Beyond Butler and Winne's (1995) discussion of some paths for exploring these issues, we know of no work on matters such as these that underlie interpretations about how measurement interventions give rise to responses.

D. TECHNICAL ISSUES

The literature on technical qualities of measures is vast and the list of possible issues to be taken up in measuring SRL is correspondingly numerous and novel. To illustrate, if trace measures are measures of ability, new work could be initiated to explore item response characteristics of trace measures as indicators of ability and difficulty. Excluding issues such as these, there remain important technical topics to be given more attention in future work on measuring SRL.

Reliability is a fundamental necessity of high quality measurements. Two methods have been applied regularly in work to date: internal consistency for measures generated by self-report and interobserver or intercoder agreement for the other measurement protocols.

Noticeable by its absence is concern for stability, the extent to which measurements do not vary over time. Stability is a difficult concept to apply to measures of SRL because, by definition, SRL is adaptive and should vary over time under certain conditions. In our view, this tension affords thinking about future work on measuring SRL in two ways. First, high stability should be observed when contexts in which SRL might be applied are homogenous. In contrast, stability should be low when contexts are heterogeneous. This tension may be helpful in bootstrapping better understandings about sampling issues in measurements of SRL. Second, when contexts vary, models of SRL lead to the prediction of high stability for a measure of "adaptiveness." However, to our knowledge, there are no such measures yet available. One possibility is a measure of conditional probability for transitions to different learning tactics (i.e., applications of metacognitive control) given metacognitive monitoring that identifies differences in context. The graph theoretic measures proposed by Winne et al. (1994) may be a starting point for work on this issue.

Another area requiring attention in measuring SRL links to Cook and Campbell's (1979) concerns about the construct validity of putative causes and effects, paralleled by Messick's (1989) focus on construct relevant versus irrelevant variance within a measurement. To date, except for correlations of SRL with achievement, there is little information kinds that can be revealed by multitrait–multimethod investigations of convergent and divergent validity (cf. Zimmerman & Martinez-Pons, 1988). As depicted in Winne and Hadwin's (1998) model, a variety of cognitive and motivational individual differences are components in an overall portrait of SRL. Multitrait–multimethod studies would help the field focus on the center of SRL and its relationships to peripheral variables. Given that measures of SRL as an event logically entail individual differences regarding beliefs and motivational variables (Pintrich, et al., 1993; Winne & Marx, 1989), it seems imperative that multitrait–multimethod studies receive quick attention.

We note that, except for the LASSI (Weinstein et al., 1987), which provides a manual plus norms based on one university sample, and the MSLQ (Pintrich et al., 1991), which also has a manual and encourages users to create local norms using quartiles, there are very few attempts to standardize and norm measures of SRL. This perhaps reflects several factors: the newness of work on measuring SRL, the field's flexibility in adopting models that guide the development of measurement protocols, and genuine questions about what would be useful norms relative to purposes for measures of SRL. The absence of standardized measurement protocols also may reflect researchers' interests in tailoring measures of SRL to context or students' developmental levels, components explicitly identified in Winne and Hadwin's (1998) model. In light of the list of issues raised so far in this section, standardizing and norming measures of SRL will be a very complex undertaking.

The LASSI (Weinstein et al., 1987) is the only measurement system that invites ipsative (within person) comparisons. Specifically, it instructs each student to draw a profile of scale scores, based on percentile transformations of raw scores relative to the LASSI's norm group, and then to compare levels of scales. Ipsative comparisons are fraught with potential difficulties, two significant ones being the typically very large standard error of an individual's scale score and the implicit suggestion that scores across scales are independent when correlations show they are not. We urge caution in this use of measurements of SRL as well as further research on how improvements might be made in this use of scores describing SRL.

E. UTILITY

Measurements are collected for purposes, and purposes can be served more or less usefully; that is, measurements have varying degrees of utility for particular purposes. The most prevalent purpose of SRL measures is description in basic research. The LASSI (Weinstein, 1987) and MSLQ (Pintrich et al., 1991) invite students to self-diagnose qualities of their approaches to learning and SRL, but formal studies of their diagnostic utility have not been done. We are not aware that any other measures of SRL have been used for formal diagnosis or evaluation in schools or training situations.

For all methods but self-report questionnaires, gathering and scoring measurements of SRL is quite resource intensive. Potential relief may be on the horizon in the form of computer technologies, such as Winne, Hadwin, McNamara, Chu, and Field's (1998) prototype notetaking system, CoNoTES. Systems such as CoNoTES can administer and score self-report questionnaires, record traces of SRL as students engage with and adapt during tasks, and use both kinds of measurements as triggers for adapting interaction with the student; for example, by presenting or withholding objectives or self-test questions. Other information to be learned and tools to use in learning, such as a find tool or a note template, also can be made available to a student based on single, profile, or pattern measurements of SRL, thereby extending protocols to adapt dynamically to a student's engagement. This kind of software also could be configured to record audio for collecting think aloud data or to present a structured interview where branches in the interview protocol were followed depending on the student's response to forced-choice items. Work on this front appears to offer considerable promise in measuring SRL as both aptitude and event.

Software systems such as CONOTES will have limited utility in the immediate future for three reasons. First, few researchers or students have access to them. Second, even if such systems are practically unobtrusive to students, the tools they provide as venues for recording SRL events constitute interventions that can alter, sometimes substantially, how students engage with tasks. Third, techniques need to be invented that validly combine information gathered through software protocols with other data gathered through currently popular methods such as portfolio assessments, performance assessments, process approaches to writing instruction, journals, and other self-assessment systems.

Whatever protocols might be practical in educational contexts, two other issues need special attention. First, teachers will need support to learn about and appropriately interpret measures of their students' SRL. Second, developmental differences need investigation with respect to how well measurement protocols work across the age spectrum. This work should address questions about developmental trajectories that bear on the models of SRL that undergird measurement protocols per se.

V. CONCLUSIONS AND FUTURE DIRECTIONS

Research on SRL and measurement protocols used in this research are relatively new and inherently intertwined enterprises. Each helps to bootstrap the other. We adopt the view that a measurement protocol is an intervention in an environment, disturbing it in a fashion that causes data to be generated. Using that data and a logic of causal inference, we infer properties and qualities of a target of measurement. Thus, measurement involves understandings about a target, its environment, and causal relationships that connect the two. Under this view, measurement is akin to model building and model testing (Cliff, 1982), and, thus, all measures of SRL are reflections of a model of SRL.

We propose that SRL has dual qualities as an aptitude and an event (Winne, 1997; Winne & Stockley, 1998). It is situated within a broad range of environmental plus mental factors and potentials, and manifests itself in recursively applied forms of metacognitive monitoring and metacognitive control that change information over time as learners engage with a task (Winne & Hadwin, 1998). Each of the seven measurement protocols we reviewed—self-report questionnaires, structured interviews, teacher judgments, think aloud measures, error detection tasks, trace methods, and observations of performance—foregrounds different components of conditions, cognitive operations, standards, and event-related change. Matching what a measurement protocol foregrounds to the purpose for measuring SRL takes a first step toward providing a basis for valid interpretations.

In our judgment, three topics about measuring SRL merit special emphasis in future work. First, too little has been achieved yet in measuring SRL as an event. Challenges in this arena are significant. Protocols are needed for collecting longitudinal measurements that span multiple brief episodes, such as activities, as well as extended periods, such as grade levels. In characterizing SRL as an event, point estimates derived from these data, such as means, are not appropriate descriptions. Methods are needed that (a) characterize temporally unfolding patterns of engagement with tasks in terms of the tactics and strategies that constitute SRL and (b) compare patterns over time to reflect regulation per se (Perry, 1998; Winne et al., 1994). In addition, work is needed on how measures of SRL as aptitude and SRL as event can be coordinated to characterize the full spectrum of SRL.

Second, triangulation across measurement protocols is too infrequent. Because each protocol generates slightly different reflections of SRL, a fuller understanding of models and methods can be achieved by using multiple measurement protocols in research. We recognize that measurements generated by different protocols may not be commensurate even if all are indicators of aptitude or of events. The challenge of commensurability affords opportunity to further understandings about technical features of scales, data, rules for aggregating data, and rules for comparing measurements. We predict that advances on these fronts will correspond to advances in modeling SRL.

Third, research into SRL and its measurement has so far included a limited range of populations, most often involving postsecondary students as participants in studies. Very little is known about young children's SRL. Until measurements are collected across the age spectrum, understandings about measurement protocols and about developmental trajectories will remain elusive.

ACKNOWLEDGMENT

Work on this chapter was supported in part by grants from the Social Sciences and Humanities Research Council of Canada to Philip H. Winne (No. 410-95-1046, #410-98-0705) and Nancy E. Perry (No. 410-97-1366).

REFERENCES

Baker, L. (1979). Comprehension monitoring: Identifying and coping with text confusions. *Journal of Reading Behavior, 11,* 365–374.

Baker, L., & Cerro, L. C. (in press). Assessing metacognition in children and adults. In G. Schraw (Ed.), *Metacognitive assessment.* Lincoln: University of Nebraska Press.

Baker, L., & Zimlin, L. (1989). Instructional effects on children's use of two levels of standards for evaluating their comprehension. *Journal of Educational Psychology, 81,* 340–346.

Boring, E. (1953). A history of introspection. *Psychological Bulletin, 50,* 169–189.

Butler, D. L., & Winne, P. H. (1995). Feedback and self-regulated learning: A theoretical synthesis. *Review of Educational Research, 65,* 245–281.

Cliff, N. (1982). What is and isn't measurement. In G. Keren (Ed.), *Statistical and methodological issues in psychology and social sciences research* (pp. 59–93). Hillsdale, NJ: Erlbaum.

Cook, T. D., & Campbell, D. J. (1979). *Quasi-experimentation: Design and analysis issues for field settings.* Chicago: Rand-McNally.

Corno, L. (1993). The best-laid plans: Modern conceptions of volition and educational research. *Educational Researcher, 22*(2), 14–22.

Ericsson, K. A., & Simon, H. A. (1984/1993). *Protocol analysis: Verbal reports as data.* Cambridge, MA: MIT Press.

Evertson, C. M., & Green, J. L. (1986). Observation as inquiry and method. In M. C. Wittrock (Ed.), *Handbook of research on teaching* (3rd ed., pp. 162–213). New York: Macmillan.

Garner, R. (1987). *Metacognition and reading comprehension.* Norwood, NJ: Ablex.

Hadwin, A. F., Winne, P. H., Stockley, D., Nesbit, J. C., & Woszczyna, C. (1997, March). *Contexts and goals as moderators of students' reports about how they study.* Paper presented at the meeting of the American Educational Research Association, Chicago, IL.

Hoge, R. D., & Butcher, R. (1984). Analysis of teacher judgments of pupils achievement levels. *Journal of Educational Psychology, 76,* 777–781.

Hoge, R. D., & Coladarci, T. (1989). Teacher-based judgments of academic achievement: A review of the literature. *Review of Educational Research, 59,* 297–313.

Howard-Rose, D., & Winne, P. H. (1993). Measuring component and sets of cognitive processes in self-regulated learning. *Journal of Educational Psychology, 85,* 591–604.

Jacobs, S. E., & Paris, S. G. (1987). Children's metacognition about reading: Issues of definition, measurement, and instruction. *Educational Psychologist, 22,* 255–278.

Many, J. E., Fyfe, R., Lewis, G., & Mitchell, E. (1996). Traversing the topical landscape: Exploring students' self-directed reading–writing–research processes. *Reading Research Quarterly, 31,* 12–35.

McKoon, G., & Ratcliff, R. (1992). Inference during reading. *Psychological Review, 99,* 440–466.

Messick, S. (1989). Validity. In R. L. Linn (Ed.), *Educational measurement* (3rd ed., pp. 13–103). New York: Macmillan.

Michell, J. (1990). *An introduction to the logic of psychological measurement.* Hillsdale, NJ: Erlbaum.

Perry, N. E. (1998). Young children's self-regulated learning and contexts that support it. *Journal of Educational Psychology, 90,* 715–729.

Perry, N. E., & Meisels, S. J. (1996). *How accurate are teacher judgments of students' academic performance?* Working paper series, National Center for Educational Statistics. Washington, DC: U.S. Department of Education, Office of Research and Improvement.

Pintrich, P. R., Marx, R. W., & Boyle, R. A. (1993). Beyond cold conceptual change: The role of motivational beliefs and classroom contextual factors in the process of conceptual change. *Review of Educational Research, 63,* 167–199.

Pintrich, P. R., Smith, D. A. F., Garcia, T., & McKeachie, W. J. (1991). *A manual for the use of the Motivated Strategies for Learning Questionnaire (MSLQ)* (Tech. Rep. No. 91-B-004). Ann Arbor: University of Michigan, School of Education.

Pintrich, P. R., Wolters, C. A., & Baxter, G. P. (1998). Assessing metacognition and self-regulated learning. In G. Schraw (Ed.), *Metacognitive assessment.* Lincoln: University of Nebraska Press.

Pressley, M., & Afflerbach, P. (1995). *Verbal protocols of reading: The nature of constructively responsive reading.* Hillsdale, NJ: Erlbaum.

Rumelhart, D. E., & Norman, D. A. (1978). Accretion, tuning, and restructuring: Three modes of learning. In J. W. Cotton and R. Klatzky (Eds.), *Semantic factors in cognition* (pp. 37–53). Hillsdale, NJ: Erlbaum.

Schraw, G. (in press). Assessing metacognition: Implications of the Buros Symposium. In G. Schraw (Ed.), *Metacognitive assessment.* Lincoln: University of Nebraska Press.

Schraw, G., & Dennison, R. S. (1994). Assessing metacognitive awareness. *Contemporary Educational Psychology, 19,* 460–475.

Schraw, G, Wise, S. L., & Roos, L. L. (in press). Metacognition and computer-based testing. In G. Schraw (Ed.), *Metacognitive assessment.* Lincoln: University of Nebraska Press.

Turner, J. C. (1995). The influence of classroom contexts on young children's motivation for literacy. *Reading Research Quarterly, 30,* 410–441.

Webb, E. J., Campbell, D. T., Schwartz, R. D., & Sechrest, L. (1966). *Unobtrusive measures.* Skokie, IL: Rand-McNally.

Weinstein, C. E. (1987). *LASSI user's manual.* Clearwater, FL: H & H Publishing.

Weinstein, C. E., Schulte, A., & Palmer, D. (1987). *LASSI: Learning and study strategies inventory.* Clearwater, FL: H & H Publishing.

Winne, P. H. (1982). Minimizing the black box problem to enhance the validity of theories about instructional effects. *Instructional Science, 11,* 13–28.

Winne, P. H. (1989). Theories of instruction and of intelligence for designing artificially intelligent tutoring systems. *Educational Psychologist, 24,* 229–259.

Winne, P. H. (1995). Inherent details in self-regulated learning. *Educational Psychologist, 30,* 173–187.

Winne, P. H. (1996). A metacognitive view of individual differences in self-regulated learning. *Learning and Individual Differences, 8,* 327–353.

Winne, P. H. (1997). Experimenting to bootstrap self-regulated learning. *Journal of Educational Psychology, 89,* 1–14.

Winne, P. H., & Field, D. (1998). STUDY: An Environment for Authoring and Presenting Adaptive Learning Tutorials (Version 3.2.5) [Computer program]. Simon Fraser University, Burnaby, BC. Canada.

Winne, P. H., Gupta, L., & Nesbit, J. C. (1994). Exploring individual differences in studying strategies using graph theoretic statistics. *Alberta Journal of Educational Research, 40,* 177–193.

Winne, P. H., & Hadwin, A. F. (1998). Studying as self-regulated learning. In D. J. Hacker, J. Dunlosky, & A. C. Graesser (Eds.), *Metacognition in educational theory and practice* (pp. 279–306). Hillsdale, NJ: Erlbaum.

Winne, P. H., Hadwin, A. F., McNamara, J. K., & Chu, S. T. L. (1998a, April). An exploratory study of self-regulating learning when students study using CoNotes2. In S. Tobias (Chair), *Metacognition: Assessment and training*. Symposium presented at the American Educational Research Association, San Diego.

Winne, P. H., Hadwin, A. F., McNamara, J. K., Chu, S. T. L., & Field, D. (1998b). CoNotes2: An *Electronic Notebook with Support for Self-Regulation and Learning Tactics* [Computer program]. Simon Fraser University, Burnaby, BC, Canada.

Winne, P. H., & Marx, R. W. (1989). A cognitive processing analysis of motivation within classroom tasks. In C. Ames and R. Ames (Eds.), *Research on motivation in education* (Vol. 3, pp. 223–257). Orlando, FL: Academic Press.

Winne, P. H., & Stockley, D. B. (1998). Computing technologies as sites for developing self-regulated learning. In D. H. Schunk and B. J. Zimmerman (Eds.), *Developing self-regulated learners: From teaching to self-reflective practice* (pp. 106–136). New York: Guilford.

Zimmerman, B. J. (1990). Self-regulated learning and academic achievement: An overview. *Educational Psychologist, 25,* 3–18.

Zimmerman, B. J., & Martinez-Pons, M. (1986). Development of a structured interview for assessing student use of self-regulated learning strategies. *American Educational Research Journal, 23,* 614–628.

Zimmerman, B. J., & Martinez-Pons, M. (1988). Construct validation of a strategy model of self-regulated learning. *Journal of Educational Psychology, 80,* 284–290.

INTERVENTIONS AND APPLICATIONS OF SELF-REGULATION THEORY AND RESEARCH

17

SELF-REGULATION AND DISTRESS IN CLINICAL PSYCHOLOGY

NORMAN S. ENDLER AND NANCY L. KOCOVSKI

York University, Toronto, Canada

The self-regulation of behavior involves establishing goals, and monitoring and evaluating behavior. If there is a discrepancy between actual behavior and goals, there is an attempt to modify behavior to eliminate this discrepancy. If goals have been achieved, a person may engage in reinforcing thoughts and/or activities (self-reinforcement).

There may be problems in aspects of the self-regulation of behavior that may contribute to distress. Goals may be too stringent or may be set at levels that an individual may not feel he or she is capable of achieving. A person may engage in perseverative self-monitoring or, at the other extreme, may disengage from or avoid self-monitoring entirely. These and other issues in the self-regulation of behavior are relevant in several areas of clinical psychology including addictive behaviors, coping with health problems, social anxiety, and depression. Strategies and techniques based on a self-regulation model of human behavior can be used for the treatment of clinical disorders and for the management of health problems.

1. INTRODUCTION

Many psychological disorders can be viewed, at least to some extent, as failures in self-regulation. Self-regulation can be defined as the psychological processes that mediate goal-directed behavior in the absence of imme-

Copyright © 2000 by Academic Press.
All rights of reproduction in any form reserved.

diate consequences (Carver & Scheier, 1986, 1999; Kanfer, 1970). This chapter reviews self-regulatory models and their relationships to several representative clinical disorders as well as relevant empirical research, so that the models may be evaluated. Furthermore, the use and potential usefulness of self-regulation in psychotherapy will be discussed.

Most psychological theories of self-regulation are based to some extent on cybernetics, a theory of automatic control systems (Carver & Scheier, 1982; Kanfer, 1975; Watson & Tharp, 1997). A simple example that illustrates the principles of cybernetic theory involves a thermostat found in any home. A thermostat is an automatic device for regulating temperature. It is set to a particular temperature (standard). A thermometer monitors the actual temperature in the home (sensor). A comparator compares the actual reading with the standard. Finally, an activator turns the heater on or off if there is a discrepancy between the actual temperature in the house and the set standard. Thus, the function of the thermostat is to regulate the temperature of the house. If the comparator determines that the temperature is lower than the standard, the activator will perform its function and turn the heater on. Once the temperature has reached the standard, the activator will turn the heater off. The comparator continually monitors the temperature in the house to determine if there is a discrepancy between the actual reading on the thermometer and the standard.

Human behavior can be viewed as being regulated in a similar fashion. We have certain standards or goals, we monitor and evaluate our own behavior to determine if they are meeting the preset goals, and, if there is a discrepancy between our standards and actual behaviors, we attempt to modify our behaviors. In describing the concept of the self, Hilgard (1949) points out that defense mechanisms and self-deception distort the view of the self before outlining two aspects of the self. These are the existence of continuous personal memories and the continual process of self-evaluation (both positive and negative). Self-appraisal forms an important part of the self-regulation of behavior in the normal self. The self, however, is not always involved in the regulatory process. The self-regulation of physiological processes do not rely on the self. For this reason, Block (1996) has argued that the term used should be autoregulation rather than self-regulation. However, in the literature, self-regulation is still the term that is usually used. Thus, self-regulation involves establishing goals, monitoring behaviors, and appraising behaviors to determine if they meet the established goals of the person. A final element in self-regulation is the reinforcement of behavior. Reinforcement may consist of thinking positive thoughts or engaging in pleasurable activities.

A large part of self-regulation theory involves eliminating the discrepancy between actual behavior and goals. Self-discrepancy theory (Higgins, 1987) differentiates between two different types of discrepancies. The first is between the actual self and the ideal self. Discrepancies of this nature have been shown to result in depression. The second is between the actual self and the ought self. Discrepancies of this nature have been shown to result in anxiety. Carver and Scheier (1999) have pointed out several differences between self-discrepancy theory and their self-regulation of behavior theory. Among these is the lack of explanatory power of self-discrepancy theory with respect to positive affect. Additionally, if there is a discrepancy between actual behavior and ideal or ought self, but there is substantial progress underway to remedy the discrepancy, negative affect should not result as discrepancy theory suggests. Higgins (1997) discusses his theory in terms of regulatory focus. According to Higgins, there are two types of self-regulation. Ideal self-regulation involves a promotion focus (e.g., accomplishment) and ought self-regulation involves a prevention focus (e.g., safety).

Discrepancy reduction is also discussed in other theories. Rogers (1954) discussed psychotherapy in terms of reducing the discrepancy between the actual self and the ideal self. The therapist provides the client with nonjudgemental, genuine, and accepting reflections of the self. A movement toward a more realistic ideal self is made, resulting in greater congruence between the actual self and the ideal self. Discrepancy reduction is also important in motivation theory. Behavior is dependent on both external stimuli and internal factors (Berlyne, 1960). The discrepancy between external information and internal cognitions induces what Berlyne has called intrinsic motivation. The person is motivated to seek ways to reduce this discrepancy. If there is no discrepancy, the external information is neglected. However, interests continually change and the standards against which behavior is evaluated change (Hunt, 1963). Hunt (1961), in discussing organism–environment interaction, notes that if there is not an appropriate "match" between schema (or cognitions) and environmental encounters, this discrepancy (analogous to cognitive dissonance) will motivate the organism to respond so as to minimize this differential.

Several disorders in clinical psychology may be partially due to or may be exacerbated by a malfunction of one or more facets of self-regulation. Individuals may set goals that are too high or that they do not believe they are capable of achieving. They may engage in perseverative self-monitoring and self-evaluation or, at the other extreme, they may cease monitoring their behavior altogether and engage in behaviors that they otherwise would not perform. Finally, individuals may not reinforce positive behaviors.

Self-regulation theory and research has been carried out in many clinical domains. Four areas have been chosen for this chapter. These are the areas in which self-regulation is most relevant. Each of these four clinical areas will be discussed in terms of each of the four aspects of self-regulation (i.e., goal setting, self-monitoring, self-evaluation, and self-reinforcement). The first section discusses self-regulatory failure and addictive behaviors. The next section also focuses on health psychology and begins by discussing the relationship between the Type A behavior pattern and self-regulation, and leads to a discussion of the use of self-regulatory principles and strategies in the treatment and management of health problems. Next, social anxiety, followed by depression, are each discussed in terms of problems with aspects of the self-regulation of behavior. Finally, implications for treatment are indicated in each section and discussed again as a separate section at the end of the chapter.

II. SELF-REGULATION AND ADDICTIVE BEHAVIORS

Addictive behaviors, ranging from excessive gambling to life-threatening disorders such as bulimia, may be viewed as failures in self-regulation. Opiate addicts have been shown to have more difficulty in self-regulatory functioning than normal controls as assessed by the Scale for Failures in Self-Regulation (Wilson, Passik, Faude, Abrams, & Gordon, 1989). This scale contains 11 items that were applied to participants' responses to the Thematic Apperception Test (TAT) by blind raters. Among the results, addicts, compared to normal controls, were found to have a poorer understanding of cause and effect relationships, displayed more confusion surrounding temporal mapping, and exhibited a greater lack of planning and a poorer anticipation of the consequences of behavior.

Many causes of failure in self-regulation have been identified. These include a reduction in the monitoring of behavior, difficulty in coping with stressors, and difficulty in focusing attention on the task at hand (Baumeister, Heatherton, & Tice, 1994; Kirschenbaum, 1987). People use various and multiple strategies for coping with stressful situations. These can be classified as task-oriented, emotion-oriented, and avoidance-oriented coping styles (Endler & Parker, 1994). Task-oriented coping (analogous to problem-focused coping) includes strategies aimed at solving the problem. Emotion-oriented coping includes strategies such as self-preoccupation or daydreaming. Avoidance-oriented coping can include responses that are a distraction from the stressful situation or a social diversion. Some strategies are more effective than others depending on the situation. However, in general, a strong positive correlation is often found between the use of emotion-oriented coping strategies and measures of psychological distress such as state anxiety. There are also individual differences in coping with stress (Endler, 1988, 1997).

Control plays an important role in coping with stress. A recent experiment in our lab investigated the effects of perceived control on psychological distress associated with a contrived stressor (an anagram task) (Endler, Speer, Johnson, & Flett, 1998). Participants with higher perceptions of control over the situation were found to use more task-oriented coping and less emotion-oriented coping, and experienced lower state anxiety (the measure of psychological distress). Thus, the perception of having control over a situation results in less psychological distress. This study also investigated the effect of experimentally produced control on levels of state anxiety and coping strategies. No effect was found on these variables. Therefore, whether or not one actually has control in their environment is not the important factor; rather, the perception of control plays an important role in coping.

Because having control over a situation usually results in less psychological distress, it would seem that control would be an important issue for individuals with addictive behaviors. Again, it is the perception of control rather than objective control that matters. Because perceptual control is associated with less distress, it is adaptive. Individuals with high perceptions of control would be more likely to effectively cope with stressful situations and hence there would be a lower probability of self-regulatory failure.

For a person to effectively self-regulate their behavior, higher order processes must override lower order processes (Baumeister et al., Carver & Scheier, 1999). Higher order processes involve more abstract long-term goals and lower order processes involve more concrete goals. For example, if an individual is addicted to alcohol, but has decided that it is time to quit that habit, the desire to have a drink would be the lower order process and the decision to stop drinking would be the higher order process. If the individual is able to overcome the desire and abstain from drinking, then the individual has effectively self-regulated his or her behavior. If the person has a drink, a failure in self-regulation has occurred. This situation also can be analyzed in terms of a self-regulatory feedback loop. The desire to stop drinking would constitute the goal. The individual would continuously monitor and appraise his or her behavior to determine if there is a discrepancy between the goal and the behavior. However, there may be a problem in each of these areas.

A. GOAL SETTING AND ADDICTIVE BEHAVIORS

A person may not establish goals or may have conflicting goals (Baumeister et al., 1994; Karoly, 1993). Confusion would result, leading to difficulty in the monitoring of behavior. The individual with the goal of not drinking alcohol also may have a conflicting goal to go out and socialize with friends on a more regular basis. The individual's friends may drink in social situations and may encourage the habit of drinking in social situations. Thus, this person is placed in a high risk and conflicting situation with respect to the original goal when attempting to achieve the conflicting goal. It may be wise to avoid socializing with these friends so as to achieve the goal of abstaining from alcohol, but, on the other hand, this would contradict the goal of increased socialization. These conflicting goals cause confusion for the individual and may result in a failure in self-regulation.

Another problem related to goal setting is the failure to disengage when a goal is unattainable (Carver & Scheier, 1999). Distress will result from the continued attempt to attain a goal that is unattainable. Disengagement may involve reducing the goal to a less demanding one or abandoning the goal altogether.

Future research should examine the goal setting behaviors of various populations of addictive behaviors. Furthermore, a comparison of goal setting behaviors relevant to the addictive behavior and goal setting in other areas should be made.

B. SELF-MONITORING AND ADDICTIVE BEHAVIORS

Second, a person may stop monitoring his or her behavior (Baumeister et al., 1994; Kirschenbaum, 1987). This is a central cause for failure in self-regulation. The individual loses self-awareness and engages in activities that he or she otherwise would not engage in. Because the person is not monitoring his or her behavior, it also is not evaluated. The person with the desire to stop drinking may binge while in such a phase.

Schupak-Neuberg and Nemeroff (1993) found evidence for this type of failure in self-regulation in a study investigating the notion of sense of self among a bulimic population. Their study compared bulimics and binge eaters on a scale (The Binging Inventory) designed by the authors to assess the extent to which individuals experience a lack of self-awareness during a binge. A binge eater engages in episodes (binges) in which enormous quantities of food are ingested. In addition to binging, a bulimic engages in purging behaviors that include vomiting or the use of laxatives or diuretics. A binge was found to be an escape from self-awareness for the bulimic group, but not for the binge eaters. Furthermore, the purpose of purging was assessed in the bulimic group and it was found to relieve negative affect. Together the binge and the purge cycle was found to serve an emotional regulatory function. Finally, compared to normals and binge eaters, bulimics were found to have greater confusion regarding sense of self. Thus, according to this study, during a binge bulimics are not monitoring and appraising their behavior, so they are, in the moment, unaware of the discrepancy between their goal (which would presumably be to achieve healthy eating habits) and their behavior (i.e., binging).

Other relevant evidence comes from the weight reduction literature. Individuals who engaged in self-monitoring were found to lose more weight than individuals who did not (Bellack, Rozensky, & Schwartz, 1974). Furthermore, it was found that self-monitoring is essential for continued weight loss after the termination of a treatment group (Perri et al.,

McAllister, 1988). Without the continued support and attention of the treatment group, the dieter may not recognize behavior that is not in accordance with his or her goal if he or she is not continually self-monitoring eating and exercise habits. Self-monitoring enhances the maintenance of weight loss after treatment, partially because of the increase in awareness of weight gain and potential relapse (Westover & Lanyon, 1990). Otherwise weight gain may go unnoticed to the point where the dieter may feel that it is too late to continue with the program. Self-monitoring is currently included in most behavioral weight loss programs (Johnson & Baggess, 1993).

It is apparent that the cessation of the monitoring of behavior is implicated in some addictive behaviors. It is unclear whether it plays a role in the onset or only in the maintenance of the addictive behavior. Future research needs to be conducted to make this clarification.

C. SELF-EVALUATION AND ADDICTIVE BEHAVIORS

Disengagement from the monitoring of behavior was shown to be implicated in some addictive behavior populations. Individuals who are not monitoring their behavior are not able to evaluate their behavior. Additionally, a person may not make the necessary changes in behavior if there is a discrepancy between his or her behavior and his or her goal. In this situation, the person sets a goal, and monitors and appraises his or her behavior, but if the behavior falls short of the goal, the individual does not react appropriately. The person may feel unable to effectively change his or her behavior, so the individual does not make any attempt to bring the behavior closer to personal goals. The person who wants to quit drinking will know that is the goal, and will monitor and appraise his or her behavior. This person will be aware that having a drink is contradicting his or her goal to quit drinking. However, when this person does have a drink, he or she will not try to eliminate the discrepancy between behavior and goals (i.e., stop drinking). Persons may feel that they do not possess the strength to accomplish this change in their behaviors.

Perceived self-efficacy, the belief that one is capable of carrying out a desired behavior (Bandura, 1977, 1997), is an important factor in self-regulation. It has been theorized that drug and alcohol addicts use substances as a means of self-regulation (Khantzian, 1990). These individuals become accustomed to using a substance for the purposes of calming themselves or relating to others, for example, and then underestimate their own ability to carry out these functions. They believe that they will not be able to achieve their goals without the use of the substance, which leads to continued substance abuse. Furthermore, the confidence in one's ability to abstain from the addictive behavior and the confidence in one's ability to recover if there is a setback are critical in the change process (Marlatt, Baer, & Quigley, 1995).

Empirical research needs to be done in this area to determine if individuals with various addictive behaviors are in fact not monitoring or evaluating their behaviors. Furthermore, it needs to be determined if individuals who are monitoring and evaluating their behaviors are concluding that they are unable to minimize the discrepancies between their desired goals and their actual behaviors.

D. SELF-REINFORCEMENT AND ADDICTIVE BEHAVIORS

The amount of self-reinforcement that an individual with an addictive behavior engages in has been theorized to play a role in the onset or the maintenance of the addictive behavior (Miller, 1987). Studies have been conducted to investigate the self-reinforcement behaviors in substance abuse and eating disorder populations. In an undergraduate population, participants indicated that they were not likely to use strategies related to self-reinforcement to control the amount of alcohol consumption. Furthermore, substance abuse patients were found to have reinforcement practices that were no different from other psychiatric groups or normal controls (Parmar & Cernovsky, 1993). Additionally, Rozensky and Honor (1984) compared the self-reinforcement and self-punishment behaviors of psychiatric patients, alcoholic patients, and nonclinical controls. These groups did not differ on self-reward; however, the alcoholic group was found to be the least self-punishing. It appears as though self-reinforcement practices of substance abuse individuals are no different than normals. Within an addiction rehabilitation population, reinforcement scores were found to be related negatively to depression (Cernovsky, 1989). Thus, frequency of self-reinforcement may have a mediating effect. Finally, therapy for bulimia, which involves modifying the self-reinforcement practices of the individual, has been shown to be effective (Mizes & Lohr, 1983).

The relationship of self-reinforcement behaviors to an addictive behavior may be dependent on which addictive behavior is in question. Therapy aimed at increasing the self-reward practices of an individual may be effective with bulimic individuals, but not with substance abuse individuals. Further research should investigate practices of self-reinforcement of various populations of individuals with addictive behaviors as well as determine if therapy aimed at increasing positive self-reinforcement is effective. It may be the case that self-reinforcement is at a similar level to normal controls; however, therapy aimed at increasing self-reinforcement may still prove to be effective.

E. IMPLICATIONS FOR TREATMENT

Self-regulation plays an important role in human adaptation to life. Rothbaum, Weisz, and Snyder (1982) outlined two processes that form adaptation. These are primary control, changing the environment to suit the self, and secondary control, changing the self to suit the environment. Self-regulation is a large component of secondary control. Having the capacity to effectively regulate one's behavior is important for becoming a well-adjusted person and adapting to the environment (Baumeister et al., 1994). Thus, learning to effectively self-regulate behavior is important for therapy.

Raising a client's belief in their self-regulatory efficacy may have an impact on their behavior (Bandura, 1997). In the eating disorder literature, this finding has been observed with bulimic participants (Schneider, O'Leary, & Agras, 1987). The greater their belief in their capability to effectively regulate their behavior, the less they engaged in purging behaviors.

In treating addictive behaviors, Kirschenbaum (1987) discussed "obsessive–compulsive self-regulation" for the prevention of self-regulatory breakdown. The term "obsessive–compulsive" traditionally is used to refer to individuals who have a disorder in which they have unwanted repetitive thoughts, images, or impulses (obsessions), and in response to these thoughts engage in repetitive, unwanted actions (compulsions). Here, the term refers to the constant and detailed self-monitoring of behavior. The intensity with which individuals with obsessive–compulsive disorder are involved with their maladaptive behavior is analogous to the intensity with which persons trying to avoid self-regulatory failure should monitor their behavior. In treating addictive behaviors, it is very important for the client to self-monitor and self-evaluate behavior so as to be aware of discrepancies between goals and actual behavior.

Relapse is an important issue in addiction. Alcohol dependence has a high rate of relapse after treatment (Litman, Eiser, & Taylor, 1979). Often, an initial lapse will lead to a complete breakdown in self-regulation and consequently relapse. An initial lapse may occur while the person is in a high risk situation. The individual may be experiencing a considerable amount of negative affect due to a variety of sources. There may be pressure from peers to engage in the unwanted habit. Once the initial lapse has occurred, it is important that the individual does not relinquish all efforts to succeed at his or her goal. The person may feel guilty about the lapse and feel that there is nothing he or she can do about it (Curry, Marlatt, & Gordon, 1987). If self-monitoring and self-evaluation continue to take place, the individual may be able to get back on track. However, the danger of the cessation of self-monitoring is paramount once a lapse has occurred. A study compared adults who were in a smoking cessation treatment group who lapsed, but then stopped smoking once again, and adults from the same group who also lapsed, but for which the lapse lead to relapse. They found that a plan to cope with an initial lapse was the important factor (Candiotte & Lichtenstein, 1981). All of the individuals who were able to avoid relapse had a plan to cope, whereas only half of the relapse group had such a plan.

Related to relapse, timing is also an important factor in self-regulation with respect to some addictive behaviors. For example, if a person is trying to diet, it is easier to refuse a bag of chips right from the original offer. It would be even easier if the dieter avoided situations where unhealthy foods were available. However, if the dieter has one chip, it will be harder and will become increasingly difficult with each chip eaten. Baumeister et al. (1994) label this factor in self-regulatory failure as psychological inertia.

The disengagement of self-monitoring and hence self-evaluation appears to be an important aspect for addictive behaviors. The impact of the role of goal setting and self-reinforcement is not as clear. Other factors such as withdrawal for substance abusers and social factors also have an impact in treatment.

III. SELF-REGULATION AND HEALTH

Self-regulatory principles have been used in the treatment or management of various health problems (in addition to the treatment of addictive behaviors discussed in the previous section). Therapies based on self-regulatory principles have been developed for use with patients with hypertension (Linden, 1988), asthma (Creer & Winder, 1986), diabetes (Wing, 1992), and chronic pain (Grunau & Craig, 1988). Additionally, such therapies have been effective with coronary heart disease patients (Clark, Janz, Dodge, & Sharpe, 1992) and for reducing Type A behavior (Suinn, 1982).

This section begins by outlining the various strategies that patients use for coping with health problems, followed by a description of the Type A behavior pattern. As in section II, each aspect of self-regulation then will be addressed separately.

As previously stated, difficulty in coping with stressors is one of the causes for failure in self-regulation (Baumeister et al., 1994; Kirschenbaum, 1987). Coping strategies for stressful situations already have been outlined. Other research has investigated specific strategies for coping with health problems. Such research has used populations of individuals with both acute health problems (e.g., colds and flus) and chronic health problems (e.g., cancer and cardiac patients). Patients use various and multiple strategies for coping with health problems. These can be classified as distraction, palliative, instrumental, and emotional preoccupation coping strategies (Endler, Parker, & Summerfeldt, 1993, 1998). Distraction strategies include thinking about other experiences, spending time with others, and engaging in activities unrelated to the illness. Palliative coping strategies are aimed at alleviating the unpleasantness of the illness and include soothing, self-care behaviors such as getting rest. Instrumental strategies are task-oriented efforts such as taking medication and actively seeking medical help. Emotional preoccupation strategies are emotion oriented and include ruminating about the health problem. As with coping with stress in general, different strategies are associated with different outcomes. Instrumental strategies are negatively correlated with psychological distress and length of hospital stay, whereas researchers have found a positive association between the use of emotion-oriented strategies and psychological distress and length of hospital stay (for reviews, see Endler & Parker, 1994, 1999). Effective coping is important to decrease the probability of failure in self-regulation.

Before looking closely at each facet of self-regulation, the Type A behavior pattern and its relationship to health will be described. Self-regulation processes have been theorized to underlie Type A behavior. Defining characteristics of this behavior pattern include heightened ambition, competitiveness, easily evoked hostility, and a rushing or hurrying component in everything that is done. Healthy individuals who exhibit Type A behavior are twice as likely to develop coronary heart disease compared to healthy Type B individuals. The hostility component of the Type A behavior pattern has been found to be the most important aspect with respect to heart disease (Matthews, 1988). The increase in the probability of heart disease associated with the Type A personality is presumably due to increased physiological arousal (Houston, 1983). Various health problems will be discussed in the following sections on the different aspects of self-regulation. Additionally, because of the association between the Type A personality pattern and coronary heart disease, Type A behavior also will be included in each of these sections. Although goal setting, self-monitoring, self-evaluation, and self-reinforcement are areas on which some treatment programs for health problems have focused, there have not been many well controlled studies to determine the efficacy of these approaches. Each section will begin with a review of the research in Type A behavior and then move on to discuss the relevance of that particular aspect of self-regulation with the management of health problems.

A. GOAL SETTING AND HEALTH

Rather than act in ways to reduce increased physiological arousal, Type A persons seem to behave in ways that maintain it. They may associate this aroused state with achievement. Type As have been found to set higher goals for themselves and are more likely to expect to attain their goals than Type Bs (Grimm & Yarnold, 1984; O'Keefe & Smith, 1988).

The use of goal setting in the management of health problems may result in better adherence to the treatment protocol and better outcome. Goal setting has been found to be effective in improving regimen adherence for diabetic patients (Delamater et al., 1991). Patients who set goals for their treatment are more likely to comply with the treatment regimen. The setting of goals may increase the patients' awareness of the desired outcome. Patients are not always clear on their illness and the recommended treatments. Setting goals may help clarify what they should do to manage their health problem most effectively. The practice of goal setting also may have its effect by increasing the patient's attention to their treatment. Because they have a goal to attain, more time may be spent monitoring and evaluating their behaviors relevant to their health problem. The efficacy of goal setting was supported in a diabetic population (Delamater et al., 1991). Future research should look into the relevance of goal setting in the management of other health problems.

Not only is the practice of goal setting important, but the level of goals that are set is an important variable with respect to health problems. Emmons (1992) examined goal setting behavior and divided participants into high-level striving and low-level striving. It was found that high-level striving was associated with higher levels of psychological distress, whereas, low-level striving was associated with higher levels of physical illness.

B. SELF-MONITORING AND HEALTH

Type A individuals tend to focus on negative feedback, which contributes to their behavior pattern and may be maladaptive (Cooney & Zeichner, 1985). It appears as if they are monitoring their behavior, but they are ruminating about negative evaluations. Rumination is not a healthy adaptive response and is associated with distress (Nolen-Hoeksema, 1991).

As for the management of health problems, setting goals may increase the likelihood of self-monitoring. Vigorous self-monitoring is an important aspect for individuals with some health problems. Treatment for type 2 diabetes can involve the careful monitoring of blood sugar levels through diet and exercise programs (Wing, 1992). Similarly, management for coronary heart disease typically also involves careful monitoring of diet and exercise. Monitoring can be important in the management of health problems in which the individual has control over some aspect of his or her illness.

C. SELF-EVALUATION AND HEALTH

Individuals with the Type A behavior pattern are less satisfied with and more critical of their performance (O'Keefe & Smith, 1988; Ovcharchyn, Johnson, & Petzel, 1981). It appears as though Type A individuals monitor and evaluate their behavior, but they set higher goals and then ruminate about discrepancies between actual behavior and goals.

Self-evaluation can affect physical and psychological health. Individuals who appraised themselves as ineffective problem solvers were found to report more psychological distress (Heppner, Kampa, & Brunning, 1987). Evaluating behavior is an important step in self-regulation. If a diabetic is supposed to monitor his or her diet, he or she must evaluate simultaneously whether his or her food intake is consistent with the treatment protocol. If there is a discrepancy between the actual food intake and the desired food intake, a change in eating habits should take place. Thus, it is important to make a change in behaviors upon the discovery of discrepancies between actual behaviors and goals. Unfortunately, in the same study (Heppner et al., 1987), individuals who appraised themselves as effective problem solvers were found to be higher on the Type A behavior pattern.

D. SELF-REINFORCEMENT AND HEALTH

Compliance with long-term medical regimens is problematic in that only half of all patients with chronic diseases adhere to their treatment protocol (Epstein & Cluss, 1982). Reinforcement for taking medication has been shown to be effective in increasing compliance (Epstein & Cluss, 1982). Compliance also was found to increase in diabetic individuals who engaged in self-reinforcement for adhering to diet and exercise programs (Heiby, Gafarian, & McCann, 1989).

Finally, Type A individuals have been found to be less self-reinforcing (Holden & Wagner, 1990). Reinforcement may involve an activity that can be engaged in or simply may be thinking positive thoughts. Gender differences have been found in this area of research. Compared to Type A females, and Type A and B males, Type B females have been found to be the most reinforcing and the least self-punishing (Holden & Wagner, 1990).

Thus, overall, Type A individuals set higher goals (which they expect to attain), are more critical of their performance, and are less likely to positively reinforce their behavior than Type Bs. The aggressive behavior of Type A persons may be viewed as an attempt to reduce the discrepancy between their preset goals and their actual performance. Implications for the treatment of Type A behavior pattern individuals will be discussed in the next section.

E. IMPLICATIONS FOR TREATMENT

Therapies based on principles from self-regulation theory have been developed for use in clients with various health problems including hypertension, asthma, and chronic pain. The appeal of self-regulation therapies for the management of health problems is that they enable patients to do something for themselves. Self-regulation therapy may be used in combination with other forms of treatment (i.e., drug therapy) or on its own. This is an especially important form of treatment for patients who do not respond to medical treatment. Most self-regulation therapies involve an effort to increase the client's awareness of behavior through self-monitoring. Relaxation techniques and biofeedback may be used to help clients become aware of different states (Linden, 1988; Shabsin & Whitehead, 1988). Other techniques involve helping the client learn effective coping strategies.

Burke (1989) outlined four basic self-regulatory tools that can be used alone or in behavior therapy to counter the stress response. As previously stated, the inability to deal with stress is a common cause for self-regulatory failure. Thus techniques to help cope with stress are very important. Cannon (1932) identified the stress response as an activation of the sympathetic nervous system that results in many bodily changes including changes in blood pressure, heart rate, and digestion (i.e., "fight or flight" response). Selye (1956) first demonstrated that constant activation of the sympathetic nervous system can lead to physiological damage and sometimes this damage can be irreversible. Tools to prevent or decrease the stress response are especially important in some health problems. For example, constant elevation in blood pressure can lead to hypertension. These self-regulatory tools are meditation, hypnosis, progressive relaxation, and biofeedback.

Meditation involves a passive attitude, a quiet environment, a body position that is associated with low muscle tension, and reduced awareness of the environment achieved through various methods including fixating on an object. Studies have shown that meditation results in relaxation (for a review, see Benson, 1975). These same elements are true of hypnosis. Additionally, in hypnosis, a practitioner typically influences the client during the state of relaxation. The efficacy of hypnosis has been under much debate. Progressive relaxation techniques also involve the elements of meditation. Additionally, the client is instructed to tense and relax different muscle groups in succession. The awareness of tension and relaxation are important for these self-regulatory tools.

Biofeedback is a method of increasing a person's awareness to smaller changes in biological functioning than normally would be noticed. The brain receives information regarding problems in the organs of the body from a feedback loop so that it can regulate the system. Normally, we are not aware of this process until certain levels of distress are reached. Physical or psychological symptoms may appear at this point. Brain wave activity (through the use of an EEG), muscle activity (through the use of an EMG), skin temperature, and sweating (GSR) are among the functions that are monitored using biofeedback. The patient is provided information regarding one of these physiological functions through auditory or visual stimuli. The client learns to change the intensity of the stimulus and thereby learns to change the biological process. The client can then monitor the process individually and make appropriate changes if necessary. Biofeedback is used for relaxation purposes and can be used in combination with progressive relaxation techniques. All of these tools can be important in decreasing stress and in combating failure in self-regulation.

Biofeedback and relaxation techniques are used to treat various health problems. Outcome studies have shown efficacy for these techniques with hypertension patients (Linden, 1988) and gastrointestinal tract disorders (Shabsin & Whitehead, 1988). Research into the use of biofeedback with pain patients has produced varied results, depending on the type of pain (e.g., headache, migraine, or back pain) and type of feedback (e.g., muscle contraction or temperature) Relaxation and coping skills training are showing potential in the treatment of pain (for a review, see Grunau & Craig, 1988). These tools also are used in therapy with Type A individuals.

Because of the association between the hostility component of Type A behavior and coronary heart disease, it is important to treat this Type A behavior pattern. However, Type A individuals have associated their behavior with achievement, so they may be reluctant to change. An unwillingness to modify behavior especially may be present in Type A individuals who do not have any symptoms of coronary heart disease. Unfortunately, sometimes symptoms of heart disease (i.e., chest pain, fatigue) go unnoticed or are mislabeled by Type A individuals (Frautschi & Chesney, 1988). Lab research has shown that Type As suppress symptoms (Carver, Coleman, & Glass, 1976) and Type As have been found to present with symptoms of myocardial infarction at a later point in their cardiac illness than Type Bs (Matthews, Siegel, Kuller, Thompson, & Varlat, 1983).

Cognitive behavior therapy (CBT) has been shown to be effective in decreasing Type A behavior (Suinn, 1982). A main component in this therapy involves training the client to self-monitor his or her behavior. Type A individuals need to pay more attention to their arousal, thoughts, and behaviors. Relaxation and biofeedback training can be used to make the client more aware of various symptoms of arousal (Suinn, 1982). The use of self-reinforcement of positive changes in behavior and thoughts may help. Type A behavior is reinforced by society and Type A individuals reinforce themselves for their achievements, which are associated with their states of arousal. The client has to recognize this pattern of conditioning that has occurred in the past and also has to be aware that it is unhealthy. Through self-monitoring and self-evaluation, Type As can become aware of discrepancies between their behaviors and their goals (i.e., less Type A behavior), and work to eliminate them. Furthermore, reinforcement of positive changes in behavior can help to reverse the previous patterns of reinforcement.

A program designed to increase patients' knowledge of the processes of self-regulation was shown to be effective for older adults with organic heart disease. Participants in this program were found to do better on measures of psychosocial functioning and had less severe symptoms (Clark, et al., 1992).

Self-management therapy programs have been developed for asthma patients (Creer & Winder, 1986; Hindi-Alexander & Cropp, 1984). Clients are first taught about their illness (e.g., breathing mechanism) and then are taught self-management skills. A main component is self-monitoring. Clients have to monitor their breathing and their asthma condition, and evaluate whether there is a problem. If there is a problem, they must come up with a solution (i.e., eliminate the discrepancy between their goal of being healthy and their current condition). Studies have shown that this is a practical method of controlling asthma, especially for children (for a review, see Creer, 1988). Asthmatic children otherwise may not recognize potentially life-threatening situations.

Thus therapy for health problems can involve learning effective coping strategies to decrease distress and subsequently decrease failure in self-regulation. In Type A behavior pattern individuals, specific aspects in the self-regulation of behavior may be addressed. Finally, in the management of health problems, specific self-regulatory tools (e.g., biofeedback) can be used.

IV. SELF-REGULATION AND SOCIAL ANXIETY

This section discusses aspects of the self-regulation of behavior that may contribute to social anxiety, one of the facets of anxiety. Anxiety has a state and a trait component. State anxiety is a transitional and emotional condition, whereas trait anxiety is a relatively stable personality character-istic (Endler & Magnusson, 1976). Spielberger's (1983) measure of trait anxiety assumes that anxiety is unidimensional and focuses on anxiety in interpersonal situations. The multidimensional interaction model states that trait (as well as state) anxiety is multidimensional and social-evaluation anxiety is one of the dimensions (Endler, 1983, 1997; Endler, Edwards, Vitelli, & Parker, 1989). Social-evaluation anxiety can be defined as anxiety that arises in situations where an individual is being observed or evaluated by others. Other labels for social anxiety are often used in the literature. Rosenberg's (1965) "evaluation apprehension" falls under the category of social-evaluation anxiety. Watson and Friend (1969) defined (and assessed) social anxiety as a combination of the experience of distress in social situations, the avoidance of social situations, and the fear of negative evaluations from others.

Self-regulation models of social anxiety state that social anxiety arises if an individual has not behaved in a manner consistent with his or her original goal (Carver & Scheier, 1986; Schlenker & Leary, 1982). Schlenker and Leary provided a self-presentation model of social anxiety. Social anxiety arises when an individual wants to make a certain impression on others, but feels that success will not occur. The amount of anxiety experienced depends on how close the person believes that he or she will come to achieving his or her goal, the reactions of others, and the importance of the interaction. Individuals assess their behavior and this assessment begins if they consider the interaction important or if they feel they are not achieving their goals. Carver and Scheier (1986) stated that human behavior is controlled by feedback loops. People have a "reference value" or anchor point for how they want to behave and they compare their behaviors to this reference. If their behavior is not acceptable, then a change occurs to make the behavior closer to the reference value or standard. This assessment and appraisal process continues. These basic self-regulatory principles have been applied to social anxiety (Carver & Scheier, 1986). The four components of self-regulation (i.e., goal setting, self-monitoring, self-appraisal, and self-reinforcement) will be discussed separately with respect to social anxiety.

A. GOAL SETTING AND SOCIAL ANXIETY

There has not been much empirical research on goal setting in socially anxious individuals, although it is part of some theories of social anxiety (Carver & Scheier, 1986; Arkin, Lake, & Baumgardner, 1986). Some people have argued that socially anxious individuals believe that others have high standards for them to meet (Rehm, 1977; Schlenker & Leary, 1982). However, Wallace and Alden (1991) found that anxious subjects did not set higher goals for themselves than nonanxious subjects and did not rate others' standards as higher than did the nonanxious group. Although it has been found that socially anxious subjects do not objectively rate others as having higher standards for them, they do seem to believe that others have high standards for them (Alden, Bieling, & Wallace, 1994; Wallace & Alden, 1991). The Socially Prescribed subscale of the Multidimensional Perfectionism Scale was used to measure the standards that the subjects believe others have for them (Hewitt & Flett, 1991). It seems that socially anxious subjects believe that others have perfectionistic standards for them, but this is not demonstrated in their objective ratings. Doerfler and Aron (1995) also found that socially anxious and normal participants did not differ in their goal setting, but the socially anxious participants, however, did not expect to achieve their goals. Thus it may be that socially anxious individuals set goals that are comparable to nonanxious people, but that they do not expect to attain their goals. They believe they lack the social efficacy necessary to meet the standards of others (Bandura, 1997).

B. SELF-MONITORING AND SOCIAL ANXIETY

Socially anxious individuals may engage in perseverative self-monitoring and self-appraisal, which may contribute to their anxiety. The tendency to be aware of oneself as a social object is measured by the Public Self-Consciousness subscale of the Self-Consciousness Scale (Fenigstein, Scheier, & Buss, 1975). Several researchers have found a correlation between public self-consciousness and social anxiety (Buss, 1980; Fenigstein et al., 1975; Lennox, 1984; Pilkonis, 1977). However, some researchers have not (Linder & Der-Karabetian, 1986). Monfries and Kafer (1993) found that the two constructs are correlated, but when the social distress and social avoidance components of the Social Avoidance and Distress (SAD) scale were separated, public self-consciousness correlated only with the social distress component. This research has relied solely on self-report. Future research should use other methods to provide confirmatory evidence of the existence of this relationship. Additionally, research should be conducted to determine if perseverative self-monitoring and self-evaluation are precursors to social anxiety, if they are factors in the maintenance of social anxiety, or if they play a role both in onset and maintenance.

C. SELF-EVALUATION AND SOCIAL ANXIETY

Socially anxious individuals may evaluate themselves negatively. Socially anxious subjects have been found to negatively evaluate their social abilities (Alden et al., 1994). Lake and Arkin (1985) found that subjects who were higher in social anxiety rated positive feedback from evaluators as less accurate than participants who were low in social anxiety. Cacioppo, Glass, and Merluzzi (1979) investigated heterosocial (dating) anxiety, using the SAD as their measure of social anxiety and male subjects in anticipation of an interaction with a female as the anxious situation. Men who were high in social anxiety produced more negative self-statements and evaluated themselves more negatively. Clark and Arkowitz (1975) also found that subjects who were high in social anxiety rated themselves more unfavorably on a social encounter and that they had lower self-esteem.

Measures of self-esteem often have been used as an indicator of self-evaluation. Jones, Briggs, and Smith (1986) found negative correlations (ranging from $-.52$ to $-.58$) between self-esteem and various measures of social anxiety. Leary also found that social anxiety is negatively correlated with self-esteem ($r = -.36$, Leary & Kowalski, 1993; $r = -.18$, Leary, 1983). There may be gender differences. Endler,

Edwards, and Vitelli (1991) found no correlation between self-esteem and social evaluation anxiety for males, but a correlation of $-.42$ for females.

As previously stated and as is evident in this section, research in social anxiety comes under many different labels. Negative correlations also have been found between shyness and self-esteem ($r = -.48$, Zimbardo, 1977; $r = -.51$, Cheek & Buss, 1981). Furthermore, in the communication apprehension literature, several researchers have found a moderately strong negative correlation (ranging from $-.48$ to $-.72$) between self-esteem and communication apprehension (McCroskey, Daly, Richmond, & Falcione, 1977; and see review by McCroskey, 1977). Communication apprehension is "an individual's level of fear or anxiety associated with either real or anticipated communication with another person or persons" (McCroskey, 1977, p. 78); a construct that may be considered to be a subtype of social anxiety (Leary & Kowalski, 1995).

Thus the negative relationship between the two constructs seems to be a stable finding. Evaluating oneself unfavorably may lead to the expectation that others will evaluate you negatively as well (Leary & Kowalski, 1995). Thus, it may be the case that low self-esteem leads to an increased fear of negative evaluations from others, which leads to increased social anxiety. Future research should investigate if the fear of negative evaluations is a mediator between low self-esteem and social anxiety.

D. SELF-REINFORCEMENT AND SOCIAL ANXIETY

Self-reinforcement is the final element in self-regulation theory (Kanfer & Karoly, 1972). Upon appraising behavior, if it meets with the preset goal, self-reinforcement may or may not take place. A low frequency of positive self-reinforcement may be an antecedent of social anxiety. Rehm and Marston (1968) placed male college students who reported social anxiety into one of three therapy conditions. The condition that is relevant to this discussion involved increasing the client's rate of self-reinforcement. The greatest improvement was found for subjects in this condition. Individuals high in social anxiety may engage in a low frequency of self-reinforcement. More studies need to be conducted in this area to draw more definite conclusions about this relationship. Related research has shown that individuals who are high in social anxiety report less positive thoughts and more negative thoughts (Bruch, Mattia, Heimberg, & Holt, 1993).

E. IMPLICATIONS FOR TREATMENT

According to the research discussed in the foregoing text, individuals who are socially anxious do not expect to attain their desired goals, tend to be more aware of themselves as social objects, have lower self-esteem, and reinforce their behavior at a lower rate compared to normal controls.

Additionally, socially anxious individuals may engage in perseverative self-monitoring and self-evaluation. Cognitive behavior therapy may be a viable option to address their cognitions regarding the expectation of not attaining their goals. The negative self-evaluations based on research asking socially anxious individuals to rate themselves, as well as correlational studies that have shown a relationship between self-esteem (as an indicator of self-evaluation) and social anxiety can be addressed in cognitive behavior therapy as well. Finally, the Rehm and Marston (1968) study, discussed before, has provided evidence for the efficacy of increasing the self-reinforcing behavior of socially anxious individuals. These are all issues that may be addressed in therapy; however, there are many other variables related to the particular individual that may affect the process and outcome of the psychotherapy.

V. SELF-REGULATION AND DEPRESSION

Similar to the preceding section on social anxiety, various aspects of the self-regulation of behavior may contribute to depression for some individuals. One of the earliest and most well-known cognitive approaches to depression is the work of Beck (1967), which stressed dysfunctional cognitions. These dysfunctional cognitions form part of the self-regulation model for depression. At the goal setting stage of self-regulation, depressed people may set unrealistically high standards; at the self-evaluation stage, depressed people may be prone to cognitive distortions; and at the self-reinforcement stage, depressed people may have low rates of positive reinforcement or alternatively may negatively reinforce their behavior (Matthews, 1977; Rehm, 1977). These areas will be discussed separately.

A. GOAL SETTING AND DEPRESSION

Beck (1967) theorized that depressed individuals set unrealistically high standards for themselves: The individual would be unable to achieve his or her goals and depression would result. It has been found by several researchers that depressed individuals have higher expectations for themselves than nondepressed individuals (Golin & Terrell, 1977; LaPointe & Crandell, 1980; Nelson, 1977). However, in a laboratory study, Nelson and Craighead (1981) investigated the difference between set goals and actual performance on a task in depressed and nondepressed participants. No differences were found. Dysphoric students have been found to set lower goals than nondysphoric students (Ahrens, Zeiss, & Kanfer, 1988). Furthermore, Kanfer and Zeiss (1983) found that depressed participants set slightly lower standards than nondepressed participants. Additionally, they found that depressed participants felt that they had higher standards than they were capable of achieving. Thus, perceived ability to attain goals may be the important factor.

Another relevant finding is that dysphoric individuals believe that others have high goals for them. Socially prescribed perfectionism is the tendency to believe (either correctly or incorrectly) that significant others have perfectionistic standards for the self. A positive association between socially prescribed perfectionism and depression has consistently been found (Hewitt & Flett, 1991, 1993; Martin, Flett, Hewitt, Krames, & Szanto, 1996). Similar to the socially anxious participants discussed previously, dysphoric participants also scored higher on the socially prescribed perfectionism measure than did controls. When asked to objectively rate the goals of others, however, their ratings also were no different than nondysphoric participants (Alden et al., 1994).

B. SELF-MONITORING AND DEPRESSION

Depressed individuals may engage in perseverative self-monitoring and self-appraisal which may contribute to and exacerbate their depression. As with socially anxious individuals, the relationship with self-consciousness has been investigated. The tendency to be aware of oneself as a social object is measured by the Public Self-Consciousness subscale of the Self-Consciousness Scale (Fenigstein et al., 1975). Kuiper, Olinger, and Swallow (1987) found that depressed participants reported higher levels of public self-consciousness than nondepressed undergraduate participants. Similarly, in a sample of undergraduate participants, Flett, Blankstein, and Boase (1987) found that public self-consciousness was a significant predictor of depression. Further support of the relationship between public self-consciousness and depression comes from a clinical study that investigated depression among a sample of pregnant women (Kitamura, Sugawara, Sugawara, & Toda, 1996). Women who were higher on a self-report measure of depression also were found to be higher on public self-consciousness.

The positive relationship between public self-consciousness and depression appears to be a stable finding. It is unclear whether depression causes an increase in self-consciousness or whether an increased level of self-consciousness predisposes one to depression. Some research has provided evidence to suggest that depression may lead to increased self-consciousness (Hull, Reilly, & Ennis, 1991), but further research needs to be done.

C. SELF-EVALUATION AND DEPRESSION

Beck (1967) stated that depressed individuals evaluate themselves negatively due to their unrealistic goal setting behavior. Although depressed people may not set goals that are higher than other individuals, they seem to set goals that they do not perceive themselves as capable of achieving.

Bandura (1977) defined self-efficacy as the perceived ability to behave in a manner consistent with achieving goals. Depressed individuals may have low self-efficacy. Depressed participants have been found to judge themselves as less self-efficacious (Kanfer & Zeiss, 1983). A large discrepancy has been found between goals set and efficacy ratings for dysphoric participants (Doerfler & Aron, 1995). However, no difference was found between the evaluation of performance between dysphoric and nondysphoric participants (Doerfler & Aron, 1995).

Another important element in the onset or maintenance of depression may be the frequency of self-appraisal. People may vary in the rate at which they evaluate their behavior. Dysphoric individuals have been found to engage in more frequent self-evaluation than nondysphoric individuals (Alden et al., 1994). Thus, a combination of negative self-evaluation and a high frequency of self-evaluation may contribute to depression. This research was conducted with undergraduate students. Further research should compare clinical populations with normal controls. Additionally, a within subjects design could be used to compare individuals while depressed and then later on when their depression has lifted.

D. SELF-REINFORCEMENT AND DEPRESSION

According to Beck (1967), depressed individuals engage in more self-criticism than normals due to their negative evaluations, which resulted from their unrealistic goal setting. This self-criticism can be classified as negative self-reinforcement. Lewinsohn (1974) postulated that depression was primarily due to a lack of positive self-reinforcement that resulted from a lack of social skills. It seems intuitive that depressed people would engage in less self-reinforcing behaviors; however, this was not confirmed empirically. Nelson and Craighead (1981) did not find a significant difference between depressed and nondepressed individuals on frequency of self-reinforcement.

Depressed individuals may benefit from therapy aimed at increasing positive self-reinforcement even though they may not be lower in the frequency of self-reinforcement than normal controls. Future research should determine the effect of therapy aimed at increasing positive self-reinforcement. Additionally, there may be a qualitative difference in the type of self-reinforcement.

E. IMPLICATIONS FOR TREATMENT

According to the research, depressed individuals do not believe that they will attain their goals. As with socially anxious individuals, cognitive behavior psychotherapy may address this issue. Also similar to socially anxious individuals, depressed individuals may engage in perseverative self-monitoring and self-evaluation, which may be addressed in psychotherapy. Within the addictive behavior research, "obsessive–compulsive self-regulation" was the recommendation for the prevention of self-regulatory failure and the attainment of goals (Kirschenbaum, 1987). Research in social anxiety and in depression seems to provide support for the assertion that "obsessive–compulsive self-regulation" may be part of the problem in socially anxious and/or depressed individuals.

Rehm (1981) provided a treatment program for depression that targets each aspect of the self-regulation process. Clients are to set attainable goals, to record experiences in such a way as to minimize the possibility of cognitive distortion, and to evaluate their behavior in the therapy session so that self-blame is discouraged and credit is given for successful behavior.

Rehm (1981) evaluated the various aspects of the self-control therapy. A self-monitoring condition, self-monitoring plus self-evaluation condition, self-monitoring plus self-reinforcement condition, a full self-control treatment condition, and a waiting list control were compared. All treatment conditions were found to be superior to the waiting list control condition; only minor differences were found between the remaining groups. Roth (1982) compared the self-control treatment with antidepressant medication treatment and found that both methods of treatment reduced depressive symptomatology, but the combination of the two approaches produced the best results. Evaluation of the participants at a 3-month follow-up showed that treatment gains were maintained. The self-control treatment approach also was compared with cognitive therapy (Thomas, Petry, & Goldman, 1987). These forms of psychotherapy were found to be equally effective in alleviating depression. Generally, good results have been obtained with the self-control treatment model (Bandura, 1997).

VI. SELF-REGULATION AND THERAPY

One of the aims of any form of psychotherapy is to enhance a client's self-regulatory behavior. Rogers (1954) emphasized the self in psychotherapy and believed that changes within the self would occur with the awareness of feelings. Successful psychotherapy involved greater acceptance of the self (i.e., greater congruence between the actual self and the ideal self). Although Rogers did not use specific, directive intervention techniques aimed at changing the self, other forms of psychotherapy use direct training in self-reinforcement and self-control (Kanfer, 1970). These concepts were discussed in the addictive behaviors section. Tools specifically aimed at improving self-regulation were discussed in the health psychology section. Cognitive behavior therapy may be effective in addressing some of the issues uncovered in self-regulation models of social anxiety and/or depression.

Tests of a self-regulatory form of therapy with different populations than discussed so far have shown that it is an effective form of treatment. A self-regulatory model of treatment was found to decrease encopretic (i.e., involuntary elimination) behaviors (Grimes, 1983). A combination of self-monitoring and self-reinforcement techniques was found to decrease hyperactive behaviors and increase academic performance in hyperactive boys (Varni & Henker, 1979). Because self-regulatory therapy has been effective in impulse control, it is thought to be well suited to the treatment of borderline personality disorder clients, although no empirical research has confirmed this assertion (Kanfer, 1970; Westen, 1991).

Skills attained in therapy are especially important when one considers that the client will eventually stop receiving therapy. It is important that a client can set attainable goals, monitor his or her behavior, and evaluate his or her behavior. If there is a discrepancy between the goal and the behavior, an attempt should be made to reduce it. Finally, the client should engage in the reinforcement of positive behaviors.

VII. SUMMARY AND CONCLUSIONS

The self-regulation of human behavior involves setting goals, and monitoring and evaluating behavior and thoughts. An attempt is made to reduce discrepancies between standards and behavior. If goals have been achieved, a person may engage in reinforcing thoughts and/or activities (self-reinforcement). Problems in the self-regulation of behavior or thoughts may result in distress. It may be that goals are set at levels that are too high or at levels that an individual does not believe he or she is capable of achieving. An individual may engage in perseverative self-monitoring and self-evaluation or, alternatively, may disengage from the monitoring of behavior. Furthermore, positive behaviors and cognitions may not be reinforced.

Several areas of clinical psychology (i.e., addictive behaviors, social anxiety, and depression) were discussed in terms of failure in self-regulation. In the addictive behaviors field, a main cause for failure in self-regulation is the disengagement of self-monitoring. An individual ceases monitoring and evaluating behavior, and engages in behaviors that deviate from goals. Therapy can involve raising a client's self-regulatory efficacy and/or having the client engage in constant and detailed self-monitoring.

Contrary to the addictive behavior research, socially anxious individuals and depressed individuals have been found to engage in perseverative self-monitoring and self-appraisal. Socially anxious and depressed persons also may set goals that they do not believe they are capable of achieving.

Furthermore, socially anxious individuals may evaluate themselves negatively and engage in less self-reinforcement. Socially anxious and/or depressed individuals may benefit from cognitive behavior therapy, where they are to set attainable goals, evaluate behavior in a therapy session so that it is done fairly, and self-reinforce positive behaviors.

Thus, principles of self-regulation theory can be used in therapy. Individuals who exhibit the Type A behavior pattern also can benefit from such self-regulatory therapy. A main component is to train the client to self-monitor behavior so as to identify states of increased arousal. Type A behavior pattern individuals may also benefit from the use of self-regulatory tools such as meditation, hypnosis, relaxation therapy, and biofeedback. These self-regulation strategies also have been shown to be effective in the management of various health problems (e.g., hypertension). Therapy based on self-regulation theory is appealing because it trains clients or patients to do something for themselves, and these skills can be used and continued after the therapy has ended.

Future research should further investigate the relevance of goal setting, self-monitoring, self-evaluation, and self-reinforcement in addictive behaviors, the management of health problems, depression, and social anxiety. Much of the research that has been done has been conducted with the use of an undergraduate population and should be replicated with clinical populations. Research in self-regulation in clinical psychology should investigate the relationship between each aspect of self-regulation (i.e., goal setting, self-monitoring, self-evaluation, and self-reinforcement) and the particular area under investigation (e.g., social anxiety). The efficacy of therapy aimed at these areas should be investigated and designed such that it is possible to determine the effects of targeting only specific aspects of self-regulation in therapy (e.g., only self-monitoring) as well as the effects of targeting all aspects of self-regulation in therapy.

ACKNOWLEDGMENT

Preparation of this article was supported, in part, by Social Sciences and Humanities Research Council Grant No. 410-94-1473 to Norman S. Endler.

REFERENCES

Ahrens, A. H., Zeiss, A. M., & Kanfer, R. (1988). Dysphoric deficits in interpersonal standards, self-efficacy, and social comparison. *Cognitive Therapy and Research, 12,* 53–67.
Alden, L. E., Bieling, P. J., & Wallace, S. T. (1994). Perfectionism in an interpersonal context: A self-regulation analysis of dysphoria and social anxiety. *Cognitive Therapy and Research, 18,* 297–316.

Arkin, R. M., Lake, E. A. & Baumgardner, A. H. (1986). Shyness and self-presentation. In W. H. Jones, J. M. Cheek, & S. R. Briggs (Eds.), *Shyness: Perspectives on research and treatment* (pp. 189–203). New York: Plenum press.

Bandura, A. (1977). Self-efficacy: Toward a unifying theory of behavioral change. *Psychological Review, 84*, 191–215.

Bandura, A. (1997). *Self-efficacy: The exercise of control.* New York: Freeman.

Baumeister, R. F., Heatherton, T. F., & Tice, D. M. (1994). *Losing control: How and why people fail at self-regulation.* San Diego, CA: Academic Press.

Beck, A. T. (1967). *Depression: Clinical, experimental, and theoretical aspects.* New York: Harper & Row.

Bellack, A. S., Rozensky, R., & Schwartz, J. (1974). A comparison of two forms of self-monitoring in a behavioral weight reduction program. *Behavior Therapy, 5*, 523–530.

Benson, H. (1975). *The relaxation response.* New York: Morrow.

Berlyne, D. E. (1960). *Conflict, arousal, and curiosity.* New York: McGraw-Hill.

Block, J. (1996). Some jangly remarks on Baumeister and Heatherton. *Psychological Inquiry, 7*, 28–32.

Bruch, M. A., Mattia, J. I., Heimberg, R. G., & Holt, C. S. (1993). Cognitive specificity in social anxiety and depression: Supporting evidence and qualifications due to affective confounding. *Cognitive Therapy and Research 17*, 1–21.

Burke, J. F. (1989). *Contemporary approaches to psychotherapy and counseling: The self-regulation and monitoring model.* Pacific Grove, CA: Brooks/Cole.

Buss, A. H. (1986). *Self-consciousness and social anxiety.* New York: W. H. Freeman.

Cacioppo, J. T., Glass, C. R., & Merlozzi, T. V. (1979). Self-statements and self-evaluations: A cognitive response analysis of heterosocial anxiety, *Cognitive Therapy and Research, 3*, 249–262.

Candiotte, M. M., & Lichtenstein, E. (1981). Self-efficacy and relapse in smoking cessation programs. *Journal of Consulting and Clinical Psychology, 49*, 648–658.

Cannon, W. B. (1932). *The wisdom of the body.* New York: Norton.

Carver, C. S., Coleman, A. E., & Glass, D. C. (1976). The coronary-prone behavior pattern and the suppression of fatigue on a treadmill test. *Journal of Personality and Social Psychology, 33*, 460–466.

Carver, C. S., & Scheier, M. F. (1982). Control theory: A useful conceptual framework for personality-social, clinical, and health psychology. *Psychological Bulletin, 92*, 111–135.

Carver, C. S., & Scheier, M. F. (1986). Analyzing shyness: A specific application of broader self-regulatory principles. In W. H. Jones, J. M. Cheek, & S. R. Briggs (Eds.), *Shyness: Perspectives on research and treatment* (pp. 173–185). New York: Plenum.

Carver, C. S., & Scheier, M. F. (1999). Themes and issues in the self-regulation of behavior. In R. S. Wyer, Jr. (Ed.), *Advances in social cognition* (Vol. 12, pp. 1–105). Mahwah, NJ: Erlbaum.

Cernovsky, Z. Z. (1989). Self-reinforcement scores of alcoholics. *Advances in Alcohol and Substance Abuse, 8*, 67–73.

Cheek., J. M. & Buss, A. H. (1981). Shyness and sociability. *Journal of Personality and social Psychology, 41*, 330–339.

Clark, J. V. & Arkowitz, H. (1975). Social anxiety and self-evaluation of interpersonal performance. *Psychological Reports, 36*, 211–221.

Clark, N. M., Janz, N. K., Dodge, J. A., & Sharpe, P. A. (1992). Self-regulation of health behavior: The "take PRIDE" program. *Health Education Quarterly, 19*, 341–354.

Cooney, J. L., & Zeichner, A. (1985). Selective attention to negative feedback in Type A and Type B individuals. *Journal of Abnormal Psychology, 91*, 110–112.

Creer, T. L. (1988). Asthma. In W. Linden (Ed.), *Biological barriers in behavioral medicine* (pp. 220–256). New York: Plenum.

Creer, T. L., & Winder, J. A. (1986). The self-management of asthma. In K. A. Holroyd & T. L. Creer (Eds.) *Handbook of self-management in health psychology and behavioral medicine* (pp. 269–303). New York: Academic Press.

Curry, S., Marlatt, G. A., & Gordon, J. R. (1987). Abstinence violation effect: Validation of an attributional construct with smoking cessation. *Journal of Consulting and Clinical Psychology, 55,* 145–149.

Delamater, A. M., Smith, J. A., Bubb, J., Davis, S. G., Gamble, T., White, N. H., & Santiago, J. V. (1991). Family based therapy for diabetic adolescents. In J. H. Johnson & S. B. Johnson (Eds.), *Advances in child health psychology* (pp. 293–306). Gainesville, FL: University of Florida Press.

Doerfler, L. A., & Aron, J. (1995). Relationship of goal setting, self-efficacy, and self-evaluation in dysphoric and socially anxious women. *Cognitive Therapy and Research, 19,* 725–738.

Emmons, R. A. (1992). Abstract versus concrete goals: Personal striving level, physical illness, and psychological well-being. *Journal of Personality and Social Psychology, 62,* 292–300.

Endler, N. S. (1983). Interactionism: A personality model, but not yet a theory. In M. M. Page (Ed.), *Nebraska Symposium on Motivation, Personality—Current theory and research* (pp. 155–200). Lincoln: University of Nebraska Press.

Endler, N. S. (1988). Hassles, health, and happiness. In M. P. Janisse (Ed.), *Individual differences, stress, and health psychology* (pp. 24–56). New York: Springer-Verlag.

Endler, N. S. (1997). Stress, anxiety and coping: The multidimensional interaction model. *Canadian Psychology, 38,* 136–153.

Endler, N. S., Edwards, J., & Vitelli, R. (1991). *Endler Multidimensional Anxiety Scales: Manual.* Los Angles, CA: Western Psychological Services.

Endler, N. S., Edwards, J., Vitelli, R., & Parker, J. D. A (1989). Assessment of state and trait anxiety: Endler Multidimensional Anxiety Scales. *Anxiety Research2,* 1–14.

Endler, N. S., & Magnusson, D. (1976). Multidimensional aspects of state and trait anxiety: A cross-cultural study of Canadian and Swedish college students. In C. D. Spielberger & R. diaz-Guerrero (Eds.), *Cross-cultural anxiety* (pp. 143–172). Washington, DC: Hemisphere.

Endler, N. S., & Parker, J. D. A. (1994). Assessment of multidimensional coping: Task, emotion, and avoidance strategies. *Psychological Assessment, 6,* 50–60.

Endler, N. S., & Parker, J. D. A. (1999). *Coping Inventory for Stressful Situations (CISS): Manual.* (2nd ed.). Toronto, Canada: Multi-Health Systems.

Endler, N. S., Parker, J. D. A., & Summerfeldt, L. J. (1993). Coping with health problems: Conceptual and methodological issues. *Canadian Journal of Behavioral Science, 25,* 384–399.

Endler, N. S., Parker, J. D. A., & Summerfeldt, L. J. (1998). Coping with health problems: Developing a reliable and valid multidimensional measure. *Psychological Assessment, 10,* 195–205.

Endler, N. S., Speer, R. L., Johnson, J. M., & Flett, G. L. (1998). *Controllability, coping efficacy, and distress.* (Research Rep. No. 245). Toronto, Canada: York University, Department of Psychology.

Epstein, L. H., & Cluss, P. A. (1982). A behavioral medicine perspective on adherence to long-term medical regimens. *Journal of Consulting and Clinical Psychology, 50,* 950–971.

Fenigstein, A., Scheier, M. F., & Buss, A. H. (1975). Public and private self-consciousness. Assessment and theory. *Journal of Consulting and Clinical Psychology, 43,* 522–527.

Flett, G. L., Blankstein, K. R., & Boase, P. (1987). Self-focused attention in test anxiety and depression. *Journal of Social Behavior and Personality, 2,* 259–266.

Frautschi, N. M., & Chesney, M. A. (1988). Self-regulation and Type A behavior. In W. Linden (Ed.), *Biological barriers in behavioral medicine* (pp. 141–162). New York: Plenum.

Golin, S., & Terrell, F. (1977). Motivational and associative aspects of mild depression and chance tasks. *Journal of Abnormal Psychology, 86,* 389–401.

Grimes, L. (1983). Application of the self-regulatory model in dealing with encopresis. *School Psychology Review, 12,* 82–87.

Grimm, L., & Yarnold, P. (1984). Performance standards and the Type A behavior pattern. *Cognitive Therapy and Research, 8,* 59–66.

Grunau, R. V. E., & Craig, K. D. (1988). Pain. In W. Linden (Ed.), *Biological barriers in behavioral medicine* (pp. 257–280). New York: Plenum.

Heiby, E. M., Gafarian, C. T., & McCann, S. C. (1989). Situational and behavioral correlates of compliance to a diabetic regimen. *Journal of Compliance in Health Care, 4,* 101–116.

Heppner, P. P., Kampa, M., & Brunning, L. (1987). The relationship between problem-solving self-appraisal and indices of physical and psychological health. *Cognitive Therapy and Research, 11,* 155–168.

Hewitt, P. L., & Flett, G. L. (1991). Perfectionism in the self and social contexts: Conceptualization, assessment, and association with psychopathology. *Journal of Personality and Social Psychology, 60,* 456–470.

Hewitt, P. L., & Flett, G. L. (1993). Dimensions of perfectionism, daily stress, and depression: A test of the specific vulnerability hypothesis. *Journal of Abnormal Psychology, 102,* 58–65.

Higgins, E. T. (1987). Self-discrepancy: A theory relating self and affect. *Psychological Review, 94,* 319–340.

Higgins, E. T. (1997). Beyond pleasure and pain. *American Psychologist, 52,* 1280–1300.

Hilgard, E. R. (1949). Human motives and the concept of the self. *American Psychologist, 4,* 374–382.

Hindi-Alexander, M., & Cropp, G. J. A. (1984). Evaluation of a family asthma program. *Journal of Allergy and Clinical Immunology, 74,* 505–510.

Holden, E. W., & Wagner, M. K. (1990). Self-regulation and type A behavior. *Journal of Research in Personality, 24,* 57–70.

Houston, B. K. (1983). Psychophysiological responsivity and the Type A behavior pattern. *Journal of Research in Personality, 17,* 22–39.

Hull, J. G., Reilly, N. P., & Ennis, L. C. (1991). Self-consciousness, role discrepancy, and depressive affect. In R. Schwarzer & R. A. Wicklund (Eds.), *Anxiety and self-focused attention* (pp. 27–40). New York: Harwood Academic Publishers.

Hunt, J. M. (1961). *Intelligence and experience.* New York: Ronald Press.

Hunt, J. M. (1963). Motivation inherent in information processing and action. In O. J. Harvey (Ed.), *Motivation and social interaction: Cognitive determinants* (pp. 35–94). New York: Ronald Press.

Johnson, W. G., & Baggess, J. T. (1993). Obesity in adults. In R. T. Ammerman & M. Hersen (Eds.), *Handbook of behavior therapy with children and adults* (pp. 393–412). Boston: Allyn & Bacon.

Jones, W. H., Briggs, S. R., & Smith, T. G. (1986). Shyness: Conceptualization and measurement. *Journal of Personality and Social Psychology, 51,* 629–639.

Kanfer, F. H. (1970). Self-regulation: Research, issues, and speculations. In C. Neuringer & J. L. Michael (Eds.), *Behavior modification in clinical psychology* (pp. 178–220). New York: Meredith Corporation.

Kanfer, F. H. (1975). Self-management methods. In F. H. Kanfer & A. P. Goldstein (Eds.), *Helping people change: A textbook of methods* (pp. 334–389). New York: Pergamon.

Kanfer, F. H., & Karoly, P. (1972). Self-control: A behavioristic excursion into the lion's den. *Behavior Therapy, 3,* 398–416.

Kanfer, R., & Zeiss, A. M. (1983). Depression, interpersonal standard setting, and judgments of self-efficacy. *Journal of Abnormal Psychology, 92,* 319–329.

Karoly, P. (1993). Mechanisms in self-regulation: A systems view. *Annual Review of Psychology, 44,* 23–51.

Khantzian, E. J. (1990). Self-regulation and self-medication factors in alcoholism and the addictions: Similarities and differences. In M. Galanter (Ed.), *Recent developments in alcoholism, Vol.8:Combined alcohol and other drug dependence* (pp. 255–271). New York: Plenum

Kirschenbaum, D. S. (1987). Self-regulatory failure: A review with clinical implications. *Clinical Psychology Review*, 7, 77–104.

Kitamura, T., Sugawara, M., Sugawara, K., & Toda, M. A. (1996). Psychosocial study of depression in early pregnancy. *British Journal of Psychiatry*, 168, 732–738.

Kuiper, N. A., Olinger, L. J., & Swallow, S. R. (1987). Dysfunctional attitudes, mild depression, views of self, self-consciousness, and social perceptions. *Motivation and Emotion*, 11, 379–401.

Lake, E. A., & Arkin, R. M. (1985). Reactions to objective and subjective interpersonal evaluation: The influence of social anxiety. *Journal of Social and Clinical Psychology*, 3, 143–160.

Lapointe, K. A., & Crandell, C. J. (1980). Relationship of irrational beliefs to self-reported depression. *Cognitive Therapy and Research*, 4, 247–250.

Leary, M. R (1983). Social anxiousness: The construct and its measurement, *Journal of Personality Assessment*, 47, 66–75.

Leary, M. R. & Kowalski, R. M. (1993). The interaction anxiousness scale: Construct and criterion-related validity. *Journal of Personality Assessment*, 61, 136–146.

Leary M. R., & Kowalski, R. M. (1995). *Social anxiety*. New York: Guilford Press.

Lennox, R. D. (1984). Public self-consciousness, social anxiety and variability of social behavior. *Psychological Reports*, 54, 911–914.

Lewinsohn, P. M. (1974). A behavioral approach in depression. In R. J. Friedman & M. M. Katz (Eds.), *The psychology of depression: Contemporary theory and research* (pp. 157–185). Washington, DC: Winston.

Linden, W. (1988). Biopsychological barriers to the behavioral treatment of hypertension. In W. Linden (Ed.), *Biological barriers in behavioral medicine* (pp. 163–192). New York: Plenum.

Linder, L. M., & Der-Karabetian, A. (1986). Social anxiety, public self-consciousness, and variability of behavior. *Psychological Reports*, 59, 206.

Litman, G. K., Eiser, J. R., & Taylor, C. (1979). Dependence, relapse, and extinction: A theoretical critique and behavioral examination. *Journal of Clinical Psychology*, 35, 192–199.

Marlatt, G. A., Baer, J. S., & Quigley, L. A. (1995). Self-efficacy and addictive behavior. In A. Bandura (Ed.), *Self-efficacy in changing societies* (pp. 289–315). Cambridge, UK: Cambridge University Press.

Martin, T. R., Flett, G. L., Hewitt, P. L., Krames, L., & Szanto, G. (1996). Personality correlates of depression and health symptoms: A test of a self-regulation model. *Journal of Research in Personality*, 31, 264–277.

Matthews, C. O. (1977). A review of behavioral theories of depression and a self-regulation model of depression. *Psychotherapy: Theory, Research and Practice*, 14, 79–86.

Matthews, K. A., Siegel, J. M., Kuller, L. H., Thompson, M., & Varat, M. (1983). Determinants of decisions to seek medical treatment by patients with acute myocardial infarction symptoms. *Journal of Personality and Social Psychology*, 44, 1144–1156.

Matthews, K. S. (1988). CHD and Type A behavior: Update on and alternative to the Booth-Kewley and Friedman quantitative review. *Psychological Bulletin*, 104, 373–380.

McCroskey, J. C. (1977). Oral communication apprehension: A summary of recent theory and research. *Human Communications Research*, 4, 78–96.

McCroskey, J. C., Daly, J. A., Richmond, V. P., & Falcione, R. L., (1977). Studies of the relationship between communication apprehension and self-esteem. *Human Communication Research*, 3, 269–277.

Miller, W. R. (1987). Techniques to modify hazardous drinking patterns. In M. Galanter, H. Begleiter, R. Deitrich, D. Goodwin, E. Gottleib, A. Paredes, M. Rothschild, & D. Van Thiel (Eds.) *Recent developments in alcoholism*, (Vol. 5, pp. 425–438). New York: Plenum.

Mizes, J. S., & Lohr, J. M. (1983). The treatment of bulimia: A quasi-experimental investigation of the effects of stimulus narrowing, self-reinforcement and self-control relaxation. *International Journal of Eating Disorders*, 2, 59–65.

Monfrious, M. M., & Kafer, N. F. (1993). Private self-consciousness and fear of negative evaluation. *Journal of Psychology, 128*, 447–454.

Nelson, R. E. (1977). Irrational beliefs in depression. *Journal of Consulting and Clinical Psychology, 45*, 1190–1191.

Nelson, R. E., & Craighead, W. E. (1981). Tests of a self-control model of depression. *Behavior Therapy, 12*, 123–129.

Nolen-Hoeksema, S. (1991). Responses to depression and their effects on the duration of depressive episodes. *Journal of Abnormal Psychology, 100*, 569–582.

O'Keeffe, J. L., & Smith, T. W. (1988). Self-regulation and type A behavior. *Journal of Research in Personality, 22*, 232–251.

Ovcharchyn, C. A., Johnson, H. H., & Petzel, T. P. (1981). Type A behavior, academic aspirations, and academic success. *Journal of Personality, 49*, 248–256.

Parmar, R. S., & Cernovsky, Z. Z. (1993). Self-reinforcement scores of psychiatric inpatients and normal controls. *Psychological Reports, 72*, 35–38.

Perri, M. G., McAllister, D. A., Gange, J. J., Johnson, R. C., McAdoo, W. G., & Nezu, A. M. (1988). Effects of four maintenance programs on the long-term management of obesity. *Journal of Consulting and Clinical Psychology, 56*, 529–534.

Pilkonis, P. A. (1977). Shyness, public and private, and its relationship to other measures of social behavior. *Journal of Personality, 45*, 585–595.

Rehm, L. P. (1977). A self-control model of depression. *Behavior Therapy, 8*, 787–804.

Rehm, L. P. (1981a). A self-control therapy program for treatment of depression. In J. F. Clarkin & H. Glazer (Eds.), *Depression: Behavioral and directive treatment strategies* (pp. 68–110). New York: Garland Press.

Rehm, L. P. (1981b). An evaluation of major components in a self-control therapy program for depression. *Behavior Modification, 5*, 459–489.

Rehm, L. P., & Marston, A. P. (1968). Reduction of social anxiety through modification of self reinforcement: An instigation therapy technique. *Journal of Consulting and Clinical Psychology, 32*, 565–574.

Rogers, C. R. (1954). Changes in the maturity of behavior as related to therapy. In C. R. Rogers & R. F. Dymond (Eds.), *Psychotherapy and personality change* (pp. 215–237). Chicago: University of Chicago Press.

Rosenberg, M. J. (1965). When dissonance fails: On eliminating evaluation apprehension from attitude measurement. *Journal of Personality and Social Psychology, 1*, 28–42.

Roth, D. (1982). A comparison of self-control therapy and combined self-control therapy and antidepressant medication in the treatment of depression. *Behavior Therapy, 13*, 133–144.

Rothbaum, F., Weisz, J. R., & Snyder, S. S (1982). Changing the world and changing the self: A two-process model of perceived control. *Journal of Personality and Social Psychology, 42*, 5–37.

Rozensky, R. H., & Honor, L. F. (1984). Self-reinforcement, locus of reward and task maintenance, and alcoholism. *Psychological Reports, 54*, 151–155.

Schlenker, B. R., & Leary, M. R. (1982). Social anxiety and self-presentation: A conceptualization and model. *Psychological Bulletin, 92*, 641–669.

Schneider, J. A., O'Leary, A., & Agras, W. S. (1987). The role of perceived self-efficacy in recovery from bulimia: A preliminary examination. *Behavior Research and Therapy, 25*, 429–432.

Schupak-Neuberg, E., & Nemeroff, C. J. (1993). Disturbances in identity and self-regulation in bulimia nervosa: Implications for a metaphorical perspective of "body as self." *International Journal of Eating Disorders, 13*, 335–347.

Selye, H. (1956). *The stress of life*. New York: McGraw-Hill.

Shabsin, H. S., & Whitehead, W. E. (1988). Psychophysiological disorders of the gastrointestinal tract. In W. Linden (Ed.), *Biological barriers in behavioral medicine* (pp. 193–220). New York: Plenum.

Spielberger, C. D. (1983). *Manual for the State-Trait Anxiety Inventory (form V)*. Palo Alto, CA: Consulting Psychologists Press.

Suinn, R. M. (1982). Intervention with Type A Behaviors. *Journal of Consulting and Clinical Psychology, 50*, 933–949.

Thomas, J. R., Petry, R. A., & Goldman, J. R. (1987). Comparison of cognitive and behavioral self-control treatments of depression. *Psychological Reports, 60*, 975–982.

Varni, J. W., & Henker, B. (1979). A self-regulation approach to the treatment of three hyperactive boys. *Child Behavior Therapy, 1*, 171–192.

Wallace, S. T., & Alden, L. E. (1991). A comparison of social standards and perceived ability in anxious and nonanxious men. *Cognitive Therapy and Research, 15*, 237–254.

Watson, D., & Friend, R. (1969). Measurement of social-evaluative anxiety. *Journal of Consulting and Clinical Psychology, 33*, 448–457.

Watson, D. L., & Tharp, R. G. (1997). Self-directed behavior: Self-modification for personal adjustment. Pacific Grove, CA: Brooks/Cole.

Westen, D. (1991). Cognitive-behavioral interventions in the psychoanalytic psychotherapy of borderline personality disorders. *Clinical Psychology Review, 11*, 211–230.

Westover, S. A., & Lanyon, R. I. (1990). The maintenance of weight loss after behavioral treatment. *Behavior Modification, 14*, 123–137.

Wilson, A., Passik, S. D., Faude, J., Abrams, J., & Gordon, E. (1989). A hierarchical model of opiate addiction: Failures of self-regulation as a central aspect of substance abuse. *Journal of Nervous and Mental Disease, 177*, 390–399.

Wing, R. R. (1992). Very low calorie diets in the treatment of Type II diabetes: Psychological and physiological effects. In T. A. Wadden & T. B. VanItallie (Eds.), *Treatment of the seriously obese patient* (pp. 231–251). New York: Guilford.

Zimbardo, P. G. (1977). *Shyness*. New York: Jove.

18

SELF-MANAGEMENT OF
CHRONIC ILLNESS

THOMAS L. CREER

Ohio University, Athens, Ohio

I. INTRODUCTION

Half a century ago, most people in the world died before the age of 50. According to the World Health Organization (1997) report, the vast majority of people now live well beyond this age, with the global life expectancy at birth reaching 65 years in 1996. Longer life can be a penalty as well as a prize, however. As life expectancy increases, so does the certainty that people will become more susceptible to chronic illness and disorders common in older age groups. The problem is of enormous proportion. Chronic illness, including circulatory diseases, cancer, and respiratory disorders, are responsible for more than 24 million deaths a year, or about half the rate of mortality in the world. The number of people aged 65 and older increased to 380 million, a 14% increase in that age group, between 1990 and 1995. Between 1996 and 2020, it is projected that the over-65 aged population will increase about 82% globally, or by about 110% in the least developed and developing countries, and by about 40% in developed countries. The problem is further accentuated when one adds those below the age of 65 who experience chronic illness. The costs of chronic health conditions are also enormous. Hoffman, Rice, and Sung (1996) reported that in the United States alone, over 45% of the population have one or more chronic conditions; their direct health care costs account for three fourths of the U.S. health care expenditures. Total costs for people with chronic conditions in 1990 amounted to $659 billion—$425 billion in direct health care costs and $234 billion in indirect costs. Marks (1996) noted that the cost of chronic illness had surpassed 60% of the $1 trillion spent on medical care in the United States.

Copyright © 2000 by Academic Press.
All rights of reproduction in any form reserved.

With few exceptions, chronic illnesses or disorders are difficult, if possible, to cure. They are less open to community action, in part because they do not spread from person to person. Every case of chronic disease represents a burden borne by an individual who, depending on circumstances, may or may not have access to treatment or support. In addition, there are many common chronic disorders, such as arthritis, diabetes, hypertension, and asthma, that simply have no cure. This stark fact, commented the World Health Organization (1997) report,

> demands a realistic response: if the majority of chronic diseases cannot as yet be cured, the emphasis must be on preventing their premature onset, delaying their development in later life, reducing the suffering that they cause, and providing the supportive social environment to care for those disabled by them. (p. 2)

The World Health Organization (1997) report acknowledges that the development of chronic diseases or disorders is seldom, if ever, due to one cause. There are many factors over which an individual has little control. These include poverty, poor reproductive and maternal health, genetic predisposition, occupational hazards, and unhealthy living and stressful working conditions. There are many lifestyle factors—smoking, heavy alcohol consumption, inappropriate diet, and inadequate physical activity —known to increase the risk of chronic illness. To some degree, these factors are within the purview of control of the well-informed and motivated individual. The World Health Organization (1997) report proclaimed that throughout the entire life span,

> opportunities exist for prevention or treatment, for cure or for care. Major efforts have also been made, and continue to be made in these fields, in promoting healthy behaviour in individuals, in attacking risk factors, in promoting health as a component of social policies, and in protecting the environment through pollution control. (p. 3)

Maximizing these opportunities for prevention will remain at the forefront of worldwide efforts to curb chronic disease. Success here can be measured by a reduction in people who cross the threshold from being healthy to having a chronic illness.

II. CHARACTERISTICS OF CHRONIC ILLNESS

Sontag (1978) began her classic essay, *Illness as Metaphor*, with the following observation:

> Illness is the night-side of life, a more onerous citizenship. Everyone who is born holds dual citizenship in the kingdom of the well and in the kingdom of the sick. Although we all prefer to use only the good passport, sooner or later each of us is obliged, at least for a spell, to identify ourselves as citizens of that other place. (p. 3)

Usually when we are ill, we know that medical treatment or the passage of time will restore us to our health. We can then escape the night side of life. Patients with a chronic illness do not have the luxury of these expectations, however. There are characteristics regarding their diseases or disorders that are always with them. They not only dictate how they live their lives, but set the parameters for any proposed treatment, including the introduction of self-management techniques. Three types of characteristics will be briefly discussed: chronic illness, psychological factors, and treatment considerations.

A. CHARACTERISTICS

Two characteristics of chronic illness merit comment:

Duration.   Verbrugge and Patrick (1995) described duration as the defining aspect of chronic illness. Once patients pass certain symptomatic or diagnostic thresholds, chronic conditions are permanent features they can expect to experience for the rest of their lives.

Rhythm of Disorder.   Although a patient with a chronic illness constantly deals with his or her condition, the rhythm of the illness itself may wax and wane. This is the case with many chronic disorders including arthritis, asthma, diabetes, cystic fibrosis, headache, and multiple sclerosis. Periods of quiescence are interspersed between exacerbations of the condition; alleviation of these episodic disease flare-ups require extra medications, additional treatment and, in extreme cases, hospitalization. The episodic nature of many chronic illnesses poses a problem for self-management in that patients will volunteer to learn these skills when symptomatic, but lose their interest once they are asymptomatic.

B. PSYCHOLOGICAL FACTORS

Two types of psychological factors deserve a brief description.

Beliefs.   When they first begin experiencing a chronic illness, patients may seek relief from a number of sources. They may visit an array of physicians or health care providers. Alternative medicine or holistic health options may be explored. Every patient harbors hope for the silver bullet that will restore him or her to good health. Gradually, however, the limits of medical knowledge become a reality. Many patients acquire the belief that nothing can be done for them or their illness. This may be accompanied by sense of hopelessness that permeates their lives. Such beliefs may become a barrier when patients are approached about becoming involved in their own treatment; they may feel themselves incapable of assuming such a role.

Other patients tend to think that any new treatment is the panacea for their problems. When it proves not to be the case, they become disillusioned. This could mean that they cease to perform self-management skills they have been taught to help control their illness.

Attitudes toward Chronic Illness.   A prevailing view is that most people with chronic illness are healthy people with a unique set of behavioral problems (e.g., Creer, Renne, & Christian, 1976; Russo & Varni, 1982). In short, they are normal people in an abnormal situation (Desquin, Holt, & McCarthy, 1994). Still, there is a lot of psychological baggage that accompanies any chronic condition; often it is reflected in the attitudes of others toward patients. A young adult with rheumatoid arthritis may be told, "Arthritis only comes when you're old. You can't have arthritis." This does not help the individual, let alone the thousands of children afflicted with juvenile rheumatoid arthritis. Alternatively, someone with asthma may be told, "Snap out of it. Asthma is all in your head." This information does not help the patient breathe any better. In another case, a patient with recurring headache hears, "Why aren't you feeling well today? You were fine yesterday." This statement does not alleviate the individual's pain. Finally, there is the premise attacked by Sontag (1978) that illness is an expression of the person with the disorder. Considering illness as a metaphor is often the cruelest blow to someone with a chronic condition. It not only generates unnecessary guilt, but it can lead to a further deterioration of hope that something can be done to alleviate the patient's condition.

C. TREATMENT CONSIDERATIONS

Two types of treatment considerations will be noted:

Degree of Control.   As noted, there are no cures for many chronic illnesses. The best that one can hope is that a condition be controlled. Establishing control over a chronic illness, whether arthritis or asthma, is often easier said than done, however. Control of a chronic disorder is a function of two sets of variables: treatment variables, such as access to appropriate medical care, and patient variables, such as ability to use self-management skills. Both sets of variables must be successfully integrated to control a chronic illness.

Uncertainty.   Uncertainty underlies the treatment received by patients with chronic illness. Whereas there is no cure for most conditions, the physician or health care professional is uncertain as to what will work to manage chronic illness in a given patient. All that can be done is to provide what appears to be the best treatment option for that patient. If it works, great; if it does not, another treatment option must be considered. A trial-and-error process of testing various treatment approaches can continue for years. Both health care providers and their patients develop a sense of uncertainty as to what will actually work for a given patient. Consequently, both patients and their health care providers may be uncertain as to whether self-management, a method that requires input from both groups, will work.

III. TREATMENT OF CHRONIC ILLNESS

The treatment and control of a chronic illness requires taking a comprehensive approach. Wagner, Austin, and Von Korff (1996) found that successful programs shared common characteristics. These components were integrated into an evidence-based model of planned health care. An overview of the five major components of the model is presented; it establishes a context for the role of self-management in the treatment of chronic illness.

A. EXPLICIT PLANS AND GUIDELINES

A common feature of effective programs for chronic illness is use of guidelines or a plan that provides an explicit outline of what need to be done for patients, at what intervals, and by whom. The use of practice protocols or guidelines, based on scientific evidence of effectiveness, permits health care professionals to "make the intellectual leap from constantly thinking and worrying about specific patients to considering all patients with specific clinical features or needs and how these needs might be met" (Wagner et al., 1996, p. 519). Examples of such guidelines include those issued for the management and control of asthma (National Asthma Education Program, 1991; National Asthma Education and Prevention Program 1997; National Heart, Lung, and Blood Institute, 1992) and diabetes (Report of the Expert Committee, 1997).

B. PRACTICE REDESIGN

Successful programs for chronic illness organize a health delivery system with a broad array of resources to meet the needs of patients who require more time and closer follow-up. Attaining these aims involves the organization of a treatment team and the allocation of tasks among them; the management of patient contact, including appointments and follow-up; and the use of other health care professionals. Such planned deviations for delivering care was referred to as practice redesign by Wagner and his coauthors (1996).

C. CLINICAL EXPERTISE

Evidence suggests that specialists have a greater knowledge of effective therapies for chronic illnesses than do generalists. Interventions that increase the expertise of physicians in general practice or that widen the availability of expertise result in better health outcomes. Conventional referral to specialists remains the dominant source of expert assistance, although Wagner et al. (1996) suggested that other models of distributed expertise, such as consultation and direction from expert teams of health care professionals, may prove more cost effective for chronic illnesses.

D. INFORMATION

Information to health care professionals about patients, their care, and their outcomes is essential in all population-based strategies for improving chronic illness care. Successful tactics are proactive in that they invite or remind patients to participate in helping to care for themselves. Specific strategies include the use of reminders, feedback, and involvement in care planning.

E. PATIENT EDUCATION

The reduction of symptoms and complications from most chronic diseases requires changes in lifestyle, as well as the development and execution of self-management competencies. All successful guidelines or chronic disease programs provide some sort of educational intervention to achieve these aims. Wagner and his colleagues (1996) concluded that four essential elements are involved, to varying degrees, in these programs. These elements are (a) collaborative problem definition by patients and their health care providers, (b) targeting, goal setting, and planning, (c) a continuum of self-management training and support services, and (d) active and sustained follow-up. These elements are essential ingredients in the self-management of chronic illness.

IV. SELF-MANAGEMENT: SETTING THE STAGE

Before a self-management program can be launched, there is a need to set the stage to initiate the procedure. In many cases, this is the most difficult challenge faced in developing and executing self-management programs for chronic illness. A number of models have been proposed for designing patient education and behavioral change programs; these various approaches have been summarized in Glanz, Lewis, and Rimer (1997). The models are often highly theoretical, however, and omit discussion of the practical problems faced in developing and conducting a self-management program for chronically ill patients. What follows is a brief summary of common problems that must be surmounted if a self-management program is to be a success.

A. SELF-REGULATION OR SELF-MANAGEMENT?

Differing models of self-regulation and self-management have been proposed over the years. Self-regulation is sometimes taken to imply that people follow self-set goals, and self-management connotes that someone follows goals set by others. There are four problems with these dichotomous definitions, however.

First, the definitions noted previously are not universally accepted. Sulzer-Azaroff and Mayer (1991) included, as part of their definition of self-management, the "self-selection of goals" (p. 597). This is identical to what was described previously herein as a definition of self-regulation. However, the definition by Sulzer-Azaroff and Mayer is representative of what one finds in searching the literature for the meanings of either self-regulation or self-management. There is considerable ambiguity and overlapping of definitions. In addition, other terms, such as self-control, self-change, self-directed behavior, and, in the case of chronic illness, self-care have been added to further muddy the water. There is a strong and growing trend to treat the terms "self-regulation," "self-management," "self-control," "self-change," and "self-directed behavior" as synonymous. As long as these terms are used interchangeably, any consideration of a distinction between self-regulation and self-management is tantamount to generating sound and fury, but little else.

Second, in the case of a chronic disease, neither of the traditional definitions of self-regulation or self-management is appropriate. This is because there is a growing practice of health care personnel and patients to set treatment goals jointly (e.g., National Asthma Education and Prevention Program, 1997). In these cases, the patient is guided neither by self-set goals nor by goals set by others. As medicine moves toward a market-driven model (Herzlinger, 1997), the practice of following treatment goals mutually established by patients and health care personnel will increase.

Third, any debate about which term to use, whether it be self-regulation or self-management, is akin to what happens in discussing how well patients do at following their physician's instructions. Here, terms such as compliance, adherence, and a new term, concordance (Mullen, 1997), are used. However, the proliferation of terms has done nothing to improve medication compliance (Creer, 1998). In anything, coining different terms for the same behavior has been a way to dance around the issue: How can we change noncompliant behavior? For this reason, investigators working with chronically ill patients have not debated the issue of which term to use, self-regulation or self-management. They have pursued more pressing issues such as trying to ameliorate the pain and suffering of patients.

Finally, if a working definition of self-management were minted to describe what happens when these techniques are applied to chronic diseases, it would read as follows:

> *Self-management* is a procedure where patients change some aspect of their own behavior. It involves processes including (a) goal selection, (b) information collection, (c) information processing and evaluation, (d) decision making, (e) action, and (f) self-reaction. Successful mastery and performance of self-management skills results in the following outcomes: (a) changes in mortality and morbidity indices of the disease; (b) improvement in the quality of life experienced by patients and those around them; and (c) the development of self-efficacy beliefs on the part of patients that they can make a contribution to the management of their disorder, in part through their becoming partners with their physicians and other health care providers to control the chronic disease or disorder.

This description is more comprehensive than other definitions, but it captures the complexity of teaching patients to perform self-management skills to help control their chronic illness.

B. RECRUITMENT OF STAFF

Perhaps the most ignored variable in setting the stage for self-management of chronic disease is recruitment of the staff who are going to conduct the program and interact, on a regular basis, with the patients. Staff members who conduct self-management programs must be skilled at interacting and communicating with patients, as well as proactive in providing constant support and reinforcement. The motivational properties of the staff can be as important, in many cases, as the program itself. Finally, successful self-management programs are conducted by staff who exhibit the qualities Rogers (1951) defined as (a) warmth, or the acceptance of the values of others without necessarily accepting all their behaviors, (b) empathy, or the ability to perceive the patients from their point of view, and (c) genuineness, or the open expression of their feelings. These qualities are not only necessary for the success of self-management programs for chronic illness (Creer, Kotses, & Reynolds, 1991), but they contribute to the maintenance of self-management skills long after the program has ended.

C. IDENTIFICATION AND REFERRAL OF POTENTIAL SUBJECTS

There is no surefire way to recruit chronically ill patients to a self-management program, but, before anyone can be recruited, potential sources of patient referrals must be identified. Creer (1983) suggested several approaches that could be taken, including personal letters to physicians, talks before local medical groups and societies, contacts with public health centers, hospitals, and health maintenance organizations, and one-on-one contacts with local physicians and health care providers. The latter approach, adapted from the successful strategies used by pharmaceutical company representatives, has proven highly effective. In a study reported by Creer and colleagues (1988) on pediatric asthma, the initial aim was to recruit 124 children for the project. Eventually, 399 children and their families participated in the program. Identification and referral of additional patients and their families by individual physicians would have continued indefinitely had the project not been terminated because of the closure of the facility where it was being conducted.

D. RECRUITMENT OF SUBJECTS

The ability to recruit and retain patients in a study is the bread and butter of self-management. Unless patients can be persuaded to volunteer to learn and perform self-management skills, any program is bound to fail. How to do it to fulfill the specific goals of a self-management program for a particular illness is another matter. Creer (1983) observed:

> Recruiting patients for any study requires a combination of interpersonal skills, patience, and, in the end, luck. The literature is riddled with reports of investigations that, beginning on a high note, gradually deteriorated because of the defection of subjects. The result is sometimes a death knell for the project or, at best, a weakening of the findings that are obtained. (p. 27)

As noted, the episodic nature of chronic illness often presents problems in subject recruitment and retention. Chronically ill patients are motivated to learn self-management skills when they experience an exacerbation of their symptoms; they are often unwilling to undergo such training when their health improves. Repeated and personal contacts by staff members, tailored for individual patients, can be used to bridge periods when patients are symptomatic or asymptomatic; these interactions also serve to prepare patients for their later acquisition of self-management skills.

E. EXPECTANCIES

Different expectancies on the part of patients and health care professionals lead to an array of difficulties. The expectancies of each group will be discussed separately.

Perceptions of Health Care Providers The goals and processes of self-management are misunderstood by the majority of physicians and health care personnel. Most are trained and experienced in using what Anderson (1995) referred to as the traditional medical model. The model suggests physicians and health care providers are responsible for diagnosing the illness and assuring that treatment is carried out as prescribed. An illustration of the model in action, continued Anderson (1995), comes in the management of the hospitalized, acutely ill patient. The patient "is viewed as passive, accepting, compliant, and dependent on the physician's medical knowledge and goodwill" (p. 413). Anderson (1995) concluded that the traditional model is inappropriate and unworkable with chronic illness, however. Using diabetes as an example, he noted:

> Patients carry out 95% or more of the daily self-care of diabetes. If such self-care merely involved taking a pill each morning, this issue might never have arisen, since taking a pill once a day is not nearly as difficult or intrusive on the patient's life as are many diabetes self-care regimens. (p. 41)

Anderson could have inserted any number of chronic illnesses, including arthritis, asthma, and HIV infections, in the place of diabetes and his statement would remain accurate.

Physicians and other health care providers are also under the illusion that there is active patient/health care provider collaboration during all phases of self-management. There is not. The confusion is reflected by the International Consensus Report on the Diagnosis and Treatment of Asthma (National Heart, Lung, and Blood Institute, 1992). It describes self-management as "guided self-management" or "co-management" between health care providers and patients. In reality, the execution of almost all self-management activities is the sole responsibility of patients. They alone collect, process, and evaluate data on themselves and their condition. They alone make decisions as to what to do on the basis of this information, and they alone initiate the action of their choice. Finally, self-reaction refers to the patient alone deciding if his or her actions were effective in helping to control his or her illness. The role of health care providers in the self-management model is limited to helping establish explicit goals and in tracking the progress of the patients (Creer & Holroyd, 1997).

The misunderstanding of what constitutes self-management is a continuing source of dismay to the medical and behavioral scientists who have developed and introduced self-management techniques for chronic illnesses. This was borne out by a recent meeting when a number of participants objected to the term, "collaborative management," used to describe the purpose of the conference (Von Korff, Gruman, Schaefer, Curry, & Wagner, 1996). It was thought that the label did not describe the reality of what happens in self-management. These experts believed that physicians and health care personnel must facilitate and reinforce the independent action of patients in performing the myriad of self-management skills they have been taught to use to control their illness. As more and more becomes known about the intricate nature of different chronic illnesses and the complex actions required to manage them, patients must assume more responsibility for the treatment of their conditions. The concerns expressed proved groundless because it was explained that the term "collaborative management" does incorporate these concerns (M. Von Korff, personal communication, January 23, 1998).

Expectations of Patients.   What is meant by self-management is no less confusing to patients. As patients and potential patients, we have been taught to leave our health care to the doctor or health care provider. The role we have assumed, suggests Anderson (1995), is akin to the interactions that take place between parents and their children rather than to what occurs between adults and adults. We are told what our problems are and how to treat them; we are repeatedly urged not to make decisions regarding our health, including whether to start exercising or to lose weight, without clearing our proposed actions with our health care provider. We not only have come to accept this advice, but many of us rely on our health care system, not on ourselves, to keep us well.

When patients enroll in a self-management program, the focus shifts dramatically: Here the patient is asked to assume a major responsibility for his or her own condition. Is this change confusing? It certainly is to many patients with a chronic illness. After being conditioned to be dependent upon a health care system for most of their lives, they are asked to become partners with their physicians by taking independent action to help manage their health. Extinguishing outdated expectations and acquiring those conducive to assuming more personal responsibility is a prerequisite to the learning and use of self-management techniques. Just how difficult this can be is illustrated by the overuse of hospital emergency rooms by many patients with a chronic illness.

Patients, particularly those with a lower income, avoid seeking regular medical care and the continuity of treatment it provides. Rather, they do nothing until they experience an exacerbation of their condition. If it becomes serious enough, they seek help at a hospital emergency room. Emergency rooms provide needed treatment, but they also reinforce continued use of their services. This pattern can be difficult to extinguish, as pointed out by Hoffmann, Broyles, and Tyson (1997). They made a primary health care provider and social services available to the parents of very low birth weight preterm infants in an effort to teach the parents to manage their children. It was found that the health care provider was not notified before 49% of the ER visits, and that mothers often did not recall what infant signs needed medical attention. Seventy-nine percent of the ER visits were delayed more than 10 hours; 24% of the ER visits resulted in admittance to the hospital.

F. RACIAL AND CULTURAL DIFFERENCES

These differences have been a barrier in conducting self-management programs for chronic illness. Characteristics of chronic illness, diversity of beliefs, differing expectations, and poor communication between patients and health care providers have served as obstacles to self-management. In addition, communication patterns (Clark, et al., 1990) and limited reading skills in low income families have presented impediments to teaching self-management skills. Weiss and Coyne (1997) described the extent of the latter problem. They reported that an estimated 40 to 44 million people, about one-quarter of the adult population in the United States, cannot understand written materials that require only a basic proficiency in reading. The average reading level among adults in the United States is no higher than eighth-grade level and, in the case of Medicaid enrollees, no higher than fifth-grade level. Poor reading levels, noted Weiss and Coyne (1997), are associated with poor health.

G. TASK DEMANDS

The chasm between health care providers and patients is often wide when it comes to considering tasks demanded of patients in self-management programs. When patients are requested to use self-management techniques to better control their chronic illness, they are often asked to perform too many activities. Anderson (1995) complained that many type II diabetic patients are unable or unwilling to carry out the tedious and often unrealistic recommendations they are given regarding weight loss and exercise. A similar situation exists with respect to asthma. A number of recommendations for the management of the disorder are incorporated in the guidelines provided for the management of asthma (e.g., National Asthma Education Program, 1991; National Heart, Lung, and Blood Institute, 1992, 1995). The numerous suggestions offered are prudent when considered individually; if combined together, however, they would overwhelm the average patient attempting to manage his or her asthma (Creer & Holroyd, 1997; Creer, Levstek, & Reynolds, 1998). In addition, observing and gathering too much information about themselves forces patients to drift toward placing the disorder at the center of their lives. This is ironical when one considers that self-management skills are designed to help a chronic illness be less of a focus for the patient.

A confusing aspect of task demands is that patients' reactions to what they are asked to do vary widely. One end of the spectrum is anchored by those patients, aptly referred to as performing "obsessive–compulsive self-regulation" by Kirschenbaum and Tomarken (1982), who display persistent self-monitoring over long periods of time. They may never miss taking a blood pressure reading or completing a daily arthritis diary; in essence their lives revolve around gathering data on themselves and their health. This creates the undesirable side effect of having their existence, as well as that of their families, revolve around their illness. At the other end of the spectrum, there are those patients who never monitor or record any information regarding themselves and their illness. This, too, is undesirable because effective self-management is dependent on accurate self-monitoring by patients. This problem was highlighted in describing difficulties encountered in placing patients on complex drug-taking regimens for HIV. Sontag and Richardson (1997) reported that many physicians refused to put some patients on regimens that required their taking medications at specific times six or more times a day, sometimes with food and sometimes without food. Why did the physicians deny patients such treatment when it could prolong the patient's lives? Because missing doses, a behavior the patients had exhibited, could lead to the HIV becoming more resistant to future treatments. This consequence, concluded the physicians, posed too great a risk for them to take.

V. PROCESSES OF SELF-MANAGEMENT

Processes of self-management are described in several sources (e.g., Ford, 1987; Holroyd & Creer, 1986; Karoly, 1993). Creer and Holroyd (1997) pointed out that although different terminology has been used, there is considerable commonality among different descriptions of self-management. Apparent differences occur because of the way specific processes are categorized, not from differences in conceptualization. Processes significant in the self-management of chronic illness include (a) goal selection, (b) information collection, (c) information processing and evaluation, (d) decision making, (e) action, and (f) self-reaction. These processes guide the discussion that follows.

A. GOAL SELECTION

Goal selection can take place only after careful preparation. Creer and Holroyd (1997) suggested two preparatory functions were necessary in goal selection: Individuals must first acquire knowledge of their chronic illness and how it can be managed. Patient education provides this information, as well as teaching patients the self-management skills they can execute to manage their condition. When patients have been taught about their illness and the role they can play in its management, specific goals can be set that, if attained, are likely to improve the health and well-being of the individual.

Goal selection is the only activity where there is true collaboration between patients and their health care providers. After goals have been discussed, negotiated, and finally determined, they should be written up and described in some sort of treatment guideline or action plan. Written action plans can be invaluable to patients when they later treat their disorder (Lieu et al., 1997). It becomes the responsibility of individual patients, however, to perform whatever self-management skills are necessary to attain the goals; physicians and other medical personnel, noted Creer and Holroyd (1997), are restricted to tracking the individual patient's behavior.

Ford (1987), Karoly (1993), and Creer and Holroyd (1997) described three positive consequences of goal selection: (a) It establishes preferences about what are desirable outcomes, (b) it increases the commitment of individuals to perform goal-relevant self-management skills, and (c) it establishes expectancies on the part of patients that trigger their effort and performance. In the case of chronic illness, goal selection can have an additional positive consequence: It establishes an objective for managing an illness that can be reached only through the collaborative efforts of patients and health care providers. Ideally, patients begin to believe that by developing specific self-management competencies, they have become partners with their physicians in managing a chronic illness (Creer & Holroyd, 1997).

B. INFORMATION COLLECTION

The basis of information collection is self-monitoring, or the self-observation and self-recording of data. Self-monitoring not only provides the foundation for self-management, but is a necessary condition for determining if goals are achieved. Self-monitoring is essential to the successful self-management of problems ranging from a chronic illness, such as asthma (Creer & Bender, 1993), to a chronic condition, such as obesity (Baker & Kirschenbaum, 1993).

Three suggestions have been offered for improving the self-monitoring of chronic illness (Creer & Bender, 1993). First, patients should monitor only phenomena that have been operationally defined as target behaviors. Anyone, including patients with a chronic illness, could be overwhelmed if asked to monitor too many categories of phenomena that constantly swirl around them. Second, when possible, an objective measure, such as use of fingerstick prothrombin times to regulate oral anticoagulation (e.g., Ansell, Holden, & Knapic, 1989) or peak flow meters to monitor airway obstruction (Creer et al., 1988), should be used to measure selected target behaviors or responses. Finally, in gathering information, it is important that individuals observe and record information only during specified periods of time as directed by their physicians or health care personnel. It is virtually impossible to perform a task, such as taking blood pressure twice daily, each day for the remainder of one's life.

C. INFORMATION PROCESSING AND EVALUATION

Patients must learn to process and evaluate the information they collect about themselves and their condition. Creer and Holroyd (1997) pointed out that five distinct steps were involved in this process.

First, patients must be able to detect any significant changes that occur in themselves. The process involves their evaluating the information they have observed, recorded, and processed about themselves. This may not be difficult when patients gather information with an objective measure, for example, a blood pressure monitor. However, when asked to monitor and process information about the subjective symptoms they experience, such as occurs with headache or chronic pain, the task may be more difficult. Here, the patient is asked to detect changes from some sort of personal baseline or adaptation level. This level is essentially private information known only to the patient. Under these circumstances, there is apt to be greater variability among patients. Some will be superb at assessing changes in themselves; others will be less skilled.

Second, to make the assessment of changes more consistent across patients, standards must be established to permit patients to evaluate the data they collect and process about themselves and their condition. Public standards have been developed for judging the severity of many chronic diseases, including hypertension, diabetes, asthma, and AIDS (Creer & Holroyd, 1997). There are fewer public criteria for evaluating the severity of other disorders, including most recurrent and chronic pain disorders. A number of attempts have been made to develop self-report and rating scales that can reliably assess the severity of these disorders. An example is provided by Holroyd and his colleagues (1996) who examined the convergent and discriminant validity of seven pain measures from three widely used self-report instruments. However, whereas information about the severity of pain is available only to the individual, the assessment of severity may be idiosyncratic only to that patient. Idiosyncratic standards may be invaluable to a patient in evaluating changes in his or her condition; however, idiosyncratic criteria vary across patients and thus are of limited value in assessing the state of a group of patients.

Third, patients must be able to evaluate, and make judgments about the data they process. Judgment making can be easy with objective data; patients can, for example, match their blood pressure readings against the objective standard that denotes what is considered as high blood pressure. Matching to standard becomes more difficult in the case of subjective symptoms. Patients must acquire and constantly refine their skill at matching their reaction to what, at the outset of their performance, may have been ambiguous and fuzzy standards (Creer & Holroyd, 1997).

Fourth, patients must learn to evaluate any changes that occur in terms of the antecedent conditions that may have led to the change, the behaviors they can perform to alter the changes, and the potential consequences of their action. An analysis of the antecedents, behaviors performed, and consequences of that action provides information necessary for making the best decision about possible courses of action that can be taken in the future.

Finally, contextual factors must be considered in processing and evaluating information about the patients' management of a chronic illness. A multidirectional interaction is constantly taking place among environmental, physical, cognitive, and behavioral elements in self-management. In addition, these factors interact with contextual variables, including setting events, establishing stimuli, and establishing operations, to influence the course of self-management of a chronic illness (Creer & Bender, 1993; Creer & Holroyd, 1997).

D. DECISION MAKING

Creer and Holroyd (1997) emphasized that decision making is a critical function in self-management: After patients collect, process, and evaluate data on themselves and their illness, they must make appropriate decisions based upon the information. Despite a growing base of data regarding medical decision making, there is a paucity of information as to how individual patients make decisions. This is ironical from two points of view: First, as noted, patients are being asked not only to make more accurate judgments about their condition, but to make more complex decisions. Second, evidence indicates that patient decision making is at the core of successful self-management. Creer (1990) found this in a study that compared a set of data from physicians, including those considered to be a gold standard group by their peers, to a set of data collected from patients regarded as a gold standard in their ability to manage pediatric asthma. The results? There were striking similarities in how both gold standard groups managed asthma. Both groups utilized effective judgment rules or heuristics in that they (a) considered each attack as a separate incident, (b) generated a number of testable treatment alternatives, (c) used their personal data base to select the most efficacious treatment strategy, (d) adjusted treatment in a stepwise manner to fit changes in severity of attacks, (e) avoided preconceived notions about attack management, (f) thought in terms of probabilities regarding their actions, and (g) avoided an overreliance on memory regarding asthma and how it should be treated. Both the gold standard patients and the gold standard physicians used advanced cognitive strategies, coupled with considerable flexibility, to process and evaluate information to generate treatment hypotheses and to make decisions regarding these hypotheses.

E. ACTION

Action involves the performance of self-management skills to control a chronic illness or health-related condition. Self-instruction, including prompting, directing, and maintaining performance, underlies whatever action is taken by individual patients. How successful patients will be is, to a major extent, a function of the instructions they provide to themselves to initiate and maintain the action they are pursuing. It is also dependent on contextual variables that may facilitate or impinge upon the performance of self-management skills.

Creer and Bender (1993) explained that self-instruction is significant to self-management in two other ways. First, control over a chronic illness requires that patients independently perform, often in a stepwise manner, the strategies they have worked out beforehand in their treatment action plan. Second, self-instruction may prompt the initiation of other strategies for coping with the illness. These may include those summarized by Karoly (1993), including attentional resource allocation, effort mobilization, planning and problem solving, verbal self-cueing, facilitative cognitive sets or expectations, stimulus control, and mental thought or cognitive control. Other strategies taken could be relaxation, self-desensitization, skill rehearsal, modeling, linking or unlinking behavioral chains, and self-reinforcement (Creer, 1997; Creer & Bender, 1993).

F. SELF-REACTION

Self-reaction refers to how individuals evaluate their performance (Bandura, 1986). On the basis of this appraisal, they can establish realistic expectations about their performance, as well as assess whether they need more training and expertise. Patients with a chronic illness also should acquire realistic expectations about the limits of self-management in helping to control their condition. They should recognize that they are unlikely to be able to use their self-management skills to control every aspect of either their behavior or their illness that they may wish to manage.

Self-efficacy influences the performance of self-management skills. Self-efficacy is the belief of patients that they can perform specific skills in a given situation (Bandura, 1977). Knowledge of self-management skills is not enough to guarantee that these skills will be used appropriately; patients must also believe they are capable of performing these skills to reach whatever goal they have helped determine for themselves. Self-efficacy arises, in part, from performance achievements; it guides and regulates future action (Creer & Holroyd, 1997). Self-reaction is not only a basic ingredient in the performance of self-management skills, but, as will be noted, is crucial to the maintenance of these skills over time.

VI. DISCUSSION

If a collage were created to depict the self-management of chronic illness, it undoubtedly would be highly diverse and abstract. Most of the assembled pieces would appear vague and ambiguous; other pieces of the collage, however, would appear quite clear. Three images incorporated into the collage would, in particular, present unifying lines and color to the composition. These topics concern (a) the development and application of self-management programs for chronic illness, (b) the recruitment and retention of patients into these programs, and, (c) the performance and maintenance of self-management skills over time. These elements would provide not only a unifying theme to the collage, but they would portray a state-of-the-art glimpse of self-management procedure as applied to chronic illness.

A. DEVELOPMENT AND APPLICATION OF SELF-MANAGEMENT PROGRAMS FOR CHRONIC ILLNESS

An Advanced MEDLINE search resulted in 681 citations to the self-management of chronic conditions, primarily chronic illness, extending back to 1971. At the beginning, several reports described attempts to use self-management procedures with problems such as smoking and weight control. With time, however, self-management techniques were applied to a broad array of chronic illnesses, including diabetes, asthma, arthritis, ataxia, chronic obstructive pulmonary disease, glaucoma, chronic pain, fibromyalgia, headache, multiple sclerosis, epilepsy, HIV infections, epilepsy, and cystic fibrosis. Even if space permitted, a detailed analysis of the findings obtained in using self-management would be premature. The data base on self-management and chronic illness is too fragmentary and preliminary to permit relevant judgments to be made on the merits of such a potentially useful approach. This is particularly the case with chronic illness in that, among the 681 cited studies, there are references not only to the nuts and bolts of self-management programs, but to a spectrum of topics. Included are discussions of patients, the application of various intervention approaches, the use of a band of self-management techniques, and the development of an array of assessment and outcome measures.

In most cases, self-management programs for chronic illness achieved many of the goals for which they were designed. They were shown to be effective, in varying degrees, in helping to control recurrent headache (Holroyd et al., 1989), multiple sclerosis (Keating & Ostby, 1996), epilepsy (Dilorio & Henry, 1995), HIV infection (Kalichman, Sikkema, Kelly, & Bulto, 1995), chronic chest pain (Payne et al., 1994), cystic fibrosis (Luder & Gilbride, 1989), fibromyalgia (Burckhardt, Mannerkorpi, Hedenberg, & Bjelle, 1994), chronic obstructive pulmonary disease (Zimmerman, Brown,

& Bowman, 1996), and adrenal insufficiency (Newrick, Braatvedt, Hancock, & Corrall, 1990). If the programs did nothing more than lead patients to become partners with their physicians in treating chronic illness, however, they would have been a success.

Many of the 681 references on self-management concern three chronic disorders: asthma, diabetes, and arthritis. There were 207 articles concerned with asthma, 128 with diabetes, and 33 with arthritis. Sometimes, but not always, recent self-management programs for these disorders were more advanced than self-management programs for other chronic illnesses. In addition, the sheer number of articles reflects that self-management is more mainstreamed into the treatment of patients with arthritis, diabetes, and asthma than may be the case with other chronic illnesses.

Although advances have been made with respect to the self-management of arthritis, asthma, and diabetes, the studies continue to reflect the embryonic state of development regarding self-management and chronic diseases. There are positive trends. For example, materials that should form the educational component of a self-management program are usually included; the materials presented are often sophisticated and incorporate various modalities for instruction, including television and computer programs. In addition, written and visual materials used in the programs are increasingly appropriate to the age, reading ability, and culture targeted by the program. There are negative trends in the cited studies, however. A major criticism is that there is an overreliance on developing the instructional component, including uses of teaching technology, to the detriment of assessing the performance of self-management skills. This is reflected in a number of studies that reported increased patients knowledge of a chronic condition, but provided no information as to whether this knowledge was actually used by patients to manage their illness. As a result, there is a schism between the two stages of acquisition and performance that has been bridged by only a few self-management programs for chronic illness.

B. RECRUITMENT AND RETENTION OF PATIENTS IN A SELF-MANAGEMENT PROGRAM

It was noted that patients often volunteer for self-management training when they are experiencing an exacerbation of their condition. Whether it be a flare-up of arthritis or asthma, they are quite willing to volunteer during periods when they are symptomatic. Later, when patients become asymptomatic, however, their interest evaporates. This poses a significant problem to those conducting self-management programs. Nowhere is the problem better embodied than with asthma. Drop-out rates from programs designed to teach patients to manage their asthma are typically high; this is particularly the case with children and their families who live in the inner city (e.g., Marwick, 1997). In one instance, the situation deteriorated to the point that the entire self-management project was aborted (Lewis, Rachelefsky, Lewis, Leake, & Richards, 1994). The situation has been a constant dilemma to those conducting such programs: they know that self-management skills greatly enhance medical treatment, but recognize that there is no way to teach patients to learn and to use these skills if they do not wish to do so.

What can be done to better recruit and retain chronically ill patients in a self-management program? Several recommendations are offered:

First, characteristics of chronic illness, psychological factors of patients with a chronic affliction, and treatment considerations must be considered in recruiting patients. Efforts to connect the initial interest of patients with their later participation in programs require considerable effort, patience, and, above all, ingenuity on the part of those conducting a self-management program. Creer, Levstek, and Reynolds (1998) pointed out that behavioral scientists have done a poor job of selling effective behavioral change techniques, including self-management. Failure to be consistently proactive and to convince patients to become partners with their health care providers has contributed to the problem.

Second, more attention must be expended to recruit a staff to conduct the program. The staff must be able not only to maintain the interest of patients in learning and performing self-management skills, but to serve as a liaison between patients and their health care providers. Thus, in addition to displaying the characteristics of warmth, empathy, and genuineness emphasized by Rogers (1951), staff members must be highly diplomatic. Above all, however, staff members must be proactive and use every personal skill they have to conduct a successful self-management program.

Third, a major problem is presented by differences in expectancies between patients and health care providers. Patients may be interested in self-management and the idea of becoming allies with their health care providers in the treatment of their illnesses. When patients discover what is actually involved in such an undertaking, however, their interest may disappear. Empowerment sounds nice in theory, but it does involve the reality of patients accepting considerable responsibility for their own health care. A number of approaches may be taken to overcome the reluctance of many patients. Changes may be produced, in part, by repeated contacts with potential subjects to explain benefits and to provide encouragement by a highly proactive staff. Despite high drop-out rates from a number of self-management programs, this is not an inevitable result; several self-management programs for asthma (e.g., Creer et al., 1988; Kotses et al., 1995), for example, experienced low drop-out rates once patients became involved in a program. In the study by Creer and colleagues (1988), recruitment of potential subjects was especially high. In part, this was because patients were sometimes contacted several times a week. This proactive approach, used with individual patients, was highly effective in recruiting and maintaining subjects in the study.

Changing the expectancies of physicians and other health care personnel may be a greater challenge for two reasons:

1. Most health care providers do not understand the rationale and modus operandi of self-management. Chronically ill patients provide most of their own care to themselves; self-management permits health care providers the opportunity to influence what the patient does but, in reality, it remains the responsibility of the patients to perform whatever behaviors they must to manage their condition.

2. When patients fail to remain involved in a program, they are blamed for their lack of participation by many health care providers. Patients are not only a victim of a chronic illness, but they are chided for failing to help themselves. In a search for a scientific rationale for their arguments, health care providers may resort to suggesting that the patients have not progressed far enough in the stages proposed by the readiness to change model (Prochaska, Norcross, and DiClemente, 1994). The rationale is that the model, developed to change behavioral habits such as smoking, has value with chronic illness. It is unlikely that this is the case. Several factors prompt this statement.

   (a) As suggested by Bandura (1997), stage theories generate a thicket of problems. "Human behavior is too multifaceted and multidimensional to be categorized into a few discrete stages," he noted (p. 412). People do not fit neatly into a few fixed stages. Categorizing behavior into stages or substages creates, in the words of Bandura (1997), "arbitrary pseudostages." Furthermore, as stressed in this chapter, what is involved in managing a chronic illness, particularly in synthesizing medical treatment and patient behaviors, is multifaceted, multidimensional, and highly complex.

   (b) In a genuine stage theory, everyone passes through the same stages. Stages cannot be skipped nor can a person be recycled back through the stages. As Bandura (1997) noted, "on close inspection, the stages-of-change scheme violates every major requirement of a stage theory: invariant sequence, qualitative transformation, and nonreversibility" (p. 414).

   (c) The stage model suggests various behavior change approaches should be used at each stage. However, cautioned Bandura (1997), suggested behavioral change techniques are often considered incompatible with one another by their proponents. He cites the concurrent use of counterconditioning and altering faulty beliefs as an example of such incompatibility.

(d) Prochaska, Redding, and Evers (1997) noted the importance of proactive recruitment in interacting with potential participants in a stage program. A similar point was made by Rimer (1997) in discussing models of health behavior. A consistent and highly proactive approach already has been shown to underlie successful self-management programs for chronic illness, particularly for arthritis (Lorig & Holman, 1993), diabetes (Glasgow, 1995), and asthma (Creer et al., 1988).

(e) There is a lack of data to support the notion that the stage model is applicable to a chronic illness (e.g., Prochaska, et al., 1997). It has, however, been useful with smoking, diet choice, cocaine use, exercise, and condom use.

(f) The stage model has focused on three of five stages that occur before introduction of self-management: precontemplation, contemplation, and preparation. Little is said about the fourth stage, maintenance, or the fifth stage, termination. Yet, as pointed out by Creer, Levstek, and Reynolds (1998), getting patients to voluntarily perform whatever skills are needed to manage their chronic illness for as long as possible is the most difficult and complex challenge faced in self-management. Whereas most need to do it for the remainder of their lives, the only termination stage with many chronic illnesses is death.

(g) Finally, and most importantly, the lack of time prohibits use of a readiness to change model. Health care professionals want to establish control over a condition as quickly as they can. They do not wish to wait until a patient decides whether or not he or she wants to perform self-management skills. For this reason, the aim is to begin teaching all patients self-management skills as soon as they are diagnosed with a chronic disease or condition.

Fourth, cultural and racial differences have been and will remain a problem in the self-management of chronic illness. However, success has been attained in many areas, including the development of educational materials appropriate for those of a lower reading level or from a different culture. In addition, there are increasing efforts by health care personnel to bridge cultural gaps (Anders, 1997). Pointers include seeking eye contact with Latino patients, but forgoing such contact with some Asian patients. As more is known about racial and cultural differences, the information undoubtedly will find its way into self-management programs.

Fifth, there is a need to consider demands made on patients. It is impossible for patients to monitor too many categories of behavior and not have their chronic illness be at the center of their lives. To be blamed for a breakdown in behavior when task demands are too high is a needless blow to patients.

Finally, anyone conducting a self-management program for a chronic illness must realize that they must do whatever it takes to make a program work. This requires taking a proactive stance toward subjects both throughout the life of a program and beyond. If it means that staff members make repeated contacts or arrangements to make certain patients attend sessions, such steps need to be taken. These steps could range from repeated personal contacts and sending a bus to pick up enrollees in a program, such as occurred in the study by Creer and co-workers (1988), to involving community agencies and leaders to reach clients. Kate Lorig, a scientist who has developed a number of programs for use with arthritis (e.g., Lorig & Holman, 1993), was successful with the latter approach, in part because she spent so much time in a community church interacting with patients (K. Lorig, personal communication, June 28, 1996). This may seem like a drastic step to take, but the success of self-management for chronic illnesses requires such dedication on the part of those conducting the programs.

C. MAINTENANCE OF SELF-MANAGEMENT SKILLS

Whereas duration is a prominent characteristic of chronic conditions, patients are likely to need to perform whatever self-management skills they are taught for the remainder of their lives. As suggested by Creer, Levstek, and Reynolds (1998), it is a monumental achievement to attain this goal. Despite some possible roadblocks in the quest for the goal, however, there are a few bright results that portend success.

First, there is an increasing recognition that, in most cases, self-management is apt to fail. Because no one does everything they should do all the time, why should we expect those with a chronic illness to be any different? The answer is that we cannot. We can, however, teach patients to realistically prepare themselves for managing failure. This is why relapse prevention, using the model proposed by Marlatt and Gordon (1980), is increasingly incorporated into self-management programs for chronic illnesses. By constantly alerting patients to several factors that could lead to relapse, including exposure to high-risk situations, failure to initiate coping responses, attributions to personal weakness, and initial relapse, patients can be taught about what factors to expect and how to manage them. The approach adds a sense of realism that was missing in early self-management programs; the presence of relapse management is likely to increase the maintenance of self-management skills over a longer duration of time.

Second, the emergence of self-efficacy as a key ingredient in the maintenance of self-management has been increasingly elucidated (Bandura, 1997). In chronic illness, it has been found to be essential in the long-term self-management of arthritis (Lorig & Holman, 1993) and asthma (Caplin, 1998; Winder, McConnaughy, Hertz, & Schork, 1997). Because of these findings, exercises to enhance self-efficacy both during and after training are being incorporated into self-management programs for chronically ill patients.

Finally, evidence is beginning to emerge that indicates that chronically ill patients do continue to perform self-management skills for a long duration of time. Lorig and Holman (1993) followed a group of patients with arthritis for a number of years. They reported that the effects of arthritis self-management lasted for 4 years without formal reinforcement. Creer and his colleagues (1988) conducted a 5-year follow-up of a random group of children who had undergone asthma self-management training. Many of the children no longer experienced asthma; those who did, however, continued to faithfully use self-management skills to control their asthma. The children and their parents reported they had remained in contact with other participants in the program. These informal contacts seemed to be sources of support and reinforcement. Finally, members of this survey group asked about specific staff members who had conducted the program 5 years earlier. They said they wanted to convey their appreciation for the training and support provided by these staff members.

Other follow-up data gathered indicate that the self-management skills taught to children since the Creer et al. (1988) publication are surprisingly resistant to change. This was noted also by Caplin (1998), who was able to contact 70% of the participants 5 years after they completed the program for adults with asthma reported by Kotses et al. (1995). Caplin (1998) found that all patients performed self-management skills to one degree or another. Some patients performed such skills as self-monitoring of daily symptoms and medications over 95% of the time. Others were less faithful, but noted that they quickly used self-management skills when symptomatic. Of additional interest was the high percentage of patients who not only reported an increased self-efficacy in performing self-management skills, but were particularly efficacious in their ability to use specific skills, particularly self-monitoring and decision making, to help them lead relatively normal lives.

VII. FUTURE DIRECTIONS AND CONCLUSIONS

Future research will be directed toward teaching more and more patients how they can help control their chronic disease. This will expand training in self-management. In addition, as pointed out earlier (Sontag, 1978), all of us inhabit the kingdoms of the well and the sick. For this reason, research will continue to emphasize how each of us can contribute to our own health. The significance of mastery of self-management skills by each of us, not just those with chronic disorders, as well as increased self-efficacy that is a consequence of such performance, cannot be overstated. In fact, Herzlinger (1997) proposed this as the cornerstone of the evolution of market-driven health care. In short, we are all going to be called upon to manage more aspects of our health in the future. To achieve this aim will require that, in one way or another, we perform and master the self-management processes outlined earlier. How the aim is attained will continue to prove fertile ground for studies by behavioral and medical scientists.

There is a caveat to such a rubicund scenario: The philosophy and implementation of self-management for the control of chronic illness will not occur unless there is a major change in the health care system, particularly the way patients are treated by health care providers. The health care system currently used in developed countries is based on a model whereby medical personnel treat patients. The role of patients, under these conditions, requires that they adhere to whatever directions are given to them, not that they become active participants in making decisions and implementing actions regarding their own care. The current system was appropriate for the treatment and management of acute diseases. As pointed out by the World Health Organization (1997), however, there has been a dramatic shift toward providing treatment and care for more and more people with an array of chronic illnesses. To successfully manage these patients requires nothing less than a revolutionary treatment paradigm for medical and behavioral science. Despite the success that has been attained, there remains a paucity of evidence that the revolution is occurring. For example, the initial set of treatment guidelines for asthma (National Asthma Education Program, 1991) were published several years ago. Yet, despite widespread dissemination of the guidelines both by the National Institutes of Health and asthma journals, Marwick (1995) pointed out that only 1 of 10 physicians in the United States knew about the guidelines, including the fact they had been published. It is likely that a similar situation exists regarding the publication of other sets of asthma guidelines used throughout the world (e.g., National Heart, Lung, and Blood Institute, 1992, 1995). Even when they have been read, there is a paucity of evidence that health care providers have integrated the guidelines into their practice. This was pointed out by Creer, Winder, and Tinkelman (1999). Their review of the evidence indicates that few physicians are willing to follow asthma guidelines that recommend that they jointly set treatment goals and cooperate in tailoring an asthma action plan for a given patient. In other words, it is business as usual when it comes to treating asthma, for example, patients are the passive recipients of whatever treatment their health care providers care to offer. Until the major hurdle posed by the current model of health care comes crashing down, progress in the implementation of self-management skills with chronic disorders will remain slow.

Still, there is hope. The self-management of chronic illnesses is still in a nascent state of development. In addition, recent findings suggest that the skills taught in self-management programs are surprisingly useful and resistant to extinction in some patients with a chronic illness. The increased self-efficacy that accompanies this performance no doubt does, as suggested by Lorig and Holman (1993), contribute to this finding. Before expecting that all patients with a chronic illness will achieve similar results, however, it is wise to remember a statement Mencken (1949) first uttered 80 years ago, but repeated numerous times: "There is always an easy solution for every human problem: neat, plausible, and wrong" (p. 443). If this statement guides future investigators, they will remain optimistic that chronically ill patients can indeed use self-management skills to lead more healthy and richer lives. At the same time, they should be realistic about the task they have undertaken and the barriers they face. Achieving success will not come easy.

REFERENCES

Anders, G. (1997, September 4). Doctors learn to bridge cultural gaps. *The Wall Street Journal*, pp. B1, B10.

Anderson, R. M. (1995). Patient empowerment and the traditional medical model. *Diabetes Care*, *18*, 412–415.

Ansell, J., Holden, A., & Knapic, N. (1989). Patient self-management of oral anticoagulation guided by capillary (fingerstick) whole blood prothrombin times. *Archives of Internal Medicine*, *149*, 2509–2511.

Baker, R. C., & Kirschenbaum, D. S. (1993). Self-monitoring may be necessary for successful weight control. *Behavior Therapy*, *24*, 377–394.

Bandura, A. (1977). Self-efficacy: toward a unifying theory of behavioral change. *Psychological Review*, *84*, 191–215.

Bandura, A. (1986). *Social foundations of thoughts and action: A social cognitive theory*. Englewood Cliffs, NJ: Prentice-Hall.

Bandura, A. (1997). *Self-efficacy: The exercise of control*. New York: Freeman.

Burckhardt, C. S., Mannerkorpi, K., Hedenberg, L., & Bjelle, A. (1994). A randomized, controlled clinical trial of education and physical training for women with fibromyalgia. *Journal of Rheumatology*, *21*, 714–720.

Caplin, D. A. L. (1998). *Variables contributing to the relapse and long-term maintenance of self-management for individuals with asthma*. Unpublished doctoral dissertation, Ohio University, Athens.

Clark, N. M., Levison, M. J., Evans, D., Wasilewski, Y., Feldman, C. H., & Mellins, R. B. (1990). Communication within low income families and the management of asthma. *Patient Education and Counseling*, *15*, 191–200.

Creer, T. L. (1983). *The self-management of a chronic physical disorder: Childhood asthma*. Athens: Ohio University.

Creer, T. L. (1990). Strategies for judgment and decision-making in the management of childhood asthma. *Pediatric Asthma, Allergy, & Immunology*, *4*, 253–264.

Creer, T. L. (1997). *Psychology of adjustment: An applied approach.* Englewood Cliffs, NJ: Prentice-Hall.

Creer, T. L. (1998). The complexity of treating asthma. *Journal of Asthma, 35,* 451–454.

Creer, T. L., Backial, M., Burns, K. L., Leung, P., Marion, R. J., Miklich, D. R., Morrill, C., Taplin, P. S., & Ullman, S. (1988). Living with asthma: Part I. Genesis and development of a self-management program for childhood asthma. *Journal of Asthma, 25,* 335–362.

Creer, T. L., & Bender, B. G. (1993). Asthma. In R. J. Gatchel & E. B. Blanchard (Eds.), *Psychophysiological disorders* (pp. 151–208). Washington, DC: American Psychological Association.

Creer, T. L., & Holroyd, K. A. (1997). Self-Management. In A. Baum, C. McManus, S. Newman, J, Weinman, & R. West (Eds.), *Cambridge handbook of psychology, health, and behavior* (pp. 255–258). Cambridge, UK: Cambridge University Press.

Creer, T. L., Kotses, H., & Reynolds, R. V. C. (1991). *A handbook for asthma self-management: A group leader's guide to living with asthma for adults.* Athens: Ohio University Press.

Creer, T. L., Levstek, D. A., & Reynolds, R. V. C. (1998). History and conclusions. In H. Kotses & A. Harver (Eds.), *Self-management of asthma* (pp. 379–405). New York: Dekker.

Creer, T. L., Renne, C. M., & Christian, W. P. (1976). Behavioral contributions to the rehabilitation of childhood asthma. *Rehabilitation Literature, 37,* 226–232, 247.

Creer, T. L., Winder, J. A., & Tinkelman, D. (1999). Guidelines for the diagnosis and management of asthma: Accepting the challenge. *Journal of Asthma, 36,* 391–407.

Desquin, B. W., Holt, I. J., & McCarthy, S. M. (1994). Comprehensive care of the child with a chronic condition. Part I. Understanding chronic conditions in childhood. *Current Problems in Pediatrics, 24,* 199–218.

Dilorio, C., & Henry, M. (1995). Self-management in persons with epilepsy. *Journal of Neuroscience Nursing, 27,* 338–343.

Ford, D. H. (1987). *Humans as self-constructing living systems: A developmental perspective on behavior and personality.* Hillsdale, NJ: Erlbaum.

Glanz, K., Lewis, F. M., & Rimer, B. K. (Eds.). (1997). *Health behavior and health education: Theory, research, and practice* (2nd ed.). San Francisco: Jossey-Bass.

Glasgow, R. E. (1995). A practical model of diabetes management and education. *Diabetes Care, 18,* 117–126.

Herzlinger, R. E. (1997). *Market-driven health care: Who wins, who loses in the transformation of America's largest service industry.* Reading, MA: Addison-Wesley.

Hoffman, C., Rice, D., & Sung, H-Y. (1996). Persons with chronic conditions. Their prevalence and cost. *Journal of the American Medical Association, 276,* 1473–1479.

Hoffmann, C., Broyles, R. S., & Tyson, J. E. (1997). Emergency room visits despite the availability of primary care: A study of high risk inner city infants. *American Journal of Medical Science, 313,* 99–103.

Holroyd, K. A., & Creer, T. L. (1986). *Self-management of chronic disease. Handbook of clinical interventions and research.* Orlando, FL: Academic Press.

Holroyd, K. A., Cordingly, G. E., Pingel, J. D., Jerome, A., Theofanous, A. G., Jackson, D. K., & Leard, L. (1989). Enhancing the effectiveness of abortive therapy: A controlled evaluation of self-management training. *Headache, 29,* 148–153.

Holroyd, K. A., Talbot, F., Holm, J. E., Pingel, J. D., Lake, A. E., & Saper, J. R. (1996). Assessing the dimensions of pain: A multitrait-multimethod evaluation of seven measures. *Pain, 67,* 259–265.

Kalichman, S. C., Sikkema, K. J., Kelly, J. A., & Bulto, M. (1995). Use of a brief behavioral skills intervention to prevent HIV infection among chronic mentally ill adults. *Psychiatric Services, 46,* 275–280.

Karoly, P. (1993). Mechanisms of self-regulation: A systems view. *Annual Review of Psychology, 44,* 23–52.

Keating, M. M., & Ostby, P. L. (1996). Education and self-management of interferon beta-1b therapy for multiple sclerosis. *Journal of Neuroscience Nursing, 28*, 350–352.

Kirschenbaum, D. S., & Tomarken, A. J. (1982). On facing the generalization problem: The study of self-regulatory failure. In P. C. Kendall (Ed.), *Advances in cognitive-behavioral research and therapy* (Vol. 1, pp. 119–200). New York: Academic Press.

Kotses, H., Bernstein, I. L., Bernstein, D. I., Reynolds, R. V. C., Korbee, L., Wigal, J. K., Ganson, E., Stout, C., & Creer, T. L. (1995). A self-management program for adult asthma. Part I. Development and evaluation. *Journal of Allergy & Clinical Immunology, 95*, 529–540.

Lewis, M. A., Rachelefsky, G., Lewis, C. E., Leake, B., & Richards, W. (1994). The termination of a randomized clinical trial for poor Hispanic children. *Archives of Pediatric and Adolescent Medicine, 148*, 364–367.

Lieu, T. A., Quesenberry, C. P., Jr., Capra, A. M., Sorel, M. E., Martin, K. E., & Mendoza, G. R. (1997). Outpatient management practices associated with reduced risk of pediatric asthma hospitalization and emergency department visits. *Pediatrics, 100*, 334–341.

Lorig, K., & Holman, H. (1993). Arthritis self-management studies: A twelve year review. *Health Education Quarterly, 20*, 17–28.

Luder, E., & Gilbride, J. A. (1989). Teaching self-management skills to cystic fibrosis patients and its effect on their caloric intake. *Journal of the American Dietary Association, 89*, 359–364.

Marks, J. S. (1996). Commentary: CDC's 50th anniversary—A chronic disease perspective. *Chronic Disease Notes & Reports, 9*, 1–4.

Marlatt, G. A., & Gordon, J. R. (1985). *Relapse prevention*. New York: Guilford Press.

Marwick, C. (1995). Inner-city asthma control campaign underway. *Journal of the American Medical Association, 274*, 1004.

Marwick, C. (1997). Helping city children control asthma. *Journal of the American Medical Association, 277*, 1503–1504.

Mencken, H. L. (1949). *A Mencken chrestomathy*. New York: Knopf.

Mullen, P. D. (1997). Compliance becomes concordance. *British Medical Journal, 314*, 691–692.

National Asthma Education Program. (1991). *Expert panel report executive summary: Guidelines for the diagnosis and management of asthma* (Publication No. 91–3042). Washington, DC: U.S. Department of Health and Human Services.

National Asthma Education and Prevention Program. (1997). *Highlights of the expert panel report 2: Guidelines for the diagnosis and management of asthma* (Publication No. 97–4051A). Washington, DC: U.S. Department of Health and Human Services.

National Heart, Lung, and Blood Institute. (1992). *International consensus report on the diagnosis and treatment of asthma* (NIH Publication No. 92–3091). Bethesda, MD: Author.

National Heart, Lung, and Blood Institute. (1995). *Global initiative for asthma* (NIH Publication No. 95–3659). Bethesda, MD: Author.

Newrick, P. G., Braatvedt, G., Hancock, J., & Corrall, R. J. (1990). Self-management of adrenal insufficiency by rectal hydrocortisone. *Lancet, 335*, 212–213.

Payne, T. J., Johnson, C. A., Penzien, D. B., Porzelius, J., Eldridge, G., Parisi, S., Beckham, J., Pbert, L., Prather, R., & Rodriguez, G. (1994). Chest pain self-management training for patients with coronary artery disease. *Journal of Psychosomatic Research, 38*, 409–418.

Prochaska, J. O., Norcross, J. C., & DiClemente, C. C. (1994). *Changing for good*. New York: Morrow.

Prochaska, J. O., Redding, C. A., & Evers, K. E. (1997). The transtheoretical model and stages of change. In K. Glanz, F. M. Lewis, & B. K. Rimmer (Eds.), *Health behavior and health education. Theory, research, and practice* (2nd ed., pp. 60–84). San Francisco: Jossey-Bass.

Report of the Expert Committee on the diagnosis and classification of diabetes mellitus. (1997). *Diabetes Care, 20*, 1183–1197.

Rimer, B. K. (1997). Models of individual health behavior. In K. Glanz, F. M. Lewis, & B. K. Rimer, (Eds.), *Health behavior and health education: Theory, research, and practice* (2nd ed., pp. 37–40). San Francisco: Jossey-Bass.

Rogers, C. R. (1951). *Client-centered therapy*. Boston: Houghton Mifflin.

Russo, D. C., & Varni, J. W. (1982). Behavioral pediatrics. In D. C. Russo & J. W. Varni (Eds.), *Behavioral pediatrics: Research and Practice* (pp. 3–24). New York: Plenum.

Sontag, D., & Richardson, L. (1997, March 2). Doctors withhold H.I.V. pill regimen from some. *The New York Times*, p. 18.

Sontag, S. (1978). *Illness as metaphor*. New York: Farrar, Straus and Giroux.

Sulzer-Azaroff, B., & Mayer, G. R. (1991). *Behavior analysis for lasting change*. New York: Holt, Rinehart, and Winston.

Verbrugge, L. M., & Patrick, D. L. (1995). Seven chronic conditions: Their impact on US adults' activity levels and use of medical services. *American Journal of Public Health, 85*, 173–182.

Von Korff, M., Gruman, J., Schaefer, J., Curry, S. J., & Wagner, E. H. (1996). *Essential elements for collaborative management of chronic illness*. Unpublished manuscript.

Wagner, E. H., Austin, B. T., & Von Korff, M. (1996). Organizing care for patients with chronic illness. *The Milbank Quarterly, 74*, 511–544.

Weiss, D. B., & Coyne, C. (1997). Communicating with patients who cannot read. *New England Journal of Medicine, 337*, 272–274.

Winder, J. A., McConnaughy, D. J., Hertz, B. S., & Schork, M. A. (1997). Self-efficacy relating to asthma improves after participation in Wheezers Anonymous (WA), adult asthma self-management program. *Journal of Allergy & Clinical Immunology, 99*, 234.

World Health Organization. (1997). *The World Health Report 1997: Conquering suffering, enriching humanity. Executive summary*. Geneva, Switzerland: World Health Organization.

Zimmerman, B. W., Brown, S. T., & Bowman, J. M. (1996). A self-management program for chronic obstructive pulmonary disease: Relationship to dyspnea and self-efficacy. *Rehabilitation Nursing, 21*, 253–257.

19

SELF-REGULATION AND ACADEMIC LEARNING

SELF-EFFICACY ENHANCING INTERVENTIONS

DALE H. SCHUNK AND PEGGY A. ERTMER

Purdue University, West Lafayette, Indiana

I. INTRODUCTION

How well students learn and perform in school depends on diverse personal, social, familial, instructional, and environmental factors (Berliner & Biddle, 1997; Steinberg, Brown, & Dornbusch, 1996; Thompson, Detterman, & Plomin, 1991). Included in this list are self-regulatory processes, which investigators believe contribute to academic motivation and learning (Meece & Courtney, 1992; Newman, 1994; Pintrich & Garcia, 1991; Schunk, 1994; Zimmerman & Martinez-Pons, 1990).

Self-regulation (or *self-regulated learning*) refers to self-generated thoughts, feelings, and actions, that are planned and systematically adapted as needed to affect one's learning and motivation (Schunk, 1994; Zimmerman, 1989, 1990, 2000, Zimmerman & Kitsantas, 1996). Self-regulation comprises such processes as setting goals for learning, attending to and concentrating on instruction, using effective strategies to organize, code, and rehearse information to be remembered, establishing a productive work environment, using resources effectively, monitoring performance, managing time effectively, seeking assistance when needed, holding positive beliefs about one's capabilities, the value of learning, the factors influencing learning, and the anticipated outcomes of actions, and experiencing pride and satisfaction with one's efforts (McCombs, 1989; Pintrich & De Groot, 1990; Weinstein & Mayer, 1986; Zimmerman, 1994).

Copyright © 2000 by Academic Press.
All rights of reproduction in any form reserved.

Self-regulation is not an all-or-none phenomenon: Rather, it refers to the degree that students are metacognitively, motivationally, and behaviorally active in their learning (Zimmerman, 1986). Students may self-regulate different dimensions of learning, including their motives for learning, the methods they employ, the performance outcomes they strive for, and the social and environmental resources they use (Zimmerman, 1994). Thus, self-regulation has both qualitative and quantitative aspects because it involves which processes students use, how frequently they use them, and how well they employ them. The hallmarks of self-regulation are choice and control: Students cannot self-regulate unless they have options available for learning and can control essential dimensions of learning (Zimmerman, 1994). Students have little opportunity for self-regulation when teachers dictate what students do, when and where they do it, and how they accomplish it.

The importance of self-regulation is underscored by research showing that self-regulated students are mentally active during learning, rather than being passive recipients of information, and exert control over setting and attaining learning goals (Pintrich & Schrauben, 1992; Schunk, 1990). In contrast, many students—including some high achievers—do not engage in effective self-regulation during learning (Weinstein & Mayer, 1986; Zimmerman & Martinez-Pons, 1990).

Students may display deficiencies in the area of self-regulation: motives (e.g., avoid activities or quit readily), methods (use ineffective strategies), outcomes (set easy goals that are not challenging), resources (not seek help when needed). These problems can arise when students lack knowledge of effective self-regulatory processes or believe that their own approaches work well enough (Fabricius & Hagan, 1984; Pressley et al., 1990). Further, training is often not given in schools due to inadequate time, space, or funding, the need for parental consent, and the widespread belief that students do not require self-regulation because achievement test scores are high (Schunk & Zimmerman, 1998a).

We believe that all students who are mentally capable of learning also are capable of self-regulating their motivation and learning. As the chapters in this volume and others make clear (e.g., Schunk & Zimmerman, 1998b), self-regulation training can be successfully implemented with diverse learners in various settings.

In this chapter, we discuss several interventions that were designed to affect students' motivation and self-regulated learning. This research focuses on influencing a key self-regulatory motive: *perceived self-efficacy*, or learners' beliefs about their capabilities to learn or perform behaviors at designated levels (Bandura, 1986, 1993, 1997). Effective self-regulation depends on students developing a sense of self-efficacy for learning and performing well (Schunk, 1994). Compared with students who doubt their learning capabilities, those with high self-efficacy are more likely to choose to engage in activities, work harder, persist longer when they encounter difficulties, use effective learning strategies, and demonstrate higher achievement (Schunk, 1994; Zimmerman & Martinez-Pons, 1990).

We initially provide an overview of a social cognitive theoretical perspective on self-regulation that highlights the role of self-efficacy. We then present nonintervention research evidence that supports theoretical predictions, after which we describe the intervention projects. We conclude with a section on future directions for self-regulation research.

II. THEORETICAL FRAMEWORK

A. SOCIAL COGNITIVE THEORY OF SELF-REGULATION

Social cognitive theory emphasizes the interaction of personal, behavioral, and environmental factors (Bandura, 1986; Zimmerman, 1994, 2000). Self-regulation is a cyclical process because these factors typically change during learning and must be monitored. Such monitoring leads to changes in an individual's strategies, cognitions, affects, and behaviors.

This cyclical nature is captured in Zimmerman's (1998, 2000) three-phase self-regulation model. The *forethought phase* precedes actual performance and refers to processes that set the stage for action. The *performance (volitional) control phase* involves processes that occur during learning and affect attention and action. During the *self-reflection phase*, which occurs after performance, individuals respond to their efforts.

B. SELF-EFFICACY AND SELF-REGULATION

Effective self-regulation depends on feeling self-efficacious for using skills to achieve mastery (Bandura, 1986, 1993; Bouffard-Bouchard, Parent, & Larivee, 1991; Schunk, 1996; Zimmerman, 1994). Learners obtain information about their self-efficacy from their performances, vicarious (observational) experiences, forms of persuasion, and physiological reactions. Students' own performances offer reliable guides for assessing self-efficacy. Successes raise efficacy and failures lower it (Zimmerman & Ringle, 1981). Students acquire efficacy information by socially comparing their performances with those of others. Similar others offer a valid basis for comparison (Schunk, 1987). Observing similar peers succeed (fail) at a task may raise (lower) observers' efficacy. Learners often receive persuasive information from teachers, parents, and others, suggesting that they are capable of performing a task (e.g., "You can do this."). Such information may raise efficacy, but can be negated by subsequent performance failure (Bandura, 1993). Students also acquire efficacy information from physiological reactions (e.g., sweating, heart rate). Symptoms that signal anxiety may convey that one lacks skill; lower anxiety may be construed as a sign of competence.

As shown in Table 1, self-efficacy operates during all phases of self-regulation. Skillful self-regulators enter learning situations with specific goals and a strong sense of self-efficacy for attaining them. As they work on tasks, they monitor their performances and compare their attainments with their goals to determine progress. Self-perceptions of progress enhance self-efficacy, motivation, and continued use of effective strategies (Ertmer, Newby, & MacDougall, 1996; Schunk, 1996). During periods of self-reflection they evaluate their progress and decide whether adaptations in self-regulatory processes are necessary. In Zimmerman's (2000) three-phase recursive model, comprising forethought, performance, and self-reflection, high self-efficacy for learning in the forethought phase becomes realized as self-efficacy for continued progress in the performance phase and self-efficacy for achievement in the self-reflection phase. The latter also sets the stage for modifying goals or setting new ones.

C. OTHER INFLUENTIAL PROCESSES

Table 1 shows that self-efficacy is not the only influence on achievement. During the forethought phase, goals, outcome expectations, and perceived value affect motivation and task engagement. *Goals* refer to what students are consciously attempting to accomplish. Goals are critical for self-regulation because they provide standards against which to gauge progress and motivate students to exert effort, persist, focus on relevant task features, and use effective strategies (Bandura, 1988; Locke & Latham, 1990; Schunk, 1990). Learners who make a commitment to pursue a goal are likely to compare their performances with their goal as they work. Positive self-evaluations of progress enhance self-efficacy and motivation (Bandura, 1988).

Of particular importance are the goal properties of specificity, proximity, and difficulty (Schunk, 1990). Motivation, learning, and self-regulation are enhanced when goals have specific performance standards, can be attained in a short time, and are of moderate difficulty. Goals that are

TABLE 1   Self-Efficacy during Phases of Self-Regulation

Forethought (pretask)	Performance (during task)	Self-reflection (posttask)
Self-efficacy	Self-efficacy	Self-efficacy
Goals	Self-monitoring	Goals
Outcome expectations	Self-perceptions of progress	Self-evaluations
Perceived value	Strategy use	Adaptations of self-regulatory
	Motivation	processes

general (e.g., do your best), distant in time, or overly easy or difficult do not motivate as well. Although long-term goals are common (e.g., read a book in 2 weeks), students benefit when they subdivide them into shorter term objectives.

Goal effects also may depend on whether the goal denotes a learning or performance outcome (Ames, 1992; Meece, 1991). A *learning goal* refers to what knowledge and skills students are to acquire; a *performance goal* denotes what task students are to complete (Dweck & Leggett, 1988; Stipek, 1996). Learning and performance goals may affect self-regulation and achievement differently, even when their properties are similar. Learning goals focus students' attention on processes and strategies that help them acquire competencies (Ames, 1992). Students who pursue a learning goal are apt to experience a sense of efficacy for attaining it and be motivated to engage in task-appropriate activities (Schunk, 1996). Efficacy is substantiated as they note task progress. In contrast, performance goals focus attention on completing tasks. Such goals may not highlight the importance of the processes and strategies underlying task completion or raise efficacy for learning. Students may not compare present and past performances to determine progress, but instead may socially compare their work with that of others. Such comparisons can lower efficacy among students who lag behind.

Outcome expectations, or the anticipated consequences of actions, are influential because students engage in activities they believe will lead to positive outcomes (Shell, Murphy, & Bruning, 1989). *Perceived value*, or students' beliefs about the incentives or purposes for learning, affects behavior because learners show little interest in activities they do not value.

Other influential processes during the performance control phase are self-monitoring, self-perceptions of progress, strategy use, and motivation. *Self-monitoring* (or *self-observation*) refers to deliberate attention to specific aspects of one's behavior. Researchers recommend assessing behaviors on such dimensions as quantity, quality, rate, and originality (Bandura, 1986; Mace, Belfiore, & Shea, 1989). Self-observation that results in self-perceptions of progress can motivate one to improve (Schunk, 1989). Self-observation is supported by self-recording, where instances of behavior are recorded along with their time, place, and frequency of occurrence (Mace et al., 1989; Zimmerman, Bonner, & Kovach, 1996).

Effective self-regulators engage in skillful strategy use during learning (Ertmer et al., 1996). Research shows that students can be taught effective strategies and that strategy use raises achievement (Pressley et al., 1990; Zimmerman & Martinez-Pons, 1990). Unfortunately, teaching a strategy does not guarantee that students will continue to use it, especially if they believe that the strategy is not as important for success as other factors (e.g., time available; Borkowski, Johnston, & Reid, 1987). Feedback about the value of the strategy and how well students are applying it can raise efficacy and motivate students to continue using it (Schunk & Swartz, 1993a). Strategy feedback promotes achievement and self-regulatory strategy use better than instruction alone (Borkowski, Weyhing, & Carr, 1988; Kurtz & Borkowski, 1987).

Motivation comes into play during performance control through the benefits of goals and self-efficacy (Meece, 1994), but in other ways as well. An important motivational factor involves students' attributions (perceived causes) of their successes and difficulties. Research supports the notion that effective self-regulators form attributions that sustain self-efficacy, effort, persistence, and learning (Schunk, 1994). Whether goal progress is deemed acceptable depends on its attribution. Students who attribute success to factors over which they have little control (e.g., luck, task ease) may hold low self-efficacy if they believe they cannot succeed on their own. If they believe they lack ability to perform well, they may judge learning progress as deficient and be unmotivated to work harder. Students who attribute success to ability, skill, effort, and effective use of strategies should experience higher self-efficacy and maintain motivation (Schunk, 1994).

During self-reflection, students engage in self-evaluation and adapt strategies as needed. Self-evaluations of learning progress and achievement substantiate students' self-efficacy and motivate them to continue to work diligently (Schunk, 1996). Low self-evaluations will not necessarily diminish self-efficacy or motivation if students believe they are capable of learning and can do so through *adaptations of self-regulatory processes*. For example, they may decide to switch to a different strategy, seek assistance, modify their goals, or make adjustments in their work environments. The recursive nature of the model is apparent when students' self-reflections on past performance lead to setting new goals and forethought about future actions (Zimmerman, 2000).

III. RESEARCH EVIDENCE

The focus of this chapter is on interventions designed to affect students' self-efficacy and self-regulation. Initially, however, we provide a brief overview of some nonintervention research that supports the hypothesized relationship of self-efficacy to self-regulation. These studies provide correlational support for the interventions that follow.

Zimmerman and Martinez-Pons (1990) explored how verbal and mathematical self-efficacy related to self-regulated learning strategies among normally achieving and gifted students in Grades 5, 8, and 11. The verbal efficacy items assessed students' perceptions of correctly defining words; mathematical efficacy examined perceived problem-solving competence.

Students read scenarios describing learning contexts and indicated the self-regulated learning methods they would use to learn. Verbal and mathematical self-efficacy correlated positively with the use of effective learning strategies (e.g., self-evaluating, goal setting and planning, keeping records, and monitoring). Gifted students displayed higher self-efficacy and strategy use than did normally achieving students; older students made greater use of self-regulated learning strategies.

Pintrich and De Groot (1990) examined relationships among self-regulation (use of metacognitive and effort management strategies), cognitive strategy use (rehearsal, elaboration, and organizational strategies), and self-efficacy for learning and performing well in class, among seventh graders in science and English. Self-efficacy, self-regulation, and cognitive strategy use were positively intercorrelated and predicted achievement.

Using high school students, Pokay and Blumenfeld (1990) explored relationships among expectancies for success (analogous to self-efficacy) in geometry, use of learning strategies (metacognitive, cognitive, and effort management), and achievement. Early in the semester, expectancies for success predicted strategy use and achievement; later on, perceived value of the learning was the best predictor of strategy use. Expectancies for success correlated positively with effort management.

The relationship of self-efficacy and self-regulation during verbal concept formation tasks among high school students was examined by Bouffard-Bouchard et al. (1991). Students with high self-efficacy for successful problem solving displayed greater performance monitoring and persisted longer than students lower in efficacy. Self-efficacy correlated positively with performance.

Zimmerman and Bandura (1994) studied the relationships among self-efficacy, goals, and self-regulation of writing among college students. Self-efficacy for writing correlated positively with students' goals for course achievement, self-evaluative standards (satisfaction with potential grades), and actual achievement. Results of a path analysis showed that self-efficacy affected achievement directly and indirectly through its influence on goals.

Tuckman and Sexton (1990) studied college students in an educational psychology course. The self-regulated learning task involved writing test items based on course lectures and text material. For each of 10 weeks, students with high self-efficacy for writing test items chose to engage in significantly more item writing than students lower in self-efficacy.

Chapman and Tunmer (1995) explored the relationship of perceptions of competence (analogous to self-efficacy) in reading and use of self-regulatory reading (e.g., letter and word identification) and comprehension strategies among children ages 5 to 7. Perceptions of competence correlated positively with comprehension strategies among older children; for younger children, perceptions of task difficulty correlated significantly with reading strategies.

Ertmer et al. (1996) examined how freshmen veterinary students with different levels of self-regulation approached learning from case-based instruction. The study employed intensive interviews designed to determine differences between high and low self-regulators.

Students enrolled in a biochemistry laboratory course that used case-based instruction were classified as high or low self-regulators. Interview data gathered on three occasions during the semester assessed students' lab goals, strategies for analyzing case studies, and perceptions of performance and progress. Motivation and self-efficacy for completing case analyses also were measured.

Students' approaches to case-based instruction were shaped by the value placed on the use of cases, types of goals and evaluation criteria used to focus learning, and ability, motivation, and self-efficacy for using self-regulatory monitoring strategies on difficult cases. High self-regulators valued case-based instruction, perceived it relevant to their needs, and felt efficacious for learning. They focused on mastering the analysis process and used self-regulatory strategies (e.g., positive self-talk, self-checking) on difficult cases.

In contrast, low self-regulators fluctuated in their perceptions of the value of the case method, as well as in self-efficacy for learning from cases. They focused on learning facts and being correct, and had difficulty adapting or inventing new strategies to meet case demands. Students acted automatically, employing habitual learning strategies (e.g., underlining, highlighting) that were not appropriate or effective on cases.

IV. INTERVENTIONS TO ENHANCE SELF-EFFICACY AND SELF-REGULATION

The preceding correlational results indicate strong support for the interrelationship of self-efficacy and self-regulation. Against this background, we now describe some research projects that were designed to enhance self-efficacy and self-regulation.

We make no attempt to discuss all intervention research relevant to our model in Table 1. Rather, we focus on how goals (forethought phase), self-monitoring and self-perceptions of progress (performance control phase), and self-evaluations of progress (self-reflection phase) affect self-efficacy and self-regulated learning. Furthermore, most of the projects we describe represent research involving situational manipulations rather than long-term interventions with program evaluation. Readers interested in the impact of other types of interventions should consult additional sources (Bandura, 1997; Schunk & Zimmerman, 1994, 1998b).

A. GOALS

Wood, Bandura, and Bailey (1990) varied task complexity and goal instructions with graduate business students during a simulated decision-making task (assigning employees to different production tasks to complete work assignments within an optimal period). Subjects were assigned to low or high task-complexity conditions based on the number of employees supervised and the degree of match between skills and job requirements. They received either a general (do your best) goal or a specific goal of raising productivity by at least 25%. They judged efficacy for attaining performance levels ranging from 30% better to 40% worse. Other measures were self-regulation (effectiveness of their managerial strategies) and performance (number of hours to complete the simulated task).

The specific goal enhanced performance in the low complexity condition, but not in the high complexity condition. During the early trials, high complexity and the specific goal produced the highest self-efficacy. Path analysis showed that self-efficacy raised performance directly and indirectly through its effect on self-regulation; the latter directly affected performance. Self-efficacy also influenced personal goal setting (the goals that subjects were striving for regardless of the assigned goal). In a related study using a similar methodology (Bandura & Jourden, 1991), self-efficacy directly affected performance and self-regulation, and had an indirect effect on performance through its effect on self-regulation. Feedback indicating progressive mastery promoted self-efficacy, high goal setting, and performance.

Zimmerman and Kitsantas (1996, 1997) found that providing process (learning) goals raised self-efficacy and self-regulation during dart throwing. Ninth- and tenth-grade girls were assigned to a process-goal condition and advised to focus on the steps in dart throwing; others were assigned to a product-goal condition and told to concentrate on their scores. Some girls engaged in self-recording (a self-monitoring strategy) by writing down after each throw the steps they accomplished properly or their throw's outcome.

In the first study (Zimmerman & Kitsantas, 1996), process-goal girls attained higher self-efficacy and performance than did product-goal girls; self-recording also enhanced these measures. These results were replicated in the second study (Zimmerman & Kitsantas, 1997); however, a shifting-goal condition was included where girls pursued a process goal, but once they could perform the steps automatically they switched to a product goal of attaining high scores. The shifting goal led to the highest self-efficacy and performance.

B. SELF-MONITORING AND PERCEPTIONS OF PROGRESS

To investigate the influence of self-monitoring on motivation and self-regulated learning, Schunk (1983) provided subtraction instruction to elementary-school children who had failed to master subtraction operations in their classes. One group (self-monitoring) reviewed their work at the end of each session and recorded the number of workbook pages they had completed. To control for the effects of monitoring generally, Schunk included a second group (external monitoring) who had their work reviewed at the end of each session by an adult who recorded the number of pages completed. In a third condition (no monitoring), children received the instructional program, but were not monitored and did not receive instructions to monitor their work.

The self- and external-monitoring conditions led to higher self-efficacy, persistence, and achievement, compared with the no-monitoring condition. The two progress-monitoring conditions did not differ on any measure. The benefits of monitoring did not depend on children's performances during the instructional sessions, because the three treatment conditions did not differ in amount of work completed. Monitoring of progress, rather than the agent, enhanced children's perceptions of their learning progress and self-efficacy for continued progress. Without monitoring, children may be less certain about how well they are learning.

Studies by Schunk and Swartz (1993a, 1993b) investigated the influence of providing students with feedback to instill perceptions of progress. Fourth- and fifth-grade children received writing instruction over 20 days that covered four types of paragraphs: descriptive (e.g., describe a bird), informative (e.g., write about something you like to do after school), narrative story (e.g., tell a story about visiting a friend or relative), and narrative descriptive (e.g., describe how to play your favorite game). During each session, children received modeled writing strategy instruction, after which they engaged in self-regulated practice. Before and after the intervention, students' self-efficacy for writing effective paragraphs and writing achievement were assessed.

There were four goal conditions: learning goal, learning goal plus progress feedback, performance goal, and general goal. The model asked learning-goal and learning-goal-plus-feedback children to pursue a goal of learning to use the strategy to write paragraphs. Performance-goal students were asked to adopt a goal of writing paragraphs; general-goal students were advised to do their best. Progress feedback was delivered periodically to individual students during the sessions. It linked strategy use with improved writing performance (e.g., "You're doing well because you followed the steps in order"). At the end of the project, all children self-evaluated their progress in using the strategy.

Across the studies, providing students with a learning goal and progress feedback led to the highest self-efficacy, motivated strategy use, and achievement. There were some benefits of providing only a learning goal. Gains were maintained after 6 weeks and generalized to types of paragraphs on which children received no instruction. Learning-goal-plus-feedback students evaluated their progress in strategy use greater than did students in the other conditions. Schunk and Swartz also found that learning-goal-plus-feedback students, compared with children in the other conditions, reported the highest writing strategy use, employed the strategy more often, and judged the strategy to be of greater value. Providing a learning goal without feedback yielded some benefits on these measures.

C. SELF-EVALUATIONS

Schunk (1996) conducted two projects in which average-achieving children received modeled explanations and demonstrations of fraction solution strategies and practice opportunities. Children judged self-efficacy for correctly solving different types of fraction problems and were tested on fractions performance before and after the intervention. Students worked under conditions involving either a learning goal (learning how to solve problems) or a performance goal (solving problems). In the first project, half of the students in each goal condition engaged in daily self-evaluation of their problem-solving capabilities. The learning goal with or without self-evaluation and the performance goal with self-evaluation conditions demonstrated higher self-efficacy, self-regulated motivation, achievement, and task orientation (desire to independently master and understand academic work), and lower ego orientation (desire to perform well to please the teacher and avoid trouble) than did the performance goal without self-evaluation condition.

In the second project, all students self-evaluated their learning progress once during the instructional program. The learning goal led to higher self-efficacy, self-regulated motivation, achievement, and task orientation, and lower ego orientation than did the performance goal. These results suggest that frequent self-evaluation of progress or competence is powerful and can override the effects of learning goals. When self-evaluation occurs less frequently, it may complement learning goals better than performance goals and exert desirable effects on self-efficacy and self-regulated learning.

Schunk and Ertmer (in press) investigated the influence of self-evaluation and goals on college students' self-efficacy, achievement, and self-reported use of self-regulation strategies. Students were pretested on

Hypercard (a computer application) self-efficacy and achievement, and on how well (competence) and how often (frequency) they performed various strategies while learning computer skills. These strategies tapped four dimensions of self-regulation (Zimmerman, 1994): motives (e.g., find ways to motivate myself to finish a lab project even when it holds little interest for me), methods (e.g., locate and use appropriate manuals when I need to accomplish an unfamiliar computer task), performance outcomes (e.g., set specific goals for myself in this course), and social/environmental resources (e.g., find peers who will give critical feedback on early versions of my projects).

All students were enrolled in a computer applications course; Hypercard was one of the units. For this study, students were assigned to one of four conditions: learning goal with self-evaluation, performance goal with self-evaluation, learning goal without self-evaluation, and performance goal without self-evaluation. At the start of each of three laboratory sessions, learning-goal students were provided with a goal of learning to perform various Hypercard tasks, which coincided with the unit objectives; performance-goal students were advised to do their work and try their best. At the end of the second session, students assigned to the self-evaluation conditions evaluated their progress in acquiring Hypercard skills. All students were posttested at the end of the project.

Providing learning goals—with or without self-evaluation—led to higher self-efficacy and strategy competence and frequency than did providing performance goals and no self-evaluation. Students who received learning goals and self-evaluation judged self-efficacy higher than did learning-goal students who did not receive self-evaluation and performance-goal students who self-evaluated. Students given learning goals without self-evaluation judged self-efficacy higher than did students given performance goals and self-evaluation. Among the self-evaluation conditions, students who pursued learning goals evaluated their learning progress greater than those who received performance goals. These results corroborate those of Schunk (1996) in showing that infrequent self-evaluation is more beneficial for self-efficacy and self-regulation in the presence of learning goals.

V. FUTURE RESEARCH ON SELF-REGULATION

The studies in the preceding section have the dual purpose of enhancing students' self-efficacy for learning and facilitating use of self-regulatory strategies. We see these ends to be complementary, although researchers need not attempt to influence both processes at once. Strictly speaking, one can address the development of self-efficacy and self-regulatory competence separately. Building efficacy requires providing students with mastery experiences, exposing them to successful models, and delivering positive feedback. Self-regulatory competence can be developed through strategy instruction, exposure to social models, or providing students with opportunities to construct strategies and test their usefulness.

Although these objectives can be addressed in isolation, we believe that because self-efficacy and self-regulation exert reciprocal effects, training programs should address both aspects. Students who possess self-regulatory skills are not apt to use them proficiently if they have doubts about their learning capabilities. Furthermore, high self-efficacy will not produce skillful self-regulation among students who lack knowledge of skills or believe that self-regulation is not beneficial. Thus, we recommend that programs designed to teach self-regulation include components to enhance students' self-efficacy for learning and implementing self-regulation skills.

Research on self-regulation has advanced tremendously in the past few years, and we expect this trend to continue. We believe that the following suggestions for research will help to further our understanding of the operation of self-regulatory processes and help to link self-regulation with educational practices.

A. INSTRUCTIONAL COMPONENTS

The studies in the preceding section primarily used social models to explain and demonstrate operations. Models are an important means of transmitting skills and strategies (Bandura, 1986; Rosenthal & Zimmerman, 1978). Models also are frequently employed in strategy instruction (Graham & Harris, 1989a, 1989b; Schunk & Swartz, 1993a, 1993b).

Alternatively, strategy instruction can be less formally structured such that teachers provide support and assistance while students construct their own strategies. This approach has been used successfully in training studies (Butler, 1998; Winne & Stockley, 1998). Forcing students to take greater responsibility for their own learning fits well with other instructional models, such as reciprocal teaching (Palincsar & Brown, 1984) and collaborative peer learning groups (Cohen, 1994; Slavin, 1995).

Research should explore the relative effectiveness of modeling and self-constructions, and especially the factors that may influence their success. For example, we might predict that strategy modeling would be more effective during initial learning when individuals' ability to construct strategies is limited, but that as students develop competence they are better able to construct effective self-regulatory sequences. There also may be developmental differences such that younger students benefit more from modeled demonstrations, but older students are able to formulate their own methods.

B. SELF-REGULATION IN CONTENT AREAS

A second suggestion is to conduct research on self-regulation in the context of content-area learning. When self-regulatory processes are linked with academic content, students learn how to apply them in a learning context. It is worthwhile to teach students how to set goals, organize their schedules, rehearse information to be remembered, and so forth, but such instruction may not generalize beyond the context in which it is provided.

We recommend that researchers conduct studies in academic settings where students are taught self-regulatory activities and how to modify them to fit different situations. These studies have the added benefit of showing students the value of self-regulation. Students who learn strategies, but feel they are not particularly useful, are not likely to use them. Linking self-regulation to actual content helps to raise the perception of value as students compare their performances with prior ones that did not have the benefit of self-regulation.

C. TRANSFER OF SELF-REGULATION PROCESSES

Embedding self-regulation processes within specific content areas brings up the issue of transfer. Although students' perceptions of the value of self-regulation strategies may increase when these strategies are integrated within regular disciplinary courses (e.g., biology, history), it is unclear whether students will then transfer these skills to other disciplinary courses (Hofer, Yu, & Pintrich, 1998). It has been argued that students' transfer of self-regulation skills across contexts, content areas, and types of academic tasks, depends on at least three factors (Pressley et al., 1990): knowing how to self-regulate, believing that self-regulation is beneficial, and possessing the skills necessary to make appropriate modifications in self-regulation processes such that they match the current situation. Research is needed to determine the extent that explicit instruction and practice in each area improves transfer.

Whether self-regulation skills are taught within a content area or as part of an adjunct course, the issue of transfer is relevant. In one case, students must transfer skills to a new content area; in the other case, transfer must occur between a "content-free" course and any number of specific content courses. What is unclear is whether one approach is more effective than the other, and if so, how specific features of the approach facilitate transfer. We recommend that researchers conduct process-oriented studies designed to determine how students think about and employ strategies they learn in one context to another setting. Researchers should consider the use of qualitative methods that involve in-depth analysis of students as they attempt to use the strategies in different courses (Hofer et al., 1998).

As the amount of information available to learners continues to increase, instructors must decide how much is reasonable to provide in any course. Instructors are beginning to seek out ways to equip their students with strategies that will enable them to locate, access, and evaluate relevant information in a self-directed manner. The question is how to balance students' need for information with the need to develop strategies to find and use information. Content-area interventions, in which instructors teach skills and embed information about the transferability to other domains, have been found to be highly beneficial for learning and transfer (Schunk & Zimmerman, 1998b).

D. SELF-REFLECTIVE PRACTICE

Finally, we recommend greater research attention be paid to self-reflective practice. This is a critical component of self-regulated learning, but to date little effort has been made to link it systematically with interventions. Self-reflective practice ought to allow students to evaluate their progress toward learning goals, alter their approach as needed, and adjust social and environmental factors to provide a setting highly conducive to learning.

Researchers might examine whether the effectiveness of self-reflection varies as a function of setting. Self-reflective practice may be more important where external evaluation is infrequent or when students encounter difficulties learning. The need for self-reflection may decline where assessment is straightforward and progress indicators are clear. Researchers also might determine ways to motivate students to engage in self-reflection on their own, such as by teaching students to treat self-reflection as any other academic task that must be planned. Such research will help us to realize the full potential of this central component of self-regulation.

VI. CONCLUSION

In this chapter we have argued that students' self-regulatory competence can be enhanced through systematic interventions that are designed to teach skills and raise students' self-efficacy for learning. We have focused on interventions involving goals, self-monitoring and perceptions of progress, and self-evaluations of progress and capabilities. We believe that research on self-regulation will enhance our understanding of achievement processes and have important implications for teaching and learning in and out of school.

REFERENCES

Ames, C. (1992). Classrooms: Goals, structures, and student motivation. *Journal of Educational Psychology, 84,* 261–271.

Bandura, A. (1986). *Social foundations of thought and action: A social cognitive theory.* Englewood Cliffs, NJ: Prentice-Hall.

Bandura, A. (1988). Self-regulation of motivation and action through goal systems. In V. Hamilton, G. H. Bower, & N. H. Frijda (Eds.), *Cognitive perspectives on emotion and motivation* (pp. 37–61). Dordrecht, The Netherlands: Kluwer.

Bandura, A. (1993). Perceived self-efficacy in cognitive development and functioning. *Educational Psychologist, 28,* 117–148.

Bandura, A. (1997). *Self-efficacy: The exercise of control.* New York: Freeman.

Bandura, A., & Jourden, F. J. (1991). Self-regulatory mechanisms governing the impact of social comparison on complex decision making. *Journal of Personality and Social Psychology, 60,* 941–951.

Berliner, D. C., & Biddle, B. J. (1997). *The manufactured crisis.* New York: Longman.

Borkowski, J. G., Johnston, M. B., & Reid, M. K. (1987). Metacognition, motivation, and controlled performance. In S. J. Ceci (Ed.), *Handbook of cognitive, social, and neuropsychological aspects of learning disabilities* (Vol. 2, pp. 147–173). Hillsdale, NJ: Erlbaum.

Borkowski, J. G., Weyhing, R. S., & Carr, M. (1988). Effects of attributional retraining on strategy-based reading comprehension of learning-disabled students. *Journal of Educational Psychology, 80,* 46–53.

Bouffard-Bouchard, T., Parent, S., & Larivee, S. (1991). Influence of self-efficacy on self-regulation and performance among junior and senior high-school age students. *International Journal of Behavioural Development, 14,* 153–164.

Butler, D. L. (1998). A strategic content learning approach to promoting self-regulated learning by students with learning disabilities. In D. H. Schunk & B. J. Zimmerman (Eds.), *Self-regulated learning: From teaching to self-reflective practice* (pp. 160–183). New York: Guilford.

Chapman, J. W., & Tunmer, W. E. (1995). Development of young children's reading self-concepts: An examination of emerging subcomponents and their relationship with reading achievement. *Journal of Educational Psychology, 87,* 154–167.

Cohen, E. G. (1994). Restructuring the classroom: Conditions for productive small groups. *Review of Educational Research, 64,* 1–35.

Dweck, C. S., & Leggett, E. L. (1988). A social-cognitive approach to motivation and personality. *Psychological Review, 95,* 256–273.

Ertmer, P. A., Newby, T. J., & MacDougall, M. (1996). Students' responses and approaches to case-based instruction: The role of reflective self-regulation. *American Educational Research Journal, 33,* 719–752.

Fabricius, W. V., & Hagen, J. W. (1984). Use of causal attributions about recall performance to assess metamemory and predict strategic memory behavior in young children. *Developmental Psychology, 20,* 975–987.

Graham, S., & Harris, K. R. (1989a). Components analysis of cognitive strategy instruction: Effects on learning disabled students' compositions and self-efficacy. *Journal of Educational Psychology, 81,* 353–361.

Graham, S., & Harris, K. R. (1989b). Improving learning disabled students' skills at composing essays: Self-instructional strategy training. *Exceptional Children, 56,* 201–214.

Hofer, B. K., Yu, S. L., & Pintrich, P. R. (1998). Teaching college students to be self-regulated learners. In D. H. Schunk & B. J. Zimmerman (Eds.), *Self-regulated learning: From teaching to self-reflective practice* (pp. 57–85). New York: Guilford.

Kurtz, B. E., & Borkowski, J. G. (1987). Development of strategic skills in impulsive and reflective children: A longitudinal study of metacognition. *Journal of Experimental Child Psychology*, *43*, 129–148.

Locke, E. A., & Latham, G. P. (1990). *A theory of goal setting and task performance.* Englewood Cliffs, NJ: Prentice-Hall.

Mace, F. C., Belfiore, P. J., & Shea, M. C. (1989). Operant theory and research on self-regulation. In B. J. Zimmerman & D. H. Schunk (Eds.), *Self-regulated learning and academic achievement: Theory, research, and practice* (pp. 27–50). New York: Springer.

McCombs, B. L. (1989). Self-regulated learning and academic achievement: A phenomenological view. In B. J. Zimmerman & D. H. Schunk (Eds.), *Self-regulated learning and academic achievement: Theory, research, and practice* (pp. 51–82). New York: Springer.

Meece, J. L. (1991). The classroom context and students' motivational goals. In M. L. Maehr & P. R. Pintrich (Eds.), *Advances in motivation and achievement* (Vol. 7, pp. 261–285). Greenwich, CT: JAI Press.

Meece, J. L. (1994). The role of motivation in self-regulated learning. In D. H. Schunk & B. J. Zimmerman (Eds.), *Self-regulation of learning and performance: Issues and educational applications* (pp. 25–44). Hillsdale, NJ: Erlbaum.

Meece, J. L., & Courtney, D. P. (1992). Gender differences in students' perceptions: Consequences for achievement-related choices. In D. H. Schunk & J. L. Meece (Eds.), *Student perceptions in the classroom* (pp. 209–228). Hillsdale, NJ: Erlbaum.

Newman, R. S. (1994). Adaptive help seeking: A strategy of self-regulated learning. In D. H. Schunk & B. J. Zimmerman (Eds.), *Self-regulation of learning and performance: Issues and educational applications* (pp. 283–301). Hillsdale, NJ: Erlbaum.

Palincsar, A. S., & Brown, A. L. (1984). Reciprocal teaching of comprehension-fostering and comprehension-monitoring activities. *Cognition and Instruction*, *1*, 117–175.

Pintrich, P. R., & De Groot, E. V. (1990). Motivational and self-regulated learning components of classroom academic performance. *Journal of Educational Psychology*, *82*, 33–40.

Pintrich, P. R., & Garcia, T. (1991). Student goal orientation and self-regulation in the college classroom. In M. L. Maehr & P. R. Pintrich (Eds.), *Advances in motivation and achievement* (Vol. 7, pp. 371–402). Greenwich, CT: JAI Press.

Pintrich, P. R., & Schrauben, B. (1992). Students' motivational beliefs and their cognitive engagement in classroom academic tasks. In D. H. Schunk & J. L. Meece (Eds.), *Student perceptions in the classroom* (pp. 149–183). Hillsdale, NJ: Erlbaum.

Pokay, P., & Blumenfeld, P. C. (1990). Predicting achievement early and late in the semester: The role of motivation and use of learning strategies. *Journal of Educational Psychology*, *82*, 41–50.

Pressley, M., Woloshyn, V., Lysynchuk, L. M., Martin, V., Wood, E., & Willoughby, T. (1990). A primer of research on cognitive strategy instruction: The important issues and how to address them. *Educational Psychology Review*, *2*, 1–58.

Rosenthal, T. L., & Zimmerman, B. J. (1978). *Social learning and cognition.* New York: Academic Press.

Schunk, D. H. (1983). Progress self-monitoring: Effects on children's self-efficacy and achievement. *Journal of Experimental Education*, *51*, 89–93.

Schunk, D. H. (1987). Peer models and children's behavioral change. *Review of Educational Research*, *57*, 149–174.

Schunk, D. H. (1989). Self-efficacy and achievement behaviors. *Educational Psychology Review*, *1*, 173–208.

Schunk, D. H. (1990). Goal setting and self-efficacy during self-regulated learning. *Educational Psychologist*, *26*, 207–231.

Schunk, D. H. (1994). Self-regulation of self-efficacy and attributions in academic settings. In D. H. Schunk & B. J. Zimmerman (Eds.), *Self-regulation of learning and performance: Issues and educational applications* (pp. 75–99). Hillsdale, NJ: Erlbaum.

Schunk, D. H. (1996). Goal and self-evaluative influences during children's cognitive skill learning. *American Educational Research Journal, 33*, 359–382.

Schunk, D. H., & Ertmer, P. A. (in press). Self-regulatory processes during computer skill acquisition: Goal and self-evaluative influences. *Journal of Educational Psychology.*

Schunk, D. H., & Swartz, C. W. (1993a). Goals and progress feedback: Effects on self-efficacy and writing achievement. *Contemporary Educational Psychology, 18*, 337–354.

Schunk, D. H., & Swartz, C. W. (1993b). Writing strategy instruction with gifted students: Effects of goals and feedback on self-efficacy and skills. *Roeper Review, 15*, 225–230.

Schunk, D. H., & Zimmerman, B. J. (1998a). Conclusions and future directions for academic interventions. In D. H. Schunk & B. J. Zimmerman (Eds.), *Self-regulated learning: From teaching to self-reflective practice* (pp. 225–235). New York: Guilford.

Schunk, D. H., & Zimmerman, B. J. (Eds.). (1998b). *Self-regulated learning: From teaching to self-reflective practice*. New York: Guilford.

Shell, D. F., Murphy, C. C., & Bruning, R. H. (1989). Self-efficacy and outcome expectancy mechanisms in reading and writing achievement. *Journal of Educational Psychology, 81*, 91–100.

Slavin, R. E. (1995). *Cooperative learning: Theory, research, and practice* (2nd ed.). Boston: Allyn and Bacon.

Steinberg, L., Brown, B. B., & Dornbusch, S. M. (1996). *Beyond the classroom: Why school reform has failed and what parents need to do*. New York: Simon and Schuster.

Stipek, D. J. (1996). Motivation and instruction. In D. C. Berliner & R. C. Calfee (Eds.), *Handbook of educational psychology* (pp. 85–113). New York: Macmillan.

Thompson, L., Detterman, D., & Plomin, R. (1991). Associations between cognitive abilities and scholastic achievement: Genetic overlap but environmental differences. *Psychological Science, 2*, 158–165.

Tuckman, B. W., & Sexton, T. L. (1990). The relation between self-beliefs and self-regulated performance. *Journal of Social Behavior and Personality, 5*, 465–472.

Weinstein, C. E., & Mayer, R. E. (1986). The teaching of learning strategies. In M. C. Wittrock (Ed.), *Handbook of research on teaching* (3rd ed., pp. 315–327). New York: Macmillan.

Winne, P. H., & Stockley, D. B. (1998). Computing technologies as sites for developing self-regulated learning. In D. H. Schunk & B. J. Zimmerman (Eds.), *Self-regulated learning: From teaching to self-reflective practice* (pp. 106–136). New York: Guilford.

Wood, R., Bandura, A., & Bailey, T. (1990). Mechanisms governing organizational performance in complex decision-making environments. *Organizational Behavior and Human Decision Processes, 46*, 181–201.

Zimmerman, B. J. (1986). Development of self-regulated learning: Which are the key subprocesses? *Contemporary Educational Psychology, 11*, 307–313.

Zimmerman, B. J. (1989). A social cognitive view of self-regulated academic learning. *Journal of Educational Psychology, 81*, 329–339.

Zimmerman, B. J. (1990). Self-regulating academic learning and achievement: The emergence of a social cognitive perspective. *Educational Psychology Review, 2*, 173–201.

Zimmerman, B. J. (1994). Dimensions of academic self-regulation: A conceptual framework for education. In D. H. Schunk & B. J. Zimmerman (Eds.), *Self-regulation of learning and performance: Issues and educational applications* (pp. 3–21). Hillsdale, NJ: Erlbaum.

Zimmerman, B. J. (1998). Developing self-fulfilling cycles of academic regulation: An analysis of exemplary instructional models. In D. H. Schunk & B. J. Zimmerman (Eds.), *Self-regulated learning: From teaching to self-reflective practice* (pp. 1–19). New York: Guilford.

Zimmerman, B. J. (2000). Attaining self-regulation: A social cognitive perspective. In M. Boekaerts, P. R. Pintrich, and M. Zeidner (Eds.), *Handbook of self-regulation* (Chap. 2). San Diego, CA: Academic Press (this volume).

Zimmerman, B. J., & Bandura, A. (1994). Impact of self-regulatory influences on writing course attainment. *American Educational Research Journal, 31*, 845–862.

Zimmerman, B. J., Bonner, S., & Kovach, R. (1996). *Developing self-regulated learners: Beyond achievement to self-efficacy*, Washington, DC: American Psychological Association.

Zimmerman, B. J., & Kitsantas, A. (1996). Self-regulated learning of a motoric skill: The role of goal setting and self-monitoring. *Journal of Applied Sport Psychology, 8*, 60–75.

Zimmerman, B. J., & Kitsantas, A. (1997). Developmental phases in self-regulation: Shifting from process goals to outcome goals. *Journal of Educational Psychology, 89*, 29–36.

Zimmerman, B. J., & Martinez-Pons, M. (1990). Student differences in self-regulated learning: Relating grade, sex, and giftedness to self-efficacy and strategy use. *Journal of Educational Psychology, 82*, 51–59.

Zimmerman, B. J., & Ringle, J. (1981). Effects of model persistence and statements of confidence on children's self-efficacy and problem solving. *Journal of Educational Psychology, 73*, 485–493.

20

TEACHER INNOVATIONS IN SELF-REGULATED LEARNING

JUDI RANDI AND LYN CORNO

Teachers College, Columbia University, New York, New York

I. INTRODUCTION

Encouraging students to take responsibility for their own learning is a loud refrain in current thinking on schooling. To help all students become "self-regulated," theory suggests the need for a better understanding of the strategies that successful students use to maintain effort and protect commitments in school. Research conducted on self-regulated learning over recent decades has made major contributions toward this goal. Although, as Part I of this handbook makes clear, there are almost as many definitions of self-regulated learning as there are lines of research on the topic, it is commonly agreed that self-regulated learners seek to accomplish academic goals strategically and manage to overcome obstacles using a battery of resources (in addition to Part I, see Schunk & Zimmerman, 1994; Zimmerman & Schunk, 1989). Self-regulation is both an aptitude for and a potential outcome of schooling.

The importance of self-regulatory potential, as both preparation for and achievement in school, is accentuated by the continuous and increasing intellectual and behavioral demands, constraints, and affordances that schools provide learners. Learning and self-management strategies appear particularly important for students to use in certain situations: when academic tasks require sustained attention, when instruction is incomplete or relatively unstructured, or when students are confronted by competing goals (Corno & Kanfer, 1993). Although some students learn to use

Copyright © 2000 by Academic Press.
All rights of reproduction in any form reserved.

self-regulatory strategies through modeling, and can be observed to work diligently on tasks both in- and outside school, their intellectual understandings of strategy use may be tacit. That is, they may not be mindful of, or able to explain, their own strategic behavior (Paris & Cunningham, 1996). Furthermore, given that many classroom environments afford few opportunities for student self-regulation even to occur, it ought not to be surprising when students fail to produce learning and self-management strategies on demand. Most students are ill prepared or insufficiently attuned to perceive opportunities for self-regulated learning when they are provided. Even students given explicit strategy instruction often do not use strategies without prompting in similar situations later on (Brown, 1994; Snow, 1992).

II. OVERVIEW

In this chapter, we consider ways that classroom teachers might provide self-regulatory opportunities and requirements for their students through tailored curricular activities. The goal is to shape a curriculum comprising some of the pieces that students will need to make deliberate, conscious use of self-regulatory strategies. The tasks of that curriculum will encourage students to add more pieces of their own. As is conventional, we review theory and research on selected classroom interventions in self-regulated learning, but we also raise questions about some of these endeavors and suggest alternatives. Most approaches to instruction in self-regulated learning are more closely attuned to the research traditions from which they arose than to the average teacher's classroom practice. Self-regulated learning might become more widespread if it is developed harmoniously within existing school curricula. Teaching for self-regulated learning also should coincide with new and more inspired ways of teaching and working with teachers. We provide some examples of what this kind of curriculum and teaching might be like.

As one example, we describe what we have learned in our collaborative efforts to develop a *curriculum-embedded* approach to teaching self-regulated learning. By curriculum-embedded, we mean that the affordances for strategic self-regulated learning were enhanced by curricular content rich with self-regulatory possibilities. This curriculum invited self-regulated learning; it gave students lots of ways to tune in to the various aspects of what it means to self-regulate. "Many ways in" is one criterion for an approach that aspires to teach self-regulated learning to more than just a few able students. As important as the examples we provide, however, is our description of the process in which we engaged to generate our curricular approach, because we learned that a collaborative innovation process between teachers and researchers can also afford a learning opportunity for those who are prepared to take advantage of it. In many ways, collaborative innovation is to traditional staff development as modern social constructivist learning theory is to behaviorism (Greeno, Collins, & Resnick, 1996). The idea of collaborative innovation in teacher development is overdue.

In sum, this chapter distinguishes our work from existing approaches to instruction in self-regulated learning in two major ways. First, it moves away from attempts to instruct students explicitly in learning or study strategies apart from subject matter curriculum (see Gall, Gall, Jacobsen & Bullock, 1990; Weinstein & Mayer, 1986). The aspects of self-regulation that affect instructional response are evidenced best by information processing regularities and patterns of strategic action that occur within the context of regular classroom curricula (Snow, 1992). Teachers can develop self-regulatory aptitude for classroom learning purposefully, by identifying ways to make these regularities and action patterns connect inherently with their curriculum and their classroom teaching environment. Principles, strategies, and modes of behavior regarding self-regulated learning can then be brought front and center in students' thinking as they work.

We present an information processing analysis of the journey tale to illustrate how integral parts of the school curriculum might be used to address this goal. As we detail later on, tailored instruction around the journey tale can provide students with several opportunities and demands for developing both an intellectual understanding of and demonstrated skills in self-regulated learning. Although others have developed instructional models for teaching self-regulatory principles and strategies within subject matter contexts, and some authors have taught self-regulation implicitly through new approaches to subject matter instruction, the evidence suggests that mindfulness and strategic application to new contexts remains a problem (Salomon & Almog, 1998; Schunk & Zimmerman, 1994). Our work seeks, in part, to address this problem.

The second major way in which our work seems to depart from that of others is our emphasis on the aforementioned process of collaborative innovation between teachers and researchers, with teachers themselves devising curricular applications (Corno & Randi, 1999). We oppose traditional models of staff development and teacher "training." Again, we shall say more about this later, but for now we note that some old lessons about how educational innovations actually find happy homes in real classrooms have still not been learned (Randi & Corno, 1997). We begin our discussion by considering content-based strategy interventions. Because this is a handbook chapter, we pay more than usual attention to details of research.

III. STRATEGY INSTRUCTION RESEARCH IN THE CONTENT AREAS

Research on self-regulated learning reviewed elsewhere in this volume has described the general kinds of learning and self-management strategies that more effective learners use, as well as the conditions under which they are most needed. More recently, research has focused on the development of instructional models for teaching self-regulatory principles and strategies to school students who might benefit most. One hope is that effective strategy use will increase students' success in specific content domains. Research also has begun to examine how students' understanding of a particular subject, as well as their interests, can influence the process of self-regulated learning (Alexander, 1995). As Snow (1992) said, "learners who are not tuned in will tune out, and ultimately turn off" (p. 27). Following this track, some recent interventions in subject area domains emphasize the subject-specific aspects of self-regulation as one means for streamlining otherwise difficult tasks. Comprehension monitoring in reading, drafting and revising in writing, and strategic estimation in mathematics represent a few examples (see, e.g., Shulman & Quinlan, 1996).

Domain-specific strategy instruction research also identifies ways teachers can incorporate models of self-regulation into regular classroom curricula. The intent is to make all students aware of the kinds of learning strategies that some students have acquired in the absence of explicit instruction and to promote their use. Strategy interventions have been conducted in several subject domains, including writing (e.g., Bereiter, 1990; Bereiter & Scardamalia, 1987; Graham & Harris, 1993), reading comprehension (e.g., Palincsar, 1986; Palincsar & Brown, 1984), literature-based reading programs (e.g., Baumann & Ivey, 1997; Collins-Block, 1993), and project-based science (Blumenfeld et al., 1991; Krajcik, Blumenfeld, Marx, & Soloway, 1994). The more successful of these interventions all have made use, to varying degrees, of an approach to instruction called *cognitive apprenticeship* to teach students cognitive skills that facilitate knowledge acquisition.

Cognitive apprenticeship is a particularly attractive means for teaching cognitive skills because it makes the covert thinking (cognitive skills) explicit through modeling and then helps students to acquire them through coaching and scaffolding. That is, it is an instructional situation that provides sufficient external support at the outset for unprepared students to perceive and use the cognitive skills in question. That external support is then faded or removed gradually, and eventually students are required to "fly solo" (Collins, Brown, & Newman, 1989). Because the initial decrease in information processing demands is made up at the end, a range of learners stand to benefit without being overly burdened or underchallenged. In apprenticed, domain-specific strategy instruction, students are scaffolded to independent use of learning strategies to acquire particular subject matter knowledge and skills.

Two research programs serve to illustrate how this kind of strategy instruction can promote the goals of the regular curriculum. First, the work done by Blumenfeld and her colleagues (Blumenfeld et al., 1991; Krajcik, et al., 1994) highlights how project-based science instruction melds strategy instruction and content area learning goals. A second promising line of research focuses on strategy instruction within reading-based literature programs. In both lines of research, children are engaged in so-called authentic tasks—in one, doing science, and in the other, reading and interpreting literature. In each case, modeling of strategies and apprenticed instruction assist learners to accomplish the goals of the curriculum.

A. STRATEGY INSTRUCTION IN STUDENT-CENTERED, PROJECT-BASED LEARNING

New visions of teaching and learning in "student-" or "learner-centered" classrooms place demands on teachers to change not only what but how their subject matter content is taught. In learner-centered classrooms, curriculum typically develops out of students' needs and interests. Students are encouraged "to formulate their own aims, to conceptualize their own problems, and to design the ways in which such problems might be addressed" (Eisner, 1991, p. 14). Although much attention has been given to redefining the role of teacher as facilitator and guide in learner-centered classrooms, there has been less attention to the ways in which student-centered instruction changes the role of the student. Research in the context of project-based science now discloses the changing role of the student in learner-centered classrooms.

In project-based science, researchers capitalize on the potential of projects as a learning tool at the same time that they recognize the need for strategy instruction to support students' efforts as active learners. In an article describing how projects afford students opportunities for learning, Blumenfeld et al. (1991) identified two essential components of projects: They (a) require a question or problem that organizes and drives related activities and (b) result in the creation of artifacts or products that address the driving question. Content goals are thus inherent in the design of the project itself. In project-based learning, strategy instruction helps students solve the problem and create the artifact representing their solution. For example, students are taught to use resources such as computers and software programs as well as printed materials, to collaborate with peers, and to work together toward solutions to problems of the sort scientists actually encounter. Self-monitoring and feedback are other aspects of self-regulation addressed directly in project-based learning. The artifacts students create, as concrete products that can be shared and critiqued, themselves provoke feedback and prompt revision. Additionally, student motivation can be addressed by providing students choice and control over the selection of problems and solutions.

Krajcik, et al. (1994) described their work with practicing teachers implementing project-based science, an integrative approach to learning science through other literacy-based means of interaction and communication. Their work with 10 middle school teachers and one elementary school science teacher involved curricular materials and a telecommunications network that teachers were encouraged to modify for their own classrooms. The researchers conversed at the outset with teachers to convey a theoretical basis for the project, to model sample activities, and to familiarize teachers with the new technology. They then videotaped teachers in their classrooms from one to four times weekly, while teachers recorded their reactions and ideas in journals. Interviews and informal work with the teachers provided additional data for case studies.

The teachers in this research gradually came around to independent functioning with project science. As the teachers developed their own, new activities, their understanding of the theoretical principles that drove their efforts reportedly increased. The researchers observed that teachers also gradually released the natural tendency toward a more prescriptive application. A great deal was learned from these case studies about the various constraints faced by practicing teachers; these authors also documented many difficulties students experienced when the responsibility for learning shifted from teacher to student in project-based science.

Although completing authentic tasks can be motivating, project-based learning often makes complex cognitive demands on students, and requires them to enlist volitional self-management strategies to accomplish their goals. Blumenfeld et al. (1991) noted that students engaged in project-based learning needed to "be far more responsible for guiding and controlling their own activities and focusing their work on the creation of artifacts over a long period of time" (p. 379). The learner's role in student-centered learning is thus more proactive, even than in some other models of "explicit teaching" (Rosenshine, 1987). Project-based learning may afford students opportunities for engaging in self-regulated learning; however, without explicit instruction in self-regulated learning strategies, some students will remain unprepared to take full advantage of the learning opportunities such projects offer.

In summary, although instruction in self-regulation was not a goal, this program of research on project-based learning highlighted the need for cognitive apprenticeship to scaffold students' strategy use. Blumenfeld et al. (1991) noted that the project-based approach to learning, in which learners construct knowledge by solving complex problems using cognitive tools, multiple sources of information, and significant others as resources is consistent with the apprenticeship model in which mentor-teachers initially provide modeling, scaffolding, and coaching, gradually increasing the learner's independence. It is important to note as well that teachers also were scaffolded to independent use of project-based science through their own collaboration with the research team providing staff development. Initially dependent on models the researchers provided, teachers later became more adept at developing their own, new activities. Thus, scaffolding seems to be a useful tool for teacher self-regulation as well as students'.

B. STRATEGY INSTRUCTION IN LITERATURE-BASED READING PROGRAMS

Other interventions in self-regulated learning draw upon the principles of cognitive apprenticeship to incorporate strategy instruction in the content areas. One such line of research focuses on strategy instruction in literature-based reading programs. As one example, Collins-Block (1993) designed a program to teach reading and thinking strategies through a literature-based curriculum. In this instructional model, students first received explicit instruction in strategy use and then applied the newly learned strategies to read literature of their own choosing. Explicit strategy instruction included "thinking guides" that depicted particular strategies in words and graphics and teacher explanations of when, where, and how to use the strategies in reference to specific readings. There were also discussions of students' successes and failures in using the strategies in guided learning situations.

It was important that students were asked to discuss how they might use these strategies with other literary materials as well as in situations outside school. These "transfer" discussions occurred before students attempted to use the "thinking guide" strategies independently. Thus, consistent with cognitive apprenticeship, models and coaching were scaffolds for students to learn particular strategies, which then were removed when students applied the strategies without teacher guidance.

Elementary students ($N = 178$) who received strategy instruction in a quasiexperimental design outperformed elementary students ($N = 174$) in a control group on standardized assessments measuring vocabulary development. Treated students also performed better in a postinstruction writing sample requiring students to describe "some important things they learned this year" (Collins-Block, 1993, p. 144). The author concluded that students who received strategy instruction were more adept at transferring the thinking and reading strategies to new situations. However, the quasi-experimental design does not ensure that group differences can be attributed to treatment.

One other example of strategy instruction in a literature-based reading program illustrates how students can be scaffolded to independent use of learning strategies. Baumann and Ivey (1997) conducted a yearlong qualitative/interpretive case study of a literature-based reading program developed and implemented by the first author. The researchers sought to determine the extent to which literacy strategy instruction could be integrated within a literature-based reading program to develop students' reading/writing skills and strategies. The program also promoted students' knowledge and appreciation of literature, and the desire to engage in reading and writing tasks independent of school-related assignments.

Baumann implemented a reading-based strategy instruction program consisting of three types of activities: (1) students read connected texts during a designated reading period when Baumann would circulate among the students, listening to them read and providing instruction as deemed necessary; (2) students received explicit instruction that introduced, reviewed, or previewed specific strategies and skills students could draw upon to understand and interpret the literature; and, (3) students engaged in extended reading and writing activities that connected the literature to their own life experiences (e.g., with sports, home, or friends). Researchers traced the progress of 13 students who remained in Baumann's second-grade class throughout the school year through participant observation, reading inventories, and reading response journals. Results documented student progress in five categories.

First, once the students tended to view reading as a natural part of their school day, their overall reading levels increased, as evidenced on reading inventories given by teachers. Second, students' engagement with literature was evidenced by an increasing willingness to respond to literature and a growing command of children's books. Third, students became more strategic in word identification; that is, they were able to identify and explain strategies they would use to decode unfamiliar vocabulary. Fourth, students used multiple strategies for comprehending text, thereby demonstrating an understanding that the purpose of reading is to acquire meaning. Fifth, students also developed fluency in writing. For example, at the end of the year, students' writing demonstrated a sense of audience not evidenced at the start of the year. The volume of student writing increased as well as the number of personal interests and experiences children included in their writing.

Although the researchers were appropriately cautious about making causal inferences from a study of this nature, they suggested that "the immersion in literature and the embedded strategy instruction created a kind of symbiotic, synergistic relationship in which each program characteristic contributed to and fed off the other" (Baumann & Ivey, 1997, p. 272). That is, the program achieved a curricular and instructional balance or harmony as children's increasing abilities to use the strategies they were taught helped to guide them through curricular content and beyond. This is precisely the sort of psychological connection between instructional situation and student-as-person that results in eventual development of aptitude for learning in a domain (Snow, 1992). In the end, having "become" readers and writers, students chose their own reading materials and writing topics. As in cognitive apprenticeship, the strategy instruction served to scaffold learners toward independent use of the reading/writing strategies for their own purposes.

In summary, unlike in previously discussed project-based science research, in the literature-based reading programs we have reviewed, strategy instruction was an explicit goal. Students were scaffolded to independent use of the strategies and primed to transfer strategies learned in one context to other similar situations in the same content domain. Although, as this research has demonstrated, domain-specific strategy instruction can provide students important scaffolds to accomplish particular kinds of tasks, most interventions in self-regulated learning thus far have failed to address the broad, underlying qualities of self-regulation that "successful" students regularly display across content domains, such as persistence, resilience, or self-reliance.

IV. STRATEGY INSTRUCTION THROUGH COLLABORATIVE INNOVATION

Educational interventions typically involve researcher-designed field studies as a means to document success; most interventions that explicitly target self-regulated learning are no different. Drawing upon what might be called basic research on self-regulated learning, researchers develop instructional models for teaching self-regulatory strategies and train teachers to implement those models. More "applied" evaluation studies then document results. The degree of flexibility teachers ultimately have in implementing or adapting the models varies from program to program. Yet, in a growing number of these research programs, as in some of those described herein, teachers' contributions are critical to both the development and implementation of the instructional model. Rather than a fully developed, instructional "script" that teachers are asked by researchers to follow, these projects actually ask teachers to take the lead in their own materials design. We have characterized this emerging class of field-based interventions in some detail elsewhere, under the label of "collaborative innovation" (Corno & Randi, 1997, 1999).

To provide background for the remainder of this chapter, we need to define collaborative innovation and briefly explain the historical context from which it derives. We also provide examples of collaborative innovation that illustrate the range and degree of teacher involvement in the design of self-regulated learning instruction. We review selected studies that involved teachers in the development of strategy instruction models, including our own work. As mentioned previously, that work has led us to our curriculum-embedded approach to teaching for self-regulated learning.

A. DEFINITION OF COLLABORATIVE INNOVATION

Collaborative innovation is a process whereby teachers and researchers work together to meld theory and practice through the construction, assessment, and documentation of new, teacher-generated curricular and instructional practices consistent with contemporary learning theory, yet carefully attuned to the individual differences of both teachers and students involved (Corno & Randi, 1997, 1999). As in traditional development and implementation research, researchers provide theory and models. However, unlike the implementation paradigm, in which researchers expect "fidelity" of implementation from teachers, in collaborative innovation, teachers are invited and encouraged to invent fresh, new practices. The researchers' role then becomes supportive and documentary, looking carefully at teachers' own efforts to create curricular and instructional innovations to determine what might be learned of a general nature for future use by others. Any "success indicators" that may be established for a particular program or model are recorded in light of that local innovation.

It follows from this line of reasoning that curricular innovations that support the development of student self-regulation and are invented by teachers in classrooms are especially appropriate targets for collaborative innovation because teachers, like their students, are afforded opportunities for self-regulated learning. In collaborative innovation, teachers' own inspirations for their work are honored by their invitation. At the same time, teachers are scaffolded by researchers or other mentors in their attempts to develop and experiment with instructional innovations before they fly solo. It is important that the innovations are not developed by those outside the classroom as in traditional research and development models (see Randi & Corno, 1997, for a comprehensive review of innovation research).

B. COLLABORATIVE INNOVATION IN RESEARCH ON SELF-REGULATION INTERVENTIONS

Collaborative innovation has been used by an increasing number of researchers in investigations of self-regulated learning (see, e.g., Guthrie & Wigfield, 1997; Perry, 1996). We describe here three studies that examine and document the teachers' role in developing learning strategy instruction.

Duffy (1993) carried out a study designed to help elementary teachers incorporate comprehension strategy instruction into their literacy curricula. Instead of providing teachers with curriculum kits, however, Duffy asked teachers to construct their own lessons. In monthly work sessions, teachers and researchers together discussed the growing body of research on elaborative reading and comprehension strategies, including theory that supported classroom implications. Duffy and his colleagues then visited teachers' classrooms twice a month to provide models, suggestions, and assistance. Their intent was not to rate the teachers' approximations or fidelity to a model, but to observe and offer suggestions that might be useful. Their data included classroom observations and teacher interviews, as well as interviews with students targeted for intensive instruction. Cases constructed for 11 teachers in four districts documented teachers' progress toward adaptive expertise in comprehension strategy instruction.

As is often the result when case studies of classroom teaching are compared, Duffy found that no two teachers were alike in their adaptations of the research on strategy instruction. To go beyond this simple finding, Duffy studied teachers' instructional practices at various points in their progress toward becoming expert strategy instructors. He constructed a theoretical continuum of progress. As a group, teachers' progress was found to be nonlinear. That is, teachers apparently visited and revisited points on Duffy's "continuum," at times asking for prescriptions and suggestions, and at other times deciding themselves what strategies to use or inventing new strategies. Duffy defined one point on his progress continuum as "creative invention"—the point at which teachers no longer followed a predefined list of strategies. They decided instead what strategies to use themselves, revised those strategies, and invented new strategies based on cues from their students. At the point of creative invention, these teachers made the innovation in question their own.

Duffy's model for this work included the professional development belief that collaborative lesson construction was better than authoritative instruction with teachers, and that part of his research team's task was to document the variety of ways teachers interpreted reading comprehension strategy instruction in their own classrooms. This is collaborative innovation, not traditional staff development with teachers, and the model of collaborative innovation Duffy and his colleagues provided teachers most likely contributed to their own progress along the continuum toward creative invention.

Another example of collaborative innovation in self-regulated learning by Coley, DePinto, Craig, and Gardner (1993), came about through graduate course work. The first author, Coley, worked with three graduate student–classroom teachers to learn how they combined and adapted reading comprehension strategies she introduced in her graduate classes. Coley did a qualitative documentation of these teachers' adaptations of "reciprocal teaching" (Palincsar & Brown, 1984) and other reading comprehension strategies. The study included first person narrative accounts by each of the three participating teachers. The narratives described how teachers adapted conventional reciprocal teaching to increase student participation and stimulate high level questioning rather than the recall questions typically observed in conventional reciprocal teaching interactions.

One teacher–author (DePinto) described how she identified several weaknesses in the traditional reciprocal teaching model by observing her particular fourth-grade students. For example, when these fourth-grade students, in small groups, engaged in the question–response dialogue characteristic of reciprocal teaching, DePinto noted that group members spent their time listening to the student who was "teacher." This interaction pattern was much the same as that repeatedly observed in traditional teacher-centered instruction—a recitation with little student talk, which DePinto wanted to avoid. She, therefore, modified the group work using "think–pair–share," a cooperative learning strategy that increases student–student interaction by requiring students to discuss a problem in pairs, after individual "think" time.

This kind of adaptation comes about when teachers' careful observations of their students "in action" lead them to identify a problem impeding the accomplishment of intended objectives. A repertoire of teaching strategies (see also Shulman's, 1986, discussion of "teaching alternatives") is then drawn upon to fix the problem. One can imagine other alternatives to think–pair–share that might provide an equally sound solution to the problem DePinto observed. The point is that teachers do detective work and tinkering all the time in their classrooms; they have to, to teach these particular students. Thus, no approach to instruction is ever implemented exactly as developers intend, and teachers' own adaptations to instructional innovations become critical components of their outcome effectiveness (Randi & Corno, 1997).

In a companion study, Marks et al. (1993) conducted a qualitative analysis of observation data from these same three teachers. They then compared the teachers' adaptations with Palincsar and Brown's original model of reciprocal teaching to generate new theory about its use in actual classrooms. This research concluded by hypothesizing that other teachers might be more likely to implement the adapted versions of reciprocal teaching that Coley et al. (1993) observed than they would the original model. The observed teachers improved upon the original model in ways that other practitioners might find adventitious. As an example of collaborative innovation, this research documented teachers' innovations with one model and recognized the unique contributions teachers themselves can make to evolving instructional theory. Put simply, when the innovation in question is attuned more closely to the classroom practice of real teachers than it is to the research tradition from which it derived, it may have greater likelihood of dissemination.

Elsewhere we have provided a detailed description of another example of collaborative innovation, namely, our own work to teach self-regulated learning within the context of secondary-level humanities curricula (see Corno, 1995; Corno & Randi, 1999). Our approach in this project was to take advantage of what designated tasks in one teacher's curriculum entailed with respect to the self-regulatory understandings, efforts, and interpretations of the particular students with which we worked. Table 1 presents a compilation of "teaching affordances," or features that we determined to be important for student learning in this project. At this point we make no claims that these five features are necessary, or even sufficient, for teaching self-regulated learning within secondary humanities. Rather, we list the components we have found most useful in our tryouts without being so specific as to preclude teachers' own permutations.

We grouped the five features into three generic tasks of teaching—setting the classroom environment, providing learning guidance, and an ongoing system of evaluation, all of which are assumed to be interrelated and dynamic. In addition, it should be noted that each of the five affordances for student self-regulated learning has been identified previously by other instructional strategy or self-regulated learning theory and research; we make no claims to originality in this list (see, e.g., other

TABLE 1   Five Features of Teaching that Afford Opportunities for Self-Regulated Learning

---

Classroom environment
  Encouraging students to meet challenges (e.g., flexible assignments allowing student choice; matching skills and opportunities)
  Community building (e.g., emphasis on collaboration; explicit instruction in cooperative and group learning skills—dividing tasks, reaching consensus, record keeping, respect for others' ideas)
Guidance
  Explicit, scaffolded strategy instruction (e.g., modeling of strategies such as planning and resource management, followed by guided enactment and eventual requirement of independent use)
Evaluation system
  Diagnostic performance evaluation (e.g., self-evaluations and peer evaluations; students taught to evaluate work against pre-determined criteria; importance of grades intentionally minimized; emphasis on specific qualitative feedback targeting improved performance)
  Curriculum-embedded assessments (e.g., instructional tasks that provide opportunities for teacher to observe and assess what students can do; tailored to student individual differences and designed to stretch students to their full potential through ongoing teacher assessment)

---

chapters in this volume). However, some useful integration is needed between our list and this complementary theory and research. The next phase of our work was undertaken, in part, to accomplish such an integration.

C. SUMMARY OF THE DISTINCTIONS BETWEEN TEACHER- AND RESEARCHER-GENERATED INNOVATIONS IN SELF-REGULATED LEARNING

Before describing our next generation of research, we take time to note some important distinctions between teacher- and researcher-generated innovations. First, our review makes it apparent that teacher-generated innovations that support self-regulated learning are qualitatively different from those developed by research teams and then "disseminated" to teachers (see also Corno, 1994). Research has found that teachers and researchers tend to plan instruction differently (Clark & Yinger, 1979). Teacher planning is a cyclical, nonlinear, process that does not move, as was once thought, from objectives to activities. Rather, teachers tend to move through successive elaborations and refinements, relying on information from their students to guide subsequent instruction. Consistent with this early research on teacher planning, teacher-designed self-regulated learning interventions are grounded in students' naive understandings and active, ongoing interpretations of classroom tasks. Taking cues from students' expressive behavior, teachers provide guidance and opportunities that take students toward more formal understanding. Instruction moves from the particular to the general and back again. This form of instruction is difficult if not impossible to "prescribe"; instructional tasks are often coconstructed by teachers and students spontaneously in classrooms. Both insight and appropriate attitudes toward self-regulated learning come about when these tasks prompt students to step back and self-observe (attitude follows behavior, rather than vice versa; see Bem, 1970). Thus, the teaching is adaptive at the microlevel; teachers are adapting instruction to the students, and students themselves are adapting to the instruction (Corno & Snow, 1986).

Also, traditional forms of instructional design would call for initial identification of learning and self-management strategies, followed by development of instructional models to teach those strategies, and then the test trial of activities in which students practice the strategies (Corno, 1977). In contrast, teacher interventions with which we are concerned tend to embed strategy instruction within tasks, setting up situations in which students need to learn strategies to succeed at the tasks (Corno & Randi, 1999). The previously described project-based strategy instruction in science (Blumenfeld et al., 1991) provides an excellent example of task-embedded strategy instruction.

Further on a hypothetical continuum of embedded strategy instruction is our own curriculum-embedded instruction, whose description we have saved for last. This form of teacher intervention draws upon the curricular analysis as an implicit model for developing students' understanding of self-regulated learning. As we illustrate, our teacher-generated intervention is grounded in literary sources that afford students opportunities for finding parallels in their own personal experiences. Unlike other literature-based strategy instruction, our curriculum-embedded strategy instruction does not prescribe sequences of strategies for accomplishing specific tasks, such as previewing a story or guiding comprehension with questions. That seems more appropriate for younger learners who are just beginning to read. Rather, we lead students to find examples in literature of strategies others have developed to move toward their desired goals, whatever those strategies and goals may be. We then ask students to identify their own goals and to articulate strategies that can direct their own efforts through tasks that are multiple and varied. Thus, our form of strategy instruction is especially appropriate at the middle-school or secondary levels, when students typically become more independent and developmentally ready to become strategic in home and school-related activities.

V. DEVELOPING A MODEL FOR TEACHING SELF-REGULATED LEARNING THROUGH STORY

Our experience teaching self-regulated learning through a humanities curriculum (Corno & Randi, 1999) led us to explore the use of story as a general model for developing self-regulated learning aptitude. For centuries, generations of parents have taught children important life lessons through story. In formal and informal settings, teachers too have used story as a universal frame in which individuals can find meaning and make sense of personal experience. Daloz (1986) claims that great teachers offer stories, not answers: "A good story is a kind of hologram of the life of an individual, a culture, or a whole species. Each of us hears in it, with ears conditioned by our own history, what we most need at the time to understand" (p. 24). The potential to guide learning seems inherent in story. Teachers of literature, in particular, always have attempted to render explicit the implicit lessons of story.

It is thus through an analysis of narrative literature or story that students might be led to articulate tacit understandings of self-regulated learning—understandings that may have come about implicitly through prior life experiences, including stories heard in school and home situations. One hypothesis is that a self-regulation analysis of narrative might provide the means for bringing self-regulated learning to a conscious level in strategy-using students; it may also be a beneficial way to introduce strategy use to novices. Again, studies suggest that many students may have acquired only tacit knowledge about the strategic aspects of "studenting," even by the time they reach higher elementary levels (Corno & Kanfer, 1993; Paris & Cunningham, 1996).

Beyond a self-regulation analysis of narrative, we suggest a general way that educators might apprentice learners into a community of "students," in the strong, purposefully strategic sense of the word. An important point is that our approach is antithetical to identifying specific strategies and teaching them in particular ways. Rather, consistent with our position on the importance of teacher innovation, the model we envision guides teachers in detecting adaptations suitable for their own classrooms and in inventing ways to teach self-regulated learning through literature of their own choosing. Finally, we hope to encourage teachers to adapt their instruction in ways that support that literature.

We began our invention with the mythical quest literature. Campbell (1949) wrote that one task of the mythical quest hero "is to return to us, transfigured, and teach the lesson he has learned of life renewed" (p. 20). Story has been said to provide a unique vehicle for taking the quest for life's meaning seriously and to be a model for teaching and learning across disciplinary boundaries (Carter, 1993). Describing the power of narrative as emblematic of human life, Witherell & Noddings (1991) wrote:

> The stories we hear and the stories we tell shape the meaning and texture of our lives at every stage and juncture. Stories and narrative, whether personal or fictional, provide meaning and belonging in our lives. They attach us to others and to our own histories by providing a tapestry rich with threads of time, place, character, and even advice on what we might do with our lives (p.1).

The quest for students of literature, then, is to follow story characters through time and place, learning lessons vicariously along the way. Social cognitive theory views observational learning as one means for acquiring a broad repertoire of self-regulatory strategies and behavior (Bandura, 1986). It then follows that literary characters who demonstrate self-regulation in pursuit of their goals might well serve as models for students, if the models' thinking and behavior are discussed and analyzed in relation to students' own lives. The formal curriculum, as Cronbach (1955) once suggested, should be structured to afford "more experiences of a certain type than nature might offer ... helping the person to draw his [or her] own conclusion more rapidly" (p. 79).

Hence, we looked to the quest literature as the source of curricular experiences that might serve as models for self-regulation. Although we chose stories from Greek and Roman quest literature, the general genre of the "journey tale" is more pervasive than that. For example, education itself has been characterized as a transformational journey comparable to the kinds of journeys stories tell (Daloz, 1986). Daloz studied the mentor–protegee relationship, conceptualizing mentors as guides along the transformational journey. Referring to the mentor as a prototype in the journey tale, Daloz described mentors as "engendering trust, issuing a challenge, providing encouragement, and offering a vision for the journey" (p. 30). As a resource, the mentor is one aspect of self-regulated learning embodied in the journey tale. We can illustrate others through a self-regulatory process analysis of the journey tale.

A. SELF-REGULATORY PROCESS ANALYSIS OF THE JOURNEY TALE

Characterized as the "monomyth" by Campbell (1949), the journey tale or "one hero story" is a literary refrain. Common to all cultures, the journey tale embodies change, learning, and growth, or movement toward goals. The journey represents a metaphorical rite of passage in which the hero undergoes the formulaic ritual of separation, initiation, and return (Campbell, 1949). That is, the hero encounters a situation in which he or she must separate from other sources of support and draw upon personal resources to accomplish a variety of goals before returning to society. In essence, the hero becomes self-regulated.

Typically, the journey begins with a clear and predetermined goal, although the best way to accomplish that goal is often purposefully left vague. Initially, with little direction, Hercules set out to retrieve the Hesperides's apples. Jason retrieved the golden fleece and Telemachos sought after his father, Odysseus. Although not all mythical goals are as elusive as the Holy Grail or the Golden Fleece, the goals tend to be more often than not just out of reach. Thus, to achieve the predetermined goal, the hero must stretch to maximum potential, and accomplish subgoals along the way. Some of the goals are inevitably in conflict—the sweet temptation must often be avoided. Gratification must be delayed. In the face of many imminent dangers, the best-laid plans must be protected. Moreover, the personal costs of the single-minded pursuit exert a strong toll on emotions. Strength and coping must win out.

As an embodiment of various aspects of self-regulated learning, the journey tale mirrors Vygotsky's (1986) zone of proximal development in which learners, guided by a mentor, strive to achieve something just beyond their reach. A North American Indian tale tells of a girl pursuing a porcupine for its quills. As she followed the porcupine to the top of a tree, the tree lengthened, and the porcupine resumed its climb. Although the girl's friends urged her to climb down, she continued, "having passed under the influence of the porcupine" (Thompson, 1929, in Campbell, 1949, p. 54). Similarly, modern volitional theory has identified a point at which the self-regulated learner "crosses the Rubicon," protecting prede-termined goals, often at any cost (Corno, 1993; Heckhausen & Kuhl, 1985). Apart from the hero's goal setting and goal protection, the affordances and constraints of the journey situation call forth the patterned responses of self-regulated learning. Once the hero is committed to goal achieve-ment, the journey takes the hero beyond known limits, separating the hero from all that is familiar and safe. At this point, the hero draws upon specific types of strategies to manage self, task, and others. These strate-gies are remarkably similar to those identified in research on self-regulated learning, for example, cognitive, motivation, or emotion control (Corno & Kanfer, 1993; Corno & Randi, 1999).

Odysseus, the wily hero of Greek myth, presents an especially clear literary example of strategic self-regulation. Renowned for his cleverness, Odysseus was a master of metacognitive control. For example, he carefully planned his escape from the Cyclops's cave, resisting his initial impulse to kill the monster and understanding that the giant alone could remove the stone that blocked the cave's entrance. Odysseus also exercised motivation and emotion control. Alone on a raft at sea, he drew upon internal resources to stay focused on his goal of homecoming, engaging in self-talk to maintain attention to task (see Vygotsky, 1978). To control emotion, he recalled prior experience in difficult situations and imagined the response of his loved ones to his eventual homecoming. In addition to self-manage-ment strategies, Odysseus controlled the task and others. He took full advantage of available resources whether they were magical herbs, various divinities, or comrades.

To make explicit the transfer from the literary journey to students' own journeys in life, parallels between the journeys of quest heroes and self-regulated individuals are not difficult to identify. In our early work embedding self-regulated learning instruction into a secondary humanities curriculum, students themselves identified what strategies the hero, Odysseus, used to persist in his efforts to return home (see Table 2).

Guided by the teacher much as quest heroes have been guided by their mentors, the students were led to (a) articulate, (b) label, and (c) catego-rize these self-regulated learning strategies (Table 1's "Explicit, scaffolded instruction"). The categories and labels assisted students in understanding the general principles underlying self-regulated learning (e.g., persistence, resilience, self-reliance). Students then applied the strategies systemati-cally to their own journeys as learners. Our present project uses a similar model to make the transfer of self-regulatory behavior explicit, but other ways may be envisioned as well (see Perkins & Salomon, 1988; Salomon & Perkins, 1989). In the next section, we describe the integrative work we did to develop and enhance our instructional model for teaching self-regulated learning through the journey tale.

Preparing Students to Perceive Self-Regulation when it Appears

One way to prepare students to perceive self-regulation within the journey tale is by cataloguing events through the eyes of the hero as learner. The journey tale describes rites of passage, initiations into communities, and forays into the unknown. Typically, the hero's noble behavior in these situations results in noticeable changes: Upon return, the hero is wiser or more experienced, often bringing back new knowledge or displaying an inner calm that others then admire. According to Campbell

TABLE 2   Examples of Student Self-Regulation Strategies[a] and Parallel Literary Examples[b]

	Covert strategies
Metacognitive control	
Planning	
Student example	Think of the first steps to take and get started right away
Literary example	Odysseus thought of what he needed to trick Polyphemus and escape from the cave
Monitoring/setting benchmarks	
Student example	Set some reachable goals
Literary examples	Odysseus had to kill the suitors before he could reclaim his place as king of Ithaca
	Odysseus took on one obstacle at a time
Evaluating goals and progress	
Student example	Check work as you go; look for feedback
Literary example	Odysseus was forced to reconsider the importance of his goal when Calypso offered him a chance for immortality
Motivation control	
Focusing/positive thinking	
Student example	Imagine doing this work well
Literary example	Odysseus imagined being home with his positive thinking wife, Penelope, and his son, Telemachus
Endurance and self-reliance	
Student examples	Give myself instruction and orders about timeliness; reward myself for hard work
Literary examples	Odysseus talked to himself while he was alone on the raft; he told himself to stay on the raft until he could swim to shore safely
Emotion control	
Visualization/mental imagery	
Student examples	Remember, I've done this kind of thing before
	Imagine being good at this
Literary examples	On Calypso's raft, Odysseus remembered the many hardships he had endured before
	After Athena showed Odysseus a vision of his success, Odysseus was ready to take on the suitors

(Continues)

TABLE 2   (*Continued*)

Overt strategies

Control of task situation
  Use of External Resources

Student examples	Gather materials and people to get the work started
Literary examples	Odysseus used a magical herb to counteract the spell of Circe

  Use of internal resources

Student examples	Streamline the task so it's easier and takes less work
	Add challenge or embellishment to make a task more fun
Literary examples	Tied to the mast, Odysseus allowed himself to hear the Sirens' song without giving up his quest for home

Others in the task setting
  Requesting help from mentors

Student examples	Ask for help from teacher
Literary examples	Odysseus had help from Athena

  Control Others in the Task Setting

Student examples	Ask kids to be quiet if they're bothering me; move to a quiet place
Literary examples	Odysseus tried to keep his men from eating the sacred cattle and incurring the anger of Helios, the sun god

[a] Self-regulation strategies are adapted from Corno & Kanfer (1993); see also Corno & Randi (1999).

[b] Literary examples were identified by students in an analysis of the literature. Labels were coconstructed by teacher and students in an activity that led students to categorize the strategies and assign labels to the categories.

(1949), these rites of initiation teach the lesson of oneness of the individual and society; the hero has been transformed to a level of emotional equanimity or "other-directedness" by encounters with rituals and central symbols of culture. Other-directedness frees the individual from self-absorption, and in so doing, paradoxically highlights those aspects of self-regulation that refer to purposeful patterns of action with respect to other persons and social situations. The wise hero realizes that orientations toward self and toward others fundamentally must be intermingled; each helps define the other (Snow, Corno, & Jackson, 1996, p. 276). Likewise, modern sociocognitive theory views learners as active constructors of knowledge. As such, learners are "imbued with powers of introspection; they [are] granted knowledge and feeling about learning, sometimes even control of it, metacognition" (Brown & Campione, 1996, p. 289). Thus active learners may be viewed as metaphorical travelers charting paths through the unknown and reflecting wisely upon their return.

Renewed interest in situated learning or learning embedded in context has prompted researchers, including anthropologists, sociologists, and linguists, to conduct careful studies of learning in situations outside school (Brown, 1994; Greeno, Collins, & Resnick, 1996). Grounding their work in this modern, situated learning theory, Brown and her colleagues designed and studied innovative classroom learning settings that replicate more natural learning situations outside school (Brown et al., 1993; Brown & Campione, 1996). According to Brown (1997), the critical elements of these new learning "communities" include agency or taking control of learning, reflection or making sense of what is learned, collaboration or interdependence, and culture or socially constructed, negotiated, and institutionalized norms. These features are embodied in a cycle of learning community activities in which students conduct research, share their expertise with others, and demonstrate their knowledge by performing a "consequential task" requiring knowledge of all aspects of the instructional unit (Brown & Campione, 1996).

The learning communities Brown and her colleagues helped to create share several features in common with the journey tale and with our interest in the preparation of students who will strive for and seek after learning. In the journey tale, mentors (or teachers) apprentice students into communities of practice. Sharing expertise, students learn the culture and discourse of the discipline from teachers and each other. Just as quest heroes are guided through trials by rituals and symbols, often returning to share their new knowledge and attitudes with others, so are students. Students work on authentic tasks, albeit not as impossible as some quest tasks. Nonetheless, students are encouraged to work at the edge of their potential or zone of proximal development (Vygotsky, 1978). As in journey tales, the goals in a learning community are just out of reach.

B. INSTRUCTIONAL MODEL FOR TEACHING SELF-REGULATED LEARNING THROUGH THE JOURNEY TALE

To teach self-regulated learning through the journey tale, then, Brown's model appears eminently suitable and readily adaptable by teachers. Brown's model also overlaps with the five features of our Table 1, a teaching environment structured to provide opportunities for self-regulated learning. The teaching environment for self-regulated learning encourages trust and risk taking through various forms of student choice, and includes a variety of ongoing self-evaluations and peer evaluations that place emphasis on improving students' work as opposed to grading it. Explicit instruction in planning, self-monitoring, and other aspects of self-regulation provides appropriate direction and guidance when students are scaffolded through pitfalls and points of decision. The ultimate performance of authentic tasks by all students in a community of learners is promoted through the coupling of school learning with students' own life experiences. That is, as a culminating learning experience and assessment, each is led to draw upon what he or she has learned through the curriculum to accomplish personal goals—goals that push beyond the boundaries of content and curriculum—thereby arriving at the journey's destination.

Among the most critical of the five elements in Table 1 is the way students are prepared to accomplish their own goals. The teacher guides students to induce and articulate; that is, to understand intellectually the principles of self-regulated learning. For example, students are led to articulate the need for goal setting, what it means to monitor their own responses to others and to situations, the various steps involved in self-management of rewards, and so on. This is done through the analysis of literary characters who exemplify the defining characteristics and patterned responses of self-regulated learners; that is, characters who are purposeful, resourceful, mindful, resilient, and, perhaps, enlightened. This guided activity models the more independent analysis of quest literature that comes later. The subsequent tasks students accomplish are designed to scaffold them toward independent use of various self-regulatory strategies, in which they might step back and observe themselves behaving as self-regulated learners. Again, these tasks are conceptualized as challenges to be met along the way of a learning journey or quest.

Following Brown et al. (1993), our approach calls for learners to embark on their learning journeys in small, multitask, groups. The learning journey is structured around cycles of (a) doing research, (b) sharing expertise, and (c) performing a consequential task. A learning community is created through collaboration and interdependence, made possible in this case by the cooperative learning jigsaw (Aronson, 1978) recommended by Brown (1997). In this form of cooperative learning, students first do research on an assigned topic in small (four to six student) groups where they become "experts." They then share their growing expertise with others in new groups formed by moving one expert from each topic group into a new group. Each new group then consists of several "experts" on the various assigned topics. Once all topic knowledge is shared, the new group accomplishes a "consequential task" that requires the integration of knowledge of all assigned topics. Individual pieces of the puzzle are thus integrated into a unified whole (a jigsaw), and what one student cannot provide for the task will be contributed by another.

Classroom Enactment

In a preliminary test of our model, the opportunity to embark on a learning journey was offered to the first author's literature class in a suburban secondary school in the Northeast; the class was comprised of 19 students in 10th, 11th, and 12th grades. We suspected this class would rise to the occasion, because students were above average in achievement; more than half (10) were ranked in the top 10% of their respective classes. Additionally, the class included five senior class officers, a student representative to the Board of Education, and a junior member of the school

Leadership Team. As further evidence that this application provided a rather optimal circumstance for students to accept our "offer," there was also a high level of participation in extracurricular activities among these students, including athletics (9), drama (3), and chorus (5).

We enacted our quest project three months into the school year after students had been acculturated into a classroom environment patterned after the description in Table 1. Although teacher assessments determined that all of these students exhibited some characteristics of self-regulated learners, at the start of the school year, the majority of the group could not articulate specific strategies they used to achieve academic success when asked (e.g., persistence, planning, prioritizing). Thus, this instructional unit was an effort to bring students' existing strategy use to a conscious level and to afford opportunities for repeated strategy use, rather than to introduce new strategies.

Consistent with Table 1, students were offered a choice from the outset —a learning opportunity. They were invited to identify strategies that quest heroes might use, strategies parallel to those that students themselves might use to be successful. As we suspected, these students agreed readily to become partners and collaborators in a community of learners in which their expertise would be acknowledged (Brown, 1997).

After accepting the challenge of our learning journey, the teacher introduced the archetype or basic story pattern of the hero's quest. Campbell (1949) described three stages in the hero's journey: (1) acceptance of a call or summons that directs the hero on his or her journey; (2) confrontations—tests of strength and wit that require the hero to draw upon available strategies and resources; and, (3) return to the community, wiser for the experience. The teacher described and exemplified each of these stages.

Students then read a quest of their choice and prepared to discuss the archetypal pattern. After they completed the reading, several students anticipated the next task and asked for the opportunity to meet with other students reading the same quest to discuss the archetype before reporting to the whole class. Students previously had participated in cooperative learning tasks and may have recognized the present task as one that would benefit from shared expertise. Perkins and Salomon (1988) called this "low road transfer," when similar situations evoke application of a previously learned repertoire. According to these authors, building in low road transfer opportunities helps prepare students for the more challenging ways to handle information to be introduced.

In their groups, students identified not only the archetypal elements, but also some of the strategies the heroes used to accomplish their goals. As students began discussing the heroes' strategies, they noted similar strategies they themselves typically used to accomplish their goals. These statements—offered by approximately one third of the class—arose without teacher prompting. For example, in one group, a student identified with the hero taking on one obstacle at a time: "I just take one day at a time." Thus, as students began to recognize similarities between the hero's learning journey and their own, the task provided an opportunity for high road transfer from a given to a new situation (Perkins & Salomon, 1988). Although not every student in the class spontaneously made high road contributions, everyone had a chance to note comments from the many who did, and so could benefit potentially (vicarious learning).

In a subsequent whole class discussion, the examples of heroes' strategies and corresponding strategies students attributed to themselves were categorized under appropriate labels the teacher provided. Here was the explicit, scaffolded strategy instruction. Table 3 presents these data.

In all, students provided 56 examples of specific self-regulated learning strategies. Some strategies were mentioned more than others. For example, all six groups identified getting help from a teacher, parent, or tutor as a form of mentoring. Each student in the groups provided at least one strategy, although many students provided more than one. Guided by the teacher, students also further explored the archetypal pattern in the quests by identifying particular elements within the call to adventure, the adventures themselves, or the hero's return. For example, some students remarked that heroes are typically offered a challenge they are free to accept or reject. This task prepared students for analyzing a quest in their own lives in a subsequent assignment.

This whole class instructional activity served as an important form of guidance provided by the teacher. The teacher relabeled the archetypal quest elements students identified, then she categorized them, and superimposed terms appropriate for describing aspects of self-regulation (e.g., the teacher relabeled a hero's mental imagery as a form of emotion control or Merlin as mentor). Students' tacit understandings were thereby rendered explicit and formalized. Thus, this approach to teaching for self-regulated learning exposed students to the discourse of the content area (i.e., the quest literature), led them to use it, and developed an intellectual understanding of self-regulation. Consistent with apprenticeship learning, this approach immersed students in the discourse of each discipline (self-regulation theory and quest literature). This type of whole-class activity, which assures that all learners have an understanding of the three assigned topics as well as a common language, has been termed *benchmarking* (Brown, 1997), and is sometimes accomplished by "crosstalk" (Brown & Campione, 1996) or whole class sharing of expertise.

Having been thus scaffolded through the self-regulation analysis of the journey tale, students were prepared to embark on a more independent journey in which they enacted self-regulatory activities for themselves. Students were assigned to six groups of three (one student was absent and not initially assigned to a group). Again, to maintain high interest and

TABLE 3 Student-Generated Examples of Self-Regulated Learning Strategies in the Quest Project Classroom[a] (N = 19 Students)

Planning
- (A) Students should plan ahead when they have a long project
- (B) Think of all the steps you need to do to finish a project
- (C) Write things down (make a list)
- (D) Manage time to get things done on time
- (E) Write down all the assignments that need to be done; time management
- (F) Plan work schedule ahead of time to make sure I do not become swamped
- (F) Plan time for getting research for a paper

Monitoring/setting benchmarks
- (A) Do one assignment at a time
- (A) Don't do more than you can handle
- (C) Do one homework assignment at a time
- (D) Set small goals; study a little every day instead of all night the day before a test
- (F) Review quizzes before tests and tests before finals

Evaluating goals and progress
- (A) Have someone check your work and proofread it
- (B) You might have to give up an activity or 'fun thing' to succeed in school; think about your real (long-range) goals
- (C) If you have plans to do something fun but you have a huge test the next day, you should study for the test
- (D) Setting priorities in order of importance in helping you succeed in life
- (E) Think about how you actually want to do on a given assignment
- (F) Give up parties for grades
- (F) Deciding whether you want to go out or do your schoolwork

Focusing/positive thinking
- (A) Imagine yourself accomplishing your goal
- (B) Imagine yourself getting good grades, doing well, having parents reward you
- (C) Thinking that you can pass a test or class
- (D) Think of your future when you try to work
- (E) If you think you can get an A, you will get an A
- (F) If you believe in yourself, you can get good grades

Endurance/self-reliance
- (A) Tell yourself you are doing well and will get a good grade
- (C) Say to yourself, 'I know I can get an A'
- (E) Studying for long periods of time
- (F) Staying on task for entire semester; no let down

Visualization
- (A) Remember how you did on this assignment before
- (C) Picture examples that you could use
- (D) Imagining how you felt the last time you received an A will help you strive to get that grade again
- (E) Flash cards, filmstrips, and videos
- (F) Flash cards and memory games

(Continues)

TABLE 3 *(Continued)*

Mentors
- (A) Ask for help from your teachers or parents
- (B) Get help from teachers, parents, friends
- (C) Going to see a teacher for extra help
- (D) Be a mentor to others; answering questions of peers when known yourself
- (D) Going to a tutor
- (E) Help from teacher or tutor
- (F) Getting tutored
- (F) Staying after school for extra help

Control others in the task setting
- (A) Try to help others
- (C) Ask people to be quiet if you are trying to concentrate
- (F) Working in groups and taking charge

External resources
- (A) Have your materials ready before you start the assignment
- (B) Use materials that you have wisely—things that you might have like flash cards and calculators
- (C) Books
- (D) Textbooks
- (E) Library, Internet

Internal resources
- (B) Live up to your potential; use your abilities to help you succeed
- (C) Remembering examples
- (D) Use creativity to make the task more fun to tackle
- (E) If you believe you can do something, if you are smart, use it to your advantage
- (F) Learning vocabulary of book before reading it
- (F) Learning vocabulary and using it later on in a paper

Sacrifice/trade-off (student-generated category)
- (B) Giving up activities that are fun to study or work on homework

[a]The category labels were provided by the teacher as a scaffold. Students generated the student strategies independently and placed the examples under the category labels as they interpreted them. Students generated the strategies A through F in a group activity. The letters A through F designate the contributions of each of the six groups.

encourage risk taking, students were allowed to select one of three assigned quests. For each quest, following Campbell, one group examined the hero's call to task and sought for evidence that the hero was setting goals and taking control of the task (e.g., accepting the call, beginning to identify resources, distinguishing among subtasks, planning appropriate courses of action). A second group explored how the hero overcame obstacles and confrontations along the way. That is, these students identified strategies the hero used to accomplish tasks (e.g., effective use of resources, taking small steps first, focusing on the task) and ways the quest hero tried to protect or enhance goals through motivation or emotion control (e.g., delaying gratification, self-talk, mental imagery). The third group focused on the hero's return. These students evaluated what the hero learned from his or her experiences in this tale (new knowledge, new attitudes) and identified which particular experiences led to various changes in the hero's behavior or attitudes (tracing chains of cause and effect). Table 4 presents our specific group tasks, designed to illustrate the "many ways in" to self-regulated learning.

The jigsaw task itself replicated a learning journey. That is, the full explication of the assigned journey tale constituted goal setting or direction. Students embarked on the journey toward goal achievement, guided

TABLE 4 Assignments for Expert Groups

As you have learned, certain archetypal patterns are readily identifiable in the monomyth or hero's quest. In this assignment, you will be asked to identify various elements of the monomyth archetype in [quest]. Discuss your assigned task in your small groups and be ready to share your small group's discussion in a new group. As in a hero's quest, you will be asked to leave your small group/community behind and embark on a "solo journey." Be sure to take careful notes from the group discussion to take along with you on your journey.

Group 1: The hero's journey is initiated typically by a call to task or summons that directs the hero on his or her solitary quest. The object of the quest is not always immediately clear to the hero. Sometimes, the hero hesitates before accepting the call. Often, the hero makes plans and preparations before embarking on his or her journey. Read the assigned quest and identify the hero's call and the goal of the quest as it is explained to the hero. You should also consider what the object of the quest may symbolize to the hero, his or her community, or both. Describe the hero's reactions to the call and any preparations he or she makes.

Group 2: The second stage of the monomyth is characterized by a hazardous journey in which the hero encounters numerous obstacles and confrontations. The hero is typically confronted with numerous temptations that threaten to take him or her off course. Describe this stage of the hero's journey, enumerate the obstacles or tasks, and explain what the hero does specifically to overcome each obstacle and temptation. Look for archetypal elements, such as guides, protective charms, and battles of wit. Remember, although the hero may be accompanied by comrades, they often do not share the hero's commitment. Note how the hero handles himself or herself and situations in which comrades may attempt to deter him or her from the goal.

Group 3: The third stage of the monomyth is the hero's return. Evaluate how the hero has changed upon his or her return. What experiences changed him or her? To what extent is the hero aware that he or she has changed? What new knowledge or understandings does he or she bring back to the community? In the hero's eyes, was achieving the goal worth the effort? Cite specific evidence from the text to support your answers to these questions. Hint: Search for answers to these questions in descriptions of the hero's reactions to the people he or she left behind when he or she embarked on the quest and these individuals' reactions to the hero upon his or her return.

---

initially by the task explication and the initial self-regulation analysis of the hero, and they ultimately flew solo in the consequential task or design of their own quest.

The final task of the learning journey served as a curriculum-embedded assessment. That is, the culminating instructional task required students to make public use of what they learned to accomplish the task. It is important from a research standpoint that these products students created also documented their understandings of both the quest literature and self-regulated learning. In this final task, students regrouped in such a way that each group had at least one expert on each aspect of self-regulated learning embodied in the quest archetype. Students were then assigned a consequential task that required them to coconstruct a contemporary learning journey tale that incorporated goal setting and task analysis, strategic self-management and task management, and an evaluation of performance (see Table 5).

Close observations of students as they worked in classroom groups to prepare the final assignment showed that each group discussed possibilities and decided on a topic for their quest. Typically, one student emerged as leader in each group; one student leader had previously identified her leadership as a way of "controlling others in the task setting." One student in each group assumed responsibility for recording an outline, discussion notes, or both. In each group, students took notes following the format of the quest archetype (i.e., call to adventure, adventures, and return). Students were reminded of the evaluation criteria as they worked on this task.

Students subsequently produced their essays in two class sessions in the computer lab. In our project, students shared their journey essays in a whole-class, crosstalk activity and discussed how the tales they wrote embodied various principles of self-regulated learning. Alternately, groups might have exchanged tales and labeled the archetypal elements and self-regulated learning principles they recognized in the tales. Certainly most teachers would provide feedback and grades as appropriate on these essays. There are many "routes" to the ends we sought.

Although the consequential task of coconstructing a contemporary learning journey required students to link what they had learned about

TABLE 5   Consequential Task

Now that you have each become "experts" on one aspect of the hero's quest, you will have the opportunity to share your expertise in a new community where your knowledge is valued as unique. As a group, write an original, contemporary "quest" that includes the archetypal elements of the monomyth. Be sure that readers can identify the elements, including the call and goals, the hazardous journey, and the return. Your hero or heroine should make use of as many self-regulated learning strategies as necessary to achieve his or her goals.

---

literature and self-regulated learning to authentic life experiences, we view this culminating task, paradoxically, as a commencement, as students' initial guided attempt at high road transfer. Once internalized, the cycles of goal and resource identification, implementation of strategies to accomplish tasks, and performance evaluation have the potential to be incorporated into all classroom (and life) learning journeys.

VI. COLLABORATIVE RESEARCH: FUTURE POSSIBILITIES

This preliminary trial with our approach provides a test under what may be ideal circumstances—one teacher and one researcher, working closely together to develop a tailored teaching and assessment protocol for developing aptitude in self-regulated learning. This occurred in a classroom with students eager and able to profit from the experience. We do not pretend to generalize from these data. Important next steps involve reaching other types of students with this approach and finding ways to bring in other teachers.

There is also a need to test the new forms of assessment we developed to evaluate student understanding of self-regulated learning. One way is to debrief students who were more and less successful on the various unit-based assessments to acquire information on their learning activities and deeper understandings of self-regulated learning. There is certainly a need for more formal assessment, including pre- and postmeasures of student self-regulation. In the present study, students enumerated the qualities they considered important for "successful students like themselves," but in an earlier study (Corno & Randi, 1999), we attempted to obtain data from a more formal preassessment. We administered a self-report measure of self-regulated learning employing a 5-point rating scale (Marzano, 1992). Invited to explain their responses in a subsequent class discussion, students said they found many items that seemed to be task specific and hard to think about in terms of general patterns of behavior. They also reported that an honest response to some items would depend on their energy levels at the time. Some students wanted to expand the 5-point scales to 10 points. In other words, this particular self-report scale did not function as developers intended. Rather, this quantitative measure highlighted some of the problems with relying on rating scales to measure student self-regulation. It was partly in response to students' musings about this scale that we came to develop our curriculum-embedded assessments.

The culminating assignment in our previously developed curriculum, for example, required students to identify a quest in their own lives, articulate their reasons for following it, and evaluate the consequences. Student essays were coded independently by each of us (see Corno & Randi, 1999).

Thus we combined the types of assessments traditionally employed by teachers with the types of measures typically employed by qualitative researchers. We believe that continued efforts along these lines will lead to the development of other forms of assessments, some combining qualitative and quantitative measures. It would be useful, for example, to obtain indicators of self-regulatory behavior as observations of students working in small groups; both discourse and the adoption of regulatory practices common to small group learning can be coded (see Corno, 1989, for one example). Ultimately, these assessments might be used not only to document student understandings, but also to validate the effectiveness of innovative teaching strategies (Greeno et al., 1997).

In keeping with the nature of this approach to teaching self-regulated learning, assessments ought to evaluate students' ability to call forth self-regulatory strategies whenever they judge a task to demand them, as well as their intellectual understandings of self-regulated learning. This kind of assessment may involve tracking individual students over time, as they engage in a variety of individual and group activities. For example, students might be observed engaged in in-class group activities unrelated to the quest literature curriculum. Alternatively, they might be observed engaged in group activities in their other classes. It would be informative to observe students as they engage in homework or independent study outside of class, in study halls, in the library, or in the computer lab. A combination of qualitative data obtained from observing students over time, in a variety of in- and out-of-class activities, together with carefully designed pre- and postmeasures of student understanding is needed to evaluate our curriculum-embedded approach for teaching student self-regulation.

One further dilemma that arises is the variety of instructional methods invited by our collaborative innovation approach for teaching student self-regulation. Traditional experimental designs rely on fidelity to treatment, but, more and more, "good" teaching is being characterized as flexible and responsive to different students and classrooms (Darling-Hammond, 1993). One explicit purpose of collaborative innovation research is to bring theory to practice in such a way that it allows teachers the flexibility to respond to individual students and class contexts. If experimental designs are to be used to evaluate these collaborative innovation programs, then measuring "fidelity to principles" rather than fidelity to treatment might be one answer to the evaluation dilemma (for a full discussion of the principles underlying our collaborative approach to teaching self-regulation, see Corno & Randi, 1999).

Our curriculum could be continually developed and evaluated, for example, by monitoring group activities closely and altering them when progress does not reach teachers' and researchers' collaboratively generated expected levels. This would not be a formal experiment with contrasting treatments; rather, it would be an evaluation in several classrooms of our general model's principles, which take on different shapes as transactions proceed. The researchers and teachers would be collaboratively involved in successive reformulations of the policies underlying teachers' improvisations. Feedback suggesting need for change would arise from records of student discourse and work samples that suggest puzzlement or misunderstanding of important aspects of self-regulation being taught or from behavioral cues such as some students' failure to use self-regulatory strategies when opportunities demand them. This cycle of ongoing assessment and revision is similar to that done by reflective teachers who attempt to make changes in their teaching practices (Randi, 1996), but without the collaboration of a researcher to document these successive changes, teachers' innovations are more likely to be viewed as idiosyncratic adaptations rather than inventive instructional improvements (Randi & Corno, 1997). The point is that a catalogue of selected classroom case studies obtained over a semester or more should demonstrate the range of adaptations that produce successful outcomes with our model, as well as suggest solutions to problems that must inevitably arise.

VII. SUMMARY

In this chapter we reviewed selected theory and research on teaching interventions in self-regulated learning. Several programs of domain-specific strategy instruction research demonstrated important gains in student learning of curricular content. Such programs also provide direction for promising new ways to teach more generic aspects of self-regulated learning.

We have been critical of most existing approaches to teaching generic strategies apart from the curriculum. Their generality is not to be assumed and their cultivation cannot be a decontextualized activity. There are good theoretical reasons to expect more effective outcomes from strategy instruction that is curriculum embedded. In addition, we argued that the method by which researchers typically develop instructional programs for teachers to implement faithfully in their own classrooms needs to be rethought. In our experience, and in much of the documented literature on educational innovations of all types, this approach often backfires completely. At best it results in teacher-adapted versions of the original innovation that vary inevitably in the extent to which they fulfill the promises developers intended (compare Corno, 1977, with Randi & Corno, 1997, for some 20 years of perspective on this problem). Researchers instead ought to be seeking ways to collaborate with teachers in the development of their own self-regulated learning innovations and then supporting their implementation and documenting results.

This chapter also outlined the features of a new, curriculum-embedded approach to teaching self-regulated learning. Our model, developed through a process of collaborative innovation, integrates our early research with work by Ann Brown and her colleagues on learning communities, and includes our self-regulation process analysis of the journey tale. The major features of Brown's approach are internally consistent with materials we designed. However, just as there are many routes to the same curricular goals, there is no theoretical reason why other teachers would have to use the same elements of Brown's model that we used (e.g., the jigsaw) as a method "du jour" to accomplish their intended self-regulatory goals (see, for another example, Scardamalia & Bereiter, 1994). Teachers' own creative license can certainly produce new ways to accomplish the general goals listed in Table 1 with students through the vehicle of literature. Our hope is that indeed will occur.

We demonstrated that the journey tale embodies the patterns of self-regulation that have been defined by psychological research; it therefore provides a good "fit" as a curricular vehicle for developing self-regulatory aptitude. To move aptitude theory into the direction of aptitude development, the kinds of connections we sought to establish between the processes of self-regulated learning as psychologists have defined them and the inherent qualities of story should be sought for other person–situation combinations as well. Such person–situation (or student–curriculum) matches are sorely needed in the conative (i.e., motivational–volitional) domain (Snow et al., 1996, Stanford Aptitude Seminar, in press). If students are to move steadily forward along the pathway from wanting to do well in school to *committing* to and ultimately *realizing* that goal, then they must be made to sample and fine tune self-regulatory processes to affordances that exist in the person–classroom situation interface (Snow, 1992, p. 29).

The rich possibilities afforded by optimal curricula still require coupling with similar, internally consistent aspects of teaching. Just as our version of Brown's learning community teaching model placed particular demands on students to display and fine tune those agentic and reflective qualities of thinking, attitudes, and behavior that define self-regulated learning, so must other new designs for teaching place demands on other aptitudes needed by students to succeed in school. Following modern situated aptitude theory (e.g., Snow, 1997; Salomon & Almog, 1998), we believe that the development of aptitude for self-regulated learning is dependent fundamentally on the learning activities that invite or demand self-regulatory responses from students within the teaching contexts to which they are exposed. Self-regulated learning logically comes about through models of self-regulation to which both teachers and students can relate and be made to emulate. We have tried to define key features of teaching environments, guidance, and evaluation systems that seem to promote this. The eventual level of expertise in self-regulated learning reached by any particular student, however, depends on how their own teachers elect to launch them toward these kinds of experiences. We look forward to new research that examines models that address the teaching of other conative aptitudes as we have addressed the teaching of self-regulation—models to which both teachers and students can relate and emulate.

REFERENCES

Alexander, P. A. (1995). Superimposing a situation-specific and domain-specific perspective on an account of self-regulated learning. *Educational Psychologist, 30*(4), 189–193.

Aronson, E. (1978). *The jigsaw classroom.* Beverly Hills, CA: Sage.

Bandura, A. (1986). *Social foundations of thought and action.* Englewood Cliffs, NJ: Prentice-Hall.

Baumann, J. F., & Ivey, G. (1997). Delicate balances: Striving for curricular and instructional equilibrium in a second-grade, literature/strategy-based classroom. *Reading Research Quarterly, 32*(3), 244–275.

Bem, D. (1970). *Beliefs, attitudes, and human affairs.* Belmont, CA: Brooks/Cole.

Bereiter, C. (1990). Aspects of an educational learning theory. *Review of Educational Research, 60,* 603–624.

Bereiter, C., & Scardamalia, M. (1987). *The psychology of written composition.* Hillsdale, NJ: Erlbaum.

Blumenfeld, P., Soloway, E., Marx, R. W., Krajcik, J. S., Guzdial, M., & Palincsar, A. (1991). Motivating project-based learning: Sustaining the doing, supporting the learning. *Educational Psychologist, 26,* 369–398.

Brown, A., & Campione, J. C. (1996). Psychological theory and the design of innovative learning environments: On procedures, principles, and systems. In L. Schauble & R. Glaser (Eds.), *Innovations in learning: New environments for education* (pp. 289–326). Mahwah, NJ: Erlbaum.

Brown, A. L. (1994). The advancement of learning. *Educational Researcher, 23*(8), 4–12.

Brown, A. L. (1997). Transforming schools into communities of thinking and learning about serious matters. *American Psychologist, 52*(4), 399–413.

Brown, A. L., Ash, D. Rutherford, M., Nakagawa, K., Gordon, A., & Campione, J. C. (1993). Distributed expertise in the classroom. In G. Salomon (Ed.), *Distributed cognitions: Psychological and educational considerations* (pp. 188–228). New York: Cambridge University Press.

Campbell, J. (1949). *The hero with a thousand faces.* Princeton, NJ: Princeton University Press.

Carter, K. (1993). The place of story in the study of teaching and teacher education. *Educational Researcher, 22*(1), 5–12.

Clark, C., & Yinger, R. (April, 1979). *Three studies of teacher planning.* Paper presented at the annual meeting of the American Educational Research Association, San Francisco.

Coley, J. D., DePinto, T., Craig, S., & Gardner, R. (1993). From college to classroom: Three teachers' accounts of their adaptations of reciprocal teaching. *Elementary School Journal, 94,* 255–266.

Collins, A., Brown, J. S., & Newman, S. E. (1989). Cognitive apprenticeship: Teaching the craft of reading, writing, and mathematics. In L. Resnick (Ed.), *Knowing, learning and instruction: Essays in honor of Robert Glaser* (pp. 453–486). Hillsdale, NJ: Erlbaum.

Collins-Block, C. (1993). Strategy instruction in a literature-based reading program. *Elementary School Journal, 94,* 139–151.

Corno, L. (1977). Teacher autonomy and instructional systems. In L. Rubin (Ed.), *Curriculum handbook: Administration and theory* (pp. 234–248). Rockleigh, NJ: Allyn & Bacon.

Corno, L. (1989). Self-regulated learning: A volitional analysis. In B. Zimmerman & D. Schunk (Eds.), *Self-regulated learning and academic achievement: theory, research, and practice* (pp. 111–142). New York: Springer-Verlag.

Corno, L. (1993). The best-laid plans: Modern conceptions of volition and educational research. *Educational Researcher, 22*(2), 14–22.

Corno, L. (1994). Student volition and education: Outcomes, influences, and practices. In D. H. Schunk & B. J. Zimmerman (Eds.), *Self-regulation of learning and performance: Issues and educational applications* (pp. 229–251). Hillsdale, NJ: Erlbaum.

Corno, L. (1995). Comments on Winne: Analytic and systemic research are both needed. *Educational Psychologist, 30*(4), 201–206.

Corno, L., & Kanfer, R. (1993). The role of volition in learning and performance. In L. Darling-Hammond (Ed.), *Review of research in education* (pp. 301–341). Washington, DC: American Educational Research Association.

Corno, L., & Randi, J. (1997). Motivation, volition, and collaborative innovation in classroom literacy. In J. Guthrie & A. Wigfield (Eds.), *Reading engagement: Motivating readers through integrated instruction* (pp. 14–31). Newark, DE: International Reading Association.

Corno, L., & Randi, J. (1999). A design theory for classroom instruction in self-regulated learning? In C. R. Reigeluth (Ed.), *Instructional design theories and models* (pp. 293–318). Mahwah, NJ: Erlbaum.

Corno, L., & Snow, R. E. (1986). Adapting teaching to individual differences in learners. In M. C. Wittrock (Ed.), *Third handbook of research on teaching* (pp. 605–629). Washington, DC: American Educational Research Association.

Cronbach, L. (1955). The learning process and text specification. In L. J. Cronbach (Ed.), *Text materials in modern education* (pp. 59–95). Urbana: University of Illinois Press.

Daloz, L. (1986). *Effective teaching and mentoring.* San Francisco: Jossey-Bass.

Darling-Hammond, L. (1993). Reframing the school reform agenda. *Phi Delta Kappan, 74*(10), 753–761.

Duffy, G. G. (1993). Teachers' progress toward becoming expert strategy teachers. *Elementary School Journal, 94*(2), 109–120.

Eisner, E. E. (1991). What really counts in schools. *Educational Leadership, 48*(5), 10–17.

Gall, M. D., Gall, J. P., Jacobsen, D. R., & Bullock, T. L. (1990). *Tools for learning: A guide to teaching study skills.* Alexandria, VA: Association for Supervision and Curriculum Development.

Graham, S., & Harris, K. R. (1993). Self-regulated strategy development: Helping students with learning problems develop as writers. *Elementary School Journal, 94*(2), 169–182.

Greeno, J. G., Collins, A. M., & Resnick, L. (1996). Cognition and learning. In D. C. Berliner & R. C. Calfee (Eds.), *Handbook of educational psychology* (pp. 15–46). New York: Macmillan.

Greeno, J. G., Plarson, P. D., & Schonfeld, A. H. (1997). *Assessment in transition: Implications for the NAEP of research on learning and cognition.* Stanford, CA: National Academy of Education.

Guthrie, J., & Wigfield, A. (1997). *Reading engagement: Motivating readers through integrated instruction.* Newark, DE: International Reading Association.

Heckhausen, H., & Kuhl, J. (1985). From wishes to action: The dead ends and short cuts on the long way to action. In M. Frese & J. Sabini (Eds.), *Goal directed behavior: The concept of action in psychology* (pp. 134–160). Hillsdale, NJ: Erlbaum.

Krajcik, J. S., Blumenfeld, P. C., Marx, R. W., & Soloway, E. (1994). A collaborative model for helping middle grade science teachers learn project-based instruction. *Elementary School Journal, 94*(5), 483–498.

Marks, M., Pressley, M., Coley, J. D., Craig, S., Gardner, R., DePinto, T., & Rose, W. (1993). Three teachers' adaptations of reciprocal teaching in comparison to traditional reciprocal teaching. *Elementary School Journal, 94,* 267–283.

Marzano, R. (1992). *A different kind of classroom.* Alexandria, VA: Association for Supervision and Curriculum Development.

Palincsar, A. (1986). The role of dialogue in providing scaffolded instruction. *Educational Psychologist, 2*, 73–98.

Palincsar, A. M., & Brown, A. L. (1984). Reciprocal teaching of comprehension-fostering and comprehension-monitoring activities. *Cognition and Instruction, 1*, 117–175.

Paris, S. G., & Cunningham, A. E. (1996). Children becoming students. In D. C. Berliner & R. C. Calfee (Eds.), *Handbook of educational psychology* (pp. 117–147). New York: Macmillan.

Perkins, D., & Salomon, G. (1988). Teaching for transfer. *Educational Leadership, 46*(1), 22–32.

Perry, N. E. (1996). *Examining relations between classroom writing environments and students' self-regulated learning.* Research proposal submitted to the Social Sciences and Humanities Council of Canada.

Pintrich, P. R., & Schrauben, B. (1992). Students' motivational beliefs and their cognitive engagement in academic tasks. In D. Schunk & J. Meece (Eds.), *Students' perceptions in the classroom: Causes and consequences* (pp. 149–183). Hillsdale, NJ: Erlbaum.

Randi, J. (1996). *From imitation to invention: The nature of innovation in teachers' classrooms.* Unpublished doctoral dissertation, Teachers College, Columbia University.

Randi, J., & Corno, L. (1997). Teachers as innovators. In B. Biddle, T. Good, & I. Goodson (Eds.), *International handbook of teachers and teaching* (pp. 1163–1221). New York: Kluwer.

Rosenshine, B. V. (1987). Explicit teaching. In D. C. Berliner & B. V. Rosenshine (Eds.), *Talks to teachers* (pp. 75–92). New York: Random House.

Salomon, G., & Almog, T. (1998). Educational psychology and technology: A matter of reciprocal relations. *Teachers College Record, 100*(2), 222–241.

Salomon, G., & Perkins, D. (1989). Rocky roads to transfer. Rethinking mechanisms of a neglected phenomenon. *Educational Psychologist, 24*(2), 113–142.

Scardamalia, M., & Bereiter, C. (1994). Computer support for knowledge-building communities. *Journal of the Learning Sciences, 3*(3), 265–283.

Schunk, D., & Zimmerman, B. (Eds.) (1994). *Self-regulation of learning and performance: Issues and applications.* Hillsdale, NJ: Erlbaum.

Shulman, L. S. (1986). Paradigms and research program in the study of teaching: A contemporary perspective. In M. C. Wittrock (Ed.), *Third handbook of research on teaching* (pp. 3–36). New York: Macmillan.

Shulman, L. S., & Quinlan, K. M. (1996). The comparative psychology of school subjects. In D. C. Berliner & R. C. Calfee (Eds.), *Handbook of educational psychology* (pp. 399–422). New York: Macmillan.

Snow, R. E. (1992). Aptitude theory: Yesterday, today, and tomorrow. *Educational Psychologist, 27*, 5–32.

Snow, R. E. (1997). Aptitudes and symbol systems in adaptive classroom teaching. *Phi Delta Kappan, 78*(5), 354–360.

Snow, R., Corno, L., & Jackson, D. (1996). Individual differences in affective and conative functions. In D. C. Berliner & R. C. Calfee (Eds.), *Handbook of educational psychology* (pp. 243–310). New York: Macmillan.

Stanford Aptitude Seminar (in press). *Remaking the concept of aptitude: Extending the legacy of Richard E. Snow.* Mahwah, NJ: Erlbaum.

Thompson, S. (1929). *Tales of the North American Indians.* Cambridge, MA: Harvard University Press.

Vygotsky, L. (1978). *Mind in society.* Cambridge, MA: Harvard University Press.

Vygotsky, L. (1986). *Thought and language.* Cambridge: MIT Press.

Weinstein, C. E., & Mayer, R. (1986). The teaching of learning strategies. In M. C. Wittrock (Ed.), *Third handbook of research on teaching* (pp. 315–327). New York: Macmillan.

Witherell, C., & Noddings, N. (1991). *Stories lives tell.* New York: Teachers College Press.

Zimmerman, B. J., & Schunk, D. H. (1989). *Self-regulated learning and academic achievement: Theory and research.* New York: Springer-Verlag.

21

SELF-REGULATION

A CHARACTERISTIC AND A
GOAL OF MATHEMATICS EDUCATION

ERIK DE CORTE, LIEVEN VERSCHAFFEL, AND
PETER OP 'T EYNDE

University of Leuven, Leuven, Belgium

I. INTRODUCTION

During the last two decades of the 20th century, important changes have emerged in mathematics education. A major shift certainly is that mathematics is no longer mainly conceived as a collection of abstract concepts and procedural skills to be mastered, but primarily as a set of human sense-making and problem-solving activities based on mathematical modeling of reality. In accordance with this view, there is now rather general agreement that the ultimate goal of student learning is the acquisition of a mathematical disposition rather than of a set of isolated concepts and skills. These shifts in the perception of mathematics as a domain and of the objectives of mathematics education are attended with a fundamental change in the conception of learning mathematics, namely, from passive and decontextualized absorption of mathematical knowledge and skills acquired and institutionalized by past generations toward active construction in a community of learners of meaning and understanding based on the modeling of reality.

This view of mathematics as an active and constructive process, which is reflected worldwide in reform documents that put forward new standards for mathematics education (e.g., Cockcroft, 1982; National Council of Teachers of Mathematics, 1989; Treffers, De Moor, & Feys, 1989), implies that learners assume control and agency over their own learning and problem-solving activities. This means that self-regulation constitutes a

Copyright © 2000 by Academic Press.
All rights of reproduction in any form reserved.

feature of effective learning and problem solving. This self-regulated conception of knowledge and skill acquisition contrasts sharply with many current educational practices in the modal mathematics classroom, where it is—mostly implicitly—assumed that regulatory activities are the responsibility of the teacher. In other words, in today's classrooms, external regulation of mathematics learning and problem solving by the teacher is the more typical situation and it prevails over self-regulation by the students. In addition, because children and youngsters apparently do not become self-regulated learners and problem solvers automatically and spontaneously, self-regulation of the processes of knowledge and skill acquisition and of problem solving is not only a major characteristic of productive learning, but it constitutes, at the same time and in itself, a main goal of a long-term learning process that, therefore, should be induced from an early age on.

From a conceptual point of view there is lack of clarity, and even confusion with respect to the concepts of metacognition and self-regulation (see also Pintrich, Wolters, & Baxter, in press; Zimmerman, 1994). In our opinion, the self-regulation of learning and problem solving is a form of action control that is characterized by the integrated regulation of cognition, motivation, and emotion (Boekaerts, 1997; Pintrich et al., in press; Snow, Corno, & Jackson, 1996). We endorse the viewpoint that self-regulation is a more comprehensive notion that, in addition to metacognitive processes, also encompasses motivational and emotional as well as behavioral monitoring and control processes (see e.g., Boekaerts, 1997; Zimmerman, 1995). We first elaborate our position by situating self-regulation in a theoretical framework of learning mathematics from instruction involving four essential components: acquiring a mathematical disposition as the ultimate goal, constructive learning processes as the road to the goal, powerful teaching–learning environments as support, and assessment as a basis for control and feedback. However, a review of the research literature shows that, until now, all the different aspects related to self-regulation of mathematics learning have not been investigated to the same degree. In the subsequent sections of this chapter, we focus on weaknesses observed in students with respect to metacognitive skills, metavolitional skills and beliefs as central aspects of a mathematical disposition, on the one hand, and attempts to develop and improve students self-regulation through systematic instructional interventions, on the other.

II. LEARNING MATHEMATICS FROM INSTRUCTION: OUTLINE OF A THEORETICAL FRAMEWORK

The extensive amount of research on mathematics learning and teaching carried out over the past two decades (see Bishop, Clements, Keitel,

Kilpatrick, & Laborde, 1996; De Corte, Greer, & Verschaffel, 1996; Grouws, 1992; Nesher & Kilpatrick, 1990; Nunes & Bryant, 1997; Steffe, Nesher, Cobb, Goldin, & Greer, 1996) has resulted in an empirically underpinned knowledge base that provides us with the building blocks for a theory of learning mathematics from instruction, that can guide the analysis of the quality and the effectiveness of educational practices, but also the design of new and more powerful teaching–learning environments for the acquisition of worthwhile pedagogical objectives. More specifically, the outcomes of this research allow us to give better answers than before to the following questions that represent four components of a theory of learning from instruction (for more detail, see De Corte, 1995a; De Corte et al., 1996):

1. What has to be learned (theory of expertise)?
2. Which kind of learning/developmental processes are necessary to attain the intended goals (theory of acquisition)?
3. What are appropriate instructional methods and environments to elicit and continue these acquisition processes in students (theory of intervention)?
4. Which types of assessment instruments are required to evaluate the degree of attainment of the intended goals (a theory of assessment)?

The general answer to the first question that has emerged from the analysis of expertise in mathematics (see, e.g., De Corte et al., 1996; Schoenfeld, 1992) is that students should acquire a mathematical disposition. Such a disposition requires the mastery of five categories of aptitude:

1. A well-organized and flexibly accessible domain-specific knowledge base involving the facts, symbols, algorithms, concepts, and rules that constitute the contents of mathematics as a subject-matter field.
2. Heuristics methods, that is, search strategies for problem solving that do not guarantee, but significantly increase the probability of finding the correct solution because they induce a systematic approach to the task.
3. Metaknowledge, which involves knowledge about one's cognitive functioning (metacognitive knowledge), on the one hand, and knowledge about one's motivation and emotions that can be used to deliberately improve volitional efficiency (metavolitional knowledge), on the other.
4. Self-regulatory skills, which embrace skills relating to the self-regulation of one's cognitive processes (metacognitive skills or cognitive self-regulation), on the one hand, and of one's volitional processes (metavolitional skills or volitional self-regulation), on the other.
5. Beliefs about the self in relation to mathematical learning and problem solving, about the social context in which mathematical

activities take place, and about mathematics and mathematical learning and problem solving.

We know from other research (see, e.g., Cognition and Technology Group at Vanderbilt, 1997) that students often possess certain knowledge and skills they cannot access or use when necessary to solve a given problem. Acquiring a mathematical disposition should help to overcome this well-know phenomenon of inert knowledge. Therefore, the integrated mastery of the different kinds of knowledge (i.e., domain specific, metacognitive, metavolitional), skills, and beliefs should result in the development of a sensitivity for occasions when it is appropriate to use them and an inclination to do so. According to Perkins (1995), this sensitivity for situations and contexts, and the inclination to follow through both are fundamentally determined by the beliefs a person holds. A person's beliefs about what counts as a mathematical context and what he or she finds interesting or important have a strong influence on the situations he or she is sensitive to and whether or not he or she engages in them. The relevance of beliefs as a component of a mathematical disposition and their impact on mathematics learning is also echoed in the *Curriculum and Evaluation Standards for School Mathematics* of the (U.S.) National Council of Teachers of Mathematics (1989): "These beliefs exert a powerful influence on students' evaluation of their own ability, on their willingness to engage in mathematical tasks, and on their ultimate mathematical disposition" (p. 233). If acquiring a mathematical disposition functions as the ultimate goal of mathematics education, the development of appropriate beliefs in students seems to be as important as mastering different kinds of knowledge and self-regulatory skills.

As far as the second question is concerned, research has led to the identification of a series of characteristics of effective (mathematics) learning processes that should be explicitly taken into account when addressing the third question about interventions. These features can be summarized in the following definition (De Corte, 1995b): Learning is a constructive, cumulative, self-regulated, goal-oriented, situated, collaborative, and individually different process of knowledge building and meaning construction. Thus, as already alluded to in the Introduction, the constructivist perspective on learning involves pupils becoming self-regulated learners and problem solvers; that is, "metacognitively, motivationally, and behaviorally active participants in their own learning processes" (Zimmerman, 1989b, p. 4; see also Boekaerts, 1997). Self-regulated learners in school are able to manage and monitor their own processes of knowledge and skill acquisition; that is, they master and apply self-regulatory learning and problem-solving strategies on the basis of self-efficacy perceptions in view of attaining valued academic goals (Zimmerman, 1989a). Skilled self-regulation enables learners to orient themselves toward new learning tasks and to engage in the pursuit of adequate learning goals; it facilitates the appropriate decision making during learning and problem solving, as well as the monitoring of an ongoing learning and problem-solving process by providing one's own feedback and performance evaluations, and by keeping oneself concentrated and motivated. It also already has been established in a variety of content domains, including mathematics, that the degree of students' self-regulation correlates strongly with academic achievement (Zimmerman & Risemberg, 1997).

As previously mentioned, the features of effective learning processes should orient inquiry that attempts to contribute to answering the third question by developing and testing a series of guiding principles for the design of powerful mathematics learning environments. In this respect, major guidelines that have emerged from the literature and are in line with the dispositional view of and the constructivist approach to mathematics learning are the following (for a more detailed discussion see De Corte et al., 1996):

1. Induce and support constructive, cumulative, and goal-oriented acquisition processes in students.
2. Enhance students' self-regulation of their own learning processes.
3. Embed learning as much as possible in authentic contexts that are rich in resources and offer ample opportunities for interaction and collaboration.
4. Allow for the flexible adaptation of instructional and emotional support, taking into account individual differences among students.
5. Facilitate the acquisition of general learning strategies and problem-solving skills embedded within the mathematics curriculum.

Finally, a theory of assessment offers methods and techniques for the construction and application of proper assessment instruments that are compatible with the new view about the objectives and the nature of mathematics learning and teaching. In this respect, strong criticisms of traditional techniques and practices of educational testing, predominantly based on the multiple-choice item format, have led to the development of alternative forms of assessments that reflect more complex, real-life or so-called authentic performances (see, e.g., Lesh & Lamon, 1992; Lester, Lambdin, & Preston, 1997; Romberg, 1995; for a critical discussion of the notion of "authentic" assessment, see Terwilliger, 1997). At the same time the need to integrate assessment with teaching and the importance of assessment instruments to yield information to guide further learning and instruction have been emphasized (see, e.g., Glaser & Silver, 1994). From the perspective of self-regulating learning, it is important in this respect to stimulate in students the development of attitudes toward and skills in assessing their own mathematical learning processes and performances.

It becomes obvious from the preceding outline of a theory of learning mathematics from instruction that the notion of self-regulation occupies a central position throughout this theory. Indeed, self-regulatory skills are a major component of the mathematical disposition as the ultimate objective of mathematics education, but self-regulation constitutes as well a key characteristic of productive mathematics learning activities and processes. The adequate use of cognitive and volitional self-regulatory skills in a specific task and instructional context depends on the subjective perception and interpretation of that dynamically changing context based on the knowledge, beliefs, skills, and strategies one possesses; that is, the different components of a mathematical disposition (see Greeno, Collins & Resnick, 1996). Specifically students' beliefs play an important role in this ongoing interpretation process, and as such have a major influence on students' problem-solving behavior. Schoenfeld (1985) pointed out that "beliefs establish the context within which resources, heuristics and control operate" (p. 45). Self-regulated mathematical learning and problem solving then can be defined basically in terms of the effective use of metacognitive and metavolitional skills, but to grasp the whole reality of self-regulated mathematical learning and problem solving, the use of these skills has to be situated against a more complex personal and contextual background (see Figure 1).

Taking this perspective on self-regulated mathematics learning into account, powerful teaching–learning environments should focus on the progressive growth and development of self-regulatory skills in students, and instruments for the assessment of those skills should be elaborated, but at the same time one should not lose sight of the powerful personal background components (i.e., beliefs, knowledge, ...) that influence the adequate use of those skills. The next section documents that research has revealed serious flaws in students with respect to the key aspects of self-regulation; that is, metacognitive and metavolitional skills. We further discuss research that shows the important influence of student beliefs on mathematical learning and problem solving. Finally, we review a series of exemplary design experiments aiming at improving self-regulation skills in students through systematic intervention.

III. STUDENTS' FLAWS IN SELF-REGULATORY SKILLS AND BELIEFS

The importance of the self-regulatory components of a mathematical disposition contrasts sharply with the research results that already were published in the 1980s that showed substantial weaknesses in many students in this respect.

STUDENT CHARACTERISTICS

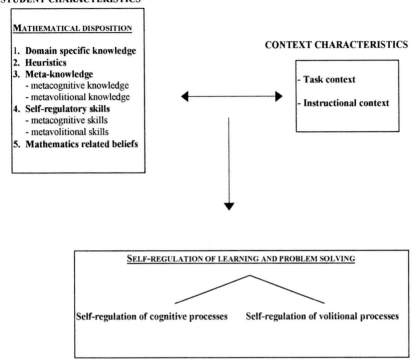

FIGURE 1   Self-regulated mathematical learning and problem solving.

A. FLAWS IN THE REGULATION OF COGNITIVE PROCESSES

The importance of self-regulation during mathematical problem solving has been very well documented in a study by Schoenfeld (1985; see also 1992). Schoenfeld videotaped high-school and college students working in pairs on unfamiliar geometry problems during 20-minute sessions, and contrasted their solution processes with those of experts in mathematics. The following task is an example of the problems used in this study: "Consider the set of all triangles whose perimeter is a fixed number P. Of these, which has the largest area? Justify your answer as best as you can" (Schoenfeld, 1985, p. 301).

The protocols of the solution processes were parsed into episodes that represented different activities: reading the problem, analyzing, exploring, planning, implementing, and verifying. Time-line graphs were used to represent the course of the solution processes visually. Figure 2 shows a representative time-line graph of an expert solving a difficult problem. This figure demonstrates clearly that regulation of cognitive activities constitutes an essential component of expert problem solving. Indeed, this expert

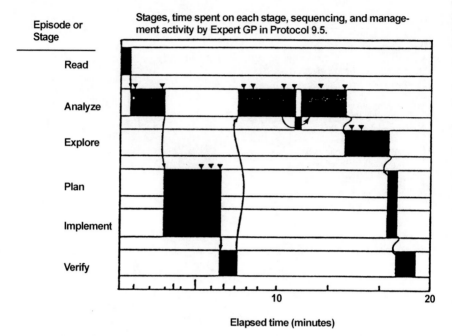

FIGURE 2   Expert mathematician solving a difficult problem. From "Mathematical problem solving," by A. H. Schoenfeld (1985). New York: Academic Press. Copyright 1985 by Academic Press. Reprinted with permission.

spent a substantial amount of time analyzing the problem in an attempt to understand what it was about and planning the solution process. Moreover, the expert continually reflected on the state of his or her problem-solving process; this is indicated in the graph by the inverted triangles that represent explicit comments during the solution process (e.g., "Hmm, I don't know exactly where to start here," followed by 2 minutes of analyzing the problem).

This expert approach is in sharp contrast to the typical problem-solving behavior that emerged from the more than 100 protocols of the student pairs. Indeed, in about 60% of the solution attempts, cognitive self-regulatory activities that are so typical of expert problem solving were totally lacking. The typical strategy in those cases is illustrated in Figure 3: reading the problem, quickly deciding to follow a certain approach, and sticking to it without considering any alternative, despite evidence that no progress was being made.

Other comparative studies of weak and skilled problem solvers of different ages—carried out not only in the United States (e.g., Lester & Garofalo, 1982; Silver, Branca, & Adams, 1980), but in distinct parts of the world—also support the crucial role of cognitive self-regulation in mathe-

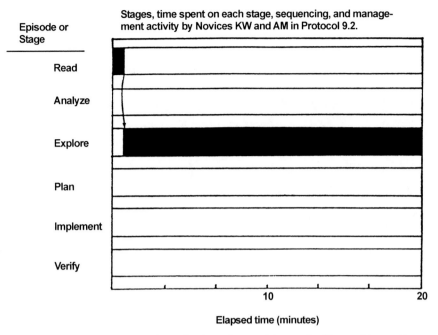

FIGURE 3 College and high school students solving unfamiliar problems. From "Mathematical problem solving," by A. H. Schoenfeld (1985). New York: Academic Press. Copyright 1985 by Academic Press. Reprinted with permission.

matics learning and problem solving. For example, Gurova (1985) analyzed the solution processes of 11-year-old Russian low and high performers on a series of difficult word problems. The high performers were much more aware of their problem-solving activities: they could explain their solution methods better, they could justify their solution strategies more appropriately, and they were more accurate in predicting which problems they had solved correctly. In his well-known studies, Krutetskii (1976) also observed differences between elementary and secondary school students of different ability levels with respect to metacognitive activities during word problem solving. Similar results were reported in the Netherlands. Nelissen (1987) found in elementary school children that good problem solvers were better in terms of self-monitoring and reflection than poor problem solvers. Overtoom (1991) registered analogous differences between gifted and average students at the primary and secondary school levels. De Corte and Somers (1982) observed a strong lack of planning and monitoring of problem solving in a group of Flemish sixth graders, leading to poor performance on a word problem test. In summary, there is abundant evidence to show that cognitive self-regulation constitutes a major aspect of skilled mathematical learning and problem solving.

B. FLAWS IN THE REGULATION OF VOLITIONAL PROCESSES

Nowadays educational researchers also acknowledge more and more the influence of motivational and emotional aptitudes next to (meta)cognitive aptitudes on mathematical learning and problem solving (see, e.g., McLeod, 1989, 1992). The self-regulation of these aspects of the learning and the problem-solving process asks for a competence to monitor and control one's volitional processes (Kuhl, 1994). This refers to the knowledge and the skills to create and support an intention until goal attainment. Students' knowledge about their motivational and emotional states and the way they influence the problem-solving process form the precondition to change the mode of one's functioning (Kuhl & Goschke, 1994). Monitoring and controlling motivational and emotional processes always implies to some extent an awareness of and knowing about these processes and their constituents. However, deliberately regulating one's volitional processes encompasses more than motivational and emotional control. Other aspects such as attention control, planning, and impulse control (i.e., environmental control, time control, inhibition of competing impulses) have to be considered also (Kuhl, 1994).

To our knowledge, until now, research has not very well documented the way in which the use of specific metavolitional skills influences the outcome of mathematical learning and problem solving. We know little about the differences between expert and novice mathematicians with respect to the self-regulation of volitional processes. However, there are some research results that point to the relevance of volitional self-regulation for mathematical learning and problem solving. A study by Seegers and Boekaerts (1993) indirectly showed how motivational control could influence the results of mathematical problem solving. They investigated the influence of more general motivational beliefs (goal orientation, attributional style, self-efficacy) on task-specific cognitions (subjective competence, task attraction, personal relevance) and emotional state, as well as the way in which these general and task-specific variables determine the willingness to invest effort (learning intention) and task performance. A group of 162 fifth and sixth graders (ages 11 and 12) was presented with a number of tests and questionnaires to measure, respectively, pupils' mathematical and reasoning ability and all the abovementioned variables. Specific questionnaires were developed to assess the three different general motivational beliefs for this age group. To measure the task-specific variables, the authors applied Boekaerts' (1987) (Quasi) On-Line Motivation Questionnaire. This questionnaire, which consists of two parts, was presented to the pupils simultaneously with a self-made mathematical problem-solving test. The first part was administered just after they glimpsed at the problems in the test, and it involved questions about task-specific cognitions, emotional state, and learning intention. The second part which measures emotional state, invested effort, result assessment, and attribution, was administered just after finishing the problems.

The results showed that motivational beliefs had only an indirect influence on mathematics performance through the task-specific appraisals and, more specifically, through the perceived competence in the task (subjective competence). Motivational beliefs also indirectly determined the learning intention and emotional state through task-specific appraisals, but there was no relationship found between learning intention and emotional state, on the one hand, and performance, on the other hand. From these results, one can infer that a high willingness to invest effort and a positive emotional state yield only positive effects on performance when they are linked with high subjective competence; this illustrates the complex way in which motivational and emotional aptitudes influence problem solving. These results as well as those from other studies done by the same research group (e.g., Vermeer, 1997) point indirectly to the relevance of motivational control as the ability to generate positive appraisals in the orientation stage of mathematical problem solving (Boekaerts, 1994). Students who are able to generate positive scenarios when confronted with a problem feel more confident and are willing to invest more effort, and as a consequence are likely to obtain better learning results.

We have discussed motivational control as one important aspect of the self-regulation of volitional processes. The other four aspects (i.e., emotional control, attention control, planning, and impulse control) may be as important, but have not received much attention yet in research on mathematical learning and problem solving. An exception is the study by McLeod, Metzger, and Craviotto (1989) on the affective reactions of expert and novice problem solvers. In a small-scale study, they interviewed four professors (experts) and four undergraduate students (novices) about their affective reactions while solving a series of mathematical problems. They came to the conclusion that both groups experienced the same emotions when they were stuck on a problem, feeling at times frustrated, aggregated, and disappointed, but whereas the novices reacted with quitting or stubbornly going on in the same way, the experts focused on staying calm and flexible. Although this exploratory study does not allow general conclusions, it illustrates that people handle emotions in different ways (emotional control) during mathematical problem solving and that this has a definite impact on their problem-solving processes and outcomes.

In summary, these and other, more general studies (see also Zimmermann & Martinez-Pons, 1986) show that students' ability to regulate certain volitional aspects of their behavior has an important influence on the course of the problem-solving process as well as on the results. Students who possess the necessary knowledge and skills to adequately regulate their volitional processes get less distracted, know when to concentrate on what, and know how to react adequately to negative appraisals or negative experiences during problem solving without falling into dysfunctional patterns of behavior (see also Boekaerts, 1992; Messick, 1987). However, much more research is needed to study the different aspects of volitional self-regulation in a more systematic and detailed way, and especially to clarify further the interactions between these volitional processes and the cognitive and metacognitive processes, and how they determine the outcome of mathematical learning and problem solving.

C. FLAWS IN STUDENTS' BELIEFS

Currently, there is a substantial amount of research that shows that a variety of beliefs that students hold are important determinants of their learning, thinking, and performance (see, e.g., Boekaerts, 1997; Pintrich, Marx, & Boyle, 1993). This is certainly also the case with respect to mathematics (see McLeod, 1992). Schoenfeld (1985) has done pioneering work in this regard:

> Belief systems are one's mathematical world view, the perspective with which one approaches mathematics and mathematical tasks. One's beliefs about mathematics can determine how one chooses to approach a problem, which techniques will be used or avoided, how long and how hard one will work on it, and so on. (p. 45)

In other words, beliefs have a very strong influence on one's approach to and effort investment in mathematical learning and problem tasks. In this respect, it is important to notice that such beliefs are not necessarily conscious, but often implicit. Schoenfeld's view on the self-regulatory impact of beliefs on mathematics learning is echoed in the *Curriculum and Evaluation Standards for School Mathematics* of the (U.S.) National Council of Teachers of Mathematics (1989) as cited previously.

In the available literature, researchers usually distinguish between three kinds of student beliefs: beliefs about the self in relation to mathematical learning and problem solving, beliefs about the social context (e.g., the mathematics class), and beliefs about mathematics and mathematical learning and problem solving (see, e.g., McLeod, 1992). The foregoing discussion of the study of Seegers & Boekaerts (1993) already revealed the important indirect influence self-beliefs (or motivational beliefs) have on mathematical problem solving. Several other researchers (e.g., Ames & Archer, 1988; Fennema, 1989; Kloosterman, 1988) also addressed the influence of self-beliefs on mathematical problem solving, often reporting gender differences in relation to differences in performance (see also Vermeer, 1997). For instance, Fennema (1989) found that "males have more confidence in their ability to do mathematics, report higher perceived usefulness, and attribute success and failure in mathematics in a way that has been hypothesized to have a more positive influence on achievement" (p. 211). Most of these studies (except Vermeer, 1997), however, do not incorporate task-specific variables and as such do not allow us to differentiate between direct or indirect effects of these beliefs.

In addition to these self-beliefs, more and more research points out that students' problem-solving behavior in a specific context is governed by their beliefs about expectations, rules, and norms that are linked with that situation. The relevance of context beliefs is illustrated indirectly by the well-known ethnomathematic studies in which everyday mathematical problem-solving activities of children and adults were contrasted with their solution strategies in a formal school context. For instance, Nunes, Schliemann, and Carraher (1993) showed that Brazilian street vendors were very skillful, quick, and accurate at calculating how much one had to pay for a number of coconuts and that they used a variety of informal, invented strategies. However, confronted with isomorphic textbook word problems, the same children used the formal, algorithmic procedures learned in school and they committed many more errors.

Finally, students' beliefs about mathematics and mathematics learning and problem solving determine in a fundamental way their problem-solving behavior. It is argued that, probably as a consequence of current educational practices, students acquire beliefs relating to mathematics that are naive, incorrect, or both, but have mainly a negative or inhibitory effect on their learning activities and approaches to mathematics problems. For instance, according to Greeno (1991), most students learn from their experiences in the classroom that mathematics knowledge is not something that is constructed by the learner, either individually or in group, but is a fixed body of received knowledge. In a similar way, Lampert (1990) characterized the common view about mathematics as follows: Mathematics is associated with certainty, and with being able to give quickly the correct answer; doing mathematics corresponds to following rules prescribed by the teacher; knowing math means being able to recall and use the correct rule when asked by the teacher; and an answer to a mathematical question or problem becomes true when it is approved by the authority of the teacher. According to Lampert (1990), those beliefs are acquired through years of watching, listening, and practicing in the mathematics classroom.

Empirical support for these claims was, for instance, reported in an article by Schoenfeld (1988) with the strange title, "When good teaching leads to bad results: The disasters of 'well-taught' mathematics courses." Schoenfeld made a year-long intensive study of one 10th-grade geometry class comprised of 20 pupils, along with periodic data collections in 11 other classes (210 pupils), involving observations, interviews with teachers and students, and questionnaires relating to students' perceptions about the nature of mathematics. The students in those classrooms scored well on typical achievement measures, and the mathematics was taught in a way that generally would be considered good teaching. Nevertheless, it was found that students acquired debilitating beliefs about mathematics and about themselves as mathematics learners, such as "all mathematics problems can be solved in just a few minutes" and "students are passive consumers of others' mathematics." It is obvious that such misbeliefs are not conducive to a mindful and persistent approach to new and challenging problems. Other strange beliefs that have been observed in pupils are that mathematics problems have one and only one right answer; formal mathematics has little or nothing to do with real thinking or problem solving; the mathematics learned in school has little or nothing to do with the real world (see, e.g., Schoenfeld, 1992).

In our own research, we also have observed that upper primary school children are affected by the belief that real-world knowledge is irrelevant when solving mathematical word problems. In the basic study (Verschaffel, De Corte, & Lasure, 1994), a paper-and-pencil test consisting of 10 pairs of problems was administered collectively to a group of 75 fifth graders (10- and 11-year-old boys and girls). Each pair of problems consisted of a standard problem (i.e., a problem that can be solved by straightforward application of one or more arithmetic operations with the given numbers; e.g., "Steve bought five planks of 2 meters each. How many 1-meter planks can he saw out of these planks?") and a parallel problem in which the mathematical modeling assumptions are problematic, at least if one seriously takes into account the realities of the context called up by the problem statement (e.g., "Steve bought four planks of 2.5 meters each. How many 1-meter planks can he saw out of these planks?"). An analysis of the pupils' reactions to the "problematic" tasks yielded an alarmingly small number of realistic responses or comments based on the activation of real-world knowledge (responding to the problem about the 2.5-meter planks with "8" instead of "10"). Indeed, only 17% of all the reactions to the 10 "problematic" problems could be considered as realistic, either because the realistic answer was given or the nonrealistic answer was accompanied by a realistic comment (e.g., with respect to the planks problem, some pupils gave the answer "10," but added that Steve would have to glue together the four remaining 0.5-meter pieces two by two).

This phenomenon of nonrealistic mathematical modeling and problem solving has been replicated in several other studies in which the same or a similar set of problematic items was administered to students from many different countries under largely the same testing conditions (for an overview, see Greer & Verschaffel, 1997). Interestingly, in some of these additional studies, interviews were carried out with some of the students, and they revealed that a significant number of students were able to articulate an awareness of a difference between conventional answers expected in the context of school mathematics and answers appropriate to real situations. One 10-year-old from a study by Greer (reported in Greer & Verschaffel, 1997) commented as follows in response to the interviewer's question as to why he did not make use of realistic considerations when solving the problematic items in the context of a school mathematics test:

"I know all these things, but I would never think to include them in a maths problem. Math isn't about things like that. It's about getting sums right and you don't need to know outside things to get sums right." Moreover, additional studies in our center (De Corte, Verschaffel, Lasure, Borghart, & Yoshida, in press), as well as by other European researchers (see Greer & Verschaffel, 1997), have shown that this misbelief about the role of real-world knowledge during word problem solving is very strong and resistant to change, and, moreover, that it is paralleled by a similar tendency among (future) teachers, as reflected by their own preferred spontaneous solutions to word problems and their way of evaluating realistic and unrealistic pupil answers. This finding supports the view that the opinions of the teachers themselves about doing and learning mathematics are at least partially responsible for the development in students of misbeliefs that have a negative impact on the regulation of their problem-solving approach and strategies.

In this section we have shown first that students' metacognitive and metavolitional skills are important self-regulatory determinants of their learning, thinking, and problem solving. Second, we pointed to the fundamental way in which students' beliefs influence their mathematical learning and problem solving. In this respect, it is striking that with respect to these aspects, the present situation in mathematics classrooms is rather bleak: many students, especially the weaker ones, lack the appropriate cognitive and volitional self-regulatory skills, and present teaching practices seem to induce in students mainly negative beliefs about mathematics as a domain and about themselves as learners of mathematics. It is useful to remark here that this unfavorable picture with respect to mathematics is not unique, but rather representative for school education today. For instance, Berry and Sahlberg (1996) studied the views about learning of 193 pupils (aged 15) in five schools in England and Finland. They took as a starting point De Corte's (1995b) model of the features of good learning as a constructive, cumulative, self-regulated, goal-oriented, situated, and collaborative process of knowledge building and meaning construction. A major finding of this investigation was that "most pupils have ideas of learning that can be described by the transmission model and are quite difficult to fit with De Corte's model .... This is to say that our pupils' ideas of learning and schooling reflect the static and closed practices of the school" (Berry & Sahlberg, 1996, p. 33). The authors add that this view of the pupil as a passive and externally regulated absorber of information is in accordance with similar findings reported by other researchers for teachers and adult students.

This state-of-the-art perspective raises the important question of whether it is possible to design and implement powerful instructional environments in which students acquire productive self-regulating strategies and develop more positive beliefs relating to learning and teaching mathematics? The next section of this chapter reviews representative examples of design studies that provide promising results in this respect.

IV. FOSTERING STUDENTS' SELF-REGULATION IN POWERFUL MATHEMATICS LEARNING ENVIRONMENTS

Notwithstanding the unfavorable picture of mathematics educational practice that emerges from the preceding section, it is the case that since the 1980s researchers have undertaken intervention studies aimed at improving students' self-regulation skills in mathematics through appropriate instruction. A number of these investigations have been conducted within the framework of a specific theoretical perspective on self-regulation and have a rather highly experimental character that focuses on the testing of hypotheses and predictions that derive from that theoretical approach. The most significant example of this kind of work is the series of studies by Schunk (1998) on the use of modeling for teaching primary school children to self-regulate the practice of mathematical skills, set up in the framework of the social–cognitive view of self-regulation. Other scholars have carried out more ecologically valid design experiments that are less closely related to a specific theoretical perspective on self-regulation, but aim at improving certain important aspects of cognitive self-regulation. As a whole, these research endeavors open perspectives for the implementation of a self-regulated conception of learning, and, as argued by Romberg (1992), the outcomes of that research call for a radical reform of mathematics learning and instruction, as well as a fundamental change in people's views and beliefs about mathematics and mathematics education. In this section we review four representative examples of the second category of studies, namely, design experiments focusing mostly on fostering students' cognitive self-regulation. These design experiment are an investigation by Schoenfeld (1985, 1992) at the college level, by Lester, Garofalo, and Kroll (1989) in seventh-grade classes, by the Cognition and Technology Group at Vanderbilt (1996, 1997) in the upper primary school, and by Verschaffel et al., (in press) with fifth graders.

A. TEACHING METACOGNITIVE AND HEURISTIC STRATEGIES IN GEOMETRY

Schoenfeld's (1985, 1992) work relating to geometry offers an excellent example of an attempt to create a powerful learning environment for teaching heuristic methods embedded in a cognitive self-regulation strategy for problem solving. The starting point of his intervention work was the observation reported earlier (see Section III.A) that metacognitive activities that constitute an essential characteristic of expert problem solving are mostly lacking in students' solution processes. Therefore, he designed a learning environment focused on the strategic aspects of problem solving. In this respect, Schoenfeld argues that it is not sufficient to teach students isolated heuristic procedures. Indeed, such heuristics are often inert, because students are unable to find and decide which heuristic is appropriate to solve the problem at hand. That is why it is necessary to teach heuristics in the context of a metacognitive strategy that supports the learner in selecting the right heuristic method to unravel and solve a given problem.

Schoenfeld (1985) elaborated such a regulatory strategy consisting of five stages:

1. Analysis oriented toward understanding the problem by constructing an adequate representation.
2. Designing a global solution plan.
3. Exploration oriented toward transforming the problem into a routine task.
4. Implementing the solution plan.
5. Verifying the solution.

According to Schoenfeld (1985), "the design stage is not really a separate phase, but something that pervades the entire solution process; its function is to ensure that you are engaged in activities most likely (as best as you can tell at that time) to be profitable. Most generally, it means keeping a global perspective on what you are doing and proceeding hierarchically" (p. 108). As such it can be viewed as the self-regulatory component par excellence of the strategy.

The exploration phase constitutes the heuristic heart of this strategy. Indeed, it is especially in transforming a problem into a routine task that heuristic methods are very helpful. However, such strategies are also useful in the problem analysis and verification stages. As an illustration, Table 1 lists a series of heuristic procedures that can be used in those three phases.

The instructional model that underlies Schoenfeld's learning environment reflects major features of the so-called cognitive apprenticeship approach to learning and teaching (Collins, Brown, & Newman, 1989). From the beginning, Schoenfeld orients his students toward the five-stage regulatory strategy as a whole, albeit in a schematic form. Then the different stages are treated consecutively, and the corresponding relevant heuristics are explained and practiced. In this respect, modeling is extensively used to demonstrate how an expert selects and applies heuristic methods. Afterward, the students are given ample opportunities to practice those methods under the guidance of the teacher, who encourages them to use certain heuristics, gives hints, provides immediate feedback, and, if necessary, helps with the execution of some parts of the strategy that the students cannot carry out independently (scaffolding). These different

TABLE 1   The Most Important Heuristics in Schoenfeld's (1985)
Problem-Solving Strategy

Analysis
   A. Draw a diagram if at all possible
   B. Examine special cases of the problem
   C. Try to simplify the problem

Exploration
   A. Consider essentially equivalent problems by replacing conditions by equivalent ones, by recombining the elements of the problem in different ways, by introducing auxiliary elements, or by reformulating the problem
   B. Try to decompose the problem in subgoals, and work on them case by case
   C. Look for a related or analogous problem where the solution method may be useful with a view to solving the new problem

Verification
   A. Check whether all pertinent data, were used and whether the solution conforms to reasonable estimates, predictions, or both
   B. Check whether the solution could have been obtained differently

forms of support and external regulation are gradually phased out as the students take over more and more agency for their problem-solving process; that is, become more and more self-regulated learners and problem solvers. In addition to modeling and whole-class teaching, Schoenfeld also uses small-group problem solving. Acting as a consultant, he regularly asks three questions during group activities:

1. What exactly are you doing? (Can you describe it precisely?)
2. Why are you doing it? (How does it fit into the solution?)
3. How does it help you? (What will you do with the outcome when you obtain it?)

Asking these questions serves two purposes: It encourages students to articulate their problem-solving strategies and it induces reflection on those activities; in other words, it stimulates and fosters cognitive regulation skills. The ultimate goal of this intervention is that students spontaneously and individually ask themselves the three questions, and in doing so regulate and monitor their own cognitive processes.

In a series of studies, Schoenfeld (1985, 1992) showed that college students can acquire the cognitive self-regulation strategy, as well as the embedded heuristics. Indeed, as a result of instruction, students' problem-solving approaches became more expertlike (see Figure 2). As reported previously, before instruction, 60% of the solution processes by students working in pairs lacked any sign of self-regulation; after the course, less than 20% of the solution attempts were of that type. The number of correct solutions increased accordingly.

Schoenfeld's approach clearly implies that self-regulatory skills and heuristics are taught. However, his learning environment is nevertheless essentially constructivist in nature. Indeed, the teacher does not impart problem solutions nor impose solution strategies, but supports students in their attempts at understanding problems, in reflecting on their methods and strategies, and in internalizing valuable self-regulation skills. In this respect, Schoenfeld's approach to the teaching of problem solving has developed in an interesting way: At present, the five stages of the control strategy delineated previously and the heuristics involved in it, are no longer taught in the same very structured and explicit way as was initially the case, but their importance and usefulness are highlighted when relevant and appropriate in the course of classroom discussions (Schoenfeld, 1987). In such an environment, student are not *learning about* mathematics, but they are *doing* mathematics. This involves learning how to use the tools of mathematics, and leads to the acquisition not only of mathematical concepts, but also of a mathematical view of the world and a sense of mathematical practice and culture (Schoenfeld, 1992). In summary, a real mathematical disposition, including cognitive self-regulation of mathematical learning and thinking, is encouraged and fostered.

B. TEACHING COGNITIVE SELF-REGULATORY SKILLS TO SEVENTH GRADERS

According to Lester et al. (1989), successful problem solving depends on five broad, interdependent categories of factors: knowledge, control, affects, beliefs, and contextual factors. In this intervention study they focus on metacognition that involves the knowledge and control one has of one's cognitive functioning. The control aspect refers to the regulation of one's cognitive processes and behavior during problem solving, and is more precisely defined as follows:

> In particular, control has to do with the decisions and actions undertaken in analyzing and exploring problem conditions, planning courses of action, selecting and organizing strategies, monitoring actions and progress, checking outcomes and results, evaluating plans and strategies, revising and abandoning unproductive plans and strategies, and reflecting upon all decisions made and actions taken during the course of working on a problem. (Lester et al., 1989, p. 4)

To explore the effect of instruction on students' cognitive self-regulation of their problem-solving processes, Lester et al. (1989) designed a learning environment that involved (1) creating opportunities for students to practice in the use of a number of valuable heuristic strategies (strategy training), (2) helping students to become more aware of the strategies and procedures they use to solve problems (awareness training), and (3) training students to monitor and evaluate their actions during problem solving (self-regulation training).

More specifically, the learning environment consisted of (1) a set of appropriate problems and tasks, and (2) a series of lesson plans with teacher roles and activities. Similar to Schoenfeld's approach, the selection of problems and teaching activities was based on a theoretical framework of skilled problem solving, encompassing a series of heuristic strategies (i.e., guess and check, look for a pattern, work backward, draw a picture, make a table, simplify the problem) embedded in an overall cognitive regulation strategy composed of four stages, namely, orientation, organization, execution, and verification (see Table 2 for a specification of the four categories). These stages correspond largely to those that occur in Schoenfeld's model (1985): analysis, exploration, implementation, and verification.

Two broad types of problems were used in the study: routine and nonroutine problems. Routine problems were typical multistep word problems intended to provide pupils with practice in translating verbal prob-

TABLE 2   A Cognitive-Metacognitive Framework for Studying Mathematical Performance[a]

Orientation: Strategic behavior to assess and understand a problem
  A. Comprehension strategies
  B. Analysis of information and conditions
  C. Assessment of familiarity with task
  D. Initial and subsequent representation
  E. Assessment of level of difficulty and chances of success

Organization: Planning of behavior and choice of actions
  A. Identification of goals and subgoals
  B. Global planning
  C. Local planning (to implement global goals)

Execution: Regulation of behavior to conform to plans
  A. Performance of local actions
  B. Monitoring of progress of local and global plans
  C. Trade-off decisions (e.g., speed vs. accuracy, degree of elegance)

Verification: Evaluation of decisions made and outcomes of executed plans
  A. Evalution of orientation and organization
     1. Adequacy of representation
     2. Adequacy of organizational decisions
     3. Consistency of local plans with global plans
     4. Consistency of global plans with goals

  B. Adequacy of performance of execution
     1. Adequacy of performance of actions
     2. Consistency of actions with plans
     3. Consistency of local results with plans and problem conditions
     4. Consistency of final results with problem conditions

---

[a]Based on the work of Lester et al. (1989).

lems posed in real-world contexts into mathematical expressions. Three kinds of nonroutine tasks were administered: problems with superfluous information, problems with insufficient information, and process problems. To solve this latter category of tasks, the problem solver needs to do something more than just translate text in a mathematical expression, apply an algorithm, or perform computations. Illustrative of this category of nonroutine problems is the following: "A caravan is stranded in the desert with a 6-day walk back to civilization. Each person in the caravan can carry a 4-day supply of food and water. A single person cannot carry enough food and water and would die. How many people must start out so that one person can get help and the others can get back to the caravan safely?" The different types of tasks were included because each kind seemed especially suited to exemplify the need for and provide practice with particular aspects of the described cognitive/metacognitive framework.

Instruction focused on solving problems in small groups, in combination with whole-class discussions, and individual assignments. During these classroom activities, the teacher had to fulfill three different, but closely related roles: (1) serve as external monitor during problem solving, (2) encourage discussion of behavior considered important for the internalization of the heuristic and cognitive regulation skills, and (3) model good executive behavior. As a more specific guideline for the teacher, a set of 10 teaching actions before, during, and after the problem-solving activity was provided, together with their purposes. Examples of these actions are the following:

— Before: Use a whole-class discussion about understanding the problem.
— During: Observe and question students to determine where they are in the problem-solving process.
— After: Relate the problem to previously solved problems and discuss or have students solve extensions of the problem.

During the intervention, a chart with problem-solving tips was presented (see Table 3) for use by the teacher and the pupils. These tips reflect in a very specific manner the major aspects of the cognitive regulation strategy.

It is obvious that the instructional model underlying Lester et al.'s learning environment shares major characteristics with the approach of Schoenfeld, especially the use of modeling good problem-solving behavior and stimulation of small-group and whole-class discussion focusing on articulation and evaluation of problem-solving processes and activities.

The instructional program was realized by one of the investigators with a regular-level and an advanced-level seventh-grade class during about 15 hours spread over 12 weeks. Before, during, and after the instruction,

TABLE 3 Problem Solving Tips[a]

Understanding the problem
  A. Read the problem carefully; often you should read it two or more times.
  B. Be sure you understand what the question is asking; ask yourself: "Do I understand what I am trying to find?"
  C. If you are not sure you understand the problem, draw a picture or a diagram of the information.
  D. Write down all the important information and the question; these are called *what I know* and *what I want to find*.

Solving the problem
  A. Explore the problem to get a good "feel" for what the problem is about.
  B. Do not do anything hard until you have tried easy ideas first; if easy things do not help, then you may need to do something more complicated.
  C. When you do not have any idea of what to do, try to make a good *guess* and then *check* it out with the important data.
  D. Use the *strategies* that you have learned; for example,

| Draw a picture | Guess and check | Look for a pattern |
| Make a table | Work backwards | Simplify the problem |

Getting an answer and evaluating it
  A. Be sure to check your work *along the way*, not just at the end; you may be able to avoid some unneccesary work by finding a mistake early.
  B. Be sure that you used all the important information.
  C. Write your answer in a complete sentence; this makes it easier to decide if the answer is reasonable.
  D. Ask yourself, "Does my answer *make sense*?"

[a] Based on the work of Lester et al. (1989).

Lester et al. (1989) employed a large set of assessment instruments, including written tests, clinical interviews, observations of individual and pair problem-solving sessions, and videotapes of classroom instruction.

The results on the written pretest and posttest, involving a set of new routine and nonroutine word problems, revealed positive effects of the learning environment on pupils' problem-solving skills. Both the regular class and the advanced class realized a considerable overall gain in total score from pretest to posttest, albeit the progress was not as great as expected. Interestingly, large individual differences were observed: although the scores of most pupils in both classes increased from pretest to posttest, the scores of a significant number of pupils remained the same or even decreased.

The results of the individual interviews before and after instruction revealed that among the four categories of activities in the cognitive regulation strategy, orientation, which refers to different types of strategic behavior to assess and understand a problem (see Table 2), had the most important effect on students' problem solving. However, no substantial differences were observed in this respect between pupils' regulatory activities before and after instruction. One explanation for this lack of effect of the learning environment is that the total time of the intervention was not long enough to produce significant changes. Moreover, problem-solving instruction was alternated with regular mathematics teaching, which reinforced pupils' "non-self-regulatory old habits" and may have been perceived as more important. Finally, the learning environment may not have been implemented with a high degree of fidelity. With regard to this latter explanation, several observations of the lessons revealed some weaknesses of the instruction and suggest, at the same time, possible improvements. First, the teachers experienced serious trouble maintaining their role of model, facilitator, and monitor in the face of classroom reality, especially when pupils had difficulties with basic aspects of the subject matter. Second, the overall quality of the thinking and the interaction in the small groups was not as high as expected.

C. THE JASPER PROJECT: ANCHORED INSTRUCTION OF MATHEMATICAL PROBLEM SOLVING

Anchored instruction has been developed by the Cognition and Technology Group at Vanderbilt (CTGV, 1997) in response to a problem observed in many students that reflects a lack of self-regulation, namely, the phenomenon of inert knowledge; that is, knowledge that is available in students' minds and can be recalled on request, but is not spontaneously accessed or applied in situations where it is relevant to solve new problems. The CTGV (1997; see also Van Haneghan et al., 1992) argued that classroom practices themselves are largely responsible for imparting inert knowledge to students. For instance, word problem solving in school typically consists of choosing the arithmetic operation to figure out the single correct answer to a mostly stereotyped and artificial problem statement. This contrasts sharply with what is going on in the real world, in which posing and defining problems—involving such cognitive regulatory activities as sense making, goal setting, planning, and decision making—are of major importance, whereas arithmetic operations serve mainly as tools to carry out a plan or to achieve a goal put forward by the problem solver. Anchored instruction has been designed as an attempt to support the acquisition of useful knowledge and skills by helping students "develop a sense of agency that allows them to identify and define problems and systematically explore solutions" (CTGV, 1997, p. 37). In other words, anchored instruction aims to foster students' self-regulation skills.

With this goal in mind, and applying videodisc technology, the starting point of anchored instruction has been the creation of rich, authentic, and interesting problem-solving contexts that can serve as the basis for the design of generative learning environments that offer students ample opportunities for self-regulated activities such as problem posing, exploration, and discovery. Although the Vanderbilt group stressed that the application of anchored instruction does not necessarily require the use of technology, they nevertheless prefer to situate instruction in video-based anchors, because the medium allows a richer, more realistic, and more dynamic presentation of information than textual material. As such, a technology-based implementation of anchored instruction makes the learning environment more powerful (Bransford, Sherwood, Hasselbring, Kinzer, & Williams, 1990). Accordingly, the Vanderbilt group has developed videodisc-based complex problem spaces that enable learners to explore and model a problem space involving mathematical problems for extended periods of time and from a diversity of perspectives; the problem spaces offer opportunities for cooperative learning and discussion in small groups, as well as for individual and whole-class problem solving. However, these videodisc-based problem spaces are only one of the components that they believe to be important. Other crucial aspects include (1) the guidance provided by an expert teacher, who organizes and designs the learning experiences, who stimulates cooperative learning and small-group as well as whole-class discussion, and who explicitly addresses the culture of the classroom, and (2) the availability to children of rich and realistic sources of information (CTGV, 1997).

The series of 12 videodiscs for mathematics instruction in the upper primary school, called *The Adventures of Jasper Woodbury*, has already become rather well known (for a description, see CTGV, 1997). In the initial videodisc of this series, called "Journey to Cedar Creek," a person named Jasper Woodbury takes a river trip to see an old cabin cruiser he is considering purchasing. Jasper and the cruiser's owner test-run the cruiser, after which Jasper decides to purchase the boat. Because the boat's running lights are inoperative, Jasper must determine if he can get the boat to his home dock before sunset. Two major questions that form the basis of Jasper's decision are presented at the end of the disc: (1) Does Jasper have enough time to return home before sunset? and (2) Is there enough fuel in the boat's gas tank for the return trip? It is obvious that these types of problems are much more authentic and realistic than the typical traditional classroom tasks, and those used in most previous investigations like the one by Lester et al. (1989) discussed above.

Underlying the Jasper series are the following seven interrelated design principles, derived from previous research and chosen because they facilitate the elicitation of specific kinds of problem-solving activities in pupils (CTGV, 1997; Van Haneghan et al., 1992).

1. Video-based presentation format: In addition to allowing a richer and more realistic presentation of information than text, the video-based format also has some advantages over real-life contexts, simply

because the latter are not always practical, efficient, and well structured, and they are often difficult to organize in a school situation.

2. Narrative format with realistic problems: The presentation of the problem in the form of a story helps pupils create a meaningful context.

3. Generative structure: By having the students themselves generate the resolution of the story, their active involvement in the learning process is stimulated.

4. Embedded data design: By having all the information needed to solve the problem embedded in the story, students are enabled to take part in problem identification, problem formation, and pattern recognition activities that traditional word problem solving does not allow.

5. Problem complexity: The problems are intentionally made complex —sometimes involving up to 15 steps—so that students learn to deal with complexity that is typical of real problems, but is mostly lacking in traditional curricula.

6. Pairs of related adventures: Triplets of related adventures provide extra practice, afford discussions about transfer, and promote analogical reasoning.

7. Links across the curriculum: Embedding information from other domains helps extend mathematical thinking to those areas and encourages the integration of knowledge.

It is obvious that these design principles contribute to creating realistic and motivating learning sites that have the potential to evoke self-regulatory activities in pupils. For instance, the generative format of the Jasper adventures means that the stories end and that the student themselves must generate the problems to be solved, which solicits strategic behavior to assess and understand a story, and planning behavior and choice of actions, respectively, called orientation and organization in the cognitive self-regulation strategy of Lester et al. (1989) (see Table 2 herein). Similar self-generated thoughts and actions are elicited by the fact that the stories and the problems are complex, that all the data needed are embedded, and that related adventures are provided.

Initial studies with the Jasper series have produced encouraging results (CTGV, 1993; Van Haneghan et al., 1992). A baseline study revealed that sixth graders who were high-achievers in mathematics were very poor in their approach to complex application problems of the kind used in the Jasper series without instruction and mediation. According to the investigators this was not too surprising, because pupils rarely have the opportunity to engage in such complex problem solving. However, a subsequent controlled teaching experiment showed that videodisc-based anchored instruction can substantially improve pupils' problem-solving processes and skills. Participants belonged to a fifth-grade class of above-average students. The first day of the experiment, the Jasper video was shown to all pupils and then they were pretested. After pretesting, pupils were assigned either to an experimental or a control group. Both groups received three additional teaching sessions. During these sessions the experimental group engaged in problem analysis, problem detection, and solution planning with respect to Jasper's trip-planning decisions, thereby intensively relying on videodisc/computer technology controlled by the instructor. In the control group, the usual teaching methods were applied to instruct students in solving traditional one- and two-step word problems that involved the same concepts as the Jasper adventure. Following instruction, pupils received two posttests—one consisting of traditional word problems and one about organizing information in the Jasper video for problem solving —and a transfer test that assessed pupils' abilities to identify, define, and solve problems presented on video similar to those posed in the Jasper series. This individually administered transfer test especially constitutes an indicator of children's cognitive self-regulation skills. The results of the study can be summarized as follows. On the traditional problems of the first posttest, the experimental pupils performed as well as the control students. In contrast to the control group, the experimental group showed significant gains from pretest to the second posttest. Most important in this context, however, are the results on the transfer test. The analysis of thinking aloud interview protocols relating to children's problem solving on video near-transfer problems showed significant transfer in the experimental group, but not in the control groups. Whereas the control children were generally unsuccessful in formulating and solving the transfer problems, the experimental pupils demonstrated great strength in identifying, stating, and solving the distance–rate–time and fuel problems embedded in the video.

Additional studies over the past 5 years have confirmed the initial positive results of anchored instruction based on the Jasper series and extended them to less skilled pupils (CTGV, 1997). For instance, a series of investigations that compared the learning and transfer outcomes of students who worked with the Jasper series with others who were taught the same concepts in the context of traditional one- and two-step word problems showed that Jasper pupils acquired a much higher ability to transfer their knowledge and skills to new, unfamiliar, and complex problems. In other words, Jasper-based learning fosters children's skills in self-regulating their problem-solving activities. Meanwhile, the results of a dissemination project in which Jasper-based anchored instruction was implemented in schools in Tennessee and nine surrounding states provided evidence that pupils not only perform better on measures of complex problem solving and attitudes to mathematics, but also on traditional standardized mathematics achievement tests. Finally, in more recent work, the Cognition and Technology Group at Vanderbilt has redesigned the Jasper series by supplementing the different adventures with analog and extension problems. It has been demonstrated already that working with these analog and extension tasks has a substantial positive impact on pupils' understanding and on their abilities to self-regulate their solution processes with respect to new, unfamiliar problem situations (Schwartz, Goldman, Vye, Barron, & the CTGV, in press).

Although the terminology that is currently in vogue in the mainstream of research on self-regulated learning is not so explicitly used in the work and writings of the Cognition and Technology Group at Vanderbilt, it is nevertheless obvious that their Jasper Project is a very advanced attempt to fundamentally change mathematical instructional practices in the direction of fostering students' self-regulation of their learning, thinking, and problem-solving processes.

D. A POWERFUL LEARNING ENVIRONMENT FOR SKILLED REALISTIC MATHEMATICAL PROBLEM SOLVING IN THE UPPER ELEMENTARY SCHOOL

Taking into account the results and conclusions of the previous design studies, as well as the findings of a teaching experiment in their own center (Verschaffel & De Corte, 1997), Verschaffel (1999) developed a learning environment for skilled realistic mathematical problem solving in upper elementary-school children. Contrary to those earlier investigations, the Verschaffel et al. (1999) learning environment was realized and tested in a typical classroom context, rather than in a somewhat exceptional instructional setting wherein the teaching was done by a researcher and/or wherein advanced computer and video technology was brought into the school. As such, this study has a still higher degree of ecological validity than the preceding ones and, therefore, documents the practical relevance and utility of the underlying research-based ideas about the central role of heuristics and cognitive self-regulation in mathematical learning and problem solving.

The aims of the Verschaffel et al. (1999) learning environment are twofold. The first aim is the acquisition of an overall cognitive self-regulatory strategy for solving mathematics application problems consisting of five stages and involving a set of eight heuristic strategies that are especially useful in the first two stages of that strategy (see Table 4). It is obvious that the five stages of this strategy for cognitive self-regulation parallel the models proposed by Schoenfeld (1985) and by Lester et al. (1989) already presented.

The second aim is the acquisition of a set of appropriate beliefs and positive attitudes with regard to mathematical problem solving, as well as

TABLE 4   The Competent Problem-Solving Model Underlying the
Learning Environment

Step 1: Build a mental representation of the problem
   Heuristics: Draw a picture
               Make a list, a scheme, or a table
               Distinguish relevant from irrelevant data
               Use your real-world knowledge

Step 2: Decide how to solve the problem
   Heuristics: Make a flowchart
               Guess and check
               Look for a pattern
               Simplify the numbers

Step 3: Execute the necessary calculations

Step 4: Interpret the outcome and formulate an answer

Step 5: Evaluate the solution

---

proper beliefs about the processes of teaching and learning it (e.g., "Mathematics problems may have more than one correct answer" or "Solving a mathematics problem may be effortful and take more than just a few minutes").

The main features of the learning environment are the following:

1. A varied set of carefully designed complex, realistic, and challenging word problems that ask for the application of the intended heuristics and self-regulatory skills that constitute the model of skilled problem solving. As an illustration of the kind of problems used in the learning environments, two examples are given in the Figures 4 and 5.

2. A series of lesson plans based on a variety of teacher and learner activities. Each new component of the metacognitive strategy is initially modeled by the teacher. Furthermore, a lesson consists of a sequence of small-group problem-solving activities or individual assignments, always followed by a whole-class discussion. During all these activities the teacher's role is to encourage and scaffold pupils to engage in and to reflect upon the kinds of cognitive and metacognitive activities involved in the model of competent mathematical problem solving. These encouragements and scaffolds are gradually withdrawn as the pupils become more competent and take more responsibility for their own learning and problem solving. In other words, external regulation is phased out as pupils become more self-regulated learners and problem solvers.

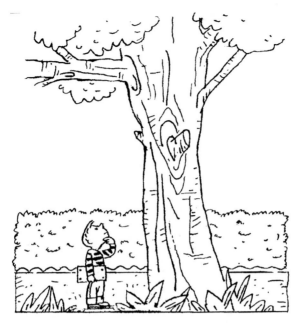

FIGURE 4 Example of a word problem used in the lesson about the heuristics "Use your real-world knowledge" (Step 1): Wim would like to attach to a branch of a big old tree. The branch has a height of 5 meters. Wim already has made a suitable wooden shelf for his swing; Now Wim is going to buy some rope. How many meters of rope will Wim have to buy?

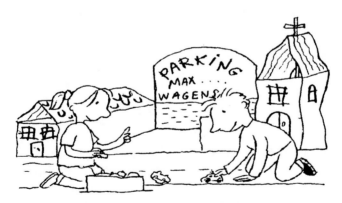

FIGURE 5 Example of a problem used in one of the project lessons: Pete and Annie are building a miniature town with cardboard. The space between the church and the town hall seems to be the perfect location for a big parking lot. The available space has the format of a square with a side of 50 cm and is surrounded by walls except for its street side. Pete already has made a cardboard square of the appropriate size. What will be the maximum capacity of their parking lot? 1. Fill in the maximum capacity of the parking lot on the banner. 2. Draw on the cardboard square how you can best divide the parking lot into parking spaces. 3. Explain how you came to your plan for the parking lot.

3. Interventions explicitly aimed at the establishment of new sociomathematical norms, resulting in a classroom climate that is conducive to the development in pupils of appropriate beliefs about mathematics and mathematics learning and teaching, and, by extension, to pupils' self-regulation of their learning. These norms relate to the role of the teacher and the pupils in the classroom (e.g., not the teacher on his or her own, but the whole class will decide which of the different learner-generated solutions is optimal after an evaluation of the pros and cons of the distinct alternatives), and about what counts as a good mathematical problem, a good solution procedure, or a good response (e.g., sometimes a rough estimate is a better answer than an exact number).

The learning environment consists of a series of 20 lessons designed by the research team in consultation and cooperation with the regular classroom teachers. Because the lessons were taught by the classroom teachers, they were prepared for and supported by implementing the powerful teaching–learning environment. With two lesson periods each week, the intervention was spread over about 3 months. Three major parts can be distinguished in the series of lessons:

1. Introduction to the content and organization of the learning environment and reflection upon the difference between a routine task and a real problem (1 lesson);
2. Systematic acquisition of the five-step regulatory problem-solving strategy and the embedded heuristics (15 lessons);
3. Learning to use the competent problem-solving model in a spontaneous and flexible way in so-called project lessons that involve more complex application problems (4 lessons).

The effectiveness of the learning environment to enhance active and self-regulated problem-solving in pupils was evaluated in a study with a pretest–posttest–retention test design. Four experimental fifth-grade classes and 7 comparable control classes from 11 different elementary schools in Flanders participated in the study. Three pretests were collectively administered in the experimental as well as the control classes: (1) a standardized achievement test (SAT) to assess fifth graders' general mathematical knowledge and skills, (2) a pretest consisting of 10 nonroutine word problems (WPT), and (3) a questionnaire aimed at assessing pupils' beliefs about and attitudes toward (teaching and learning) mathematical word problem solving (BAQ). Also, pupils' WPT answer sheets for each problem were analyzed carefully, looking for evidence of the application of one or more of the heuristics embedded in the problem-solving strategy. Also these collective pretests, three pairs of pupils of equal ability from each experimental class were asked to solve five nonroutine application problems during a structured interview. The problem-solving processes of these dyads were video-registered, and afterward analyzed by means of a self-made schema for assessing the intensity and the quality of pupils' cognitive self-regulation activities. While the intervention took place in the experimental classes, the control classes followed the regular math program. By the end of the intervention, parallel versions of all collective pretests (SAT, WPT, and BAQ) were administered in all experimental and control classes. The answer sheets of all pupils were scrutinized again for traces of the application of heuristics, and the same pairs of pupils from the experimental classes as prior to the intervention were subjected again to a structured interview that involved parallel versions of the five nonroutine application problems used during the pretest. Major expectations were that as a result of acquiring the self-regulatory problem-solving strategy, the experimental pupils would significantly outperform the control children on the WPT, and that this would be accompanied by a significant increase in the use of heuristics; furthermore it was anticipated that the frequency and the quality of the self-regulation activities in the dyads would substantially grow. Three months later a retention test—a parallel version of the collective WPT used as pretest and posttest—was also administered in all experimental and control classes. To assess the implementation of the learning environment by the teachers of the experimental classes, a sample of four representative lessons was videotaped in each experimental class and analyzed afterward to get a so-called implementation profile for each experimental teacher.

The results of this study can be summarized as follows. First, although no significant difference was found between the experimental and control groups on the WPT during the pretest, the former significantly outperformed the latter during the posttest, and this difference in favor of the experimental group continued to exist on the retention test. However, it should be acknowledged that in the experimental group, pupils' overall performance on the posttest and retention tests was not as high as anticipated (i.e., the pupils of the experimental classes still produced only about 50% correct answers on these tests). Second, in the experimental group there was a significant improvement in pupils' beliefs about and attitudes toward (learning and teaching) mathematical problem solving, while in the control group there was no change in pupils' reactions to the BAQ from pretest to posttest. Third, although there was no difference between the pretest results on the SAT between the experimental and the control group, the results on the posttest revealed a significant difference in favor of the former group, indicating some transfer effect of the intervention toward mathematics as a whole. Fourth, a qualitative analysis of the pupils' response sheets for the WPT revealed a dramatic increase from pretest to posttest and retention test in the manifest use of (some of) the heuristics that were specifically addressed and discussed in the learning environment; in the control classes there was no difference in pupils' use of heuristics between the three testing moments. In line with this result, the videotapes of the problem-solving processes of the dyads revealed substantial improvement in the intensity and the quality with which the pairs from the experimental classes applied certain—but not all—(meta) cognitive skills that were specifically addressed in the learning environment. Both findings are indicative of a substantial increase in pupils' ability to self-regulate their problem-solving processes. Fifth, although there is some evidence that pupils of high and medium ability benefited more from the intervention than low-ability pupils, the statistical analysis revealed at the same time that all three ability groups contributed significantly to all the abovementioned positive effects in the experimental group. This is a very important outcome, because it suggests that through appropriate intervention, the cognitive self-regulatory skills of the weaker children can be improved also. Finally, the positive effects of the learning environment were not observed to the same extent in all four experimental classes. Actually, in one of the four classes there was little or no improvement on most of the process and product measures. Analysis of the videotapes of the lessons in these classes indicated substantial differences in the extent to which the four experimental teachers succeeded in implementing the major aspects of the learning environment. For three of the four experimental classes, there was a good fit between the teachers' implementation profiles, on the one hand, and their pupils' learning outcomes, on the other hand.

In this intervention study a set of carefully designed application problems, a varied series of highly interactive teaching methods, and an attempt to change the sociomathematical classroom norms were combined in an attempt to create a powerful learning environment that focuses on the development of a mindful and self-regulated cognitive approach toward mathematical modeling and problem solving. The findings indicate that this intervention can have significant positive effects on different aspects of pupils' mathematical modeling ability, on their cognitive self-regulation of and performance in problem solving, and on their beliefs about (learning and teaching) mathematics. However, as already mentioned, the effects were not as strong as expected; therefore, the results warrant less optimistic conclusions with respect to the possibility of changing and improving educational practice easily and quickly.

E. LOOKING BACK TO THE FOUR DESIGN EXPERIMENTS

All four design experiments have reported positive outcomes—albeit in different degrees—in terms of students' performance. It is now interesting to ask in retrospect explicitly to what degree there are similarities among the four projects with respect to the aspects of self-regulation they have addressed and with regard to the instructional models underlying the learning environments.

Concerning the first issue, it was mentioned at the outset of this section that the design experiments focus mainly on students' cognitive self-regulation. In three out of the four interventions, acquiring cognitive self-regulation was elaborated in terms of learning an overall metacognitive strategy consisting of a four- to five-step systematic approach to problem solving. It already has been mentioned that these strategies of Schoenfeld (1985), Lester et al. (1989), and Verschaffel et al. (in press) are very similar. Looking back at the results and contrasting the strategies with what happens in traditional mathematics classrooms, it seems to us that—without underestimating the significance of the strategy as a whole —the crucial self-regulatory components in the three approaches are the first steps. Although different terms are used in the three intervention studies, the regulatory activities of problem solving in the first two stages come more or less to the same thing, namely, strategic behavior aimed at understanding the problem by constructing a good representation of what it is about, and, thereafter, designing or making a solution plan that involves the use of cognitive strategies such as heuristics. For instance, in the study by Verschaffel et al., we have seen that after the intervention the spontaneous, self-regulated use of the heuristics taught in the first and second stage of the overall metacognitive strategy increased significantly in the experimental pupils. In accordance with this observation, Lester and his colleagues reported that orientation, the first phase of their strategy, had the most important effect on pupils' problem solving. The work of Schoenfeld has shown that in his learning environment students' problem-solving approach becomes more expertlike; as shown in Section III.A of this chapter, the major differences between novices and experts relate precisely to analysis of the problem and to solution planning. The Jasper project does not use a cognitive regulation strategy similar to the three other investigations. However, in their learning environment, the Vander-bilt group stresses precisely the same two cognitive self-regulatory skills when they argue that pupils "should develop a sense of agency that allows them to identify and define problems and systematically explore solutions" (CTGV, 1997, p. 44). With respect to the first aspect—problem analysis and understanding—they even go a step further by accentuating the importance of problem generating, and they heavily stress "the importance of helping students learn to plan, a process that involves generating subgoals necessary to solve complex problems." (CTGV, 1997, p. 65)

The instructional models that underlie the learning environment of the four projects also share major components. In fact, the three main charac-teristics of the learning environment developed by Verschaffel et al. are also largely reflected in the other interventions:

- Except for Schoenfeld's project, the other three use more realistic and challenging tasks than the traditional textbook word problems (the fact that this feature is less prominent in Schoenfeld's study probably has to do with the fact that he focuses on the teaching of geometry at the college level).
- All four projects apply a comparable variety of teaching methods and learner activities, including modeling of strategic aspects of problem solving by the teacher, guided practice with coaching and feedback, problem solving in small groups, and whole-class discussion focusing on evaluation and reflection concerning alternative solutions as well as different solution strategies. It is important in view of fostering cognitive self-regulation that in all interventions, external regulation is progressively withdrawn as students' competence increases.
- Finally, and related to the previous characteristic, all interventions create a classroom climate that is conducive to the development in pupils of appropriate beliefs about mathematics and mathematics learning and problem solving, and to active, self-regulated learning and problem solving.

As mentioned in the introductory paragraph of this section, Schunk (1998) has carried out a series of intervention studies that are more experimental in character than the four projects reported. It is nevertheless interesting to compare his instructional model with the learning environments of those four design experiments. The basic features of Schunk's (1998) intervention are modeled demonstrations, guided practice, self-regulatory training (e.g., goal setting, strategy use), and independent/self-reflective practice. Although these aspects are very convergent with the design experiments, there are apparently a number of important differences. First, whereas in Schunk's interventions the organization of self-regulatory activities happened in the context of learning basic arithmetic skills (e.g., subtraction, division, fractions, ...), the major objective of the four abovementioned design experiments was to enhance the development of a set of cognitive and self-regulatory skills for complex problem solving. In the second place, Schunk's (1998) interventions were implemented in a context "similar to that in which much mathematics instruction takes place in American elementary schools" (p.144). This seems to imply that traditional mathematics tasks and problems were used in an also traditional classroom context and climate. With regard to the teaching methods used in Schunk's intervention program, no mention is made of small-group work, which is a major component in all four design experiments described. It seems to us that for future researchers who undertake intervention studies within the framework of a specific theoretical approach to self-regulation it might be useful to cooperate with scholars who set up more comprehensive design experiments.

V. CONCLUSIONS AND FUTURE DIRECTIONS FOR RESEARCH

In this chapter we have elucidated the importance and centrality of self-regulation in the context of the prevailing new conception of school mathematics, namely, as a major objective of mathematics education, on the one hand, and as a crucial characteristic of effective mathematics learning, on the other. However, this importance contrasts sharply with the many observations that demonstrate that students of different ages show serious shortcomings in the various self-regulatory aspects of a mathematical disposition, more specifically, in their metacognitive and metavolitional skills. In addition, they are affected by naive and incorrect beliefs about mathematics, mathematics learning, and problem solving that are not conducive to the development of self-regulation skills. In the preceding section we presented evidence that these weaknesses should not necessarily occur and develop in students, and, if they do, that they probably can be remedied. Indeed, a series of design experiments, in which new, research-based learning environments were implemented in real classrooms, indicate that such interventions can have significant favorable effects on students' cognitive self-regulation skills as well as on their mathematics-related beliefs. A comparison of the instructional models that underlie the interventions in those experiments led us to the identification of a rather coherent set of principles for the design of powerful learning environments. These principles relate to the nature of the tasks and problems presented to the pupils, the kinds of powerful instructional activities embedded in the learning environment, and the sociomathematical norms that determine the classroom culture and climate.

Notwithstanding the latter positive conclusion, major questions for continued research remain. First of all, this chapter illustrates that some aspects of self-regulated mathematics learning have so far not, or at least not sufficiently, been addressed. This is especially the case for the metavolitional skills, but also for the beliefs about oneself as a mathematics learner, which have an important impact on the development of pupils' self-regulation. However, even those aspects that have been studied are in need of further inquiry aimed at a better understanding of the most crucial processes involved in regulating learning and problem solving effectively and at tracing the development of regulatory processes in children and young adults. For instance, by comparison, we were able to identify major self-regulatory components in the overall metacognitive strategies used in three design experiments. However, future research is needed to further unravel the skills and processes involved in regulating problem understanding and solution planning. In this respect, Zimmerman (1994) has argued rightly that the explanatory power of the construct of self-regulation is still rather restricted, that many of the self-regulatory processes that have been proposed, such as cognitive self-monitoring, are subtle and covert, and that major constructs that relate to self-regulation are conceptually overlapping.

The fact that a number of intervention studies have been carried out with respect to mathematics meets a recommendation that was made in the literature (Schunk & Zimmerman, 1994). These investigations show convincingly that by immersing students in a new, powerful learning environment, it is possible to foster their cognitive self-regulation skills. We even were able to identify a set of common components in those environments that relate to the nature of the problems, the instructional activities, and the classroom culture. However, the holistic design and implementation of these complex learning environments do not allow us to trace the relative significance of the different components in accounting for the observed positive effects. Therefore, there is also a strong need for studies that are intent on unravelling how and under what specific instructional conditions students become self-regulated learners in a more precise way. What are the crucial elements in the learning environment that help and support students in learning to manage and monitor their own processes of knowledge building and skill acquisition? In other words, how can the transition from external to self-regulation most effectively be enhanced? Also relative to this issue is the important question concerning the interaction between domain-specific knowledge and competence, on the one hand, and self-regulation, on the other: Does (successful) regulation of mathematics learning and problem solving require a certain level of mathematical competence? (Alexander, 1995).

REFERENCES

Alexander, P. A. (1995). Superimposing a situation-specific and domain-specific perspective on an account of self-regulated learning. *Educational Psychologist, 30*, 189–193.

Ames, C., & Archer, J. (1988). Achievement goals in the classroom: Students' learning strategies and motivation processes. *Journal of Educational Psychology, 80*, 260–267.

Berry, J., & Sahlberg, P. (1996). Investigating pupils' ideas of learning. *Learning and Instruction, 6*, 19–36.

Bishop, A. J., Clements, K., Keitel, C., Kilpatrick, J., & Laborde, C. (Eds.). (1996). *International handbook of mathematics education: Part 1 & 2*. Dordrecht, The Netherlands: Kluwer.

Boekaerts, M. (1987). Situation specific judgments of a learning task versus overall measures of motivational orientation. In E. De Corte, H. Lodewijks, R. Parmentier, & P. Span (Eds.), *Learning and instruction* (pp. 169–179). Oxford/Leuven: Pergamon Press/Leuven University Press.

Boekaerts, M. (1992). The adaptable learning process: Initiating and maintaining behavioural change. *Applied Psychology: An International Review*, *41*, 377–397.

Boekaerts, M. (1994). Action control: How relevant is it for classroom learning? In J. Kuhl & J. Beckmann (Eds.), *Volition and personality: Action versus state orientation* (pp. 427–435). Seattle, WA: Hogrefe & Huber.

Boekaerts, M. (1997). Self-regulated learning: A new concept embraced by researchers, policy makers, educators, teachers, and students. *Learning and Instruction*, *7*, 161–186.

Bransford, J. D., Sherwood, R. S., Hasselbring, T. S., Kinzer, C. K., & Williams, S. M. (1990). Anchored instruction: Why we need it and how technology can help. In D. Nix & R. Spiro (Eds.), *Cognition, education, and multimedia. Exploring ideas in high technology* (pp. 115–141). Hillsdale, NJ: Erlbaum.

Cockroft, W. H. (1982). *Mathematic counts*. (Report of the Committee of Inquiry into the Teaching of Mathematics in Schools). London: H. M. Stationery Office.

Cognition and Technology Group at Vanderbilt. (1993). Anchored instruction and situated cognition revisited. *Educational Technology*, *33*(3), 52–70.

Cognition and Technology Group at Vanderbilt. (1996). Looking at technology in context: A framework for understanding technology and education research. In D. C. Berliner & R. C. Calfee (Eds.), *Handbook of educational psychology* (pp. 807–840). New York: Macmillan.

Cognition and Technology Group at Vanderbilt. (1997). *The Jasper Project. Lessons in curriculum, instruction, assessment, and professional development*. Mahwah, NJ: Erlbaum.

Collins, A., Brown, J. S., & Newman, S. E. (1989). Cognitive apprenticeship: Teaching the craft of reading, writing and mathematics. In L. B. Resnick (Ed.), *Knowing, learning and instruction. Essays in honor of Robert Glaser* (pp. 453–494). Hillsdale, NJ: Erlbaum.

De Corte, E. (1995a). Fostering cognitive development: A perspective from research on mathematics learning and instruction. *Educational Psychologist*, *30*, 37–46.

De Corte, E. (1995b). Learning theory and instructional science. In P. Reiman & H. Spada (Eds.), *Learning in humans and machines. Towards an interdisciplinary learning science* (pp. 97–108). Oxford, UK: Elsevier Science Ltd.

De Corte, E., Greer, B., & Verschaffel, L. (1996). Mathematics teaching and learning. In D. C. Berliner & R. C. Calfee (Eds.), *Handbook of educational psychology* (pp. 491–549). New York: Macmillan.

De Corte, E., & Somers, R. (1982). Estimating the outcome of a task as a heuristic strategy in arithmetic problem solving: A teaching experiment with sixth graders. *Human Learning: A Journal of Practical Research and Applications*, *1*, 105–121.

De Corte, E., Verschaffel, L., Lasure, S., Borghart, I., & Yoshida, H. (1999). Real-world knowledge and mathematical problem solving in upper primary school children. In J. Bliss, R. Säljö, & P. Light (Eds.), *Learning sites: Social and technological contexts for learning*. Oxford, UK: Elsevier Science Ltd.

Fennema, E. (1989). The study of affect and mathematics: A proposed generic model for research. In D. B. McLeod & V. M. Adams (Eds.), *Affect and mathematical problem solving: A new perspective* (pp. 205–219). New York: Springer-Verlag.

Glaser, R., & Silver, E. (1994). Assessment, testing, and instruction. In L. Darling-Hammond (Ed.), *Review of research in education* Vol. 20, (pp. 393–419). Washington, DC: American Educational Research Association.

Greeno, J. G., (1991). A view of mathematical problem solving in school. In M. U. Smith (Ed.), *Toward a unified theory of problem solving. Views from the content domains* (pp. 69–98). Hillsdale, NJ: Erlbaum.

Greeno, J. G., Collins A. M., & Resnick, L. B. (1996). Cognition and learning. In D. C. Berliner & R. C. Calfee (Eds.), *Handbook of educational psychology* (pp. 15–46). New York: Macmillan.

Greer, B. & Verschaffel, L. (Eds.). (1997). Modelling reality in mathematics classrooms [Special issue]. *Learning and Instruction, 7*, 293–397.

Grouws, D. A. (Ed.) (1992). *Handbook of research on mathematics teaching and learning.* New York: Macmillan.

Gurova, I. L., (1985). De reflectie op het eigen handelen tijdens het oplossen van rekenopgaven bij schoolkinderen [Reflection on one's own activity during the solution of arithmetic tasks]. In L. Verschaffel & M. Wolters (Eds.), *Zes Sovjetrussische bijdragen over vraagstukkenonderwijs en cognitieve ontwikkeling* [Six Soviet contributions about word problem instruction and cognitive development] (Internal Rep. No. 30, pp. 15–30). Leuven, Belgium: Katholieke Universiteit Leuven, Afdeling Didactiek.

Kloosterman, P. (1988). Self-confidence and motivation in mathematics. *Journal of Educational Psychology, 80*, 345–351.

Krutetskii, V. A. (1976). *The psychology of mathematical abilities in school children.* Chicago: University of Chicago Press.

Kuhl, J. (1994). A theory of action and state orientations. In J. Kuhl & J. Beckmann (Eds.), *Volition and personality: Action versus state orientation* (pp. 9–46). Seattle, WA: Hogrefe & Huber.

Kuhl, J., & Goschke, T. (1994). A theory of action control: Mental subsystems, modes of control, and volitional conflict-resolution strategies. In J. Kuhl & J. Beckmann (Eds.), *Volition and personality: Action versus state orientation* (pp. 93–124). Seattle, WA: Hogrefe & Huber.

Lampert, M. (1990). When the problem is not the question and the solution is not the answer: Mathematical knowing and teaching. *American Educational Research Journal, 27*, 29–63.

Lesh, R., & Lamon, S. J. (Eds.). (1992). *Assessment of authentic performance in school mathematics.* Washington, DC: American Association for the Advancement of Science.

Lester, F. K., & Garofalo, J. (1982). *Metacognitive aspects of elementary school students' performance on arithmetic tasks.* Paper presented at the annual meeting of the American Educational Research Association, New York.

Lester, F. K., Garofalo, J., & Kroll, D. L. (1989). *The role of metacognition in mathematical problem solving: A study of two grade seven classes* (Final report, NSF project MDR 85-50346). Bloomington: Indiana University, Mathematics Education Development Center.

Lester, F. K., Lambdin, D. V., & Preston, R. V. (1997). A new vision of the nature and purposes of assessment in the mathematics classroom. In G. D. Phye (Ed.), *Handbook of classroom assessment: Learning, adjustment, and achievement* (pp. 287–319). San Diego, CA: Academic Press.

McLeod, D. B. (1989). The role of affect in mathematical problem solving. In D. B. McLeod & V. M. Adams (Eds.), *Affect and mathematical problem solving: A new perspective* (pp. 20–36). New York: Springer-Verlag.

McLeod, D. B. (1992). Research on affect in mathematics education: A reconceptualization. In D. A. Grouws (Ed.), *Handbook of research on mathematics teaching and learning* (pp. 575–596). New York: MacMillan.

McLeod, D. B., Metzger, W., & Craviotto, C. (1989). Comparing experts' and novices' affective reactions to mathematical problem solving: An exploratory study. In G. Vergnaud (Ed.), *Proceedings of the Thirteenth International Conference for the Psychology of Mathematics Education* (Vol. 2, pp. 296–303). Paris: Laboratoire de Psychologie du Developpement et de l'Education de l'Enfant.

Messick, S. (1987). Structural relationships across cognition, personality and style. In R. E. Snow & J. F. Marshall (Eds.), *Aptitude, learning, and instruction Vol. 3: Conative and affective process analyses* (pp. 35–75). Hillsdale, NJ: Erlbaum.

National Council of Teachers of Mathematics (1989). *Curriculum and evaluation standards for school mathematics.* Reston, VA: National Council of Teachers of Mathematics.

Nelissen, J. M. C. (1987). *Kinderen leren wiskunde: Een studie over constructie en reflectie in het basisonderwijs* [Children learning mathematics: A study on construction and reflection in elementary school children]. Gorinchem, The Netherlands: Uitgeverij De Ruiter.

Nesher, P., & Kilpatrick, J. (Eds.). (1990). *Mathematics and cognition: A research synthesis by the International Group for the Psychology of Mathematics Education* (ICMI Study Series). Cambridge, UK: Cambridge University Press.

Nunes, T., & Bryant, P. (Eds.). (1997). *Learning and teaching mathematics: An international perspective*. Hove, UK: Psychology Press.

Nunes, T., Schliemann, A. D., & Carraher, D. W. (1993). *Street mathematics and school mathematics*. Cambridge, UK: Cambridge University Press.

Overtoom, R. (1991). *Informatieverwerking door hoogbegaafde leerlingen bij het oplossen van wiskundeproblemen* [Information processing by gifted sutdents in solving mathematical problems]. De Lier, The Netherlands: Academisch Boeken Centrum.

Perkins, D. (1995). *Outsmarting IQ. The emerging science of learnable intelligence*. New York: The Free Press.

Pintrich, P. R., Marx, R. W., & Boyle, R. A. (1993). Beyond cold conceptual change: The role of motivational beliefs and classroom contextual factors in the process of conceptual change. *Review of Educational Research, 63*, 167–199.

Pintrich, P. R., Wolters, C. A., & Baxter, G. P. (in press). Assessing metacognition and self-regulation. In G. Schraw (Ed.), *Metacognitive assessment*. Lincoln: University of Nebraska Press.

Romberg, T. A. (1992). Mathematics learning and teaching: What we have learned in ten years. In C. Collins & J. N. Mangieri (Eds.), *Teaching thinking: An agenda for the 21st century* (pp. 43–64). Hillsdale, NJ: Erlbaum.

Romberg, T. A. (Ed.). (1995). *Reform in school mathematics and authentic assessment*. Albany: State University of New York.

Schoenfeld, A. H. (1985). *Mathematical problem solving*. New York: Academic Press.

Schoenfeld, A. H. (1987). What's all the fuss about metacognition? In A. H. Schoenfeld (Ed.), *Cognitive science and mathematics education* (pp. 61–88). Hillsdale, NJ: Erlbaum.

Schoenfeld, A. H. (1988). When good teaching leads to bad results: The disasters of "well-taught" mathematics courses. *Educational Psychologist, 23*, 145–166.

Schoenfeld, A. H. (1992). Learning to think mathematically: Problem solving, metacognition, and sense-making in mathematics. In D. A. Grouws (Ed.), *Handbook of research on mathematics learning and teaching.* (pp. 334–370). New York: Macmillan.

Schunk, D. H. (1998). Teaching elementary students to self-regulate practice of mathematical skills with modeling. In D. H. Schunk & B. J. Zimmerman (Eds.), *Self-regulated learning: From teaching to self-reflective practice* (pp. 137–159). New York: Guilford.

Schunk, D. H., & Zimmerman, B. J. (1994). Self-regulation in education: Retrospect and prospect. In D. H. Schunk & B. J. Zimmerman (Eds.), *Self-regulation of learning and performance: Issues and educational applications* (pp. 305–314). Hillsdale, NJ: Erlbaum.

Schwartz, B. L., Goldman, S. R., Vye, N. J., Barron, B. J., & the Cognition and Technology Group at Vanderbilt. (in press). Using anchored instruction to align everyday and mathematical reasoning, The case of sampling assumption. In S. Lajoie (Ed.), *Reflections on statistics: Agendas for learning, teaching and assessment in K–12*. Hillsdale, NJ: Erlbaum.

Seegers, G., & Boekaerts, M. (1993). Task motivation and mathematics in actual task situations. *Learning and Instruction, 3*, 133–150.

Silver, E. A., Branca, N., & Adams, V. (1980). Metacognition: The missing link in problem solving. In R. Karplus (Ed.), *Proceedings of the Fourth International Congress of Mathematical Education* (pp. 429–433). Boston, MA: Birkhäuser.

Snow, R. E., Corno, L., & Jackson, D., III. (1996). Individual differences in affective and conative functions. In D. C. Berliner & R. C. Calfee (Eds.), *Handbook of Educational Psychology* (pp. 243–310). New York: Macmillan.

Steffe, L. P., Nesher, P., Cobb, P., Goldin, G. A., & Greer, B. (Eds.) (1996). *Theories of mathematical learning*. Mahwah, NJ: Erlbaum.

Terwilliger, J. (1997). Semantics, psychometrics, and assessment reform: A close look at "authentic" assessments. *Educational Researcher, 26*(8), 24–27.

Treffers, A., de Moor, E., & Feys, E. (1989). *Proeve van een nationaal programma voor het reken-wiskundeonderwijs op de basisschool. Deel 1. Overzicht einddoelen.* [Towards a national mathematics curriculum for the elementary school. Part 1. Overview of the general goals]. Tilburg The Netherlands: Zwijssen.

Van Haneghan, J., Barron, L., Young, M., Williams, S., Vye, N., & Bransford, J. (1992). The Jasper series: An experiment with new ways to enhance mathematical thinking. In D. F. Halpern (Ed.), *Enhancing thinking skills in the sciences and mathematics* (pp. 15–38). Hillsdale, NJ: Erlbaum.

Vermeer, H. J. (1997). *Sixth-grade students' mathematical problem-solving behavior: Motivational variables and gender differences.* Leiden: UFB, Leiden University.

Verschaffel, L., & De Corte, E. (1997). Teaching realistic mathematical modeling in the elementary school: A teaching experiment with fifth graders. *Journal of Research in Mathematics Education, 28,* 577–601.

Verschaffel, L., De Corte, E., & Lasure, S. (1994). Realistic considerations in mathematical modeling of school arithmetic word problems. *Learning and Instruction, 4,* 273–294.

Verschaffel, L., De Corte, E., Lasure, S., Van Vaerenbergh, G., Bogaerts, H., & Ratinckx, E. (1999). Learning to solve mathematical application problems: A design experiment with fifth graders. *Mathematical Learning and Thinking, 1*(3).

Zimmerman, B. J. (1989a). A social cognitive view of self-regulated academic learning. *Journal of Educational Psychology, 81,* 329–339.

Zimmerman, B. J. (1989b). Models of self-regulated learning and academic achievement. In B. J. Zimmerman & D. H. Schunk (Eds.), *Self-regulated learning and academic achievement: Theory, research, and practice* (pp. 1–25). New York: Springer-Verlag.

Zimmerman, B. J. (1994). Dimensions of academic self-regulation: A conceptual framework for education. In D. H. Schunk & B. J. Zimmerman (Eds.), *Self-regulation of learning and performance: Issues and educational applications* (pp. 3–21). Hillsdale, NJ: Erlbaum.

Zimmerman, B. J. (1995). Self-regulation involves more than metacognition: A social–cognitive perspective. *Educational Psychologist, 30,* 217–221.

Zimmerman, B. J., & Martinez-Pons, M. M. (1986). Development of a structured interview for assessing student use of self-regulated learning strategies. *American Educational Research Journal, 23,* 614–629.

Zimmerman, B. J., & Risemberg, R. (1997). Self-regulatory dimensions of academic learning and motivation. In G. D. Phye (Ed.), *Handbook of academic learning: Construction of knowledge* (pp. 105–125). San Diego, CA: Academic Press.

22

SELF-REGULATION INTERVENTIONS WITH A FOCUS ON LEARNING STRATEGIES

CLAIRE ELLEN WEINSTEIN,*
JENEFER HUSMAN,†
AND DOUGLAS R. DIERKING*

*University of Texas, Austin, Texas
†University of Alabama, Tuscaloosa, Alabama

Since ancient times we have tried to understand and harness our ability to identify, reflect upon, and take actions to control our own thoughts, feelings, emotions, actions, and destinies. This past quarter century has witnessed incredible progress in our understanding of diverse aspects of self-regulation. This book is a testament to our progress and many important aspects of self-regulation that have been identified and studied (e.g., motivational and cognitive management strategies), and many of the contexts in which it can be used (e.g., adult, mathematics, and reading education; effort management programs) are discussed. The purpose of this chapter is to address self-regulation in relation to the acquisition, use, and control of students' learning strategies. Learning strategies include any thoughts, behaviors, beliefs, or emotions that facilitate the acquisition, understanding, or later transfer of new knowledge and skills. We briefly describe a model of strategic learning that demonstrates the relationships among students' learning strategy knowledge, learning strategy skills, and self-regulation, as well as other variables that significantly impact learning and achievement. We also describe a sample of the interventions that have

Copyright © 2000 by Academic Press.
All rights of reproduction in any form reserved.

been developed to help college-level students become more strategic learners; highlighting a highly successful program developed at the University of Texas at Austin. We start with a historical overview of some of the research and development work that has focused specifically on understanding or modifying the acquisition, use, and control of learning strategies. This overview helps to explain how researchers have come to understand the self-regulatory processes involved in strategy use.

I. HISTORICAL OVERVIEW

In the early 1970s, the information processing model of cognition (Simon, 1979b) was proposed as a viable way to conceptualize cognitive processes and products. With the establishment of this model (or, perhaps more accurately, family of models), the cognitive revolution (see Simon, 1979a, for a review) was in full swing and the early battles were being fought. Within this new field of cognitive psychology, a consensus was growing among researchers that thoughts or mental processes could be studied and understood directly. This work led to an evolving focus on information processing research and models that emphasized that cognition was something that could be controlled through cognitive and metacognitive processes (Brown, Collins, & Duguid, 1989; Flavell, 1979; Garner, 1987; Pressley & McCormick, 1995), particularly in academic and training learning contexts (Wang, 1983; Weinstein, 1978).

II. LEARNING STRATEGIES CAN BE MODIFIED OR LEARNED

One of the first practical applications of these new information processing theories was in the area of memory strategies that could be used in educational settings (Wood, 1967). Research on mnemonics and advances in our understanding of associative networks (Wang, 1983; Weinstein, 1978) paved the way for researchers to investigate different types of training that could be used to improve students' paired-associate learning (e.g., Danner & Taylor, 1973). The model of what it meant to be a learner was shifting from viewing the learner as a passive receptacle for knowledge to the leaner as an active, self-determined individual who processes information in complex ways (Weinstein, Underwood, Wicker, & Cubberly, 1979). This shift in thinking led to development of the concept of planful and self-directed "cognitive strategies" (Weinstein, 1978; Weinstein et al., 1979). This shift and the ideas and concepts that have been derived from it have been cited among the major accomplishments in instructional research in the last 30 years (Rosenshine, 1995). In particular, the conceptualization of cognitive strategies is seen as a critical development in both instructional research and educational psychology, because knowing about and using learning strategies is a major factor for discriminating between low achieving students and those who experience success (Alexander & Murphy, 1998; Pintrich & De Groot, 1990; Weinstein, Goetz, & Alexander, 1988). One of the most important findings in the early strategy literature was that cognitive learning strategies represent a mutable factor in promoting academic achievement for students (Pintrich, Brown, & Weinstein, 1994; Weinstein, 1978).

Using cognitive learning strategies involves the intentional manipulation of information by the learner through processes such as repetition, elaboration, or reorganization of the material in such a way that the new information is able to be stored in the learner's associative network and accessed for retrieval. Weinstein and her colleagues (Weinstein & Meyer, 1991) further defined cognitive learning strategies as including the following three critical characteristics: they are goal-directed, intentionally invoked, and effortful.

As researchers learned more about cognitive strategies, they became interested in answering the following questions: Are they modifiable? Can we teach students how to improve their repertoire of learning strategies and will this affect their academic achievement? In an early study in this area, Weinstein (1978) demonstrated that cognitive strategies could, in fact, be modified through instruction. After a 6-week training program, junior high school students improved their learning performance for both laboratory (e.g., paired-associate word lists) and everyday learning tasks (e.g., a shopping task). In the early 1980s, a large number of researchers began investigating the effectiveness of specific memory strategies, such as mnemonics and categorization strategies (e.g., Bean, Inabinette, & Ryan, 1983). Many of these studies, which examined the effectiveness of strategy use, were investigating strategies that students had learned largely on their own, rather than those that they had learned from planned direct instruction. Several researchers also investigated how strategies spontaneously developed in children (e.g., Bjorklund & Zeman, 1983; Wade, Trathen, & Schraw, 1990). Although it did seem that strategies could develop spontaneously, their development was dependent on students' exposure to effective models of the use of specific strategies and to environments that provided opportunities for practice. However, many students did not have exposure to effective memory strategy use, and even when they did, not all students took advantage of the information provided to them in their environment (Bielaczyc, Pirolli, & Brown, 1995).

Only recently have effective programs focusing on learning to learn been developed, and most of these are at the college level under the rubric of "developmental education." Developmental education focuses on helping college students succeed and excel in their postsecondary studies by deepening their prior knowledge in critical subject areas (e.g., mathematics), helping them to develop effective and efficient reading skills, or helping them to develop more effective learning and study strategies (e.g., the course to be described later at the University of Texas and programs offered through learning centers at many institutions). Over time, many developmental education programs at the college and university level have shifted their focus to developing students' self-regulation and strategic learning strategies and skills in a variety of areas related to student success and retention to graduation (e.g., DuBois, 1995; Hattie, Biggs, & Purdie, 1996; Lipsky & Ender, 1990; Weinstein et al., 1997).

III. THE NATURE OF STRATEGIES AND STRATEGY INSTRUCTION

Although the importance of providing strategy instruction is clear from the work described in this and other chapters in this volume, how to go about providing strategy instruction is less clear and less well established. Many researchers are developing integrated approaches to examine strategic and self-regulated learning (e.g., Boekaerts, 1997; Pintrich, Marx, & Boyle, 1993; Weinstein et al., 1997). Many of the topics that are part of these integrated systems and are critical to strategy instruction (e.g., motivation) are more thoroughly described in other chapters within this volume. We only briefly discuss these areas and their importance to learning strategy instruction.

The primary goal of strategy instruction is to help students become "good strategy users" or "good thinkers" (Pressley, Borkowski, & Schneider, 1987; Pressley, Forrest-Pressley, Elliott-Faust, & Miller, 1985; Pressley & McCormick, 1995). One thing we mean when we say "good strategy user" is a student who possesses three kinds of knowledge about strategies: declarative, procedural, and conditional. Declarative knowledge is simply knowing about a variety of strategies (Paris, Lipson, & Wixson, 1983); for example, what does summarizing in your own words mean? Procedural knowledge is knowing how to use these strategies (Anderson, 1990; Garner, 1990); for example, knowing *how* to summarize in your own words and being able to do so effectively. Acquiring these two types of knowledge implies very different types of instruction. Students may obtain declarative knowledge about strategies by simply being told about them. However, these students will need hands-on practice with these strategies in order to learn *how* to use them. I may know the components of a three-part essay, but I had to create many essays before I felt that I knew how to write one. Acquiring conditional knowledge about strategies also requires a specialized type of instruction. Conditional knowledge is knowing when (and when not) to use particular strategies (Paris et al., 1983). Students need to know the strengths and weaknesses, or costs, of using different strategies. Some strategies are applicable in some situations and not others, although the conditions might look the same on the surface. For example, mind mapping (mapping out relationships within the content being studied) is an excellent method for learning important material or material that is very complex or difficult for a student. However, mind mapping is a very time-intensive strategy and cannot be used for all of a student's learning needs. Therefore, for students to be effective in their use of any given strategy, they must first obtain conditional knowledge about when that strategy might or might not be effective. A good base of conditional knowledge can provide the foundation for transfer of strategy knowledge and skills to new situations (Garner, 1990; Paris et al., 1983).

IV. TYPES OF LEARNING STRATEGIES AND THEIR RELATIONSHIP TO OTHER STRATEGIC LEARNING COMPONENTS

An early taxonomy of learning strategies was provided by Weinstein and Mayer (1986). In this taxonomy, five categories were delineated: rehearsal, elaboration, organization, comprehension monitoring, and affective strategies. Three of the categories represent strategies that operate directly on the information to be learned to aid in acquisition and organization of the information. The remaining two categories represent strategies that provide metacognitive and affective support for learning.

Strategies that aid in acquisition and organization of information can be applied to both basic and complex learning tasks. Basic learning tasks involve rote or verbatim memorization or learning. Complex learning tasks involve higher-level conceptual or content learning. For both basic and complex learning tasks, one of three types of strategies, either rehearsal, elaboration, or organization, can be used to master information, depending on the learner's purpose in acquiring the information.

Rehearsal strategies are used to select and encode information in a verbatim manner. Rehearsal strategies that are used for basic learning tasks involve recitation or repetition of information. Rehearsal strategies used for complex or content learning tasks include copying material, taking notes, and underlining or marking texts. Elaboration strategies are used to make information meaningful and to build connections between information given in the learning material and a learner's existing knowledge. Elaboration strategies for basic learning tasks include creating mental imagery and using mnemonic techniques to associate arbitrary information to personally meaningful knowledge. Elaboration strategies for complex learning tasks include strategies that manipulate the information by paraphrasing, summarizing, creating analogies, relating the new information to prior knowledge, questioning, and trying to teach the information to another person. Organizational strategies are used to construct internal connections among the pieces of information given in the learning material. Organizational strategies for basic learning tasks include sorting or clustering related information based on common characteristics or relationships. Organizational strategies for complex learning tasks include outlining or diagramming the information and creating spatial relationships using strategies such as networking.

In addition to the strategies the learner uses to interact directly with the learning material, Weinstein and Mayer proposed two types of support strategies that could be used to enhance the acquisition of knowledge. Comprehension monitoring strategies and affective control strategies were thought to work in concert with the previously defined strategies for both basic and complex learning tasks. Comprehension monitoring strategies are metacognitive strategies used to assess the learner's understanding of the learning material and to executively control the use of acquisition and organizational strategies. Comprehension monitoring strategies include self-questioning, error detection, and problem solving.

Affective and support strategies are used to help focus the learner's attention and maintain the learner's motivation. Affective and support strategies include positive self-talk, anxiety reduction, and time management.

As can be seen in the Weinstein and Mayer (1986) taxonomy, as well as more recent conceptual work by other researchers, the use of cognitive strategies does not occur in isolation. Self-regulated and strategic learning involve integrated processes. The invocation and use of cognitive learning strategies is connected to other aspects of self-regulation such as motivation and metacognition (Paris & Cunningham, 1996; Pressley & McCormick, 1995). For example, from both empirical and anecdotal evidence it is clear that knowing what strategies to use and knowing how to use them is not enough. Students must want to use them and must maintain that desire throughout the learning task. To use cognitive learning strategies effectively, students must be able to manage the amount and direction of their effort, must be motivated to engage in the task, and must be volitional in their use of strategies (Corno, 1994).

The kinds of goals students have also impacts their strategy choice (Paris & Cunningham, 1996). Strategy use must be goal directed. This aspect of strategic learning has two implications. Goals are required so that strategic learners have a reference point to use for continued self-evaluation. The types of goals they set also may impact the kinds of strategies they select and the way they implement them (Pintrich, 1989).

V. MODEL OF STRATEGIC LEARNING

Broadly defined, students' learning strategies include any thoughts, behaviors, beliefs, or emotions that facilitate the acquisition, understanding, or later transfer of new knowledge and skills. In the past, researchers and educational program developers usually have focused on one or a subset of topics within this broad definition, such as cognitive elaboration strategies or student motivation. Current work is more purposefully examining the interaction among two or more components or factors related to the acquisition and use of learning strategies. This change is a result of increasing understanding of the nature of student learning and school achievement at all educational levels. Like most areas of self-regulation, it is the interaction among varying factors that results in successful learning and transfer of new knowledge and skills. The components and factors that seem to have the greatest impact on students' acquisition and use of learning strategies are summarized in a model developed by Weinstein (Weinstein, Husman, and Dierking, in press), which is an extension of an earlier model developed by Weinstein and Mayer (1986). This model focuses on variables that impact strategic learning, that is, learning that is goal driven. Weinstein's model of strategic learning (Weinstein et al., in press) has at its core the learner: a unique individual who brings to each learning situation a critical set of variables, including his or her personality, prior knowledge, and school achievement history. Around this core are three broad components that focus on factors that, in interaction, can tremendously influence the degree to which students set and reach learning and achievement goals. These three components are referred to as skill, will, and self-regulation (see Figure 1). Both the components and the interactive nature of the model are discussed further in Section VIII, which describes the strategic learning course at the University of Texas at Austin.

VI. TYPES OF STRATEGY INSTRUCTION AND THEIR EFFECTIVENESS

Several researchers have reviewed the literature available on programs designed to teach cognitive learning strategies. (When searching this literature, it is important to note that most developmental educators describe their programs that provide instruction in cognitive strategies as "study skills programs"; Hattie et al., 1996.) Simpson, Hynd, and Burrell (1997) created a program classification as a starting point for evaluating the effectiveness of particular types of strategy instruction. In our discussion of this classification scheme we highlight one of the most important criteria for evaluating the success of cognitive strategy instruction. That is,

Model of Strategic Learning

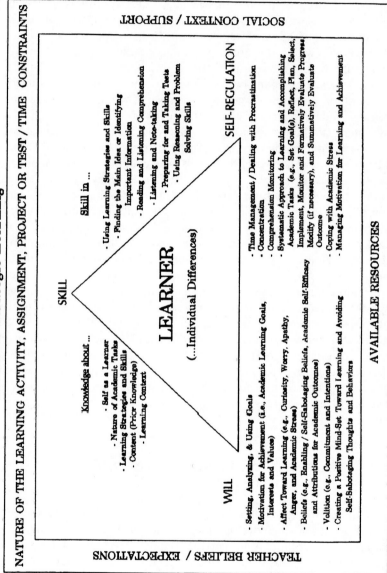

NATURE OF THE LEARNING ACTIVITY, ASSIGNMENT, PROJECT OR TEST / TIME CONSTRAINTS

SOCIAL CONTEXT / SUPPORT

TEACHER BELIEFS / EXPECTATIONS

AVAILABLE RESOURCES

SKILL

Knowledge about ...

- Self as a Learner
- Nature of Academic Tasks
- Learning Strategies and Skills
- Content (Prior Knowledge)
- Learning Context

Skill in ...

- Using Learning Strategies and Skills
- Finding the Main Idea or Identifying Important Information
- Reading and Listening Comprehension
- Listening and Note-taking
- Preparing for and Taking Tests
- Using Reasoning and Problem Solving Skills

LEARNER
(...Individual Differences)

WILL

- Setting, Analyzing, & Using Goals
- Motivation for Achievement (i.e., Academic Learning Goals, Interests and Values)
- Affect Toward Learning (e.g., Curiosity, Worry, Apathy, Anger, and Academic Stress)
- Beliefs (e.g., Enabling / Self-Sabotaging Beliefs, Academic Self-Efficacy and Attributions for Academic Outcomes)
- Volition (e.g. Commitment and Intentions)
- Creating a Positive Mind-Set Toward Learning and Avoiding Self-Sabotaging Thoughts and Behaviors

SELF-REGULATION

- Time Management / Dealing with Procrastination
- Concentration
- Comprehension Monitoring
- Systematic Approach to Learning and Accomplishing Academic Tasks (e.g., Set Goal(s), Reflect, Plan, Select, Implement, Monitor and Formatively Evaluate Progress Modify (if necessary), and Summatively Evaluate Outcome)
- Coping with Academic Stress
- Managing Motivation for Learning and Achievement

©C.E. Weinstein 1994

FIGURE 1   The Model of Strategic Learning. © C. E. Weinstein, 1994.

what is the degree to which students transfer the strategies and skills they learn to other contexts they encounter in academic settings, following their participation in a learning strategies course? This question is central for researchers and for both policymakers and educators concerned about the feasibility and practicality of providing strategy instruction. If transfer to other academic coursework and future learning tasks does not occur, these programs are of little value to the students or the institution.

Simpson et al. (1997) divided academic assistance programs into five general categories. The first category includes learning-to-learn courses that are semester-long, for-credit courses that are developmental in nature rather than deficit oriented. These courses are based on conceptual work in psychology and education (e.g., see the other chapters in this volume), and tend to focus on assisting students to become self-regulated learners by developing a repertoire of learning strategies that they can modify and adapt to novel situations. Learning-to-learn courses tend to be more process oriented as well. Students are encouraged to identify and utilize appropriate strategies based on the learning conditions they experience in the other courses they are taking concurrently with the learning-to-learn course. Such an orientation appears to enhance transfer because students develop an awareness of the conditions associated with a given academic task and then select the strategies that best fit the conditions, their goals, and their relevant prior knowledge and skills. Learning-to-learn courses have been demonstrated to increase grade-point averages, retention, and graduation rates significantly (Weinstein, 1994; Weinstein et al., 1997). This type of strategy instruction also has been referred to as adjunct instruction, because it is presented as an adjunct to the usual content-area courses (Weinstein, 1994; Weinstein & Meyer, 1994).

Simpson et al.'s second category is supplemental instruction or paired courses. Like learning-to-learn courses, these are generally developmental in nature and involve the embedding of strategic learning concepts (learning and study strategies) within the content of a specific course or in supplemental sessions (e.g., labs and small group seminars). As a result, these programs promote academic success in relation to a specific course or subject matter, and are less likely to be transferred to other courses. These programs appear to impact the grades obtained within the specific course positively, but do not seem to have much impact on the grades achieved in other courses (Simpson et al., 1997).

The third category is required programs for underprepared students. This category includes summer interventions and bridge programs (between high school and college). These programs are generally required for certain groups of first year students who are considered to be at risk for being underprepared for college. The summer or bridge programs generally focus on reading, writing, and more traditional study skills to prepare students for the coming academic year. Unfortunately, these programs are likely to result in much less transfer of learning strategies due to the lack of concurrent course work in which to practice using the strategies and due to the time lag between when the strategies are learned in the summer and when they can be applied in the fall.

Simpson's fourth category is approaches integrating reading and writing. These programs are sometimes known as writing-to-learn or writing-across-the-curriculum programs, and are generally process- (as opposed to product-) oriented programs. The format of these programs varies, but typically it involves courses where a writing course is paired with a reading or content course. Writing courses also may be embedded within learning strategies or other courses. The goal of these programs is to enhance the writing proficiency of students as well as to enhance performance in the content area course. These programs have not demonstrated consistent results (Ackerman, 1993).

Simpson's fifth and last category includes learning assistance centers that provide a wide variety of services, such as self-paced and small group skill-specific programs to improve reading, writing, and various study skills as well as tutoring in specific subject areas. Students make use of these usually brief stand-alone services as they feel the need. Whereas each of the services provided by the centers is generally independent of the others, there is no overarching learning theory or conception guiding the provision of the services. Due to the varied offerings and the student-initiated nature of these programs, very little quantitative data on their impact on academic achievement and transfer are available.

It seems that the learning-to-learn end of Simpson's continuum has the greatest potential for positively impacting academic performance and transfer of skills as demonstrated through cumulative grade-point average, retention, and graduation. Learning-to-learn programs tend to be process-oriented programs that provide students with conditional knowledge as well as declarative and procedural knowledge. They also tend to provide a range of strategies and a self-regulation process to manage their application across varying academic challenges.

Another method that has been used to help students develop effective learning strategies within the context of a content area course is called the metacurriculum (Weinstein & Meyer, 1994). Instructors who use the metacurriculum provide direct instruction concerning motivational, self-regulatory, and cognitive strategies as it specifically relates to their content area (see Entwistle & Tait, 1992, for examples). Embedding the instruction within the context of a class provides an opportunity for immediate and authentic use of learning strategies. In their review of learning skills interventions, Hattie et al. (1996) found that learning skills courses were most successful when they were taught in context. This finding is consistent with other data on situated cognition (Brown et al., 1989). These findings make a strong case for the incorporation of strategy instruction into teacher training programs. Teachers need to be able to effectively show their students how to learn course material most effectively. Although it is clear that this form of instruction can be an effective way to help students develop strategies within a domain, it is not clear that it is the most effective way to provide strategy instruction to all students in varying contexts. There are both pragmatic problems and conceptual problems with relying on the metacurriculum for all strategy instruction. The pragmatic problems are due to the fact that many instructors (particularly at the postsecondary level) feel that they have too little time to cover the course material, much less provide strategy instruction as well. The conceptual problems arise from the transfer issues raised earlier. Although some students are able to effectively transfer what they learn in a specific course to other novel situations, this seems to require a deep understanding of the strategies and how to use them (Salomon & Perkins, 1989). Students who have experienced consistent modeling of strategic learning and have a rich prior knowledge base of both strategies and content information may need only strategy instruction imbedded in a content course. However, for students who are considered at risk for failure or low performance in school, it is much more likely that they have less experience and prior knowledge about strategies, and require more practice and instruction. This kind of practice, for all practical proposes, can be provided only in a separate, or adjunct, course.

VII. IMPORTANT COMPONENTS OF ADJUNCT COURSES

Based on the research and applied literature, there are several components that seem to be needed for an adjunct course to be successful. The first is that there must be ample opportunity to practice using the strategies on authentic tasks. Students not only need to understand that strategies exist, they also need to know how to use them. It is not enough for students to be told to apply a strategy any more than it is enough simply to be told to ride a bicycle. At first learning how to ride a bicycle may seem cumbersome and difficult. However, over time, if we are provided with opportunities to practice, we can become proficient. It is the same with strategies. With guided practice and feedback we can become proficient enough at using a strategy that it becomes invisible to us and we are able to focus fully on learning the content.

The second component is that to enhance transfer, cognitive strategy instruction needs to be taught using a model (Hadwin & Winne, 1996). According to Sternberg and Frensch (1993), there are four mechanisms of transfer that, taken together, have critical implications for learning-to-learn courses. The first mechanism is encoding specificity, in which the retrieval of information from memory is dependent on the manner in which the information was encoded. Information that is encoded as context specific or self-contained is likely to be accessed within that context. Students in a learning-to-learn course need to complete assignments that require them to apply components of the model to a variety of contexts. Stahl, Simpson, and Hayes (1992) suggested that having students practice the strategies being learned on real course work from other classes results in more natural strategy transfer.

The second mechanism is organization, which refers to how the information is organized in memory. Information that is organized within a clear framework and is connected to prior knowledge is likely to facilitate retrieval of that information (Alexander & Judy, 1988). Therefore, strategic learning courses should encourage students to become involved in actively seeking to organize information into a format that is meaningful to the students themselves. With a framework in mind, the learner can identify which information is important or critical for them to focus on and which information is of secondary importance or just supporting details. This is also one of the reasons why it appears to be helpful to use a conceptual model in a learning strategies course.

Sternberg and Frensch's third mechanism for transfer is discrimination, which refers to the tagging of information as relevant or irrelevant to a novel situation. If the instructor provides a model for the students to use to organize the information they are learning, the students can use the model to help them discriminate between relevant and irrelevant information in novel situations, thus improving transfer (Salomon & Perkins, 1989).

The fourth mechanism is set, which is how the learner mentally approaches a problem or learning task; that is, whether or not the learner is planning to transfer or use what he or she is are learning. To maximize the transfer of information presented in adjunct learning-to-learn courses to courses the students will participate in during the rest of their academic experience, the students need to know how helpful the strategies are and how they have helped others who are similar to them. The students need to value and feel efficacious about using those strategies (Pintrich & Schunk, 1996; Schunk & Zimmerman, 1994).

VIII. THE NATURE AND IMPACT OF A COURSE IN STRATEGIC LEARNING AT THE UNIVERSITY OF TEXAS

The course we describe was originally developed by Weinstein in 1977. A major purpose of this course is to provide learners with an awareness of the range of learning strategies and techniques available to them, the conditions that influence the selection and application of strategies (i.e., when to use which strategy), and a process for managing and evaluating the application process. Thus, this course addresses not only the declarative and procedural knowledge of learning strategies, but also the conditional knowledge by teaching students how to assess the learning situation and identify which strategies or techniques most likely will produce the desired outcome within the constraints and resources (personal and contextual) of any given situation.

One critical aspect of this course is that Weinstein's Model of Strategic Learning (Weinstein et al., in press) is at its center. The development of interventions specifically designed to help students become more strategic, successful learners is a relatively new phenomenon. Although interventions have been developed for late elementary, middle, and high school students, the most extensive interventions have been developed for postsecondary students.

An underlying concept of the Model of Strategic Learning is that learners need to be aware of elements from all four major component areas of the model: skill, will, self-regulation, and the academic environment. The use of a model in the design of a course and the direct teaching of that model helps the students to make the necessary abstractions for transfer to occur (Salomon & Perkins, 1989; Stahl et al., 1992).

The course begins with an overview of an outline version of the model. This provides students with a glimpse of the larger picture of the various factors that impact their academic performance. Throughout the course the students are not only taught specific strategies, they are also taught how the strategies fit together and interact with the other elements and larger components in the model. It is the interactions among components from all four areas (skill, will, self-regulation, and the academic environment) that are crucial for strategic learning, transfer of learning, and ultimately students' academic success, retention, and graduation (Hadwin & Winne, 1996).

Prior to the introduction of the model, the students are given extensive assessment instruments, including a reading battery and the Learning and Study Strategies Inventory (Weinstein, Schulte, and Palmer, 1987). The Learning and Study Strategies Inventory (LASSI) is used in this course to provide students with diagnostic and prescriptive information for each of the 10 scales, which include aspects from the skill, will, and self-regulation components of the Model of Strategic Learning.

Within the skill component, knowledge about oneself as a learner, knowledge about different academic tasks, and knowledge about context is assessed. Knowledge about oneself as a learner is important because it is a key step toward metacognitive awareness (a critical feature of strategic learning) (Pintrich, Wolters, & Baxter, in press) and the ability to think strategically about learning. This includes knowing one's strengths and weaknesses as a learner and one's attitude, motivation, and anxiety level toward learning. This provides crucial information for conditional knowledge, because it cues learners to areas where they may anticipate problems in a given situation so that they may plan to avoid or minimize those problems.

Another element of the skill component is knowledge about different types of academic tasks, which includes an understanding of what is required to successfully complete a given academic task (e.g., writing a term paper), that is, the steps to be taken and how much time should be required. This directly impacts conditional knowledge by clarifying what needs to occur to reach a desired outcome.

Knowledge about the learning context is also a critical factor for strategic learners in terms of both their understanding of the academic environment and their instructor's beliefs and expectations, as well as their perception of the instrumentality of a course. For example, how will their performance in a particular course be evaluated and how will that evaluation impact them? How does the content of the course relate to their future academic, personal, or occupational goals? By providing instruction about these aspects of strategic learning and linking them to the effective use of cognitive learning strategies, the students obtain valuable conditional knowledge. By recognizing the importance of the information a course contains for their future goals, students may understand more readily the need to learn about and use strategies that are more effective for long-term retrieval (Husman & Lens, 1999). This implies that learners know which strategies are helpful to them for long-term retrieval of information. This is where the learning strategies element of the skill component of the Model of Strategic Learning comes in.

Knowledge and skill acquisition strategies that help to build bridges between what learners already know, the new things they are trying to learn, and how they could potentially apply the course content to current or future academic situations are used to increase knowledge of context as well as the participants' level of understanding of the course content. Such strategies help to build meaning for learning and encourage students to learn in such a way that their new knowledge will be easier to recall and use (Pressley & McCormick, 1995). If students understand the conditional knowledge necessary to successfully use and manipulate a strategy, they are more likely to acquire and transfer the strategy to new situations (Paris et al., 1983). Students in the learning-to-learn course are taught declarative, procedural, and conditional knowledge about three general types of knowledge acquisition strategies: rehearsal, elaboration, and organization. During the semester (approximately 14 weeks with 3 hours of class per week) students are provided with opportunities to apply these strategies to specific course content in their other classes. Providing students with the opportunity to apply strategy instruction to actual course material is considered critical for both acquisition of strategy knowledge and transfer to new situations (Hadwin & Winne, 1996; Rosenshine, Meister, & Chapman, 1996; Simpson et al., 1997; Stahl et al., 1992). Specifically, after the students have considered their academic goals for the semester through class assignments and assessments and have considered their own academic strengths and weaknesses, they are provided with an overview of the information processing theory that is the basis for the strategy instruction. After the students have developed some degree of theoretical understanding for why strategies work, how they can help them, and how knowledge acquisition strategies fit into the model of strategic learning, they are required to complete a class assignment. This class assignment requires the students to use two new learning strategies while they are studying for another class and report on the strategies' effectiveness. By requiring the students to engage in using and evaluating these new strategies, the students get valuable experience and practice. By providing the students with an understanding of both information processing theory and how knowledge of strategies fit into the model of strategic learning, the students are better able to transfer what they learn to courses outside of those they use during the practice assignment.

Knowledge about strategies and knowledge of the contexts the strategies are to be used in are, of course, not enough. The students must also want to use the strategy. Students must be aware of their goals and how those goals impact their academic performance (Hadwin & Winne, 1996). As we said previously, strategies are simply tools used in the service of goals. How the strategies will be used or whether they will be used at all is determined in large part by the students' goals and their motivational orientation (Pintrich, 1989). Before strategy instruction can begin, students must first examine their goals and their motivation for being in school. Therefore, the first few weeks of the course are devoted to examining the will component of the model. This component includes elements such as motivation for attending college or taking a particular course, setting, analyzing, and using goals, anxiety about performing well in learning situations, and attitude toward learning and the degree to which education is valued. These are all-important variables for initial learning and subsequent transfer to other course work. Motivation and attitude toward learning are also closely related to knowledge of context. The instrumentality that the learner perceives for the course content affects his or her motivation for actively participating and the value he or she places on the course (Eccles, 1983; Husman, 1998; Husman & Lens, 1999). In addition to the perceived value of a course, the presence and types of students' goals for the class can have a significant effect on the degree to which they are strategic in their learning in the course (Heyman & Dweck, 1992; Pintrich, 1989). Students who are performance oriented and motivated primarily by extrinsic factors (e.g., grades) tend to use surface-level strategies (e.g., rehearsal strategies), whereas students who are motivated by their enjoyment of the learning process tend to use deeper strategies (e.g., elaboration strategies). The course helps students to develop and examine their goals in the first few weeks of the course through both direct instruction and completion of an extensive project. By helping students become aware of the relationship between their goals and their academic achievement, students learn that they can consciously control their own thoughts and behaviors. The process of regulating motivation and strategy use creates a bridge to the self-regulation component of the model.

From the self-regulation component of the model, the systematic approach to learning plays a crucial role in contributing to academic success and enhancing retention and graduation rates. This approach cues students to consider all aspects of the model in planning for and completing academic tasks. Throughout the learning-to-learn course, students use this approach on projects involving material and assignments from other courses they are taking concurrently. This provides them with opportunities to practice transferring their use of this self-regulatory technique. Briefly, the systematic approach to learning involves eight steps:

1. Setting a goal
2. Reflecting on the task and one's personal resources
3. Developing a plan
4. Selecting potential strategies
5. Implementing strategies
6. Monitoring and formatively evaluating the strategies and one's progress
7. Modifying the strategies if necessary
8. Summatively evaluating the outcomes to decide if this is a useful approach for future similar tasks or if it needs to be modified or discarded for future use

The middle of the course is focused on providing training in specific learning strategies that the students are then encouraged to use in their other courses as part of the projects involving the systematic approach. This provides the students with the practical experience of applying strategies in different contexts while maintaining a metacognitive awareness about their activities and the success or problems they encounter.

The last portion of the course is devoted to reintegration of the components and elements of the model. The purpose of this is to emphasize for the student the heuristic nature of strategic learning and assist the student to understand the interactive nature of the model. Both the initial introduction of the model and the final reintegration of the parts of the model provide the students with the tools they can use to make mindful abstractions about the course. The issues involved in transfer are also directly emphasized.

Salomon and Perkins' (1989) concept of high-road transfer, particularly forward-reaching high-road transfer, and their concept of "mindful abstraction" seem to fit quite well with the tenets of Weinstein's Model of Strategic Learning as well as other conceptions of self-regulated learning. In each of these conceptions the learner is metacognitively aware that the information being learned has potential current and future applications outside of the original learning context. Salomon and Perkins (1989) stated that the main characteristic of the high road to transfer is the mindful generation of an abstraction during learning. This abstraction then can be applied in the future to a new problem or situation. The mechanism by which this takes place is the deliberate process of separating cognitive elements from the context in which they were learned and considering them for application in quite different contexts.

Research and evaluation data for this course have been obtained in a number of ways. From semester evaluations of the pre- and postdata on the Nelson Denny Reading Test (Brown, Bennett, and Hanna, 1981) and LASSI scores, it was found that students evidenced highly significant gains on these measures. However, given the importance of transfer issues in cognitive process learning contexts, data concerning the long-term effects of the course will be highlighted. The question addressed with this study was what impact the course had on students' subsequent GPAs and retention at the university over a 5-year period. The most interesting data concerning transfer data appears in the fifth-year followup statistics. Approximately 55% of the students who entered in 1990 and did not take the strategic learning course graduated after 5 years; this statistic has remained about the same for a number of years. However, despite significantly lower SAT scores and significantly lower motivation scores on the LASSI Motivation Scales, approximately 71% of the students who successfully completed our course (primarily those who did not drop out or fail due to excessive absences) graduated after 5 years. This 16-point difference is a dramatic finding that supports the long-term retention effects of an intervention in learning strategies. In addition, the cumulative GPAs for these students were higher than for the general population. These data offer strong support for the importance and impact of developmental education that emphasizes learning strategies for students at risk for academic failure or low achievement.

IX. FUTURE DIRECTIONS FOR LEARNING STRATEGIES RESEARCH

We have come a long way in our understanding of learning strategies and their role in strategic, goal-driven learning. However, we still have crucial issues and questions that need to be addressed both for our conceptual understanding of the processes and variables involved and for building a more solid foundation for the development of applications at all educational levels and in diverse educational settings, both in and out of formal school environments. For example, there is a need for more research that investigates the development and use of learning strategies and processes by young children and early teenagers. What are the precursors of effective strategy use? How can we facilitate the development of these skills at differing ages? What can we do to help teachers incorporate learning-to-learn activities into their classroom teaching? We also need to investigate further the nature of transfer of cognitive skills. How do we facilitate high-level transfer across tasks and content areas? How do we help students learn to cue themselves to transfer strategies? We need more refined models that learners can use to help them identify the most critical skill, will, and self-regulation elements they must consider in a given learning situation. How can we help them learn to take more control of their own learning processes and outcomes? Finally, we need to investigate the changing nature of learning in computer and distance learning environments, and the implications for both the roles played by learning strategies and the design of these learning environments.

This list is not in any way meant to be exhaustive, but it is reflective of the vibrant nature of the field of self-regulation and the critical needs we face in preparing for the learners and learning demands of the 21st century.

REFERENCES

Ackerman, J. M. (1993). The promise of writing to learn. *Written Communication, 10*(3), 334–370.

Alexander, P. A., & Judy, J. E. (1988). The interaction of domain specific and strategic knowledge in academic performance. *Review of Educational Research, 58*, 375–404.

Alexander, P. A., & Murphy, P. K. (1998). The research base for APA's learner-centered psychological principles. In N. M. Lambert & B. L. McCombs (Eds.), *How students learn: Reforming schools through learner-centered education* (pp. 25–60). Washington, DC: American Psychological Association.

Anderson, J. R. (1990). *Cognitive psychology and its implications* (3rd ed.). New York: Freeman.

Bean, T. W.; Inabinette, N. B., & Ryan, R. (1983). The effect of a categorization strategy on secondary students' retention of literary vocabulary. *Reading Psychology, 4*, 247–252.

Bielaczyc, K., Pirolli, P. L., & Brown, A. L. (1995). Training in self-explanation and self-regulation strategies: Investigating the effects of knowledge acquisition activities on problem solving. *Cognition and Instruction, 13*(2), 221–252.

Bjorklund, D. F., & Zeman, B. R. (1983). The development of organizational strategies in children's recall of familiar information: Using social organization to recall the names of classmates. *International Journal of Behavioral Development, 6*, 341–353.

Boekaerts, M. (1997). Self-regulated learning: a new concept embraced by researchers, policy makers, educators, teachers, and students. *Learning and Instruction, 7*(2), 161–186.

Brown, J. S., Collins, A., & Duguid, P. (1989). Situated cognition and the culture of learning. *Educational Researcher, 18*(1), 32–42.

Brown, J. T., Bennett, J. M., & Hanna, G. (1981). *Nelson–Denny Reading Test Forms E and F.* Chicago: Riverside.

Corno, L. (1994). Student volition and education: Outcomes, influences, and practices. In D. H. Schunk & B. J. Zimmerman (Eds.), *Self-regulation of learning and performance* (pp. 229–251). Hillsdale, NJ: Erlbaum.

Danner, F. W., & Taylor, A. M. (1973). Integrated pictures and relational imagery training in children's learning. *Journal of Experimental Child Psychology, 16*, 47–54.

DuBois, N. F. (1995, April). *An eight minute paper on fostering student learning.* Paper presented at the American Educational Research Association, San Francisco.

Eccles, J. (1983). Expectancies, values, and academic behaviors. In J. T. Spence (Ed.), *Achievement and achievement motives.* San Francisco: Freeman.

Entwistle, N. J., & Tait, H. (1992). Promoting effective study skills. In P. Cryer (Ed.), *Learning actively on one's own.* Sheffield, UK: CVCP Universities' Staff Development and Training Unit.

Flavell, J. H. (1979). Metacognition and cognitive monitoring: A new area of cognitive-developmental inquiry. *American Psychologist, 34*(10), 906–11.

Garner, R. (1987). *Metacognition and reading comprehension.* Norwood, NJ: Ablex.

Garner, R. (1990). *Children's use of strategies in reading.* Hillsdale, NJ: Erlbaum.

Hadwin, A. F., & Winne, P. H. (1996). Study strategies have meager support. *Journal of Higher Education, 67*(6), 692–715.

Hattie, J., Biggs, J., & Purdie, N. (1996). Effects of learning skills interventions on students learning: A meta-analysis. *Review of Educational Research, 66*(2), 99–136.

Heyman, G. D., & Dweck, C. S. (1992). Achievement goals and intrinsic motivation: Their relation and their role in adaptive motivation. *Motivation and Emotion, 16*(3), 231–245.

Husman, J. (1998). *The effects of perceptions of the future on intrinsic motivation.* Unpublished dissertation, University of Texas at Austin.

Husman, J. & Lens, W. (1999). The role of the future in student motivation. *Educational Psychologist, 34*, 113–125.

Lipsky, S. A., & Ender, S. C. (1990). Impact of a study skills course on probationary students' academic performance. *Journal of the Freshmen Year Experience, 2*, 5–17.

Paris, S. G., & Cunningham, A. E. (1996). Children becoming students. In D. C. Berliner & R. C. Calfee (Eds.), *Handbook of educational psychology* (pp. 117–146). New York: Macmillan.

Paris, S. G., Lipson, M. Y., & Wixson, K. K. (1983). Becoming a strategic reader. *Contemporary Educational Psychology, 8*, 293–316.

Pintrich, P. R. (1989). The dynamic interplay of student motivation and cognition in the classroom. *Advances in motivation and achievement: Motivation enhancing environments* (Vol. 6, pp. 117–160). Greenwich, CT JAI Press.

Pintrich, P. R., Brown, D. R., & Weinstein, C. E. (Eds.). (1994). *Student motivation, cognition, and learning: Essays in honor of Wilbert J. McKeachie.* Hillsdale, NJ: Erlbaum.

Pintrich, P. R., & De Groot, E. V. (1990). Motivational and self-regulated learning components of classroom academic performance. *Journal of Educational Psychology, 82*(1), 33–40.

Pintrich, P. R., Marx, R. W., & Boyle, R. A. (1993). Beyond cold conceptual change: The role of motivational beliefs and classroom contextual factors in the process of conceptual change. *Review of Educational Research, 63*(2), 167–199

Pintrich, P. R., & Schunk, D. H. (1996). *Motivation in education: Theory, research, and applications.* Englewood Cliffs, NJ: Prentice-Hall.

Pintrich, P. R., Wolters, C. A., & Baxter, G. P. (in press). Assessing metacognition and self-regulated learning. In G. Schaaw (Ed.) *Metacognitive Assessment*. Lincoln: University of Nebraska Press.

Pressley, M., Borkowski, J. G., & Schneider, W. (1987). Cognitive strategies: Good strategy users coordinate metacognition and knowledge. *Annals of Child Development*, *4*, 89–129.

Pressley, M., Forrest-Pressley, D., Elliott-Faust, D. L., & Miller, G. E. (1985). Children's use of cognitive strategies, how to teach strategies, and what to do if they can't be taught. In M. Pressley & C. J. Brainerd (Eds.), *Cognitive learning and memory in children* (pp. 1–47). New York: Springer-Verlag.

Pressley, M., & McCormick, C. B. (1995). *Advanced educational psychology for educators, researchers, and policymakers*. New York: Harper Collins.

Rosenshine, B. (1995). Advances in research on instruction. *The Journal of Educational Research*, *88*(5), 262–268.

Rosenshine, B., Meister, C., & Chapman, S. (1996). Teaching students to generate questions: A review of the intervention studies. *Review of Educational Research*, *66*(2), 181–221.

Salomon, G., & Perkins, D. N. (1989). Rocky roads to transfer: Rethinking mechanisms of a neglected phenomenon. *Educational Psychologist*, *24*(2), 113–142.

Schunk, D. H., & Zimmerman, B. J. (1994). *Self-regulation of learning and performance: Issues and educational applications*. Hillsdale, NJ: Erlbaum.

Simon, H. A. (1979a). Information processing models of cognition. *Annual Review of Psychology*, *30*, 363–396.

Simon, H. A. (1979b). *Models of thought*. New Haven, CT: Yale Univ. Press.

Simpson, M. L., Hynd, D. R., Nist, S. L., & Burrell, K. I. (1997). College academic assistance programs and practices. *Educational Psychology Review*, *9*(1), 39–87.

Stahl, N. A., Simpson, M. L., & Hayes, C. G. (1992). Ten recommendations from research for teaching high-risk college students. *Journal of Developmental Education*, *16*, 2–10.

Sternberg, R. J., & Frensch, P. A. (1993). Mechanisms of transfer. In D. K. Detterman & R. J. Sternberg (Eds.), *Transfer on trial: Intelligence, cognition and instruction*. Norwood, NJ: Ablex.

Wade, S. E., Trathen, W., & Schraw, G. (1990). An analysis of spontaneous study strategies. *Reading Research Quarterly*, *25*, 147–166.

Wang, A. Y. (1983). Individual differences in learning speed. *Journal of Experimental Psychology: Learning, Memory, & Cognition*, *9*(2), 300–311.

Weinstein, C. E. (1978). Elaboration skills as a learning strategy. In H. G. O' Neil, Jr. (Ed.), *Learning strategies*. New York: Academic Press.

Weinstein, C. E. (1994). Strategic learning/strategic teaching: Flip sides of a coin. In P. R. Pintrich, D. R. Brown, & C. E. Weinstein (Eds.), *Student motivation, cognition, and learning: Essays in honor of Wilbert J. McKeachie* (pp. 257–273). Hillsdale, NJ: Erlbaum.

Weinstein, C. E., Goetz, E. T., & Alexander, P. A. (1988). *Learning and study strategies: Issues in assessment, instruction, and evaluation*. New York: Academic Press.

Weinstein, C. E., Hanson, G., Powdrill, L., Roska, L., Dierking, D., Husman, J., & McCann, E. (1997, March). *The design and evaluation of a course in strategic learning*. Paper presented at the meeting of the National Association of Developmental Educators, Denver, CO.

Weinstein, C. E., Husman, J., & Dierking, D. (in press). Strategic learning. In C. E. Weinstein & B. L. McCombs (Eds.), *Strategic learning: The merging of skill, will, and self-regulation in academic environments*. Hillsdale, NJ: Erlbaum.

Weinstein, C. E., & Mayer, R. E. (1986). The teaching of learning strategies. In M. C. Wittrock (Ed.), *Handbook of research on teaching*. (3rd ed., pp. 315–327). New York: Macmillan.

Weinstein, C. E., & Meyer, D. K. (1991). Cognitive learning strategies and college teaching. *New directions for teaching and learning*, *45*, 15–26.

Weinstein, C. E., & Meyer, D. K. (1994). Teaching and assessment of learning strategies. In T. Husen & T. N. Postlethwite (Eds.), *The international encyclopedia of education* (2nd ed., pp. 335–340). Oxford, UK: Pergamon.

Weinstein, C. E., Schulte, A., & Palmer, D. R. (1987). *The Learning and Studies Strategies Inventory*. Clearwater, FL: H & H Publishing.

Weinstein, C. E., Underwood, V. L., Wicker, F. W., & Cubberly, W. E. (1979). Cognitive learning strategies: Verbal and imaginal elaboration. *Cognitive and affective learning strategies* (pp. 45–75). New York: Academic Press.

Wood, G. (1967). Mnemonic systems in recall. *Journal of Educational Psychology, 58*(6), 1–27.

23

SELF-REGULATION

DIRECTIONS AND CHALLENGES
FOR FUTURE RESEARCH

MOSHE ZEIDNER,* MONIQUE BOEKAERTS,[†]
AND PAUL R. PINTRICH[‡]

*University of Haifa, Mt. Carmel, Israel
[†]Leiden University, Leiden, The Netherlands
[‡]University of Michigan, Ann Arbor, Michigan

This handbook was designed to present the current state of the field of self-regulation, providing foundations of knowledge for the development of a more comprehensive understanding of self-regulation theory, research, and applications. The chapters in this book reflect recent advances in conceptualization, methodology, research, individual differences, and areas of application, and represent some of the best contemporary thinking and research on key facets of self-regulation. The work in this book represents current perspectives in the area of self-regulation and some of the contemporary ways in which changes in this domain have taken place. The contributing authors summarize and discuss important themes and issues, raising critical questions and providing some of today's best guesses about the answers. Many of the people blazing the trail to those answers over the past two decades have contributed their insights to this book.

To those who came of age professionally during the late 1970s and afterward, the concept of self-regulation is a natural and organic part of the landscape of psychology and education. However, this was not always the case. The vast majority of work in this field has occurred over the past 15 years or so, with self-regulation now the subject of intense professional interest and scrutiny. Research in the area of self-regulation has proliferated in the past few years, and synthesizing scholarship in this sprouting domain is quite a substantial task, the scope of which is evidenced by the

Copyright © 2000 by Academic Press.
All rights of reproduction in any form reserved.

number and variety of chapters in this book. Today, after a virtual explosion of work in this area, the topography of research and theory pertaining to self-regulation has changed in a number of ways.

Although this book covers considerable terrain, many additional questions remain unanswered. Presently, a good number of issues, from the conceptual, to the methodological, to the philosophical, remain unresolved. The refinement of self-regulation models, research, and applications appears to be an important goal for scientific psychology in the 21st century. To advance this goal, we wish to point out several overarching issues that need to be addressed in future research efforts in this area. (In the following discussion, references relate to handbook authors and chapters, unless otherwise indicated by asterisk.)

I. DEVELOPING A TRACTABLE CONCEPTUAL FOUNDATION AND CONSISTENT NOMENCLATURE OF SELF-REGULATION CONSTRUCTS

To facilitate communication among researchers in the self-regulation domain, a tractable conceptual foundation and taxonomy for self-regulation constructs needs to be systematically developed. At present, there is considerable confusion in the literature with respect to the criterial attributes of self-regulation, its key components, and related constructs from the same semantic domain. As noted by a number of contributors to this volume, there are almost as many definitions and conceptions of self-regulation as there are lines of research on the topic. Thus, the term has been used in somewhat different ways by researchers in different subfields, and various terms have been used to denote the same concept (e.g., self-regulation, self-control, self-management, problem solving, behavioral control, mood control, self-regulated learning).

It is unclear whether the concepts provided by prevalent theory and analytic techniques are both molar and molecular enough to cover all the important theoretical needs presently in the domain of self-regulation. Thus, above the main components, there also might be a need for compound constructs. Indeed, it is becoming clearer by the day that both broad, sweeping, higher-order constructs (e.g., self-regulation) as well as narrower constructs (e.g., self-regulated learning) and lower-order constructs (e.g., metacognitive strategies, self-observation, automaticity) need to be represented in the research. A principal advantage of lower-order concepts is that they often have clearer psychological referents, because the psychological clarity of individual differences dimensions often seem to vary inversely with the breadth of the dimension. Thus, lower-order categories often carry certain specialized and situational meanings that are not captured in the higher-order factors.

Although contributors to this volume differ in their specific perspectives on self-regulation and employ slightly different terminologies, the commonalities that exist among conceptualizations appear to be greater than the uniquenesses. A casual glance at the various chapters in the handbook (e.g., Brownlee, Leventhal, & Leventhal, Carver & Scheier, Jackson, MacKenzie, & Hobfoll, Matthews, Schwean, Campbell, Saklofske, & Mohamed, Shapiro & Schwartz, and Maes & Gebhardt) suggests that authorities view self-regulation as a systematic process of human behavior that involves setting personal goals and steering behavior toward the achievement of established goals. For example, both Zimmerman and Schunk and Ertmer conceptualize self-regulation from a social-cognitive perspective in terms of a multiphasic process in which self-generated thoughts, affects, and actions are planned and cyclically adapted as needed to attain personal goals. Similarly, Maes and Gebhardt define self-regulation as a sequence of actions, steering processes, or both, intended to attain personal goals. Matthews and his co-workers view self-regulation as a generic umbrella term for the set of processes and behaviors that support the pursuit of personal goals within a changing external environment.

Furthermore, there appears to be some consensus among contributors that self-regulation involves *cognitive, affective, motivational,* and *behavioral* components that provide the individual with the capacity to adjust his or her actions and goals to achieve desired results in light of changing environmental conditions. Contributors concur that self-regulatory behavior involves a feedback loop that serves to decrease the discrepancy between ideal and desired behavior (see chapters by Zimmerman, Carver & Scheier, and Vancouver). Overall, definitions and conceptualizations of self-regulation that appear in the various chapters of the handbook tend to embody the basic ingredients of goal setting, steering process and strategies, feedback, and self-evaluation (e.g., see models put forth by Endler and Kocovski, Brownlee et al., Demetriou, Pintrich, and Carver & Scheier). As suggested by Creer, apparent differences occur among contributors because of the way they tend to categorize specific processes, rather than from different conceptualizations.

In particular, the concept of self-regulation needs to be more sharply differentiated from related constructs in the same semantic domain (self-control, self-management, coping, adjustment, etc.). As pointed out by Creer, a myriad of terms (self-control, self-change, self-directed behavior) have proliferated recently to "further muddy the water." A number of contributors to this volume (e.g., De Corte, Verschaffel, and Op 't Eynde, Matthews et al., and Brownlee et al.) point out that major constructs that relate to self-regulation (metacognition, volition, planning) overlap each other and also overlap related domains (e.g., transactional theories of personality and stress; Matthews et al.). We now briefly highlight a number of overlaps among concepts in the self-regulation literature that are in need of further clarification.

To begin with, the distinction between the two grand concepts of *self-regulation* and *self-management* is rather fuzzy. Self-regulation is sometimes taken to imply that people follow self-set goals, whereas self-management is taken to imply that people follow goals set by others. However, as noted by Creer, there appears to be no clear demarcation among the terms, and the preceding distinction is not universally accepted.

There is also some confusion regarding the concepts of *regulation* and *self-regulation*. Brownlee et al. propose that to distinguish between the two constructs, we need to know whether the goal originated in the external world or internal world (i.e., the social environment versus the self system), and whether the person sees its origin as being internal or external. Thus, when a person is setting a goal or defining a relevant procedure, he or she is self-regulating; otherwise, his or her behavior is being externally or "other regulated."

The distinction between *self-regulation* and *metacognition* is also somewhat unclear from the literature; there is considerable ambiguity and overlapping of definitions (cf. Demetriou, Pintrich). Metacognition is commonly construed as the awareness individuals have of their personal resources in relation to the demands of particular tasks, along with the knowledge they possess of how to regulate their engagement in tasks to optimize goal-related processes and outcomes. According to Demetriou, self-regulation may be viewed as the more comprehensive term, embracing both metacognitive knowledge and skills, as well as motivational, emotional, and behavioral monitoring and control processes. However, there is little consensus on the nature of the relationship among these terms.

The also seems to be considerable conceptual overlap between the concepts of *coping* and *self-regulation*. As pointed out by Matthews et al., the various processes employed in negotiating a goal in self-regulation are akin to the basic processes described when coping with a stressor. These include appraisal of the potential threat a situation poses to the person, its related emotional reactions, and the various procedures, mental actions, and overt actions taken to manage the problem and the feelings it evokes.

Brownlee et al. draw an important distinction between *self-regulation* and *regulation of the self*. They propose that self-regulation becomes regulation of the self when the problem-solving process focuses upon the self and leads to its reorganization and redefinition. In the case of regulation of the self, a component of the self is the focus of problem solving (redefinition of old identities, the creation of new ones, the addition or remodeling of existent procedures for managing the self, and illness threats) Furthermore, these authors point to the conceptual overlap between *self-regulation* and *problem solving* (Brownlee et al.). Both self-regulation and problem solving involve the extended process of setting goals, applying strategies, monitoring, evaluation, and reinforcement. Thus, the question arises, "When should a process be called self-regulation and when should it simply be termed problem solving?" The answer to this question is awaiting further conceptualization and research.

In sum, self-regulation, as well as a number of concepts in the same semantic domain are "fuzzy" concepts and need to be defined more definitively and used more consistently by researchers and practitioners in the field. This confusion among concepts stems, in part, from the division of modern behavioral science into numerous subareas of specialization, each with its unique nomenclature and somewhat idiosyncratic use of the self-regulation construct. Furthermore, the fragmentation and disparate, but overlapping, lines of research within the self-regulation domain have made any attempt at furthering our knowledge an arduous task. Indeed, consistent nomenclature and taxonomy have been virtually impossible for many years because little coherence exists among theory and measures of self-regulation and other conative constructs

II. CLARIFYING SELF-REGULATION STRUCTURE AND PROCESSES

Self-regulation is currently seen as involving a number of integrated microprocesses, including goal setting, strategic planning, use of effective strategies to organize, code, and store information, monitoring and metacognition, action and volitional control, managing time effectively, self-motivational beliefs (self-efficacy, outcome expectations, intrinsic interest, and goal orientation, etc.), evaluation and self-reflection, experiencing pride and satisfaction with one's efforts, and establishing a congenial environment (Zimmerman; Schunk & Ertmer, Pintrich).

A major goal for future research is to identify the specific elements and distinct steps in the process of self-regulation (see Rheinberg, Vollmeyer, & Rollett). Overall, the limited number of components or facets that comprise many models of self-regulation, typically three to five cyclical phases or elements (Vancouver cites three; Carver & Scheier identify four; Winne & Perry cite three to four), while they do represent the law of parsimony, they may represent only a fraction of the total number of phases or facets in the structure and morphology of self-regulation. Although the principles of parsimony should be endorsed whenever applicable, the evidence often points to relative complexity rather than simplicity (e.g., see Vancouver's probing discussion of Power's perceptual control mode or Carver & Scheier's discussion of chaos and catastrophe perspectives on self-regulation). Thus, future models may need to be less simplistic and more complex than current models, incorporating dynamic concepts and additional structural components into the model (cf. Kuhl's chapter, for example).

Although there is little agreement on what a goal is, there is agreement on the critical role of goals in the structure and morphology of self-regulation. However, experts currently fail to agree on the number or the configuration of components involved in the self-regulation process. Thus, a casual glance at the chapters in this book shows that there is little consensus regarding the status of constructs such as metacognition or metamonitoring, self-awareness, automaticity, self-efficacy, self-evaluation, self-reinforcement, and self-reaction. For example, some contributors to this book include self-reinforcement in their models (e.g., Zimmerman; Endler & Kocovski), whereas others do not (e.g., Carver & Scheier). Whereas some models posit the existence of a metamonitoring system or process (e.g., Carver & Scheier), others do not see the need to do so (e.g., Vancouver; Zimmerman).

The role of a number of constructs in the self-regulation process, such as self-efficacy and affect, is somewhat ambiguous. Accordingly, some contributors (e.g., Creer; Zimmerman, Schunk & Ertmer) view self-efficacy as an integral part of the self-regulation process. As pointed out by Creer, knowledge of self-regulation skills is simply not enough to guarantee that these skills will be used appropriately; persons must also believe that they are capable of performing these skills to reach whatever goals they determine for themselves. Thus, the beliefs about one's capabilities to organize and implement actions are necessary to attain designated performance and, according to Zimmerman, are an integral component of the self-regulation process. Other contributors (Endler & Kocovski), while viewing self-efficacy as an important factor in self-regulation, do not view it directly as an element or facet of self-regulation.

An intriguing question for future research on the structure and process of self-regulation is, "How should we deal with emotions or affect?" Some experts (e.g., Brownlee, et al., Carver & Scheier, Shah & Kruglanski, Weinstein, Husman, and Dierking, Pintrich, and Zimmerman) view emotion as part and parcel of the self-regulatory process. Zimmerman views affective reactions, such as doubts and fears about specific performance contexts, as an integral part of the forethought phase of self-regulation. Furthermore, models proposed by various contributors (e.g., Carver & Scheier and Shah & Kruglanski) relate affect to goal promotion. Thus, if a goal is promoted, positive affect results; if a goal is blocked or prevented, negative affect results. By contrast, other models (e.g., particularly the TOTE models surveyed by Vancouver) do not assign a functional role to affect. A related issue that has not been sufficiently addressed in the literature is, "What are the effects of positive mood on performance? Does positive mood lead to coasting and withdrawal of effort or to investment of effort in the task?" (cf. the treatment of affect in self-regulation by Carver & Scheier.)

Current cybernetic or TOTE models (see Vancouver's chapter) have paid particular attention to *negative* feedback loops, a key component of self-regulation processes. Future research needs to pay more attention to positive feedback loops. As pointed out by Shapiro and Schwartz, positive loops engender heterostasis, leading to change, growth, and development. Negative feedback loops, by contrast, engender homeostasis—a stable state that a living organism strives to maintain by keeping vital parameters within viable bounds. Presumably, a system needs a reasonable balance between positive and negative feedback loops.

III. MAPPING OUT THE NOMOLOGICAL NETWORK

A major problem in exploring the self-regulation construct is mapping out the pattern of interrelationships between self-regulation and related individual difference constructs, and the underlying processes to which they relate. Whereas research has examined the nature of the association between self-regulation and a selected number of individual difference variables (e.g., self-efficacy, optimism, and anxiety; see chapters by Carver & Scheier, Matthews et al., and Zimmerman), we know relatively little about the relationships between self-regulation (and its key components) and other variables, such as intelligence, extroversion, openness to experience, or conscientiousness.

Furthermore, whereas we have a body of research on the environmental determinants and outcomes of self-regulation in such areas as education (see Zimmerman and Boekaerts & Niemivirta) and health (see chapters by Maes & Gebhardt, Brownlee, et al., and Shapiro & Schwartz), other environments (family, social, religious, political, military) need to be carefully mapped out as well. Clearly the construction of a valid nomological network that maps self-regulation onto key environmental and personal (cognitive, affective, conative) variables is critical to further our understanding of self-regulation.

To map out the nomological network, it might be useful to employ a facet-analytic approach to investigate the interface of self-regulation and relevant constructs by constructing a matrix with self-regulation components represented by rows (j) and related variables or components in the nomological network represented by columns (k), where the entire two-dimensional matrix ($j \times k$), or Cartesian space, represents the domain of discourse for any future integrative attempt. A third facet—area of application (school, social, occupation, health, etc.)—may be added to form a three-faceted cubic model for examining the much needed mapping of variables. Indeed, tentative mapping of the domain may suggest entire areas that are uncovered by present research; these lacunae need to be identified and systematically researched. Even quite loose, provisional classification structures might help guide exploration and provide a useful framework to which to pin individual data as they accumulate.

Researchers interested in dynamic interactions between self-regulation and other constructs will need to look at the reciprocal effects of self-regulation and other variables, say intelligence, in the course of development and day to day manifestations. Thus, poor self-regulated learning skills may constrain the development of a person's intellectual ability, which, in turn, impedes the development of self-regulatory skills. If what interests us is how self-regulation and another variable, say intelligence, interact to impact on a third variable, say leadership, we may need to consider synergistic interactions, that is, where the presence of one variable (say self-regulation) potentiates the effects of the other (say IQ) on some criterion performance (e.g., leadership). In this form of interaction, the effects of both factors on the third variable are greater than the sum of each.

IV. CONSTRUCTION OF MORE REFINED MODELS

How best to model self-regulation is one major area that future research needs to address Because self-regulation is viewed as a sequence of activities or processes designed to attain personal goals, any model of self-regulation should contain a concept of personal goals along with the steering processes used to attain personal goals. The handbook chapters tend to be based on the more prevalent models of self-regulation, including social cognitive models (Zimmerman; Schunk & Ertmer), cybernetic control (TOTE) models (Carver & Scheier; cf. Vancouver), and expectancy models (Rheinberg et al.). The social-cognitive perspective and the control perspectives are the most prevalent models represented in this handbook. In addition, some novel perspectives, such as dynamic models (cf. Carver & Scheier and Kuhl) are discussed by contributors. Sociocultural and discourse models are not represented in this handbook.

An intriguing question for future thought is, "Should we stick with current models of self-regulation or perhaps shift away from these models and develop higher-order paradigmatic models?" Might it not be fruitful to examine alternative paradigms and conceptualize self-regulation in novel ways? One possible direction for future research is to construct more elaborate and refined processual models (theories) of self-regulation that allow us to make focused predictions of the relationship between self-regulation and other conative, affective, and cognitive factors as they unfold over time. The optimal approach to the study of self-regulation is to construct tenable models of self-regulation, arrange experimental conditions to test deductions (hypotheses) from these models, and interpret results cautiously in the light of the models being tested. In addition, future models need to consider the effects of divergent environments and contexts that may interact with personal variables to impact on self-regulation.

V. REFINING MEASUREMENT OF SELF-REGULATION CONSTRUCTS

It is evident that a sine qua non for the development of a sound knowledge base for furthering theory and applications in this area is the use of reliable and valid measures. Thus, one important goal for future research in this area is modeling relationships through more complex measurement models. The particular measures we use to gauge a given construct are particularly important, because they may impact strongly upon the outcomes of our research. Unfortunately, measurement methods currently in use to assess some of the more "slippery" self-regulation constructs (e.g., metaregulation, automaticity, open and closed feedback loops, and feedback control levels) are not always optimal in assessing the various components of self-regulation.

A major task for future research is to determine the optimal "grain size," that is, the unit of metric to measure components of self-regulation, and how best to integrate variables defined in quite different "grain sizes" into a coherent self-regulation model of human behavior (see Winne & Perry's in-depth discussion of this issue). As pointed out by Winne and Perry, the self-regulation components of tactic and strategy reflect differences in grain size; the latter are larger grains because they involve decision making to select among alternative tactics. The time span is another variant of a grain size: self-regulation conceptualized as an *event* occupies a very brief span. By contrast, self-regulation conceptualized as an aptitude is theorized to be enduring, at least over the course of a single research investigation that may span several weeks.

As pointed out by Matthews et al., current research relies heavily on self-report measures. Thus, more observational and performance measures relevant to self-regulation processes and outcomes are urgently needed. Because there is a fundamental problem with using self-reports and survey methods to demonstrate dynamic processes, we sorely need better ways to operationalize the self-regulation construct so that the processual nature of self-regulation is captured. Fortunately, a number of promising ways to measure the different components of self-regulation as they unfold over time are being developed and refined. For example, by employing computer simulations of different aspects of behavior (e.g., vocational, health, educational), we may be able to assess various components of the self-regulatory process "on line." Also, analyses of the protocols of "think-aloud" procedures, in which subjects describe exactly what goes through their minds when self-regulating during a given task, might be useful for examining the subjects' phenomenological perceptions and understanding of different aspects of self-regulation. Additional techniques that may be useful for studying adaptive self-regulatory processes are study of experts who are known for their self-discipline and success, clinical studies of individuals experiencing self-regulatory dysfunctions, and experimental research on personal methods of control during demanding cognitive tasks (see Zimmerman).

Much akin to the state–trait distinction found in personality research, self-regulation may be conceived of as an *aptitude* or trait (i.e., a relatively enduring mental attribute of a person that predicts future behavior) or as an *event* or state (i.e., transient state in a large, longer process that unfolds over time). However, these two facets or forms of self-regulation are not clearly differentiated in measurement or research (see Winne and Perry). Thus, there is a need to better differentiate aptitude measures of self-regulation from event-related measures of self-regulation. As pointed out by Winne and Perry, when studying self-regulation as a state or an event, point estimates derived from these data (such as means) are not appropriate descriptions. Instead, methods are needed that characterize temporally unfolding patterns of engagement with tasks in terms of the tactics and strategies that constitute self-regulation, over time. In addition, work is needed on how measures of self-regulation, as aptitude and as event, can be interleaved to characterize the full spectrum of self-regulation.

Further attention needs to be given to the issue of *validity* of self-regulation measures. A number of cognitive, motivational, affective, and behavioral variables are components in an overall portrait of self-regulation. Multitrait–multimethod studies would help focus on the center of self-regulation and its relationships to contributing peripheral variables (see Winne and Perry's discussion). To date, however, there is little information of the kind that would be revealed by multitrait–multimethod investigations of convergent and divergent validity. Furthermore, additional work on the practical or diagnostic validity of self-regulation measures is also sorely needed. Beyond description for purposes of basic research, few measures have been used for formal diagnosis and evaluation in educational, occupational, and health contexts. Given that few formal studies of the diagnostic utility of measures of self-regulation have been done, assessing the discriminant validity of components of self-regulation in differing criterion groups would be most welcome.

The issue of reliability of self-regulation measures also deserves further work. Two methods of assessing reliability traditionally have been applied in self-regulation research: internal consistency reliability for measures generated by self-report and interobserver reliability for measurement protocols (Winne and Perry). Unfortunately, very little attention has been given to the issue of stability of self-regulation measures. Stability is a difficult concept to apply to measures of self-regulation, mainly because self-regulation, by definition, is adaptive and should vary over time under certain conditions.

Furthermore, few attempts have been made to *standardize* and norm measures of self-regulation. This perhaps reflects the newness of work on measuring self-regulatory components and processes, the field's flexibility in adopting models that guide the development of measurement protocols, and genuine questions about what would be useful norms relative to purposes for measures of self-regulation.

VI. IMPROVING RESEARCH METHODOLOGY

Clearly, the processual nature of self-regulation and the dynamic inter-action among its component parts requires sophisticated methodology to capture the essence of self-regulatory processes as they unfold over time. Unfortunately, much of the current research methodology in the area of self-regulation has employed simplistic experimental designs or traditional correlational methods, which may not capture the dynamic and transac-tional process of self-regulation optimally. In particular, these methods are insufficient to validly test some of the more complex models found in many applied areas. Although recent advances in design and analysis are ripe for application to the self-regulation domain, there are currently few concrete examples of research that capitalizes on the power of such methods as dynamic modeling, structural equation modeling, partial order scalogram analyses, and higher-order linear models. Various contributors (Carver & Scheier; Kuhl) believe that now we can apply dynamic concepts and models to the area of self-regulation, the reason being that now we can handle the mathematical intricacies of nonlinear, dynamic, and bidirec-tional relationships. This is exemplified by contemporary models of deter-ministic chaos, catastrophe theory, and synergetics. By employing more sophisticated analytic techniques to research self-regulation constructs, we should greatly elucidate the dynamic interactive roles of these concepts.

Furthermore, self-regulation research would benefit from capitalizing on the complimentarities of methods in actual research. Nomothetic and ideographic designs, interindividual and intraindividual methods, quantita-tive and qualitative (the phenomenology of self-regulation), and experi-mental, correlational, and naturalistic descriptions are needed to investi-gate different research questions and hypotheses. The *triangulation* of research operations via complimentary designs, ranging from survey to multivariate experimental, to longitudinal designs, would be useful to tap different research questions. It would also be worthwhile to try out alternative methods and measures from a utilitarian and eclectic perspec-tive, seeking to identify and explore functional complimentarities. Triangulation across measurement protocols is infrequent (see Winne & Perry). Because each protocol generates a slightly different reflection of self-regulation, a fuller understanding of models and methods can be achieved by using multiple measurement protocols in research. However, as researchers move out into the real world, the different methods certainly need to be adopted to the specific contexts under consideration. For example, if we want to know more about the dynamics of the self-regulatory process in a given educational or occupational setting, a quasi-experimental design might be the most useful protocol.

In addition to the construction of valid measures and research designs, we need to develop appropriate *statistical techniques* to analyze the dynamic and transactional (interactive) nature of self-regulatory processes optimally. Simple correlational or even simple experimental designs, emphasized by self-regulation researchers at the expense of more appropriate multivariate and longitudinal designs, are inadequate for providing a better understanding of the self-regulation process. Although the interrelationships between self-regulatory components and related variables have been conceptualized generally and investigated as linear ones, the nature of the relationship, in fact, may be curvilinear (i.e., the linear correlation might be null, even if there is some substantial correlation). In addition, when self-regulation is employed as a predictor of some criterion variable in a regression equation, we also need to look at multiplictive functions, introducing both linear and quadratic functions of self-regulation as they impact on criterion performance. For example, if successful performance in tennis is a curvilinear function of self-regulation, with highest attainments at mid levels of self-regulation, self-regulation should be accompanied by the same variable *squared* in the regression equation predicting performance. An additional point to consider is that the magnitude or direction of the relationships explored may change across time, context, cultural group, or gender (see Jackson et al.).

Long-term research, employing longitudinal research methodology, and focusing on the development and training of self-regulation is in order. Presently, there is little long-term research aimed at development of self-regulated skills in student populations. A real experiment in which students receive instruction that promotes self-regulation throughout their schooling remains to be performed. Thus, no one yet has evaluated the hypothesis that a schooling career immersed in high quality instruction aimed at promoting self-regulation would, in fact, produce much better self-regulated learners than typical elementary-grades instruction.

In addition, more adequate sampling of variables is urgently needed in self-regulation research. It is necessary to select variables strategically to thoroughly cover the self-regulation domain. Studies often have sufficed with a few components and a small sample design, and, consequently, are flawed because of inadequate sampling of both variables and number of subjects. Only by strategically selecting subjects, variables and settings can we expect to thoroughly cover the self-regulation domain and the facets of units, observations, and settings. In addition, future research needs to examine the consistency of self-regulatory processes across time and situations. Thus, it is presently unclear to what degree there is one set of self-regulatory processes across domains; perhaps the structure and processes of self-regulation are the same across various domains.

As noted by a number of authors (Winne & Perry and Endler & Kocovski), research into self-regulation has so far has included a limited range of populations. Postsecondary students and college students are most often participants in studies; hence, very little is known about young children's self-regulatory strategies in social and learning spheres. Until measurements are collected across the age spectrum, fully understanding measurement protocols and developmental trajectories will remain elusive. In addition, most research has been conducted from a Western perspective and on middle-class Western populations; relatively little research has been conducted on ethnic minority groups or individuals in non-Western cultures (see Jackson et al.).

Finally, the bulk of the data that relates self-regulation to other variables is of a correlational nature, so that the direction of causality in the association is indeterminate. Although the nature of the causal flow of direction in the observed relationships between self-regulation and other constructs has been conceptualized and interpreted in a variety of different ways, perhaps the most productive form of association is that of reciprocal determinism, with self-regulation and other key personal and environmental variables showing a bidirectional relationship.

VII. EXPLORING INTERACTIONS BETWEEN ENVIRONMENT AND SELF-REGULATION

Person–situation interactionist perspectives have now largely superseded the old person versus situation debates; most researchers agree that behaviors are largely a function of the interaction among person and situational characteristics. Clearly, some situational characteristics (e.g., a traffic light) are sometimes powerful enough to regulate and produce consistency of behavior across many persons. Also, some personal characteristics (e.g., self-regulation) are sometimes powerful enough to produce consistency of behaviors across situations. As we consider interactions involving self-regulation and the environment, we need to be clear on the models being used and interpreted. The interaction between self-regulation and other variables may take many forms and may reflect different hypotheses about particular types of interactive effects and mechanisms presumed to be operative. Following Hettema and Kenrick*

(1992), we briefly point out six different forms of self-regulation–environment interaction that might be considered:

1. Person–environment matching, when relatively consistent characteristics of a person, that is, highly efficient and powerful self-regulatory processes, are assumed to suit that person for relatively consistent characteristics of situations (e.g., working as a surgeon, pilot, electrical engineer, or accountant), and vice versa, to prove a mesh.

2. Choices of environment by persons to suit their own self-regulatory skills (e.g., a student trying to self-regulate to limit tobacco consumption chooses to dine in the nonsmoking area of a restaurant).

3. Choice of persons by environment, as in most selection systems (e.g., using high goal setting and self-efficacy to choose members of an elite army unit).

4. Transformation of environment by persons to suit their own personal goals for self-regulation (e.g., removing all high-fat cheeses from the refrigerator to maintain one's diet).

5. Transformation of person by the environment, as in learning new self-control procedures or acquiring self-regulated learning skills in the classroom through explicit instruction and modeling.

6. Self-regulation–environment transaction—reciprocal interactions over time that change both persons and situations to attain a mesh.

In keeping with current cognitive-social models of self-regulation and the notion of reciprocal determinism, it is the latter approach that we believe is the most suitable for conceptualizing the person–situation interaction in self-regulation research. Accordingly, when a person is self-regulating to achieve a set goal, that person's behavior impacts upon the environment, which in turn, becomes the input function used to further self-regulate behavior.

Recent thinking in the area of self-regulation emphasizes the importance of taking contextual variables into consideration in models of self-regulation (see Brownlee et al.). Context operates at several levels, from the role of language (label of problem or reference point) through cultural myths and causes of particular situations, and established strategies for handling or managing problems. Problem solving and self-regulation are bounded by these contextual factors. Thus, future research in the area of self-regulation needs to pay greater attention to sociocultural factors and incorporate these factors into the model.

Jackson et al. underscore that the concepts on which self-discrepancy theories are based (standards, reference points, etc.) derive from culturally based notions of acceptable behavior and are rooted in socially based roles. Future definitions need to consider the communal components of models, because individual behaviors are nested within a wider collectivistic context. Future research would be served well by incorporating themes from communally based theories and investigating what strategies individuals use to establish a balance between achieving goals that are beneficial for themselves and others. Future research should also examine the impact of self-set goals versus external standards or cultural norms on various facets of the self-regulation process.

VIII. ACQUISITION AND TRANSMISSION OF SELF-REGULATORY SKILLS

As noted by Matthews et al., an important question for future research focuses on the vehicles of transmission of self-regulatory skills—an issue we presently know very little about. Thus, an important question for future consideration is whether self-discovery of self-regulatory skills suffices, or whether we need special training methods to inculcate and teach skills?

Although it is possible to develop self-regulatory competence by personal discovery, this path is often tedious and frustrating, and limited in its effectiveness. Zimmerman's chapter nicely illustrates how modeling and instruction serve as a primary vehicle through which parents, teachers, and communities socially convey self-regulatory skills. Thus, self-regulatory skills can be acquired from and are sustained by social as well as self sources of influence. However, the social-cognitive hypothesis that self-regulation of learning develops initially from social modeling and progresses through increasing levels of self-directed functioning needs further validation. The various phases in Zimmerman's model of self-regulatory skill acquisition, namely, observational, modeling, self-control, and self-regulation phases, need to be empirically validated and better differentiated.

Schunk and Ertmer urge researchers to conduct more research on self-regulation in the context of different content area domains. This is because self-regulatory processes are linked with content domains, and individuals learn how to apply them in a given learning or applied domain. Clearly, contexts determine, to some measure, what self-regulatory skills might be most useful. Embedding self-regulation processes within specific content areas brings up the issue of transfer. Thus, a key issue for future research relates to the transfer of self-regulatory skills from one situation to the next. At present, it is unclear whether persons will transfer skills from one content area to another or one disciplinary domain to another. What skills are necessary so that students make appropriate modifications in self-regulatory processes so that they match the current situation? Researchers need to conduct process-oriented studies to determine how students think about and employ the strategies they learn in one context to another setting. Individuals may need to be taught self-regulatory skills and activities in different applied or learning setting and how to modify them to fit different applied areas or situations. Thus, additional studies need to be conducted to understand when self-regulatory skills are deemed to be useful by students. These skills need to be linked to particular contexts.

IX. EXAMINING DEVELOPMENTAL DIFFERENCES IN SELF-REGULATORY SKILLS

Future research needs to carefully look at the development of self-regulatory skills across time. Thus, we need to understand how biology and aging (maturation, senescence) change both the self-regulatory processes (goal setting, monitoring, feedback control, self-evaluation, etc.) and the effects of self-regulatory skills. How do biological and age changes affect the inputs, representation, procedures, and errors in self-control? Does the pattern of relationship between self-regulation and other components grow weaker or stronger over the years?

As mentioned, Zimmerman's social-cognitive model posits that people acquire self-regulatory skills, mainly through observation, imitation, self-control, and self-regulation. This model does not assume that all phases are measured in sequence. Are different components of self-regulation managed in sequence? Do they show differential growth over time? Do they have similar age functions? These and other nagging questions need to be addressed in future research.

As suggested by Schunk and Ertmer, there may be developmental differences in acquisition and instruction of self-regulatory skills. Younger students may benefit more from modeled demonstrations, whereas older students may be able to formulate their own methods. Alternatively, we might predict that strategy modeling would be more effective during initial learning, when individual's ability to construct strategies is limited; as students develop competence, they may be better able to construct self-regulatory strategies.

X. EXAMINING INDIVIDUAL DIFFERENCES IN SELF-REGULATORY SKILLS

We need to find ways to integrate research on individual differences with research on the development of self-regulatory components in individuals in the context of differential distributions and trajectories of development. As noted by Matthews et al., the assessment of individual differences in self-regulation could be immeasurably improved. Differential psychologists, who focus on measures taken at one or two points in time, can only speculate about developmental trends in self-regulation. By contrast, developmentalists focus on the development of self-regulation trends, but usually measure no individual differences except age. Yet, the best way to understand both individual differences and individuality may be in the context of development, whereas development may be interpreted best in the context of differential distributions and trajectories of development.

Furthermore, little research has focused on self-regulatory processes (inputs and representations of goals, self-regulatory procedures, monitoring, and self-assessment) in different demographic and sociocultural subgroups in the population. Do males and females differ in the use of and efficiency of self-regulatory processes? If so, in what domains? Are there meaningful social class differences in the process and efficiency of self-regulation? Do different sociocultural groups differ in their self-regulatory processes?

In addition, we need to better understand the role of cultural actors in self-regulatory processes. For example, do people with traditional beliefs self-regulate differently from their modern counterparts? Do people in collectivistically oriented cultures self-regulate differently or more efficiently than those living in modern individually oriented cultures. Are the goals and procedures the same?

XI. APPLICATIONS

There is little doubt that self-regulation plays a central role in influencing performance in a wide array of applied areas (school and academic performance, health, occupational behavior, etc.). Thus, over the years, a variety of conative factors, such as self-regulation, have been used jointly in various practical domains. In fact, it is at the applied or clinical level that the greatest amount of integration of self-regulatory and other variables takes place by necessity. For example, the clinical or school psychologist may assess a child's poor school achievement by gathering data on the child's intelligence, self-regulated learning skills, learning style, motivation, anxiety, and academic self-concept (as well as social behavior, physical and health status, and home environment) so as to arrive at a diagnosis and prescription of the most appropriate intervention program. Thus, the psychological practitioners' task is to develop a comprehensive and integrated description of the person by employing precise measurement strategies and continuously referencing the theory and research that describes the interrelationships among the various conative and intellective factors examined. Given that such an integration is not always explicit from the literature or measures available, clinicians may be required to make this integration on their own, that is, at an intuitive level.

Unfortunately, we know very little about considerations practitioners bring to bear in making decisions based on the integration between conative constructs, such as self-regulation, and ability constructs. For example, how does the school psychologist, probation officer, personnel officer, or health provider combine information on a person's self-regulatory skills to make decisions that are of major importance to the individual and society as a whole? Systematic observations, in-depth interviews, self-observation and monitoring, single-subject design research, and protocol analysis are needed in a wide array of practical domains to shed light on this needed area.

In addition, a most worthwhile effort would be to conduct an intensive and careful analysis of individual cases, contrasting those individuals who are extremely high or low on self-regulation so as to identify qualitative differences between individuals. Such an analysis would provide avenues for understanding what it means to be exceptionally high or low in self-regulation (cf. Zimmerman). For example, one method that may be used is to study the biographies of individuals who are high on self-regulation; this information will allow us to spread a broader methodology. In addition, cross-partitioning individuals by specific self-regulatory and other factors would help the development of useful typologies in various domains.

We need to learn how best to promote self-regulation in different areas and how to motivate or influence people to self-regulate to achieve important behavioral objectives (e.g., managing study time, maintaining healthy behaviors, and adhering to a medicinal regimen). Thus, we need to learn how best to help people who need to self-regulate, such as the obese, those who abuse alcohol and drugs, parents who mistreat children, and adults who abuse their spouses.

More knowledge is needed on how best to develop and foster self-regulation skills in social microcosms that are not themselves systematically regulated (e.g., classrooms, hospitals, and homes). It may be especially hard to induce lawful behavior when the microcosm is in flux. Thus, we need to deal with the self as being reinforced and changed by the social milieu in which the self is operating. In addition, research needs to identify the various impediments to successful self-regulation, as well as the reasons for failure of self-regulatory processes

XII. TRAINING AND PROMOTION OF SELF-REGULATORY CONCEPTS

A major reason for attempting to understand the nature of self-regulation and its determinants and consequences is the belief that more complete awareness of its nature might go far to stimulate thinking about ways to promote more adaptive self-regulatory aptitudes, practices, and interventions. We need to learn how best to promote an individual's self-regulatory learning skills at various developmental stages, from nursery school children through college and adult lifelong learning. A number of chapters in this book (e.g., Creer on promoting self-regulation in the area of chronic disease and Weinstein et al. on promoting students' learning skills and habits) have provided some concrete guidelines for promoting self-regulatory skills in these areas.

There is an increasing recognition, according to Creer, that in many applied cases, self-regulation is apt to fail. By constantly alerting individuals, say chronically ill patients, to several factors that could lead to relapse, including exposure to high risk situations, failure to initiate responses, attributions to personal weakness, and initial relapse, patients can be taught about what factors to expect and how to manage them. Indeed, defensive inferences that may undermine successful adaptation, include helplessness, procrastination, task avoidance, cognitive disengagement, and apathy.

In researching the effects of instruction and self-regulation interventions, it is important to identify components that are responsible for the effects. As pointed out by De Corte et al., although some investigations show convincingly the possibility to foster self-regulation in students, they do not allow us to identify which components of the learning environments that were designed and implemented account for the observed effects. Therefore, there is a need for studies that set out to unravel how and under what specific instructional conditions individuals become efficient self-regulators. What are the crucial elements in the learning environment that help and support students in learning to manage and monitor their own processes of knowledge building and skill acquisition? Research shedding light on the specific parameters of treatment programs responsible for outcomes is urgently needed (Endler & Kocovski) to determine the effects of a specific aspect of self-regulation in therapy (e.g., goal setting, self-reinforcement), as well as the cumulative effects of targeting all aspects of self-regulation in therapy.

As pointed out by Schunk and Ertmer, little effort has been made to link self-reflective practices to interventions. Researchers need to determine whether the effectiveness of self-reflection varies as a function of setting. Is self-reflective practice more important when external evaluation is infrequent or students encounter difficulties? How should students be motivated to engage in self-reflection on their own, such as by teaching students to treat self-reflection as any other academic activity that must be planned? Another important question for future research is, "When are self-regulatory skills particularly important?" Randi and Corno hypothesize about some conditions in which skills are important, such as when instruction is incomplete, when a challenging task requires sustained attention, or when a person is confronted by competing goals. These hypotheses need to be tested empirically.

Clearly, we want to foster and promote self-regulation when it is adaptive for the individual and social context under consideration. Thus, we need to learn how to distinguish between adaptive and maladaptive self-regulation. This requires us to identify situations where self-regulation may interfere with the achievement of important goals (e.g., excessive self-regulation that involves obsessive or compulsive behavior). A case in point: Say we want to foster a creative and spontaneous learning or work environment. Excessive self-regulation may take people out of the flow of behavior, causing them to resist the affordances of the spontaneous and creative environment; thus, the effect of self-regulation is violated. Moreover, if a person is self-regulating to a negative goal or standard, we might want to reestablish goals or break this self-regulatory pattern (rather than promote self-regulation). Unfortunately, it is unclear exactly what constitutes an "excessive" or "insufficient" amount of self-regulation or whether or not too much self-regulation is as deleterious as insufficient self-regulation.

Unfortunately, many of the current applications are not based on sound conceptual or theoretical framework. Thus, additional research is needed on optimal ways to construct and implement interventions designed to train and promote functional self-regulatory skills within specific domains of application (alcohol consumption, substance abuse, weight reduction, etc.). The critical components of the intervention process need to be identified and practical guidelines are needed to determine the specific conditions for the promotion of self-regulatory skills.

In sum, additional research is needed to achieve a sound knowledge base for self-regulation theory, research, and applications. By bringing all the contributors together in this handbook, we hope to have come closer to developing some theoretical consensus regarding the construct of self-regulation, as well as seeing where there may be important conceptual disagreements across areas. We hope that this type of intellectual dialogue has refined the construct of self-regulation to some extent and that future research directions are now more clearly mapped out.

REFERENCE

Hettema, P. J., & Kendrick, D. T. (1992). Models of person–situation interactions. In G. V. Caprara & G. L. Van Heck (Eds.), *Modern personality psychology: Critical reviews and directions* (pp. 393–417). New York: Harvester Wheatsheaf.

INDEX

reactions to life stress, 182–187
reductionistic theories, 258
refining measurement of constructs,
    757–759
regulation or, 752
reinterpretation of familiar phenomena,
    149–150
research evidence, 636–638
role of intention in, 253–274
versus self-control, 115
self-efficacy and, 633–634
self-management or, 752
self-monitoring and perceptions of
    progress, 640–641
self-reflective practice, 645
self system in, 393–407
self-understanding and, 227–237
explaining development of, 237–244
social and environmental influences, 24–26
social anxiety and, 584–588
social cognition and, 175
social-cognitive theory, 633
social components of, 276–280
structure and process of, 753–755
as a systems concept, 256–257
techniques and limitations, 257–258
training and promotion of concepts,
    766–768
traits and cognitive stress processes,
    177–182
traits and stable individual differences in,
    176–177
transfer of processes, 644–645
triadic definition, 13–15
Self-regulation and Concentration Test for
    Children, 158
Self-regulation constructs, tractable concep-
    tual foundation and consistent nomen-
    clature, 750–753
Self-Regulative Executive Function, Wells
    and Matthews, 174, 178, 180–181
Self-regulatory function, dysfunctions in, 13
Self-regulatory learning, classroom enact-
    ment, 672–679
Self-regulatory phases, cyclic, 16
Self-regulatory process analysis, use of the
    journey tale, 667–671
Self-regulatory skills
    acquisition and transmission of, 763–764
    cognitive, teaching to seventh graders,
        705–709
    developmental differences in, 764
    development of, 28–32

individual differences in, 764–765
Self-regulatory systems
    internal views of, 24
    structure of, 15–24
Self-reinforcement
    addictive behaviors and, 576
    depression and, 590
    health behavior, 581
    social anxiety and, 587
Self-relaxation, 138
    neurobiological basis of, 133–134
Self-relevance of arguments, 152–153
Self-report questionnaires, measuring self-
    regulated learning, 542–545
Self-representation
    attitude change, 150–154
    development of, 232–234
    implicit, 130
Self-rewards, 25
Self-satisfaction, 23
Self system, 393–407
    goals and problem solving strategies,
        394–398
    redefining and reorganizing, 398–402
Self-transformation, 177, 179
Self-understanding
    development of, 227–237
    organization and development, 209–251
Self versus other generated goals, self-
    regulation as, 370
Sensitive dependence on initial conditions
    catastrophe theory, 72–73
    dynamic systems theory, 66–67
Social adaptation, three-level hierarchical
    structure, 223–224
Social anxiety, 185
    goal setting and, 585–586
    implications for treatment, 587–588
    self-evaluation and, 586–587
    self-monitoring and, 586
    self-regulation and, 584–588
    self-reinforcement and, 587
Social cognition, self-regulation and, 175
Social-cognitive framework, application to
    aggressive behavior, 193–199
Social cognitive model, self-regulation, 24
Social cognitive theory, I/O psychology,
    324–326
Social comparison processes, elements of
    feedback loop, 46
Social components, self-regulation models,
    276–280